DATE DUE

DIFFICULT DIAGNOSES IN DERMATOLOGY

Edited by

Mark Lebwohl, M.D.

Assistant Professor
Department of Dermatology
Mount Sinai School of Medicine
of the City University of New York

Clinical Director
Department of Dermatology
Mount Sinai Medical Center
New York, New York

CHURCHILL LIVINGSTONE
New York, Edinburgh, London, Melbourne 1988

Library of Congress Cataloging-in-Publication Data

Difficult diagnoses in dermatology

  Includes bibliographies and index.
  1. Skin—Diseases—Diagnosis. I. Lebwohl, Mark.
[DNLM: 1. Skin Diseases—diagnosis. WR 140 D5693]
RL72.D54   1988   616.5′075   87–25675
ISBN 0–443–08460–2

Distributed in the United Kingdom by Churchill Livingstone, Robert
Stevenson House, 1–3 Baxter's Place, Leith Walk, Edinburgh EH1 3AF,
and by associated companies, branches, and representatives throughout
the world.

Accurate indications, adverse reactions, and dosage schedules for drugs
are provided in this book, but it is possible that they may change. The
reader is urged to review the package information data of the
manufacturers of the medications mentioned.

Copy Editor: *Margot Otway*
Production Designer: *Melanie Haber*
Production Supervisor: *Jane Grochowski*

Printed in the United States of America

First published in 1988

To Madeleine, Andy, and Eve,
whose presence I sorely missed
during the many hours of writing and editing.

CONTRIBUTORS

Bernard R. Adelsberg, M.D.
Chief, Division of Allergy and Immunology, Department of Medicine, Nassau County Medical Center, East Meadow, New York

Jeffrey D. Bernhard, M.D.
Associate Professor of Medicine, Department of Dermatology, University of Massachusetts Medical School; Director, Division of Dermatology, and Director, Phototherapy Center, University of Massachusetts Medical Center, Worcester, Massachusetts

Virginia L. Chen, M.D.
Clinical Instructor, Department of Dermatology, Mount Sinai School of Medicine of the City University of New York, New York, New York

Andrea Dunaif, M.D.
Assistant Professor, Departments of Medicine and of Obstetrics-Gynecology and Reproductive Science, Mount Sinai School of Medicine of the City University of New York, New York, New York

Michael Fisher, M.D.
Professor and Head, Division of Dermatology, Department of Medicine, Albert Einstein College of Medicine of Yeshiva University, New York, New York

Raul Fleischmajer, M.D.
Professor and Chairman, Department of Dermatology, Mount Sinai School of Medicine of the City University of New York, New York, New York

Jonathan L. Halperin, M.D.
Associate Professor of Clinical Medicine, Mount Sinai School of Medicine of the City University of New York; Director of Clinical Services, Division of Cardiology, Mount Sinai Medical Center, New York, New York

Dorie Hankin, M.D.
Assistant Professor, Department of Pediatrics, Albert Einstein College of Medicine of Yeshiva University, New York, New York; Coordinating Pediatrician, Blythedale Children's Hospital, Valhalla, New York

James Herndon, Jr., M.D.
Associate Clinical Professor, Department of Dermatology, University of Texas Health Science Center at Dallas Southwestern Medical School, Dallas, Texas

Robert E. Jordon, M.D.
Professor and Chairman, Department of Dermatology, University of Texas Medical School at Houston; Director, Cutaneous Immunopathology Unit, The University of Texas Health Science Center at Houston, Houston, Texas

Susan Katz, M.D.
Assistant Professor, Department of Medicine, Division of Dermatology, Albert Einstein College of Medicine of Yeshiva University, New York, New York

Mark Lebwohl, M.D.
Assistant Professor, Department of Dermatology, Mount Sinai School of Medicine of the City University of New York; Clinical Director, Department of Dermatology, Mount Sinai Medical Center, New York, New York

Dominick J. Ligresti, M.D.
Clinical Instructor, Department of Dermatology, Mount Sinai School of Medicine of the City University of New York, New York, New York

Nelson Lee Novick, M.D.
Associate Clinical Professor, Department of Dermatology, Mount Sinai School of Medicine of the City University of New York, New York, New York

David S. Orentreich, M.D.
Clinical Instructor, Department of Dermatology, Mount Sinai School of Medicine of the City University of New York, New York, New York

Norman Orentreich, M.D.
Clinical Professor, Department of Dermatology, New York University School of Medicine, New York, New York

Amy S. Paller, M.D.
Assistant Professor, Departments of Dermatology, Pediatrics, and Immunology, Rush Medical College of Rush University; Head, Section of Pediatric Dermatology, Rush-Presbyterian-St. Luke's Hospital, Chicago, Illinois

Robert G. Phelps, M.D.
Assistant Professor, Departments of Dermatology and Pathology, Mount Sinai School of Medicine of the City University of New York; Director of Dermatopathology, Mount Sinai Medical Center, New York, New York

Shirley Press, M.D.
Assistant Professor, Department of Pediatrics, University of Miami School of Medicine; Director, Pediatric Emergency Service, Jackson Memorial Hospital, Miami, Florida

Philip G. Prioleau, M.D.
Assistant Professor, Departments of Medicine and Pathology, Cornell University Medical College, New York, New York

Rhonda E. Rand, M.D.
Clinical Instructor, Department of Dermatology, University of California, Los Angeles, UCLA School of Medicine, Los Angeles, California

Bijan Safai, M.D.
Professor, Department of Medicine, Division of Dermatology, Cornell University Medical College; Chief, Dermatology Service, Department of Medicine, Memorial Sloan-Kettering Cancer Center, New York, New York

W. Mitchell Sams, Jr., M.D.
Professor and Chairman, Department of Dermatology, University of Alabama in Birmingham School of Medicine, Birmingham, Alabama

Lawrence Schachner, M.D.
Associate Professor, Departments of Dermatology and Pediatrics, and Director, Division of Pediatric Dermatology, University of Miami School of Medicine, Miami, Florida

Mathew Varghese, M.D.
Instructor, Department of Medicine, Division of Dermatology, Cornell University Medical College; Assistant Attending Physician, New York Hospital–Cornell Medical Center, New York, New York

Eric Vonderheid, M.D.
Associate Professor, Department of Dermatology, Temple University School of Medicine, Philadelphia, Pennsylvania

George B. Winton, LTC, M.D.
Assistant Chief, Dermatology Service, Department of Medicine, Walter Reed Army Medical Center, Washington, D.C.

PREFACE

Successful dermatologic treatment begins with accurate diagnosis. However, the proliferation of previously undescribed syndromes, new diagnostic criteria, and innovative tests can make diagnosis an increasingly formidable task. The clinician must be able to decide when to obtain specimens for electron microscopy or immunofluorescence, when to perform phototesting, when to patch test, and when to photopatch test. An ever-increasing number of serologic tests for a rapidly expanding array of diseases and syndromes faces the practicing physician, and through this maze the patient must be led to the correct diagnosis.

Difficult Diagnoses in Dermatology attempts to simplify the diagnosis of the disorders reviewed. The diagnosis is sometimes obvious—for example, in a patient with vasculitis who presents with palpable purpura. However, the search for underlying causes and associated symptoms can be extraordinarily difficult. The systematic approach outlined in each chapter should help the physician identify significant elements of the history and physical examination and should facilitate selection of appropriate diagnostic tests. Each chapter contains a section and/or table entitled ''Approach to the Patient'' which lists easy-to-follow steps that can be used to direct the patient's work-up in a simple and orderly fashion.

So that each condition is thoroughly reviewed, some disorders are intentionally covered in more than one chapter. Graft-versus-host disease, for example, is reviewed with the pseudosclerodermas and is also discussed in the chapters dealing with chronic generalized erythroderma and neonatal erythrodermas. Similarly, since the ichthyosiform eruptions reviewed in Chapter 13 are included also in the differential diagnosis of neonatal erythrodermas, they are discussed in Chapter 12 as well.

Many disorders worthy of inclusion have undoubtedly been omitted, and many of the diagnoses reviewed are only occasionally or, in some cases, rarely encountered. Nevertheless, when particularly problematic cases are seen, it is hoped that *Difficult Diagnoses in Dermatology* will serve as a useful reference for the practicing dermatologist.

Mark Lebwohl, M.D.

ACKNOWLEDGMENTS

To my family, friends, and colleagues, whose support and understanding have helped me during the completion of this book, I want to extend my heartfelt thanks. In particular, I want to thank Kay Feick, Gay Megherian, and Carmen Rodriguez for their constant assistance in typing, photocopying, making phone calls, checking references, and generally aiding in the preparation of *Difficult Diagnoses in Dermatology*. I am also indebted to Marta Kilgour for her meticulous review of the manuscript and to Beth Kaufman Barry and Margot Otway of Churchill Livingstone for their editorial assistance.

Most importantly, I want to thank Dr. Raul Fleischmajer, without whose assistance and support this book would not have been written. His guidance has shaped my career and I shall forever be indebted to him.

CONTENTS

Vasculitis

W. Mitchell Sams, Jr.

The group of clinical diseases known as *vasculitis* share the histologic feature of transmural inflammatory cell infiltrate, accompanied by fibrinoid necrosis and having a probable immune complex pathogenesis. The various clinical forms of this necrotizing vasculitis may occur in a variety of vessels of differing sizes and differing locations. Small postcapillary venules are involved in hypersensitivity (allergic) vasculitis, medium-sized arteries in polyarteritis nodosa, and large vessels in giant cell arteritis. The major syndromes can be viewed as representing clinical expressions of an immunopathologic process with differing systemic manifestations. The best example of this is the vasculitis associated with hepatitis B antigenemia, which may present as hypersensitivity vasculitis, hypocomplementemic vasculitis, or polyarteritis nodosa. The cutaneous lesions that occur with all forms of vasculitis may represent only a dermatologic problem, a minor secondary component of an unrelated systemic disease, or a manifestation of a severe and potentially fatal systemic form of vasculitis.

CLASSIFICATION

The most widely accepted classification utilizes six major and several minor categories (Table 1-1). Those diseases classified as *hypersensitivity vasculitis* are relatively benign and involve primarily small vessels of the skin, although some patients may have systemic involvement as well. *Rheumatic vasculitis* deserves special distinction as a category because of its close association with such diseases as systemic lupus erythematosus and rheumatoid arthritis. The *polyarteritis nodosa* group is distinct because of the medium-sized muscular arteries that are usually involved. The *granulomatous diseases* may in some cases begin as typical vessel wall inflammation with polymorphonuclear leukocytes, but soon progress to the development of granulomata, often involving distinct vessels within specific organs. The granulomatous vasculitides tend to be far more malignant than the other forms.

PATHOGENESIS

It is likely that most, if not all, the forms of necrotizing vasculitis are due to an immune complex pathogenesis. The evidence for this includes (1) the typical neutrophilic infiltrate, (2) the presence of granular immunoreactants, (3) the anticomplementary activity of the sera, (4) the presence of hypocomplementemia, (5) the detection of circulating immune complexes, and (6) the positive histamine trap test. The evidence for an immune complex pathogenesis is most conclusive for hypersensitivity vasculitis as this is the form on which most of the

Table 1-1. Classification of Vasculitis

Hypersensitivity vasculitis
    Typical hypersensitivity vasculitis (leukocytoclastic vasculitis)
    Variant forms of hypersensitivity vasculitis
        Henoch-Schönlein purpura
        Hypocomplementemic (urticarial) vasculitis
        Mixed cryoglobulinemia
        Serum sickness
Rheumatic vasculitis
    Rheumatoid arthritis
    Systemic lupus erythematosus
    Others: Sjögren's syndrome, polymyositis, scleroderma
Polyarteritis nodosa
    Classic polyarteritis nodosa
    Cutaneous polyarteritis nodosa
Granulomatous vasculitis
    Allergic granulomatous angiitis (Churg-Strauss syndrome)
    Wegener's granulomatosis
    Lymphomatoid granulomatosis
Giant cell arteritis
    Temporal arteritis
    Takayasu's disease
Miscellaneous cutaneous forms of vasculitis
    Erythema elevatum diutinum
    Erythema nodosum
    Behçet's syndrome
    Others

studies have been conducted. It is well recognized that neutrophils comprise the inflammatory infiltrate both within the vessel wall and in the area immediately surrounding the vessel, which is accompanied by leukocytoclasia (nuclear dust) as the neutrophils die. Studies by Gower et al.[1] demonstrate that lesions produced by intradermal injection of histamine must be 18 to 36 hours old to demonstrate typical neutrophilic infiltrates. Lesions either younger or older than this are likely not to show characteristic histopathologic changes. Similarly, Gower et al. demonstrated that the characteristic granular immunoreactants (usually IgG, IgM, and C3) are most likely to be present in lesions less than 6 hours old. As the lesions age, the immune complexes are phagocytized and rapidly disappear, so that virtually none are present by 24 hours. A number of studies have demonstrated that the serum from patients with acute vasculitis has the ability to bind complement, which suggests that immune complexes are present. This has been confirmed by the fre-

quent finding of low serum complement levels in these patients and by detection of circulating immune complexes. The histamine trap test consists of intradermal injection of histamine in a patient with active vasculitis. If the serum contains high levels of circulating complexes, these might be expected to rapidly deposit within the histamine-dilated vessel wall, and in fact this is exactly what Braverman and Yen[2] and Gower et al.[1] have demonstrated occurs, with maximum deposition approximately 1 hour following histamine injection.

Thus, the immune complex pathogenesis of vasculitis can be summarized as follows. Following exposure to an antigenic stimulus, antibodies, usually of the IgG or IgM class, are formed and complex with the antigen in the circulation. This complex may circulate without causing any difficulty until something happens to the vessel wall, such as vasodilatation or trauma, at which time the complex becomes bound to the vessel wall and the Fc portion of the immunoglobulin molecule binds complement and initiates the complement cascade. Subsequent elaboration of the potent chemotactic factor C5a attracts neutrophils into the vessel wall. Tissue injury occurs as the activated neutrophils phagocytize the immune complexes and thereby release destructive proteolytic enzymes, including elastase and collagenase. The resulting inflammation, necrosis, and hemorrhage appear clinically as palpable purpura when they occur in the skin. Factors that favor deposition of immune complexes within the vessel wall include formation of the immune complexes in slight antigen excess, an intermediate size of the complexes (approximately 19 S), and the increased vascular permeability.

PRESENTATION

Hypersensitivity (Allergic or Leukocytoclastic) Vasculitis

Patients with hypersensitivity vasculitis typically present with sharply demarcated and clearly defined lesions of palpable purpura, pre-

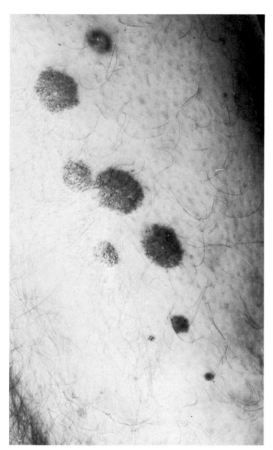

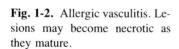
Fig. 1-1. Allergic vasculitis. Early lesions of palpable purpura on the lower extremities.

dominantly on the lower legs, although lesions may occur to a lesser extent on other parts of the body. With continued development lesions may coalesce to produce large areas of purpura, and some areas may become necrotic to produce hemorrhagic blisters or even ulcers (Figs. 1-1 and 1-2). Small lesions are usually asymptomatic while larger or ulcerated lesions may become painful. Some patients may note malaise, myalgias, arthralgias, and fever. When other organs are involved, symptoms may include abdominal pain or melena from involvement of the gastrointestinal tract, frank arthritis from joint involvement, and occasional peripheral neuropathy. In these patients in particular the kidneys are likely to be involved, as evidenced by proteinuria and microscopic hematuria. It is this constellation of symptoms, including the skin lesions of palpable purpura, arthritis, abdominal pain, and glomerulitis, that is characteristic of Henoch-Schönlein purpura. This disease usually occurs in the spring of the year and is most frequently preceded by an upper respiratory infection in children. It appears that IgA, the immunoglobulin associated with mucosal surfaces, plays a distinct role in the immunopathogenesis of Henoch-Schönlein purpura. IgA may combine with an antigen in the upper respiratory tract, leading to formation of

Fig. 1-2. Allergic vasculitis. Lesions may become necrotic as they mature.

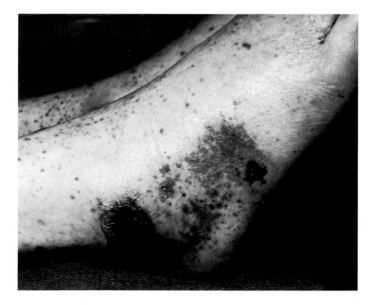

circulating immune complexes, which are then deposited in the vessel walls to activate the complement cascade, as described earlier.

HYPOCOMPLEMENTEMIC VASCULITIS

Hypocomplementemic, or urticarial, vasculitis is a subtype that has been recognized only in recent years. Patients present with recurrent urticaria, transient arthralgias, hypocomplementemia, and an elevated erythrocyte sedimentation rate. The individual lesions of urticaria characteristically persist for 24 to 36 hours rather than resolving within a few hours, as occurs with ordinary allergic urticaria. Fever, abdominal pain, lymphadenopathy, and glomerulonephritis may also occur.

ESSENTIAL MIXED CRYOGLOBULINEMIA

The syndrome of essential mixed cryoglobulinemia is characterized by recurrent dependent purpura, weakness, arthralgias, and often glomerulonephritis.[4] The mixed cryoglobulins are usually composed of a polyclonal IgG and a monoclonal IgM (rarely IgA) having specificity for the Fc portion of IgG, that is, having rheumatoid factor activity. Vasculitic manifestations most frequently occur in this "essential" form of mixed cryoglobulinemia although there may be an association with a wide variety of diverse disorders, including infections, connective tissue vascular diseases, lymphoproliferative disorders, and chronic inflammatory states. Some patients may have cold urticaria, Raynaud's phenomenon, peripheral neuropathy, and hepatosplenomegaly. Immune-complex-mediated renal damage occurs in approximately 50 percent of patients.

SERUM SICKNESS

Serum sickness, the prototypic form of immune complex vasculitis, is rarely seen now in its classic form, as horse serum is injected into humans in recent years only for snake antivenom. Serum-sickness-like reactions to various drugs are far more commonly observed, most notably with penicillin. Clinical manifestations begin 7 to 10 days following exposure with the abrupt onset of fever and arthralgias, followed by headache and meningismus, abdominal pain, paresthesias, and glomerulonephritis. Urticaria rather than palpable purpura is the usual skin manifestation.

Rheumatic Vasculitis

Vasculitis can often be an important clinical feature of the connective tissue diseases, primarily rheumatoid arthritis and systemic lupus erythematosus.[5] Vasculitis may also occur, although much less frequently, in association with progressive systemic sclerosis, dermatomyositis, particularly in children, and Sjögren's syndrome. Vessels of virtually all sizes may be involved, the manifestations ranging from cutaneous palpable purpura or infarcts to potentially lethal widespread systemic vasculitis.

RHEUMATOID VASCULITIS

Rheumatoid vasculitis is found most often in patients who have longstanding severe disease with high titers of IgA rheumatoid factor, a form not usually detected by standard rheumatoid arthritis latex fixation techniques.

SYSTEMIC LUPUS ERYTHEMATOSUS

Systemic lupus erythematosus may involve cutaneous vasculitis in up to 2 percent of patients; the most common lesion is palpable purpura, others being ulcers, hemorrhages beneath the nails, and necrotic digital infarcts.[6] Cutaneous involvement may herald small vessel vasculitis in other organs, particularly the central nervous system and viscera, in which case it is associated with a poor prognosis.

Polyarteritis Nodosa

Polyarteritis nodosa is characterized by widespread vasculitis of small to medium-sized arteries, with predictably lethal consequences without treatment.[7] Like the other forms of vasculitis, it is probably mediated by immune complexes and has a well-recognized association with certain antigens, most notably the hepatitis B surface antigen. The disease may involve virtually any organ system although it has a strong predilection for renal and visceral vasculature, with a tendency to spare the spleen and lungs. Cutaneous lesions may occur in as many as 50 percent of the patients and may include painful subcutaneous nodules, ulcers, palpable purpura, or urticaria.

The cutaneous form of polyarteritis is more benign and lesions are localized primarily in medium-sized muscular arteries of the lower extremities. Patients present with palpable tender subcutaneous nodules and a livedo reticularis pattern (Fig. 1-3). Fever, arthralgias, and myalgias frequently accompany the acute phase of the disease.

Granulomatous Vasculitides

There are several forms of vasculitis classified as granulomatous vasculitis, the common denominator among them being the histologic feature of intravascular and extravascular formation of granulomas in association with the vasculitis. In all forms there is multisystem involvement and skin manifestations are frequent.

ALLERGIC GRANULOMATOUS ANGIITIS (CHURG-STRAUSS SYNDROME)

Allergic granulomatous angiitis is a rare form of systemic vasculitis, which was originally distinguished from polyarteritis nodosa in 1951 by Churg and Strauss.[8] Its characteristic features include adult onset asthma, pulmonary involvement, and peripheral eosinophilia. The skin is involved in up to 60 percent of the pa-

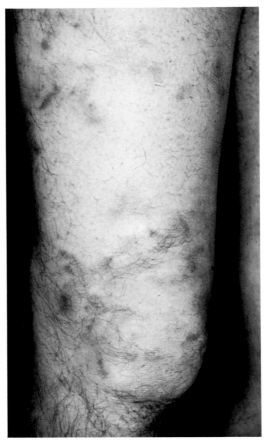

Fig. 1-3. Cutaneous polyarteritis nodosa. Livedo pattern of lower legs. Tender, deep nodules are frequent within the pattern.

tients, the lesions being palpable purpura, cutaneous infarcts, and/or subcutaneous nodules. Characteristic histopathologic granulomas and an eosinophilic cellular infiltrate are often found on biopsy of the skin nodules.

The heart, liver, and gastrointestinal tract may be involved, just as they are occasionally in polyarteritis nodosa, but renal disease is very infrequent.

WEGENER'S GRANULOMATOSIS

Wegener's granulomatosis is characterized by necrotizing granulomatous vasculitis of both the upper and lower respiratory tracts, glomerulonephritis, and a rather generalized small vessel vasculitis.[9] The characteristic histopathologic features of fibrinoid necrosis of small arteries and veins associated with granulomas are best seen in the pulmonary lesions.

The most frequent initial complaints are recurrent sinusitis, persistent rhinorrhea, and nasal mucosal ulcerations accompanied by fever, malaise, and weight loss. As many as 50 percent of patients may have skin lesions characterized as cutaneous infarcts, ulcerations, hemorrhagic blisters, purpuric papules, and/or generalized urticaria (Fig. 1-4). A skin biopsy of one of these lesions will frequently show a leukocytoclastic vasculitis rather than the granulomatous involvement.

Glomerular disease, seen clinically as hematuria and proteinuria, may occur in up to 80 percent of patients, and renal biopsy will reveal a focal necrotizing glomerulonephritis. Pulmonary involvement is invariable, with x-ray findings of solitary or multiple poorly marginated nodular densities.

LYMPHOMATOID GRANULOMATOSIS

Lymphomatoid granulomatosis was recognized as distinct from Wegener's granulomatosis in 1972 by Leibow et al., who observed granulomatous vasculitis with a pleomorphic cellular infiltrate more characteristic of the lymphoproliferative diseases.[10] Small arteries and veins are affected in an angiocentric pattern, with atypical lymphocytes and histiocytes.

The disease primarily involves the pulmonary tract, with cough, dyspnea, or pleuritic chest pain accompanied by fever, malaise, and weight loss. Skin lesions may occur in up to 50 percent of patients as nodules, cutaneous infarcts, chronic ulcers, or indolent plaques. Skin biopsy may often be diagnostic. Renal involvement is less frequent than in some of the other forms of granulomatous vasculitis, and the central nervous system may be involved as well.

Giant Cell Vasculitis

TEMPORAL ARTERITIS

Temporal arteritis, which is also called *giant cell* or *cranial arteritis,* is a well-recognized form of vasculitis involving one or more branches of the carotid artery. It is seen most commonly in older individuals, with presenting symptoms that include headache, scalp tenderness, and visual impairment. It is frequently accompanied by polymyalgia rheumatica, in which there is aching pain and stiffness of the

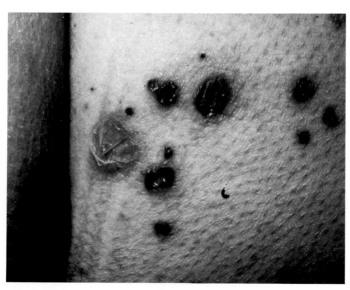

Fig. 1-4. Wegener's granulomatosis. The most common skin lesion is a cutaneous infarct leading to ulceration.

proximal muscles of the neck and shoulders and the hip girdle.[11]

Skin lesions can occur in the form of necrosis and eventually ulceration of the overlying skin. Biopsy of the involved artery reveals intimal thickening and giant cell formation. Prompt treatment with systemic corticosteroids is indicated because of the severity of the pain and because of the likelihood of blindness.

TAKAYASU'S DISEASE

Takayasu's disease is a rare form of vasculitis primarily affecting medium- to large-sized arteries, particularly the aortic arch and branches. It has no cutaneous manifestations.[12]

APPROACH TO THE PATIENT: EVALUATION OF CUTANEOUS VASCULITIS

The first part of any evaluation for vasculitis is histologic confirmation of the suspected disease, and since skin lesions are so technically easy to biopsy, one should begin with them when present. In the case of allergic vasculitis it has become increasingly clear that the process is so dynamic that any lesion less than about 18 hours or more than 36 hours old will not yield typical results. Clearly, it is often difficult to determine the exact age of any individual lesion, and this makes selection quite difficult. In some patients a biopsy for direct immunofluorescence may be helpful, as it will characteristically show granular deposition of immunoreactants, particularly C3, but the lesions for direct immunofluorescence must be less than

6 hours old, as the immune complexes are rapidly phagocytized and removed.

Once the diagnosis has been established, it is necessary to determine the extent of the disease. Symptoms relative to specific organs and the appropriate screening tests are listed in Table 1-2. In the case of allergic vasculitis it is more frequent to find that there is no systemic organ involvement, whereas in the other forms of vasculitis that have been discussed previously patients may present with widespread systemic involvement.

Since numerous other diseases may be associated with vasculitis, it is important to ask specific questions relating to symptoms caused by these diseases and to obtain appropriate screening tests, as indicated in Table 1-3.

Furthermore, there are a number of other possible causes of vasculitis, such as exposure to foreign proteins, to a variety of chemicals, and to any one of numerous drugs, some of which are listed in Table 1-4. Usually, these causes are more difficult to incriminate, particularly in the case of drugs and medications. Clearly, any suspected drug should be discontinued, and the only way to prove its involvement is by rechallenge, an ethically and medically unacceptable testing procedure.

MANAGEMENT

Hypersensitivity Vasculitis

If there is no associated demonstrable disease or any suspected causative chemical or drug agent, the physician is faced with management of patients suffering from hypersensitivity vas-

Table 1-2. Approach to the Patient: Vasculitis Evaluation—
Internal Organ Involvement

Organ	Sign	Test
Gastrointestinal tract	Bleeding	Stool guaiac
Kidneys	Glomerulitis	Urinalysis
Joints	Arthritis	—
Nerves	Neuropathy	Nerve conduction
Lungs	Hemoptysis	Chest x-ray
	Dyspnea	
Heart	Arrhythmias	Electrocardiogram
	Congestive heart failure	

**Table 1-3. Approach to the Patient: Vasculitis Evaluation—
Associated Conditions and Screening Tests**

Condition	Test
Streptococcal infection	Throat culture and antistrepto-lysin-O titer
Lupus erythematosus	Antinuclear antibody
Hemolytic anemia	Complete blood count
Hodgkin's disease	Chest x-ray
Cryoglobulinemia	Serum cryoglobulins
Macroglobulinemia	Serum protein electrophoresis
Myeloma	Serum protein electrophoresis
Rheumatoid arthritis	Rheumatoid factor
Hypocomplementemic vasculitis	Serum complement
	Erythrocyte sedimentation rate
Hepatitis	Hepatitis antigens

culitis in a way that will bring relief of the disease without unnecessary side effects. Clearly, if there is compromise of normal function of any organ, whether that organ be the kidney or the skin, aggressive therapy such as use of corticosteroids and/or cytotoxic agents may be appropriate. For instance, function of the skin may be compromised when the involvement is so extensive and the number of infarctive and ulcerative lesions so great that pain, secondary infection, or loss of normal protective function of the skin limits the patient's normal activities. The most benign and apparently effective agent in some patients is colchicine, 0.6 mg 2 to 3 times daily. Although this treatment is not effective in all patients, it is effective in a sufficient number and its side effects are so minimal that it is appropriate as a trial. If the disease is quite severe and acute in onset, it is probably reasonable to administer predni-sone in a dose of 1 to 1.5 mg/kg/day for the first 5 to 7 days and then to taper the prednisone over the ensuing 2 to 3 weeks. It is usually not necessary to become involved in long-term prednisone therapy.

Since dapsone has been described as being effective in an unusual form of cutaneous vasculitis called erythema elevatum diutinum, it might be an appropriate drug to try but its toxicities must be recognized.

Rheumatic Vasculitis

The treatment of the vasculitis associated with rheumatic diseases is obviously treatment of the underlying disease.

**Table 1-4. Approach to the Patient:
Vasculitis Evaluation—Causes Other
Than Disease**

Foreign protein
    Horse serum (snakebite antivenom)
    Hyposensitization antigen
Chemicals
    Insecticides, weed killers
    Petroleum products
Drugs
    Aspirin
    Phenacetin
    Sulfonamides
    Penicillin
    Phenothiazines
    Iodides

Polyarteritis Nodosa

Without aggressive treatment of polyarteritis nodosa overall long-term survival is very poor, the majority of deaths occurring from progressive renal failure or visceral infarction. Aggressive treatment with corticosteroids alone or in combination with cytotoxic agents such as cyclophosphamide or azathioprine has induced long-term remissions with a 5-year survival of 50 to 80 percent.

Granulomatous Vasculitides

The use of aggressive cytotoxic agents, particularly cyclophosphamide 1 to 2 mg/kg/day, has frequently been demonstrated to reverse what were formerly fatal diseases.

Giant Cell Vasculitis

Systemic corticosteroids constitute the therapy of choice and in the case of temporal arteritis should be instituted promptly to prevent severe complications, particularly blindness.

REFERENCES

1. Gower RG, Sams WM Jr, Thorne EG, et al: Leukocytoclastic vasculitis: sequential appearance of immunoreactants and cellular changes in serial biopsies. J Invest Dermatol 69:477, 1977
2. Braverman IM, Yen A: Demonstration of immune complexes in spontaneous and histamine-induced lesions and in normal skin of patients with leukocytoclastic vasculitis. J Invest Dermatol 64:105, 1975
3. McDuffie FC, Sams WM Jr, Maldonado J, et al: Circulating immune complexes in cutaneous vasculitis: detection of Clq and monoclonal rheumatoid factor. J Clin Invest 64:1652, 1979
4. Meltzer M, Franklin EC, Elias K, et al: Cryoglobulinemia: a clinical and laboratory study. Am J Med 40:828, 1966
5. Glass D, Soter N, Schur PH: Rheumatoid vasculitis. Arthritis Rheum 19:950, 1976
6. Estes D, Christian CL: The natural history of systemic lupus erythematosus by prospective analysis. Medicine (Baltimore) 50:85, 1971
7. Cupps TR, Fauci AS: The Vasculitides. WB Saunders, Philadelphia, 1981
8. Churg J, Strauss L: Allergic granulomatosis, allergic angiitis, and periarteritis nodosa. Am J Pathol 27:277, 1951
9. Fauci AS, Wolff SM: Wegener's granulomatosis. Medicine (Baltimore) 52:535, 1973
10. Leibow AA, Carrington CB, Friedman PJ: Lymphomatoid granulomatosis. Hum Pathol 3:457, 1972
11. Hunder GG, Allen GL: Giant cell arteritis: a review. Bull Rheum Dis 29:980, 1978
12. Judge RD, Currier RD, Gracie WK, et al: Takayasu's arteritis and the aortic arch syndrome. Am J Med 32:379, 1962

2

Systemic Sclerosis (Scleroderma) and Pseudosclerodermas

Raul Fleischmajer
Mark Lebwohl

SYSTEMIC SCLEROSIS (SCLERODERMA)

Scleroderma, or *systemic sclerosis,* is a connective tissue disorder characterized by vascular damage and severe fibrosis. Although the disease was initially recognized by its striking skin changes, it later became obvious that it represents a systemic disturbance affecting various organ systems, notably the lungs, gastrointestinal tract, heart, and kidneys. The disease has a predilection for females over males in a ratio of 3:1, and it affects all races and all ages, although it is more common during the third and fourth decades of life. The cause of scleroderma remains unknown. However, three hypotheses have been proposed to explain its pathophysiology, namely: (1) it is an autoimmune response, perhaps to a connective tissue antigen; (2) the primary event is vascular damage secondary to a cytotoxic factor; and (3) it is a derangement in collagen metabolism.[1] The clinical picture of scleroderma is quite distinct, although in the past few years two clinical subsets have been identified that may carry different prognoses. In addition, there is some evidence of a possible relationship between scleroderma and other connective tissue disorders such as mixed connective tissue disease, dermatomyositis, Sjögren's disease, lupus erythematosus, and, more recently, diffuse fasciitis with eosinophilia and the chronic graft-versus-host reaction.

Classification and Diagnostic Criteria

Most patients with systemic sclerosis reveal a rather distinct clinical picture, particularly with respect to the skin involvement. Thus, an extensive study by the Subcommittee for Scleroderma Criteria, sponsored by the American Rheumatism Association, found that only one major criterion was necessary for the diagnosis of systemic sclerosis, namely, proximal scleroderma. *Proximal scleroderma* is defined as tightness, thickening, and nonpitting induration of the fingers and of the skin proximal to the metacarpophalangeal or metatarsophalangeal joints. Other parts of the extremities, face, neck, or trunk (thorax or abdomen) can be affected, and the condition is usually bilateral

Table 2-1. Classification of Scleroderma

Systemic scleroderma
    CREST (calcinosis cutis, Raynaud's phenomenon, esophageal involvement, sclerodactyly, and telangiectasia)
    Diffuse scleroderma
Localized scleroderma
    Morphea
    Generalized morphea
    Linear scleroderma
Overlap syndromes
    Mixed connective tissue disease
    Diffuse fasciitis with eosinophilia
    Chronic graft-vs.-host disease
    Chemically induced scleroderma

and symmetrical and almost always includes sclerodactyly. In the absence of proximal scleroderma, the diagnosis can also be confirmed if two out of three minor criteria are present, namely: (1) sclerodactyly; (2) digital pitting scars of the fingertips or loss of substance of the distal finger pad; and (3) bilateral basilar pulmonary fibrosis.[2] On the basis of the morphology and pattern of skin involvement, clinical picture, and serology, it is possible to identify several scleroderma subsets, as outlined in Table 2-1. We shall briefly review the diagnostic criteria for each subset.

SYSTEMIC SCLERODERMA

Two subsets have been identified in systemic sclerosis:

CREST (calcinosis, Raynaud's phenomenon, esophageal involvement, sclerodactyly, and telangiectasia) identifies a common subset, which usually carries a more benign prognosis. This form usually reveals a positive antinuclear antibody (ANA) in a fine-speckled pattern, which

by chromosomal spread has been shown to stain the centromere region.[3] However, the syndrome may not be complete, and this may be related to the duration of disease. Furthermore, the benign prognosis should be qualified, since many patients with CREST develop pulmonary disease, and some have serious complications such as pulmonary arterial hypertension and biliary cirrhosis.

Diffuse scleroderma is characterized by diffuse skin involvement and appears to carry a poor prognosis since these patients frequently develop severe pulmonary and kidney disease. Many of these patients have a positive SCL-70 antibody, and they are usually centromere-negative[4] (Table 2-2).

LOCALIZED SCLERODERMA

Localized scleroderma affects all ages although it is frequently seen in children. The disease usually lasts from 2 to 5 years and most lesions resolve, leaving atrophy of the skin. There is no Raynaud's phenomenon, sclerodactyly, or internal involvement except for muscle atrophy, usually secondary to skin induration. About 50 percent of localized sclerodermas have a positive ANA (homogeneous or nucleolar pattern), but centromere, SCL-70, nuclear ribonucleoprotein (nRNP), Sm, and SS-B are negative.[5]

Morphea presents itself as indurated, well-circumscribed plaques, usually 1 to 5 cm in diameter and having ivory white color, sometimes surrounded by an erythematous halo known as a *lilac ring*. Lesions may occur on the trunk or extremities. Morphea may be ac-

Table 2-2. Systemic Sclerosis

Type	Dermatologic Features	Laboratory Findings
CREST	Calcinosis, Raynaud's phenomenon, sclerodactyly, telangiectases	Antinuclear antibody = positive Anticentromere antibody = positive (50 to 96%)
Diffuse	Diffuse skin involvement	Antinuclear antibody = positive Anticentromere antibody = negative anti-SCL-70 antibody = positive (34%)

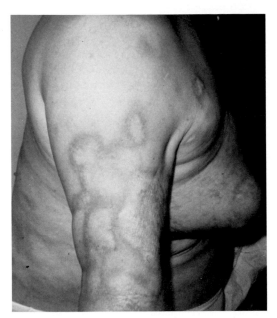

Fig. 2-1. Generalized morphea. Note indurated plaques surrounded by a "halo ring."

companied by *atrophoderma,* which consists of soft patches that are slightly depressed and hyperpigmented and have prominent superficial veins due to dermal atrophy. It appears that atrophoderma is not preceded by skin induration so it is not the end stage of a morphea plaque.

Generalized morphea is the most severe form of localized scleroderma and may affect large parts of the skin, particularly the trunk and extremities. The lesions consist of large, markedly indurated, ivory-colored plaques, 5 to 10 cm or more in diameter, surrounded by an erythematous halo (Fig. 2-1). Usually face, neck, hands, and toes are spared. This form may cause severe muscle atrophy of the extremities. In females breasts are usually involved, but the periareolar area is not affected and thus becomes prominent.

Linear scleroderma is frequently seen in children and has a band morphology usually affecting the arms, legs, side of the face, and scalp (coup de sabre). This is a self-limited disease but may cause serious disfigurement and functional impairment, particularly when it affects the hands and feet (Table 2-3).

Overlap syndromes comprise a number of conditions that closely resemble or overlap with systemic sclerosis. This is particularly true for mixed connective tissue disease (MCTD), diffuse fasciitis with eosinophilia, chronic graft-versus-host disease, and chemically induced sclerodermas. They will be discussed in the section on pseudosclerodermas.

Clinical Picture

Most patients with systemic sclerosis have skin induration accompanied by pulmonary and/or gastrointestinal involvement. It is very rare to have "scleroderma sine scleroderma," as has been described in isolated reports.

SKIN

Skin involvement occurs in about 90 percent of patients with systemic sclerosis. Initially they develop nonpitting edema involving the face and hands, which may last for about 3 months. This edematous stage is missed by many patients. If this stage is present as the initial event, systemic sclerosis is difficult to diagnose and should be differentiated from contact dermatitis, angioedema, nephrotic syndrome, dermatomyositis, and trichinosis. The edema is followed by severe skin induration, which may be restricted to the fingers (sclerodactyly) or develop into the acrosclerotic or diffuse form (Fig. 2-2). Raynaud's phenomenon, consisting of sudden pallor (paroxysmal vasospasm) and/or cyanosis, is present in about 95 percent of patients and may precede the onset of systemic sclerosis by many years. These episodes are

Table 2-3. Localized Scleroderma

Type	Dermatologic Features
Morphea	Single or multiple round patches with peripheral halo
Generalized morphea	Multiple confluent patches, no sclerodactyly
Linear scleroderma	Bandlike morphology

Laboratory findings for all three types: antinuclear antibody, positive (50–72%); anticentromere antibody, negative; SCL-70 antibody, negative.

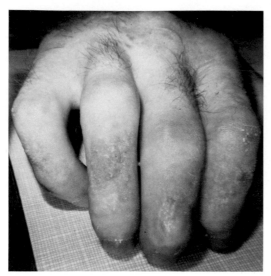

Fig. 2-2. Systemic sclerosis. Acrosclerosis and marked ischemia.

usually induced by cold exposure or by emotional stress and affect the hands and feet, although they have been described on the tip of the nose, the tongue, and the knees. Severe Raynaud's phenomenon may eventually result in spontaneous finger amputations, particularly in those affected by the CREST syndrome. About 10 percent of patients develop calcinosis cutis, and this finding is especially prominent in patients with the CREST syndrome. Calcium nodules and plaques develop on the volar aspect of the phalanges of the fingers, forearms, in the olecranon bursa, and in the prepatellar area (Fig. 2-3). Calcinosis cutis rarely may occur in morphea. Frequently, calcium deposits result in inflammation and ulcerations and drainage, which may be painful and become secondarily infected. There is no systemic treatment for calcinosis cutis, and the plaques sometimes have to be removed surgically.

Telangiectases are very common and may occur in the form of mats or linear dilated vessels. They are most frequently seen on the face, lips, and palms; however, they can occur in the oral mucosa and in the intestinal tract, suggesting Rendu-Osler-Weber disease. The cause of the telangiectasia is not known although an increased uptake of [³H]thymidine by endothe-

lial cells has been demonstrated.[6] Some patients, particularly blacks, develop a striking symmetrical depigmentation affecting the forehead near the hairline, clavicular areas, chest, abdomen, and flanks (Fig. 2-4). Hyperpigmentation may occur but it is less common.

A rather rare manifestation of scleroderma is the appearance of multiple widespread nodules associated with acrosclerosis. The nodules are usually 5 to 10 mm in diameter, dome-shaped, skin-colored, and indurated. The histology reveals severe dermal fibrosis.

GASTROINTESTINAL TRACT

It is estimated that 90 percent of patients with systemic sclerosis have esophageal involvement, which is characterized by dysphagia, dyspepsia, and reflux esophagitis. Barium swallow with fluoroscopic examination is not sensitive enough to detect esophageal hypomotility. A ciné-esophagram is more sensitive and has the additional advantage that it can also detect hiatus hernia and other complications, such as peptic esophagitis and esophageal strictures second-

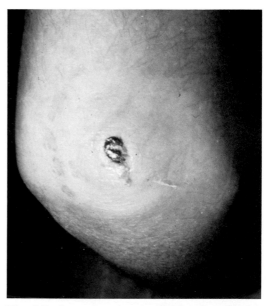

Fig. 2-3. Systemic sclerosis. Calcinosis cutis with ulceration.

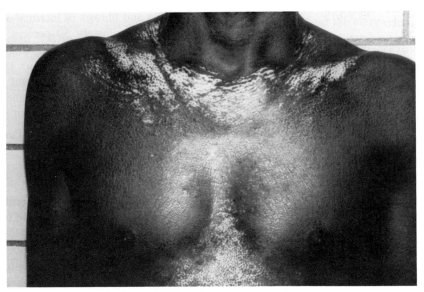

Fig. 2-4. Systemic sclerosis. Symmetrical depigmentation.

ary to gastric fluid reflux. However, the most sensitive technique to detect early esophageal hypomotility is esophageal manometry. Malabsorption and steatorrhea may occur secondarily to bacterial overgrowth and respond well to tetracyclines. Constipation, ileus, and colonic diverticuli are less common. A small percentage of patients, particularly those with the CREST syndrome, develop primary biliary cirrhosis.

LUNGS

Lung involvement is characterized by dyspnea (the most frequent complaint), coughing, and sputum production. Patients may also complain of hemoptysis and pleuritic chest pain. There is localized or diffuse fibrosis, and roentgenograms reveal changes ranging from linear or nodular densities to diffuse mottling and honeycombing, frequently affecting the bottom third of both lungs. Most recently, open-lung biopsies, gallium-67 scanning, and bronchoalveolar lavage have revealed that interstitial fibrosis is also accompanied by an inflammatory reaction consisting of macrophages, lympho-

phages, and polymorphonuclear leukocytes.[7] Pulmonary function studies are usually abnormal and reduction in gas exchange seems to be the initial change, although a restricted pattern is not uncommon. This may be seen in both the CREST and the diffuse form.[8] There is usually poor correlation between the severity of reduction in carbon monoxide diffusing capacity and x-ray fibrosis.[8] However, a severe reduction in gas exchange may be a predictive factor for mortality. Thus, patients with a gas-diffusing capacity less than 40 percent of the predicted value had a 9 percent 5-year survival while those above 40 percent of the predicted value had a 75 percent 5-year survival.[9] The most serious complication is pulmonary arterial hypertension, which can be seen in association with the CREST syndrome (50 percent) and the diffuse form (33 percent).[10] Noninvasive studies may be helpful in detecting significantly elevated pulmonary arterial pressures. A reduction in diffusing capacity below 43 percent of the predicted value combined with chest x-rays and electrocardiographic findings can correctly identify 75 percent of patients with pulmonary hypertension.[10]

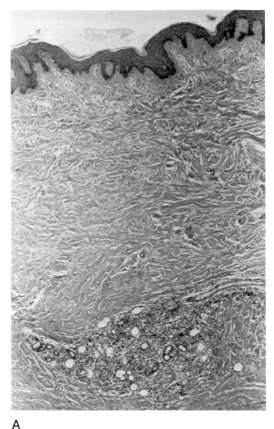

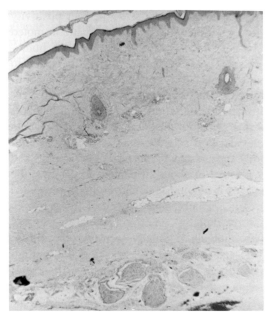

B

Fig. 2-5. Systemic scleroderma. (**A**) Inflammatory stage showing mononuclear cell infiltrates invading eccrine sweat glands. (**B**) Severe fibrosis of dermis and subcutaneous tissue.

A

Scleredema

Scleredema is a benign disease of the connective tissue, which may closely simulate systemic sclerosis. It has a sudden onset, is rapidly progressive, and is characterized by marked induration of the skin. This disease affects all ages and all races and seems to be more preva-

Table 2-4. Pseudosclerodermas

Scleredema
Mixed connective tissue disease
Diffuse fasciitis with eosinophilia
Chronic graft-versus-host disease
Chemically induced scleroderma
Progeria
Werner's disease
Porphyria cutanea tarda
Carcinoid syndrome
Phenylketonuria
Papular mucinosis
Melorheostosis

lent among females. The onset may be preceded by an infection of viral or bacterial origin, such as influenza, measles, mumps, scarlet fever, tonsillitis, pharyngitis, otitis, furunculosis, erysipelas, and impetigo. Skin induration may be preceded by low-grade fever, malaise, myalgia, and arthralgia. The skin induration is symmetrical and usually confined to the back of the neck and upper back, although it may affect the face, trunk, and extremities. However, fingers and toes are not involved, and there is no Raynaud's phenomenon, telangiectasia, or ulcerations. The skin has a woodlike consistency and is tightly bound to underlying structures. The involved areas are usually of normal skin color but occasionally mild erythema may be present. Although the disease is usually restricted to the skin, internal involvement has been observed, consisting of hydrarthrosis, pleural and pericardial effusions, macroglossia, and muscle involvement, including the pharynx and heart muscles. In children, nonspecific cardiac findings have been described, including gallops, ST depression, T wave inversion, and carditis secondary to rheumatic fever. Scleredema preceded by an infection, which frequently occurs in children, is a self-limited disease and usually undergoes spontaneous resolution in 6 months to 2 years. However, more recently a new syndrome affecting adults was recognized, which consists of obesity, insulin-dependent or latent diabetes mellitus accompanied by hyperinsulinism, scleredema, and a high incidence of cardiovascular disease. These patients are usually severe diabetics, resistant to antidiabetic therapy.[26] This form of scleredema persists indefinitely even if the diabetes mellitus is under control. There have also been some reports of adult scleredema associated with a monoclonal gammopathy of the IgG-κ or IgG-λ types with no evidence of multiple myeloma.

The histology reveals marked thickening of the dermis with thick collagen bundles separated by large interfascicular spaces, which sometimes may contain hyaluronic acid. Occasionally, an inflammatory reaction consisting mostly of lymphocytes, histiocytic cells, and plasma cells may be present. There is no treatment for scleredema.

Mixed Connective Tissue Disease

MCTD has been regarded as a distinct entity by some, while others regard it as a clinical variant of lupus erythematosus (see Ch. 3). There may be some overlapping between MCTD and scleroderma. Raynaud's phenomenon, accompanied by persistent enlargement of the fingers without skin induration, is usually seen in MCTD. In our experience both disorders may be distinguished by the serologic profile since ANAs against nuclear ribonucleoprotein at high titers are rare in systemic sclerosis. However, one should be aware that patients with MCTD may eventually develop systemic sclerosis.

Diffuse Fasciitis with Eosinophilia (Eosinophilic Fasciitis)

In 1975 Shulman[27] described an apparently new syndrome characterized by painful swelling followed by severe skin induration and a striking peripheral blood eosinophilia. Age of onset has ranged from childhood to 88 years, and the disease appears to be more prevalent in males.[28] Onset may be preceded by trauma or unusual physical exertion and usually involves extremities, although it may also involve the trunk, neck, hands, and feet. Clinically some patients present with a condition resembling morphea while others may show acrosclerosis. The skin is indurated and tightly bound to underlying structures and may reveal a puckered or "peau d'orange" appearance (Fig. 2-6). These patients usually do not have Raynaud's

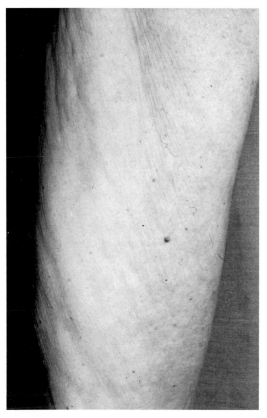

Fig. 2-6. Diffuse fasciitis with blood eosinophilia. Puckering of the forearm.

phenomenon or internal manifestations suggestive of systemic sclerosis. Other manifestations reported are flexion contractures involving small and large joints, carpal tunnel syndrome related to flexor tenosynovitis, and occasional development of an oligoarticular synovitis. The most frequent laboratory abnormalities are severe peripheral eosinophilia, usually ranging from 10 to 50 percent, elevated erythrocyte sedimentation rate, and hypergammaglobulinemia. Rheumatoid factor and ANAs are usually negative. Complement levels are normal. The histology initially reveals cellular infiltrates consisting of lymphocytes, plasma cells, and sometimes eosinophils, affecting the lower dermis, fat, and particularly the deep fascia. As the disease progresses, the inflammatory phase is followed by severe fibrosis (Fig. 2-7). The prognosis appears to be good and skin induration may resolve spontaneously or following oral corticosteroid therapy.

The pathogenesis of diffuse fasciitis remains unknown. It is not known whether it represents a distinct entity or is part of the scleroderma complex. In this regard it is noteworthy that transient peripheral eosinophilia, tissue eosinophilia, and deep fascia thickening may occur in scleroderma. Since the description by Shulman there have been several cases of diffuse fasciitis associated with severe hematologic disorders. These disorders consisted usually of aplastic anemia of unknown origin, but thrombocytopenia, myeloproliferative disorders, Hodgkin's disease, and overt leukemia have also been reported. This group of cases, which apparently represents a distinct subset from the other cases of diffuse fasciitis, carries a poor prognosis since most of the patients succumb to bleeding complications or sepsis. The cause of the aplastic anemia and thrombocytopenic purpura is unknown, although Weltz et al. demonstrated antiplatelet antibodies and a circulating inhibitor of autologous and homologous erythroid stem cells.[29] In addition, Hoffman et al.[30] showed that the IgG fraction obtained from their patient inhibited growth of committed granulocytic and erythroid progenitor cells. Circulating immune complexes have also been

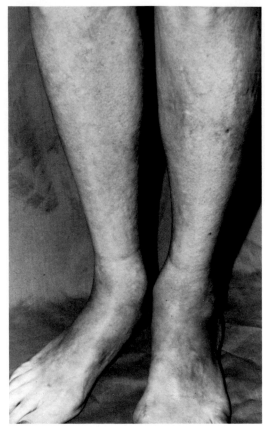

Fig. 2-7. Diffuse fasciitis with blood eosinophilia. Severe skin induration of the lower extremities.

demonstrated.[31] Although it appears that diffuse fasciitis with eosinophilia and bone marrow aplasia may represent an immunologic response, the exact mechanism remains to be disclosed.

Chronic Graft-Versus-Host Disease

Allogeneic bone marrow transplantation is frequently used for the treatment of certain leukemias, aplastic anemia, and some immunodeficiency diseases. Acute graft-versus-host disease (GVHD) can develop 10 to 40 days after transplantation and is characterized by a morbilliform or scarlatiniform eruption, hepatitis, diarrhea, and lymphopenia. Other cutaneous manifestations are purpura, hyperpigmentation, and

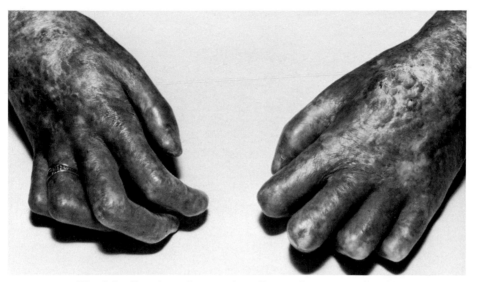

Fig. 2-8. Chronic graft-versus-host disease. Severe acrosclerosis.

toxic epidermal necrolysis. Patients who survive 3 or more months following a bone marrow transplant may develop chronic GVHD. This syndrome consists of Sjögren's syndrome, lichen planus-like lesions affecting the skin and oral mucosa, a maculopapular rash, cholestatic liver disease, and striking sclerodermoid skin changes.[32,33] These patients may show acrosclerosis to diffuse skin induration, which may result in severe flexion contractures of hands, feet, and knees and cause severe disability (Fig. 2-8). Sclerodermatous lesions may be accompanied by large telangiectases and hypo- and hyperpigmentation resembling poikiloderma (Fig. 2-9). Raynaud's phenomenon, however, is usually not present. The skin pathology reveals features of both acute GVHD and scleroderma, namely, lymphocytic infiltration of the basal cell layer and around blood vessels, vacuolization of basal cells, and fibrosis of the dermis and subcutaneous tissue. IgM is found at the dermoepidermal junction, and IgM, IgA, and C3 are present in the dermal blood vessels.[34] Scleroderma-like lesions have also been induced in experimental animals following bone marrow transplantation. The development of scleroderma and Sjögren's syndrome during chronic GVHD suggests an immune reaction whereby the donor lymphocytes may be activated by a host connective tissue component, although at present this hypothesis remains purely speculative.

Chemically Induced Scleroderma

Scleroderma-like lesions have been described in persons with certain occupations, following the administration of certain medications and, more recently, following the ingestion of adulterated oil. Scleroderma-like illness has been described in workers exposed to gaseous vinyl chloride prior to its polymerization to polyvinylchloride (solid). This syndrome consists of Raynaud's phenomenon, sclerodermatous skin changes involving hands and forearms, and osteolytic and sclerotic lesions of bone. The fingers may reveal pseudoclubbing and hands may appear pink or blue.[35] Osteolysis usually occurs in finger bones although it has been described in bones of the feet, ulna, radius, and sacroiliac joints. The skin histology reveals interstitial edema with positive metachromatic material, homogenization of collagen, perivascular cellular infiltrates consisting mostly of lymphocytes, and medial hypertrophy and intimal fibrosis of small arteries. Wide-field capillaroscopy reveals dilated capillary loops intermingled with

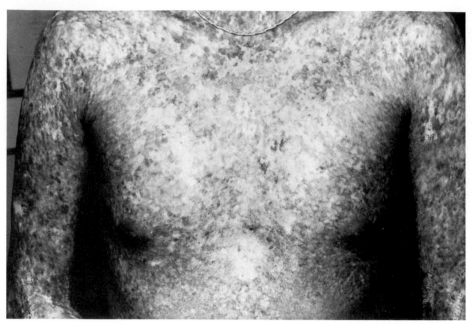

Fig. 2-9. Chronic graft-versus-host disease. Poikiloderma showing depigmentation, atrophy, and large telangiectases.

avascular areas, as described in true systemic sclerosis.[36] Since only about 3 percent of workers develop the disease, a predisposing factor in addition to vinyl chloride exposure may be involved. The systemic nature of the disease suggests that the portal of entry may be the lungs rather than the skin.

Systemic sclerosis may be 5 to 17 times more common among underground miners, stone masons, and other workers exposed to silica dust.[37] The clinical picture is similar to that found in other cases of systemic sclerosis and includes acrosclerosis, Raynaud's phenomenon, dysphagia, arthralgia, calcinosis, kidney disease, and a high incidence of pulmonary fibrosis. Some patients also reveal positive ANAs of different patterns. Silicosis with scleroderma has been observed mostly in males.

Several drugs have also been associated with scleroderma-like syndromes. Bleomycin is an antineoplastic antibiotic obtained from the fermentation of *Streptomyces verticillus,* a strain of Actinomycetales. This drug is used for the treatment of squamous cell carcinomas (except for lung), lymphosarcomas, Hodgkin's disease,

and embryonal cell carcinoma of the testis. One of the main side effects of bleomycin administration is pulmonary and skin fibrosis. These patients develop nodules or plaques and, occasionally, generalized skin induration. Some patients also develop Raynaud's phenomenon. Other cutaneous reactions consist of linear hyperpigmentation, alopecia, nail changes, vesiculation, and pruritus. The skin induration occurs on the hands and may result in severe disability and eventual gangrene of the digits as seen in scleroderma.[38] The histology reveals dense collagen bundles and focal areas of collagen homogenization, especially around blood vessels and adnexal structures. The disease is self-limited and may resolve spontaneously within 2 months after therapy is discontinued.

Pentazocine (Talwin) is an analgesic that, given by injection, may cause local or diffuse cutaneous sclerosis and/or ulcerations. Patients so affected may be drug or alcohol abusers and have a high incidence of personal or family history of diabetes mellitus. Cutaneous induration of a woody consistency occurs 2 weeks to 3 years after the first injection.[39] Fibrosis may affect skin, subcutaneous tissue, and muscle and may be accompanied by superficial ulcers and calcinosis of fat and muscle. Laboratory data are essentially negative except for an elevation in the erythrocyte sedimentation rate.

Cosmetic surgical procedures that involve injection of a foreign substance (usually for breast augmentation) may induce in some patients a syndrome closely resembling scleroderma. In a study of four cases the materials injected were paraffin, silicone, and other less well-defined substances.[40] The clinical picture consisted of Raynaud's phenomenon, skin induration ranging from sclerodactyly and morphea to acrosclerosis and widespread involvement, arthralgia, arthritis, polymyositis, esophageal dilation, pulmonary fibrosis, and Sjögren's syndrome. The interpretation of this so-called adjuvant disease is difficult, since under similar circumstances other patients developed lupus erythematosus, rheumatoid arthritis, Sjögren's disease, polymyositis, and MCTD.[41] However, immunologic factors may be operative.

In May 1981 the ingestion of illegally sold denatured rapeseed oil, mostly in the northwest area of Madrid, resulted in an outbreak of a new clinical syndrome that reached epidemic proportions and is known as the toxic oil syndrome (TOS). It is estimated that about 18,000 persons were affected, and by December 1982 there were 336 deaths, mostly due to noncardiogenic pulmonary edema and thromboembolic complications.[42,43] The syndrome began with an acute stage characterized by fever, eosinophilia, exanthematous rash, pruritus, malaise, myalgia, arthralgia, dyspnea, and noncardiogenic edema. During the second month patients developed a diffuse papular eruption and edema of the face and limbs, which initially was soft but later became progressively more indurated. This stage suggested a toxic or allergic reaction. The pathology consisted of damaged endothelial cells of small blood vessels and perivascular infiltrates consisting of lymphocytes, histiocytes, occasional eosinophils, and neutrophils. Plasma cells were usually absent. Vascular lesions involved arterioles, veins, and medium-sized arteries. The skin also

revealed mucinous deposits. The chronic stage of the TOS, which developed in some patients over a period of several months, consisted of peripheral neuropathy, muscle atrophy, skin tightness simulating scleroderma, xerostomia, xerophthalmia of the sicca type, pulmonary hypertension, and, less frequently, Raynaud's phenomenon, esophageal hypomotility, and development of autoantibodies. Thus, there were several features similar to those described in systemic sclerosis. Further follow-up revealed marked atrophy of facial subcutaneous tissue, simulating a form of lipodystrophy. In addition, patients developed flexion contractures of fingers and palms, with marked fibrosis and muscle atrophy. The skin histology during the chronic or sclerodermatous stage is not clear, but there appears to be fibrosis of the dermis. Medium-sized arteries also revealed subintimal fibrosis, resulting in marked narrowing of the lumen. Fibrosis was also demonstrated in nerves, skin, arteries, salivary glands, and pancreas but not in the lungs.

Progeria (Hutchinson-Gilford Disease)

Progeria is a rare autosomal recessive disorder characterized by premature aging, accelerated atherosclerosis, and sudden death at a very early age. The onset takes place at age 6 to 12 months and the disease affects both sexes equally. The clinical picture consists of dwarfism, craniofacial disproportion, high-pitched voice, prominent joints, thin bones, small clavicles, coxa valga, and defective ossification of the skull.[44] The facial features are so distinct that most patients look alike and reveal a small face, recessed chin, prominent nasal cartilage, and nasolabial and circumoral cyanosis. There is general atrophy of muscle and subcutaneous tissues. The scalp veins are prominent. There is diffuse alopecia, atrophy of the skin, and dystrophy of the nails. Severe skin induration may be present on the abdomen, upper thighs, and gluteal areas. Histology shows fibrosis of the dermis and subcutaneous tissue. There is no sexual maturation, but intelligence is apparently normal. The prognosis is poor, since most patients die during the second decade of life from coronary thrombosis secondary to atherosclerosis. The etiology of progeria is unknown, although progeric fibroblasts are regarded as models for premature senescence since in vitro they show decreased growth capacity; reduced mitotic activity, DNA synthesis, and cloning efficiency; and deficient DNA repair following exposure to ionizing radiation.

Werner's Disease

Werner's disease, also known as progeria of the adult, is transmitted as an autosomal recessive trait and is characterized by premature aging accompanied by accelerated atherosclerosis. The onset usually occurs shortly after adolescence. There is no sex predilection, more than one sibling may be affected, and there is frequently consanguinity between parents.[45,46] The patients reveal short stature, typical facies with a beak-shaped nose, premature canities, baldness, wrinkling of the skin, hyper- and hypopigmentation. In addition, these patients develop scleroderma-like changes involving the upper and lower extremities. The skin appears smooth, glossy, and tightly bound. On the lower extremities skin induration may be accompanied by severe ischemia, ulcers, and eventually gangrene. The rest of the clinical picture consists of juvenile cataracts, diabetes mellitus, hypogonadism, high-pitched or husky voice, vascular calcification, and early myocardial infarction. Roentgenographic findings include osteoporosis, small bone structure, metastatic calcifications of soft tissue, foot deformities, osteomyelitis-like lesions, osteoarthrosis, and spondylosis deformans.[47] There is a high incidence of neoplasia. Laboratory data may reveal hyperglycemia, hypercholesterolemia, and an increase in low-density lipoproteins and serum uric acid. Werner's fibroblasts also show features of premature senescence related to defective production of histocompatibility antigens and abnormalities in protein synthesis.[48]

Porphyria Cutanea Tarda

Porphyria cutanea tarda (PCT) is a disturbance in pyrrole metabolism affecting the liver. Although the disease is usually acquired, a heritable form transmitted in an autosomal dominant fashion was recently discovered.[49] The most common causative agents of PCT are estrogens, oral contraceptives, iron overload, alcoholism, and hexachlorobenzene (an insecticide). PCT has also been found in association with lupus erythematosus.[50] The porphyrin abnormality is due to a decrease in uroporphyrinogen decarboxylase activity, resulting in an increase in urinary uroporphyrins and fecal coproporphyrins.

The cutaneous manifestations consist of hypertrichosis, photosensitivity expressed by the appearance of bullous lesions, scarring of hands and forearms, and eventual development of scleroderma-like lesions that may resemble morphea, linear scleroderma, or acrosclerosis (Fig. 2-10). Skin induration may start in exposed parts of the body such as the face, "V" of the neck, and back and is frequently accompanied by a yellowish hue secondary to hyperkeratinization. The histology reveals sclerosis of the dermis, homogenization of collagen, cellular inflammatory infiltrates, and reduction in skin appendages. The cause of the sclerosis is unknown, although it may be related to a phototoxic reaction.

Carcinoid Syndrome

Carcinoids are metastasizing tumors derived from the granular (Kulchitsky) cells of the crypts of Lieberkühn of the intestine. They usually develop in the appendix, although they may be found in the jejunum and ileum and, rarely, in the bronchi. Functioning carcinomas release large amounts of 5-hydroxytryptamine (seroto-

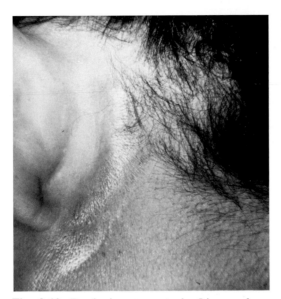

Fig. 2-10. Porphyria cutanea tarda. Linear sclero-derma-like lesion behind ear.

nin), which causes a syndrome characterized by dyspnea, coughing and wheezing, diarrhea, and fibrosis of the pulmonary and tricuspid valves and inferior vena cava. This syndrome is more common in patients who have liver metastases. The cutaneous manifestations of carcinoid tumors are paroxysmal flushing, pellagra, cutaneous metastases, and scleroderma-like plaques. The skin induration usually occurs in the lower extremities and consists of erythema, edema, and thickening and tightening of the skin.[51] Acrosclerosis and Raynaud's phenomenon have not been found in association with carcinoid tumors. Skin biopsies reveal fibrosis and mononuclear cell infiltrates. It has been suggested that serotonin may be responsible for the skin induration.

Phenylketonuria

Phenylketonuria (PKU) is an autosomal recessive disease, and it is estimated that 1 in 50 persons is an asymptomatic heterozygous carrier. This disease is the cause of profound mental retardation. In this disorder phenylala-

nine accumulates owing to a deficiency of phenylalanine hydroxylase, the enzyme responsible for conversion of phenylalanine to tyrosine. Since tyrosine is essential for the synthesis of melanin, patients with PKU frequently have fair skin, blue eyes, and blond hair. Eczema and scleroderma-like lesions have also been described in PKU. The sclerodermatous lesions resemble plaquelike or guttate morphea, usually develop during the first 2 years of life and involve the buttocks, thighs, and lower legs. The skin induration may become generalized, but hands and feet are usually spared.[52] Flexion contractures of the knees are frequently noticed. These patients do not develop systemic manifestations of scleroderma, and the skin induration may subside following a diet restricted in phenylalanine. The cause of the skin induration is not known although an impairment in tryptophan metabolism has been suggested.

Papular Mucinosis

Papular mucinosis, also known as *lichen myxedematosus,* is a rare disease characterized by three distinct features: a chronic papular lichenoid eruption, the presence of mucin in the dermis, and paraproteinemia. A clinical variant in which the disease is more generalized and accompanied by erythema and sclerosis is referred to as *scleromyxedema.* This disease affects adults 30 to 70 years old and has no sex predilection. Patients present with a lichenoid eruption consisting of dome-shaped papules, which are skin-colored or red, are 2 to 4 mm in diameter, and may show a linear arrangement. The areas most frequently affected are the dorsum of the hands and fingers, axillary folds, and extensor surfaces of arms and legs. On the face the coalescence of papules, particularly on the glabella, may give a leonine appearance. There are no subjective symptoms except for mild pruritus. Although the disease affects primarily the skin, other manifestations can occur, including severe proximal myopathy, inflammatory polyarthritis, central nervous system symptoms resembling acute organic brain syndrome, esophageal aperistalsis, and hoarseness. The disease is frequently associated with a paraproteinemia consisting of myeloma-like serum globulin of the IgG type, predominantly λ, although κ light chains have also been reported.[53,54] Association of papular mucinosis with multiple myeloma is rare if it occurs at all. The pathology reveals an increase in fibroblasts, which appear plump and stellate and are accompanied by dermal fibrosis. The most striking feature is the presence of a mucinous material between collagen bundles, which is susceptible to hyaluronidase digestion. This disease runs a chronic course, usually persisting indefinitely, but the prognosis for long-term survival is good.

Melorheostosis

Melorheostosis is a rare acquired disorder of bone, which affects children and adolescents, has no sex predilection, and is usually progressive during the period of active growth. The diagnosis is made by roentgenographic examination, which reveals linear hyperostosis, usually involving the cortical area of an extremity bone.[55] These patients develop vascular lesions and linear scleroderma. The vascular lesions are glomus tumors, hemangiomas, and lymphangiectasias. The etiology of this disorder remains unknown.

APPROACH TO THE PATIENT

Differentiation of systemic sclerosis from localized forms of scleroderma is critical because of the serious systemic complications and prognostic implications of the former condition (Table 2-5). A history of Raynaud's phenomenon and symmetrical involvement of the digits on physical examination is very strongly suggestive of a diagnosis of systemic sclerosis. Isolated plaques suggest a diagnosis of morphea, and widespread involvement that spares the hands and feet is characteristic of generalized morphea.

Table 2-5. Approach to the Patient

History
 Raynaud's phenomenon, dysphagia, dyspnea, dry eyes, exposure to polyvinyl chloride or silica dust
Medical history
 Diabetes, bone marrow transplant, breast augmentation
Medications
 Bleomycin, pentazocine (Talwin)
Family history
 Progeria, Werner's disease, porphyria cutanea tarda, phenylketonuria

Physical Examination
 Sclerodactyly, fingertip scars or ulcerations, induration, "lilac ring," telangiectasia, calcinosis, hyper- and hypopigmentation

Laboratory Investigation
Initial screen
 Complete blood count + differential, blood urea nitrogen, creatinine, creatine phosphokinase, urinalysis, antinuclear antibody, skin biopsy, chest x-ray
In-depth examination
 Scleroderma: (capillary microscopy), ciné-esophagram or esophageal manometry, carbon monoxide diffusing capacity, electrocardiogram
 Eosinophilic fasciitis: biopsy down to fascia
 Scleredema: glucose tolerance test
 Porphyria cutanea tarda: Wood's lamp examination of urine, 24-hour urinary porphyrins
 Carcinoid: urinary 5-hydroxyindoleacetic acid
 Phenylketonuria: urine screen or serum phenylalanine
 Papular mucinosis: skin biopsy, serum protein electrophoresis
 Melorheostosis: bone x-rays of affected extremity

The pseudosclerodermas are usually easily distinguished from systemic sclerosis as well. While hand involvement can occur in eosinophilic fasciitis, the eosinophilia is striking and Raynaud's phenomenon is usually absent. Biopsy of skin down to fascia overlying muscle will show a characteristic inflammatory infiltrate of the fascia. Raynaud's phenomenon and hand involvement can occur in the chemically induced sclerodermas, but these should be easily diagnosed by eliciting a history of exposure to the offending chemical or medication. Similarly, a history of bone marrow transplantation should suggest a diagnosis of chronic graft-versus-host disease. Induration of the skin of the posterior neck and upper back with noteworthy sparing of the fingers and absence of Raynaud's phenomenon should make the clinician suspect a diagnosis of scleredema, especially in a diabetic patient. Differentiation of MCTD from systemic sclerosis can be particularly difficult since Raynaud's phenomenon and scleroderma-tous skin changes can occur. Concomitant signs of lupus or dermatomyositis should suggest this diagnosis, and high titers of antibodies to ribonucleoprotein distinguish it from systemic sclerosis.

Family history is seldom of benefit in the pseudosclerodermas, but progeria, Werner's disease, and phenylketonuria are inherited in an autosomal recessive fashion. A history of affected siblings or cousins should therefore be sought when these diseases are suspected. In all three disorders Raynaud's phenomenon and hand involvement are uncommon. The craniofacial features of progeria are so distinctive that this diagnosis is easily made. Werner's disease depends on the recognition of a constellation of clinical features, including cataracts, early alopecia and canities, diabetes, accelerated atherosclerosis, premature wrinkling, and leg ulcers. Phenylketonuria should be suspected in a patient with sclerodermatous skin changes, fair skin, and mental retardation. Definitive diagnosis is established by the demonstration of elevated blood levels of phenylalanine. Alternatively, a simple screening test can be performed by adding a few drops of ferric chloride solution to the urine. In patients with phenylketonuria the urine will turn green, demonstrating the presence of phenylpyruvic acid.

Porphyria cutanea tarda can also be inherited in an autosomal dominant fashion, although most cases are acquired as a result of exposure to substances such as estrogens or alcohol. The presence of hypertrichosis, photosensitivity, bullous lesions, or scarring of the hands should alert the clinician to the possibility of this diagnosis. Sclerodermatous lesions usually resemble morphea and although acrosclerosis can rarely occur, Raynaud's phenomenon is absent. Wood's lamp examination of the urine shows a pinkish red fluorescence, in contrast to the green-yellow appearance of normal urine. Addition of a few drops of hydrochloric or acetic acid to the urine intensifies the fluorescence. Demonstration of elevated 24-hour urinary por-

phyrins is diagnostic. In unusual instances quantitative analysis of fecal or plasma porphyrins is necessary.

Sclerodcrma-like induration of the lower extremities can occur in the carcinoid syndrome as well. Raynaud's phenomenon and acrosclerosis are absent. If other symptoms, such as paroxysmal flushing and a pellagra-like photosensitive eruption, are present, urinary levels of 5-hydroxyindoleacetic acid should be determined.

Diffuse infiltration of the skin in papular mucinosis (scleromyxedema) can result in indurated plaques, although the more common papular lesions are not usually confused with scleroderma. Skin biopsy is diagnostic, and alcian blue stains at pH 2.5 with hyaluronidase digestion shows the dermal mucin to be hyaluronic acid. Serum protein electrophoresis (and if negative, immunoelectrophoresis) should be performed in patients with papular mucinosis since in nearly all cases there is an associated paraproteinemia.

Finally, radiographs of an extremity bone underlying a plaque of linear scleroderma will, rarely, demonstrate the presence of melorheostosis.

In summary, clinical features of the scleroderma-like disorders usually enable the clinician to suspect the correct diagnosis. Investigative efforts can then be directed towards the appropriate condition, and work-up, as outlined in Table 2-5, can be pursued.

ACKNOWLEDGMENT

This study was supported by NIH grants AM27608 and AM07376.

REFERENCES

1. Fleischmajer R, Perlish JS, Duncan M: Scleroderma. A model for fibrosis. Arch Dermatol 119:957, 1983
2. American Rheumatism Association Diagnostic and Therapeutic Criteria Committee, Subcom-

mittee for Scleroderma Criteria: Preliminary criteria for the classification of systemic sclerosis (scleroderma). Arthritis Rheum 23:581, 1980

3. Fritzler MJ, Kinsella TD: The CREST syndrome: a distinct serologic entity with anticentromere antibodies. Am J Med 69:520, 1980

4. Douvas AS, Achten M, Tan EM: Identification of a nuclear protein (Scl-70) as a unique target of human antinuclear antibodies in scleroderma. J Biol Chem 254:10514, 1979

5. Takehara K, Moroi Y, Nakabayashi Y, Ishibashi Y: Antinuclear antibodies in localized scleroderma. Arthritis Rheum 26:612, 1983

6. Fleischmajer R, Perlish JS: [^{3}H]-Thymidine labeling of dermal endothelial cells in scleroderma. J Invest Dermatol 69:379, 1977

7. Rossi GA, Bitterman PB, Rennard ST, et al: Evidence for chronic inflammation as a component of the interstitial lung disease associated with progressive systemic sclerosis. Am Rev Respir Dis 131:612, 1985

8. Steen VD, Owens GR, Fino GJ, et al: Pulmonary involvement in systemic sclerosis (scleroderma). Arthritis Rheum 28:759, 1985

9. Peters-Golden M, Wise RA, Hochberg MC, et al: Carbon monoxide diffusing capacity as predictor of outcome in systemic sclerosis. Am J Med 77:1027, 1984

10. Ungerer RG, Tashkin DP, Furst D, et al: Prevalence and clinical correlates of pulmonary arterial hypertension in progressive systemic sclerosis. Am J Med 75:65, 1983

11. Traub YM, Shapiro AP, Rodnan GP, et al: Hypertension and renal failure (scleroderma renal crisis) in progressive systemic sclerosis. Review of a 25-year experience with 68 cases. Medicine (Baltimore) 62:335, 1983

12. Follansbee WP, Curtiss EI, Rahko PS, et al: The electrocardiogram in systemic sclerosis (scleroderma). Study of 102 consecutive cases with functional correlations and review of the literature. Am J Med 79:183, 1985

13. Wynn J, Fineberg N, Matzer L, et al: Prediction of survival in progressive systemic sclerosis by multivariate analysis of clinical features. Am Heart J 110:123, 1985

14. Osial TA Jr, Whiteside TL, Buckingham RB, et al: Clinical and serologic study of Sjögren's syndrome in patients with progressive systemic sclerosis. Arthritis Rheum 26:500, 1983

15. Resnick D, Scavulli JF, Goergen TG, et al: Intra-articular calcification in scleroderma. Radiology 124:685, 1977

16. Bernstein RM, Steigerwald JC, Tan EM: Association of antinuclear and antinucleolar antibodies in progressive systemic sclerosis. Clin Exp Immunol 48:43, 1982

17. Tan EM: Antinuclear antibodies in scleroderma. Int J Dermatol 20:569, 1981

18. Catoggio LJ, Bernstein RM, Black CM, et al: Serological markers in progressive systemic sclerosis: clinical correlations. Ann Rheum Dis 42:23, 1983

19. Tuffanelli DL, McKeon F, Kleinsmith DM, et al: Anticentromere and anticentriole antibodies in the scleroderma spectrum. Arch Dermatol 119:560, 1983

20. Fleischmajer R, Perlish JS, Shaw KV, Pirozzi DJ: Skin capillary changes in early systemic scleroderma. Arch Dermatol 112:1553, 1976

21. Fleischmajer R, Perlish JS, Reeves JRT: Cellular infiltrates in scleroderma skin. Arthritis Rheum 20:975, 1977

22. D'Angelo WA, Fries JF, Masi AT, Shulman LE: Pathologic observations in systemic sclerosis (scleroderma). Am J Med 46:428, 1969

23. Fleischmajer R, Dessau W, Timpl R, et al: Immunofluorescence analysis of collagen, fibronectin, and basement membrane protein in scleroderma skin. J Invest Dermatol 75:270, 1980

24. Fleischmajer R, Perlish JS, Krieg T, Timpl R: Variability in collagen and fibronectin synthesis by scleroderma fibroblasts in primary culture. J Invest Dermatol 76:400, 1981

25. Fleischmajer R, Pollock JL: Progressive systemic sclerosis. Pseudoscleroderma. Clin Rheum Dis 5:243, 1979

26. Fleischmajer R, Faludi G, Krol S: Scleredema and diabetes mellitus. Arch Dermatol 101:21, 1970

27. Shulman LE: Diffuse fasciitis with eosinophilia: a new syndrome? Trans Assoc Am Physicians 88:70, 1975

28. Fleischmajer R, Jacotot AB, Shore S, Binnick S: Scleroderma, eosinophilia and diffuse fasciitis. Arch Dermatol 114:1320, 1978

29. Weltz M, Salvado A, Rosse W, et al: Humoral suppression of hematopoiesis in eosinophilic fasciitis. (Abstract). Blood, suppl., 52:218, 1978

30. Hoffman R, Dainiak N, Sibrack L, et al: Antibody-mediated aplastic anemia and diffuse fasciitis. N Engl J Med 300:718, 1979

31. Seibold JR, Rodnan GP, Medsger TA Jr, et al: Circulating immune complexes in eosinophilic fasciitis. Arthritis Rheum 25:1180, 1982

32. Masters R, Hood AF, Cosini AB: Chronic cuta-

neous graft-vs-host reaction following bone marrow transplantation. Arch Dermatol 111:1526, 1975

33. Gratwhol AA, Haralampos M, Moutsopoulos M, et al: Sjögren-type syndrome after allogeneic bone-marrow transplantation. Ann Intern Med 87:703, 1977

34. Spielvogel RL, Goltz RW, Kersey JH: Scleroderma-like changes in chronic graft-versus-host disease. Arch Dermatol 113:1424, 1977

35. Harris DK, Adams WGF: Acro-osteolysis occurring in men engaged in the polymerization of vinyl chloride. Br Med J 3:712, 1967

36. Maricq HR, Johnson MN, Whetstone CL, LeRoy EC: Capillary abnormalities in polyvinyl chloride production workers. Examination by in vivo microscopy. JAMA 236:1368, 1976

37. Rodnan GP, Benedek TG, Medsger TA Jr, Cammarata RJ: The association of progressive systemic sclerosis (scleroderma) with coal miners' pneumoconiosis and other forms of silicosis. Ann Intern Med 66:323, 1967

38. Cohen IS, Mosher MB, O'Keefe EJ, et al: Cutaneous toxicity of bleomycin therapy. Arch Dermatol 107:553, 1973

39. Palestine RF, Millns JL, Spigel GT, et al: Skin manifestations of pentazocine abuse. J Am Acad Dermatol 2:47, 1981

40. Kumagai Y, Abe C, Shiokawa Y: Scleroderma after cosmetic surgery. Four cases of human adjuvant disease. Arthritis Rheum 22:532, 1979

41. Kondo H, Kumagai Y, Shiokawa Y: Scleroderma following cosmetic surgery ("adjuvant disease"). p. 135. A review of nine cases reported in Japan. In Black CM, Myers RW (eds): Systemic Sclerosis (Scleroderma). Gower Medical Publishing Ltd., New York, 1985

42. Noriega AR, Gomez-Reino J, Lopez-Encuentra A, et al: Toxic epidemic syndrome study group. Toxic epidemic syndrome, Spain, 1981. Lancet 2:697, 1982

43. Kilbourne EM, Rigau-Perez JG, Heath CW, et al: Clinical epidemiology of toxic-oil syndrome. Manifestations of a new illness. N Engl J Med 309:1408, 1983

44. Fleischmajer R, Nedwich A: Progeria (Hutchinson-Gilford). Arch Dermatol 107:253, 1973

45. Fleischmajer R, Nedwich A: Werner's syndrome. Am J Med 54:111, 1973

46. Epstein CJ, Martin GM, Schultz AL, Motulsky AG: Werner's syndrome. Medicine (Baltimore) 45:177, 1966

47. Zucker-Franklin D, Rifkin H, Jacobson HG: Werner's syndrome. An analysis of ten cases. Geriatrics 23:123, 1968

48. Goldstein S, Singal DP: Alteration of fibroblast gene products "in vitro" from a subject with Werner's syndrome. Nature 251:719, 1974

49. Benedetto AV, Kushner JP, Taylor JS: Porphyria cutanea tarda in three generations of a single family. N Engl J Med 298:358, 1978

50. Cram DL, Epstein JH, Tuffanelli DC: Lupus erythematosus and porphyria. Arch Dermatol 108:779, 1973

51. Zarafonetis CJD, Lorber SH, Hanson SM: Association of functioning carcinoid syndrome and scleroderma. Am J Med Sci 236:1, 1958

52. Jablonska S, Stachow A, Suffczynska M: Skin and muscle indurations in phenylketonuria. Arch Dermatol 95:443, 1967

53. Osserman EF, Takatsuki K: Role of an abnormal, myeloma-type, serum gamma globulin in the pathogenesis of the skin lesions of papular mucinosis (lichen myxedematosus). J Clin Invest 42:962, 1963

54. McCarthy JT, Osserman E, Lombardo PC, Takatsuki K: An abnormal serum globulin in lichen myxedematosus. Arch Dermatol 89:446, 1964

55. Soffa DJ, Sire DJ, Dodson JH: Melorheostosis with linear sclerodermatous skin changes. Radiology 114:577, 1975

3

Cutaneous Lesions in Connective Tissue Diseases

Raul Fleischmajer
Mark Lebwohl

In 1941 Klemperer and his associates introduced the concept of "collagen diseases." These authors suggested that there is a group of disorders that have in common a collagen alteration, which can involve various organ systems such as the skin, lung, heart, and kidney. From a pathologic viewpoint the common denominator for collagen diseases was the presence of fibrinoid degeneration in the connective tissue. Under the heading of collagen diseases the following disorders were grouped together: lupus erythematosus, dermatomyositis, scleroderma, rheumatoid arthritis, and polyarteritis nodosa. At present it is generally acknowledged that the above diseases do not represent primarily a collagen abnormality, but the concept of systemic diseases involving mesenchymal tissues appears to hold true even if the pathophysiology of these disorders may be quite unrelated. True collagen diseases have already been identified and involve mutations of collagen genes, as is seen in osteogenesis imperfecta and various forms of Ehlers-Danlos syndrome. Connective tissue diseases are frequently associated with cutaneous lesions, some of which may be quite specific and thus provide the clinician with an important clue to the diagnosis of a complicated syndrome. The diagnosis of a connective tissue disorder is facilitated by recognition of the cutaneous manifestations, a thorough clinical examination, and proper interpretation of the laboratory data, particularly when specific antibodies accompany the disease process (Table 3-1). In this chapter we will discuss juvenile rheumatoid arthritis, rheumatoid arthritis, lupus erythematosus, dermatomyositis, and mixed connective tissue disease. Scleroderma and pseudosclerodermas are described in Chapter 2.

JUVENILE RHEUMATOID ARTHRITIS (STILL'S DISEASE)

Juvenile rheumatoid arthritis (JRA) is a disease that usually affects children under the age of 16. The clinical picture may vary, but the common denominator is arthritis of one or more joints that lasts for at least 6 weeks. Three clinical forms have been identified: arthritis with systemic onset; polyarticular disease not accompanied by systemic manifestations; and a milder form, known as *pauciarticular* or *oligoarticular,* in which the articular involvement may be restricted to five joints or less.

When it occurs with acute onset, JRA has

Table 3-1. Antinuclear Antibodies:
Patterns of Fluorescence

Pattern	Associated Disease
Particulate	Mixed connective tissue disease Systemic lupus erythematosus (SLE) Scleroderma
Homogeneous	Any connective tissue disease High titers usually in SLE
Peripheral	SLE (active)
Speckled	CREST, Raynaud's phenomenon (anticentromere antibody)
Nucleolar	Scleroderma (high titers) Raynaud's phenomenon

(Data from Gilliam JN, Cohen SB, Sontheimer RO, Moschella SL: Connective tissue diseases. p. 1087. In Moschella SL, Hurley HJ (eds): Dermatology. WB Saunders, Philadelphia, 1985.)

Table 3-2. Juvenile Rheumatoid
Arthritis

Age of onset
   16 years or less
Clinical picture
   Arthritis
   Fever
   Hepatosplenomegaly
   Myalgia
   Lymphadenopathy
   Serositis
Cutaneous manifestations
   Maculopapular rash
   Subcutaneous rheumatic nodules
   Vasculitis
Laboratory data
   Nonspecific
   Rheumatoid factor usually negative
   Positive antinuclear antibody (25%)

no sex predilection and is characterized by systemic symptoms, namely, high intermittent fever, myalgia, serositis (pericarditis, pleuritis, or peritonitis), hepatosplenomegaly, and generalized lymphadenopathy. The polyarthritis appears later and may undergo spontaneous resolution or progress to chronic deformities (Table 3-2).

The cutaneous lesions are rather characteristic, occur in 30 to 50 percent of patients, and consist of an evanescent eruption, which appears during late afternoon or early evening and is usually accompanied by fever spikes[1] (Fig. 3-1). The lesions are maculopapular, salmon to red in color, and usually nonpruritic and appear on the trunk, face, and extremities, including palms and soles. The histology is nonspecific and only reveals mild edema and lymphohistiocytic perivascular infiltrates. Subcutaneous nodules, similar to those reported in adult rheumatoid arthritis, have been described in the feet, pretibial areas, and scalp. Vasculitis may occur but is rather rare. The lesions may show pallor in the center, and mild trauma may

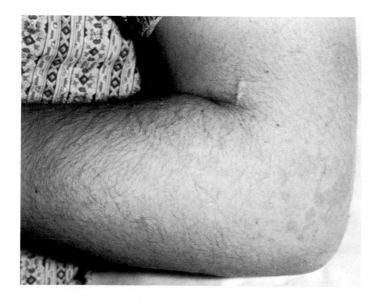

Fig. 3-1. Juvenile rheumatoid arthritis. Maculopapular lesions.

induce a Koebner phenomenon. The skin rash may last for days or weeks or may persist for years.

The polyarticular form without prodromal or systemic manifestations reveals a clinical picture similar to that of the adult form of rheumatoid arthritis, with involvement of multiple symmetrical joints, usually affecting the metacarpophalangeal and interphalangeal joints. This form usually affects girls, and the prognosis is more severe. Typically the pauciarticular form involves large joints, such as elbows, knees, and ankles, and is frequently associated with chronic iridocyclitis. Cutaneous manifestations are not prominent in the latter two forms of JRA.

A rare seronegative polyarthritis in adults resembles systemic onset JRA and has many similar features, including the salmon-colored, morbilliform rash. Subcutaneous nodules have not been reported in adult onset Still's disease.

Laboratory data in JRA are not specific and usually reveal an increased erythrocyte sedimentation rate and leukocytosis. An increased incidence of HLA-B27 was found in patients predisposed to develop ankylosing spondylitis. The rheumatoid factor (RF) is usually negative although some studies showed that positivity of RF increases with the age of the patient.[2] Antinuclear antibodies are positive in about 25 percent of patients, usually in females and at low titers.[2]

RHEUMATOID ARTHRITIS

Rheumatoid arthritis is a disabling disease, which affects approximately 1 to 3 percent of the adult population of the United States. The disease is characterized by an intense inflammatory reaction of articular tissues, although other tissues may also be affected, particularly the skin. Rheumatoid arthritis is frequently associated with skin manifestations, some of which are rather characteristic and may have important clinical and diagnostic implications. Furthermore, the severity of skin lesions may parallel the activity of the underlying disease. Many of the cutaneous lesions show cellular infiltrates as well as deposition of complement and immunoglobulins, which suggests that these lesions may be the result of an immune response. The disease has a predilection for smaller joints but also affects bone, muscle, fascia, ligaments, and tendons. Criteria for diagnosis are morning stiffness, pain on motion, or tenderness; swelling of at least one joint; cutaneous nodules over bony prominences, extensor surfaces, or near joints; characteristic roentgenographic changes; positive RF; and synovial pathology and fluid consistent with rheumatoid arthritis.

Cutaneous involvement is common and can be divided into three forms: subcutaneous nodules, rheumatoid vasculitis, and miscellaneous lesions[3] (Table 3-3). Subcutaneous nodules, frequently referred to as rheumatoid nodules, are rather characteristic for rheumatoid arthritis and are present in about 20 percent of patients. These lesions usually occur in the subcutaneous tissue although they may invade adjacent structures such as the periosteum, fascia, or tendons. They range in size from a few millimeters to 5 cm in diameter, and they usually occur in areas of friction or trauma, namely, elbows, extensor surfaces of forearms, metacarpophalangeal and interphalangeal joints, ischial tuberosities, and sacrum. Similar nodules have been described in the vocal cords, sclerae, lungs, heart, muscle, splenic capsule, peritoneum, and

Table 3-3. Rheumatoid Arthritis

Age of onset
    Adult life
Clinical picture
    Polyarthritis
Cutaneous manifestations
    Subcutaneous nodules
    Vasculitis
        Digital infarcts
        Necrotizing venulitis
        Ulcers
        Pyoderma gangrenosum (?)
    Miscellaneous
Laboratory data
    Rheumatoid factor
    Increased erythrocyte sedimentation rate
    Increased platelet count
    Positive antinuclear antibodies in some subsets
    Serum complement normal except with active
        vasculitis
    HLA-DR4

nervous system.[4] The histology reveals three distinct areas: an inner zone of fibrinoid degeneration, a surrounding zone of elongated, histiocytic-type cells in palisade arrangement, and an outer zone of vascularized granulation tissue and chronic inflammatory cells. A vasculitis probably precedes the development of a rheumatoid nodule. Immune complexes containing the RF, autologous IgG, and complement have been described within rheumatic nodules. These lesions have to be differentiated from gouty tophi, amyloid nodules, ganglions, epidermoid cysts, xanthomas, reticulohistiocytosis, and subcutaneous granuloma annulare.[3] Most patients with subcutaneous nodules show high RF titers. The RF is usually an IgM but could also be an IgG or IgA antibody that has specificity against constant domains of autologous immunoglobulins. The association of subcutaneous nodules, vasculitis, and RF at high titers carries a serious prognosis.

Rheumatoid vasculitis is frequently associated with rheumatoid arthritis and usually occurs in patients with long-standing severe active erosive arthritis with high RF titers. This vasculitis usually develops in patients with HLA-DR4.[5] Deposition of immune complexes appears to play an important role in the development of these vascular lesions, which may involve small and medium muscular arteries, postcapillary venules, and capillaries. The most common manifestations of rheumatoid vasculitis are splinter hemorrhages and digital infarcts. These lesions may be found in the nail folds, finger pulp, and nail edges and occasionally may progress to gangrene. Ulcers and livedo reticularis involve small or medium-sized arteries or veins, while purpuric papules (palpable purpura) and hemorrhagic bullae and urticaria (acute necrotizing vasculitis) involve postcapillary venules. Patients with large vessel involvement have a serious prognosis, since they frequently develop visceral infarctions, coronary arteritis, cerebral vasculitis or widespread mononeuritis multiplex due to involvement of vasa nervorum. Vasculitic ulcers usually occur in patients with subcutaneous nodules and high titers of RF. They are sharply marginated, deep, and sometimes very painful and have a tendency to heal slowly. They may be preceded by purpuric or macular lesions. Ulcers are often associated with Felty's syndrome, which consists of a triad of rheumatoid arthritis, splenomegaly, and leukopenia. In addition, pyoderma gangrenosum, with or without vasculitis, has been described in rheumatoid arthritis. These lesions consist of sharply marginated ulcers with a distinctive purple-red areola and an undermined border. Blood vessel disease may also be secondary to cryoglobulinemia and a hyperviscosity syndrome due to elevated concentrations of macromolecular polymers of IgG RF.[6] Sjögren's syndrome (failure of lacrimal and salivary gland secretion), occurs in about 10 percent of patients. Other cutaneous manifestations in rheumatoid arthritis are Raynaud's phenomenon, skin atrophy, amyloidosis, lipoid nodules, bullous lesions (bullous pemphigoid, cicatricial pemphigoid, dermatitis herpetiformis), granuloma annulare, yellow nail syndrome, and livid palms accompanied by hyperhidrosis.[3]

LUPUS ERYTHEMATOSUS

Lupus erythematosus (LE) represents one of the best documented disorders of autoimmunity. A broad spectrum of autoantibodies have been recognized that have diagnostic as well as pathogenetic implications. On the basis of the clinical picture, cutaneous manifestations, and serologic profiles, three distinct clinical subsets have been identified, namely, acute, subacute, and chronic LE (Tables 3-4 and 3-5).

Acute Lupus Erythematosus

Acute LE represents the most severe form of the disease. The clinical picture consists of fever, malaise, arthralgia or arthritis, lupus nephritis, pericarditis, pleuritis, hepatospleno-

Table 3-4. Clinical Subsets of Lupus Erythematosus

Clinical Subset	Diagnostic Laboratory Findings
Acute LE	

Facial erythema (butterfly)
    Generalized erythematous plaques
    Morbilliform rash
	Positive antinuclear antibodies
	Anti-ds DNA
	Anti-Sm
	Low complement

Subacute LE	

Annular
    Discoid
    Psoriasiform
	Positive antinuclear antibodies
	Anti-SSA/Ro and anti-SSB/La
	HLA-DR3

Chronic LE	

Discoid (localized or generalized)
    Hypertrophic
    Lupus profundus
	Positive antinuclear antibodies (30%, low titers)

megaly, lymphadenopathy, and central nervous system involvement characterized by peripheral neuropathy, seizures, and organic brain disease. Skin lesions are present in about 25 percent of the patients and consist of a typical butterfly rash or a more generalized morbilliform or plaquelike eruption involving light-exposed and nonexposed parts of the body (Fig. 3-2). The lesions are erythematous, edematous, and non-scarring, appear suddenly, may last for hours to days, and resolve spontaneously, sometimes leaving residual postinflammatory hyperpigmentation. The acute edematous stage is sometimes precipitated by sunlight exposure. The widespread reaction may simulate a drug reaction, erythema multiforme, or toxic epidermal necrolysis.[5] Acute LE may be accompanied by a variety of nonspecific cutaneous manifestations, including vasculitis (palpable purpura, gangrene), livedo reticularis, subcutaneous nodules, alopecia, mucous membrane lesions, pigmentary abnormalities, calcinosis cutis (rare), hypocomplementemic urticarial vasculitis, and Raynaud's phenomenon. Acute LE usually is accompanied by active disease, and this can be corroborated by laboratory findings. These patients have a positive antinuclear antibody (ANA) test at high titers with homogeneous or peripheral pattern, positive double-stranded DNA, positive Sm antibodies, low serum complement levels, high sedimentation rate, anemia, leukopenia, hypergammaglobulinemia, proteinuria, and hematuria. The lupus band test is 98 percent positive in involved skin and 75 percent positive in uninvolved skin.[7]

Subacute Lupus Erythematosus

Subacute LE (also called subacute cutaneous LE) is a clinical subset characterized by typical skin lesions and a distinct serologic profile and carries a better prognosis than the acute type. The clinical picture consists of photosensitivity, arthritis, arthralgias, fever, malaise, myalgias, pleuritis, and Raynaud's phenomenon. There is a low incidence of renal and central nervous system disease. These patients frequently present with a widespread symmetrical skin eruption, usually affecting the neck, trunk, and

Table 3-5. The 1982 Revised Criteria for Classification of Systemic Lupus Erythematosus[a]

Criterion	Definition
1. Malar rash	Fixed erythema, flat or raised, over the malar eminences, tending to spare the nasolabial folds
2. Discoid rash	Erythematous raised patches with adherent keratotic scaling and follicular plugging; atrophic scarring may occur in older lesions
3. Photosensitivity	Skin rash as a result of unusual reaction to sunlight, by patient history or physician observation
4. Oral ulcers	Oral or nasopharyngeal ulceration, usually painless, observed by a physician
5. Arthritis	Nonerosive arthritis involving 2 or more peripheral joints, characterized by tenderness, swelling, or effusion
6. Serositis	a) Pleuritis—convincing history of pleuritic pain or rub heard by a physician or evidence of pleural effusion or b) Pericarditis—documented by ECG or rub or evidence of pericardial effusion
7. Renal disorder	a) Persistent proteinuria greater then 0.5 g/day or greater than 3+ if quantitation not performed or b) Cellular casts—may be red cell, hemoglobin, granular, tubular, or mixed
8. Neurologic disorder	a) Seizures—in the absence of offending drugs or known metabolic derangements (e.g., uremia, ketoacidosis, or electrolyte imbalance) or b) Psychosis—in the absence of offending drugs or known metabolic derangements (e.g., uremia, ketoacidosis, or electrolyte imbalance)
9. Hematologic disorder	a) Hemolytic anemia—with reticulocytosis or b) Leukopenia—less than 4,000/mm^3 total on two or more occasions or c) Lymphopenia—less than 1,500/mm^3 on two or more occasions or d) Thrombocytopenia—less than 100,000/mm^3 in the absence of offending drugs
10. Immunologic disorder	a) Positive lupus erythematosus cell preparation or b) Anti-DNA: antibody to native DNA in abnormal titer or c) Anti-Sm: presence of antibody to SM nuclear antigen or d) False-positive serologic test for syphilis known to be positive for at least 6 months and confirmed by *Treponema pallidum* immobilization or fluorescent treponemal antibody absorption test
11. Antinuclear antibody	An abnormal titer of antinuclear antibody by immunofluorescence or an equivalent assay at any point in time and in the absence of drugs known to be associated with ''drug-induced lupus'' syndrome

[a] The proposed classification is based on 11 criteria. For the purpose of identifying patients in clinical studies, a person shall be said to have systemic lupus erythematosus if any 4 or more of the 11 criteria are present, serially or simultaneously, during any interval of observation.

(Tan EM, Cohen AS, Fries JF et al: The 1982 revised criteria for the classification of systemic lupus erythematosus (SLE). Arthritis Rheum 25:1271, 1982. Reprinted from ARTHRITIS AND RHEUMATISM Journal, copyright 1982. Used by permission of the American Rheumatism Association.)

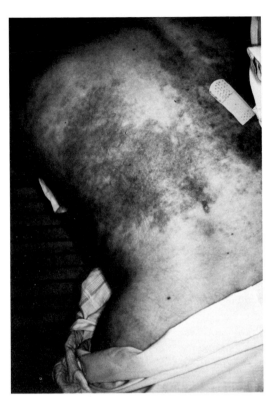

Fig. 3-2. Acute lupus erythematosus. Erythematous lesions on the back.

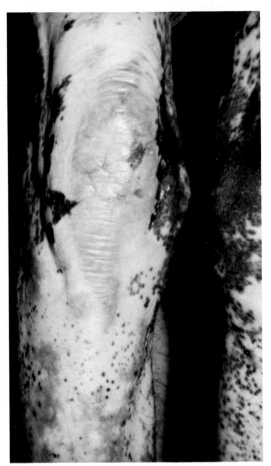

Fig. 3-3. Subacute lupus erythematosus. Psoriasiform lesions and marked depigmentation in a patient with concomitant vitiligo.

arms. The lesions are erythematous and scaling, and may be psoriasiform or annular. They resolve without residual scarring[7] (Fig. 3-3). In addition, nonspecific cutaneous lesions have been described such as alopecia, livedo reticularis, vasculitis, discoid atrophic lesions, sclerosis, and telangiectases. The lupus band test is 50 percent positive in involved skin but only 30 percent positive in uninvolved skin. A high percentage of patients (about 75 percent) will have a positive ANA test if a sensitive substrate such as KB or Hep-2 tumor cells is used.[7] On the other hand, the ANA is usually negative if rodent kidney or liver is used.[8] The pattern of immunofluorescence is usually homogeneous or particulate. Double-stranded DNA antibodies are much less common in these patients (15 to 20 percent) as compared with the acute clinical subset, and, when present, they are of low titers and are not accompanied by significant hypocomplementemia. Patients with subacute LE have a high incidence of SSA-Ro antibodies;[9] RF and SSB-La antibodies are less frequent, while antibodies against extractable nuclear antigens (ribonucleoprotein and Sm) are only occasionally found in these patients. It has also been shown that the B cell alloantigen HLA-DR3 is frequently associated with subacute LE, particularly in those patients with annular lesions.[10] Recently, a transient form of subacute

LE was recognized in newborn infants. These children present with discoid or annular lesions and circulating SSA-Ro and SSB-La antibodies, which presumably are transferred transplacentally from the mother to the fetus. The onset takes place at 1 week to 3 months of age. The skin lesions usually occur in sun-exposed areas and disappear in about 6 months when the Ro and/or La antibodies become negative, which suggests a direct relationship between the development of skin lesions and the presence of these antibodies. The mothers of these patients may have LE or some other connective tissue disease.[11,12] Neonatal lupus is the most common cause of congenital heart block in infants.[12] The heart damage may be permanent and appears to be related to the SSA-Ro antibody. These antibodies have also been found in association with Raynaud's phenomenon with vasculitis and in acute LE and C2 deficiency.

Chronic Lupus Erythematosus

Chronic LE is usually restricted to the skin and carries a good prognosis. It is also known as *chronic discoid LE,* although this is a poor term since discoid lesions may occur in neonatal LE and acute LE. The lesions have a predilection for light-exposed areas such as the head and neck, although they may be generalized and involve the trunk, arms, and plantar and palmar surfaces. These lesions are usually sharply marginated and consist of erythema, hypo- or hyperpigmentation, follicular plugging, and atrophy. Scalp lesions usually result in permanent alopecia. Mucous membrane involvement occurs in approximately 15 percent of patients and may result in ulcerations. Approximately 10 percent of patients with chronic LE may develop systemic involvement, manifested by fever, fatigue, arthralgia, sun sensitivity, vasculitis, and cutaneous manifestations of acute LE.

Lupus panniculitis is another clinical expression of chronic LE, although it is much less common than the discoid form. The lesions usually involve the head, arms, chest, buttocks, and thighs and consist of deep dermal or subcutaneous inflammatory nodules, which eventually cause deep depressions. Immunoglobulins and complement may be detected in the blood vessels of the deep dermis but may be absent in the dermoepidermal junction. About 70 percent of patients with lupus panniculitis have discoid lesions, and about 50 percent of these patients may have some systemic involvement.[13]

Hypertrophic discoid LE is a variant of the discoid form and is characterized by thick hyperkeratotic lesions with a verrucous appearance similar to hypertrophic lichen planus, keratoacanthomas, or psoriasis. However, in general these patients have other lesions with features of the discoid type. The lupus band test in chronic LE is positive in involved skin in 80 percent of patients and about 20 percent positive in uninvolved areas. Patients with only cutaneous involvement may have a positive ANA at low titers (about 30 percent).[14] A small percentage may have a biologic false positive test for syphilis, positive rheumatoid factor, slight depression in serum complement, a modest leukopenia, and an elevation of gamma globulins. Conversion of chronic to systemic LE should be suspected in patients with positive ANA at high titers, unexplained anemia, significant leukopenia, marked hypergammaglobulinemia, or a positive lupus band test in normal unexposed skin.[15]

POLYMYOSITIS/DERMATOMYOSITIS

Polymyositis is an inflammatory myopathy of proximal muscles, frequently accompanied by a variety of cutaneous manifestations. There are no well-defined clinical subsets as seen in LE, but Bohan and Peter[16] identified five subsets that correlate reasonably well with current clinical experience (Table 3-6). The most common subset is polymyositis alone, in which the only manifestation is muscle involvement. Dermatomyositis, the second most frequent group, shows myositis plus a variety of skin manifestations. The third group refers to the association

Table 3-6. Polymyositis-Dermatomyositis

Group 1—Polymyositis
Group 2—Dermatomyositis
Group 3—Dermatomyositis or polymyositis and internal malignancies
Group 4—Childhood dermatomyositis: (a) adult-like subset, (b) vasculitic subset
Group 5—Overlap group

of polymyositis or dermatomyositis with internal malignancies. The fourth group is childhood dermatomyositis, while the fifth group refers to other connective tissue diseases associated with this syndrome.

The polymyositis starts with pain or tenderness, is symmetrical, and affects proximal muscles of extremities, but it also may involve the limb girdle and anterior neck flexors. This is accompanied by dysphagia due to involvement of pharyngeal (distal) or palatal (proximal) muscles; dyspnea due to diffuse interstitial fibrosis;

aspiration pneumonia secondary to muscle weakness; glomerulonephritis; weight loss; malaise; and fever. About 25 percent of patients may complain of symmetrical generalized arthralgias, often involving the hands, wrists, knees, or ankles. Cardiac disease is not uncommon and may occur as myocarditis or pericarditis. Myocarditis may cause arrhythmias and, eventually, congestive heart failure.

Dermatomyositis is accompanied by several cutaneous lesions, some of which have diagnostic implications. Early in the disease there may be periorbital edema that simulates contact dermatitis, the nephrotic syndrome, or trichinosis. This may be accompanied by a butterfly rash that simulates LE, although the erythema is usually light pink and referred to as *heliotrope* (Fig. 3-4). Perhaps the most distinct cutaneous finding in dermatomyositis is the presence of Gottron's sign, which consists of erythematous macules and papules, with or without scaling,

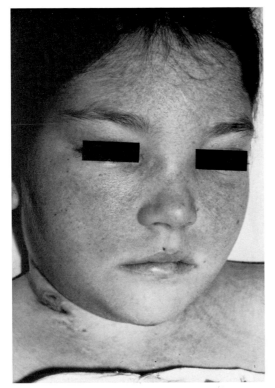

Fig. 3-4. Dermatomyositis. Malar erythema.

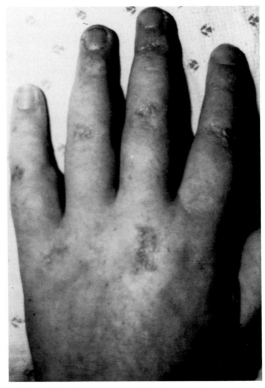

Fig. 3-5. Dermatomyositis. Gottron's papules.

localized on the knuckles (Fig. 3-5). This sign is said to be pathognomonic for dermatomyositis. Poikilodermatous changes consisting of erythema, scaling, telangiectases, and atrophy may be seen on the upper chest, back, neck, face, and limbs. Erythema and telangiectases of the nail fold and thickening of the cuticle have also been described in dermatomyositis. Other manifestations, although uncommon, include Raynaud's phenomenon, photosensitivity, and sclerodactyly (Table 3-7).

The association of internal malignancies and polymyositis-dermatomyositis remains a controversial subject.[16] Malignancies have been observed in adults above the age of 35 years, and the incidence varies from 15 to 50 percent of the patients. Most of the reported tumors were adenocarcinomas, including primary malignancies of the stomach, colon, nasopharynx, breast, lung, ovary, and uterus. In a few well-documented cases, the dermatomyositis disappeared following removal of the tumor, but a relapse caused the dermatomyositis to reappear. There is an equal sex distribution in those patients with associated carcinomas. Adult patients with dermatomyositis should be subjected to a comprehensive history, physical examination, and routine laboratory and radiologic studies.

Dermatomyositis of childhood has a rather characteristic clinical picture and a well-defined pathology. The clinical picture is similar to that of adults except for a higher incidence of calcinosis, which may affect skin, muscle, or both. There is, however, a more acute form associated with vasculitis, described by Banker and Victor.[17] This fulminating form is accompanied by abdominal pain, hematemesis and melena, and is frequently associated with gastrointestinal ulcerations, perforations, and death. One of our patients revealed several ulcerations involving the skin (Fig. 3-6). The pathology reveals an inflammatory process of small blood vessels, proliferation of the intima, and thrombosis. Recently, antibodies against coxsackie B virus were demonstrated in childhood dermatomyositis. Mortality is very high in the vasculi-

Table 3-7. Dermatomyositis: Cutaneous Lesions

Heliotrope erythema
Gottron's papules
Poikiloderma
Periorbital edema
Nailfold alterations
    Telangiectasia
    Cuticular hypertrophy
Photosensitivity
Calcinosis
Cutaneous vasculitis
    Infarcts
    Nodules
    Ulcers

tic type, but the prognosis is rather good in children without vasculitis.

Myositis has been found in association with various connective tissue disorders, including scleroderma, LE, rheumatoid arthritis, and Sjögren's syndrome.[18] These overlap syndromes seem to be more common in females,[19] while association with internal malignancies is rare or nonexistent. There are no specific diagnostic tests for polymyositis or dermatomyositis. The diagnosis is usually confirmed by an increase in serum muscle enzymes, particularly aldolase and creatine phosphokinase (CPK); increase in urinary creatine; and characteristic changes in

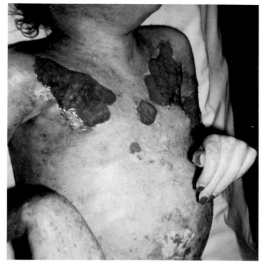

Fig. 3-6. Infantile dermatomyositis. Vasculitic type.

the electromyogram. ANA and RF may be positive, particularly in the overlap group. Muscle biopsy reveals degeneration of muscle fibers, lymphocytic infiltrates, necrosis, and interstitial fibrosis.

MIXED CONNECTIVE TISSUE DISEASE

Mixed connective tissue disease (MCTD) is regarded by some as an entity characterized by clinical overlapping of LE, polymyositis, scleroderma, and occasionally rheumatoid arthritis. The most distinct finding is the presence of high titers of an antibody against nuclear ribonucleoprotein (nRNP) which gives an ANA with a speckled pattern while other antibodies to extractable nuclear antigens are usually absent. The clinical picture usually consists of polyarthralgia, Raynaud's phenomenon with swollen hands (Fig. 3-7), sclerodactyly, esophageal hypomotility, pulmonary disease, and inflammatory myositis. Anti-DNA antibodies may be present, usually at low titers, and serum complement may be depressed, but Sm antibodies are absent. Other features of LE, such as

serositis, leukopenia, anemia, and skin rashes, may be present.[20,21] Other clinical manifestations in association with high antibody titers against nRNP are myocarditis and trigeminal neuropathy. On the other hand, progressive severe kidney disease and central nervous system disease are infrequent in MCTD. Other clinical studies suggest that MCTD is probably not a disease entity, since high antibody titers to nRNP may be seen with systemic LE, polymyositis, or systemic sclerosis. In the experience of these authors, however, the association of anti-nRNP antibodies and systemic scleroderma has been rather low.

APPROACH TO THE PATIENT

Diagnosis of connective tissue diseases often depends upon the recognition of elaborate symptom complexes, with supporting physical findings and laboratory examinations (Table 3-8).

Table 3-8. Approach to the Patient

History
   Arthralgias, morning joint stiffness, photosensitivity, Raynaud's phenomenon
Medications
   Hydralazine
   Procainamide

Physical Examination
   Skin lesions, joint swelling, muscle weakness

Laboratory Investigation
Initial screen
   Erythrocyte sedimentation rate, complete blood count with differential and platelets, antinuclear antibodies, serum protein electrophoresis, rheumatoid factor
In-depth examination
   Lupus: Antibodies to double-stranded DNA, Sm antigen, SSA-Ro and SSB-La antigens; skin biopsy, lupus band test; urinalysis, VDRL, complement, LE cell preparation, electrocardiogram (neonatal lupus), blood urea nitrogen, creatinine
   Rheumatoid arthritis: synovial fluid analysis, joint x-rays
   Dermatomyositis: aldolase, creatine phosphokinase, urinary creatine, electromyogram, muscle biopsy
   Mixed connective tissue disease: Antibody to nuclear ribonucleoprotein

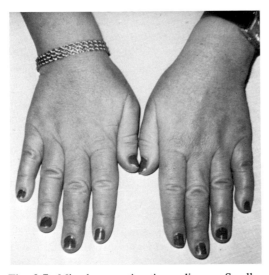

Fig. 3-7. Mixed connective tissue disease. Swollen hands and Raynaud's phenomenon.

A history of joint swelling or pain and morning stiffness are characteristic features of rheumatoid arthritis. It should be noted, however, that arthritis can also occur in JRA, lupus, and MCTD. Similarly, Raynaud's phenomenon can occur in rheumatoid arthritis, but it is sufficiently common in lupus that it used to be one of the diagnostic criteria for that disease and is a routine finding in patients with scleroderma. Photosensitivity remains a diagnostic criterion for lupus but is a nonspecific finding that is present in many conditions. One can often elicit a history of proximal muscle weakness from patients with dermatomyositis, although muscle weakness can also affect patients with MCTD. In advanced cases patients may be unable to climb steps, comb their hair, or arise from a prone position.

Because many of the signs and symptoms of connective tissue diseases are nonspecific, elaborate combinations of criteria have been established for the diagnosis of particular diseases. In addition to the items in a patient's history elaborated above, a medical history is particularly important in lupus since a number of drugs are known to cause lupus-like syndromes.

On physical examination particular attention should be directed to the joints. Cutaneous lesions can be associated with each of the connective tissue diseases, as detailed previously in this chapter.

Laboratory evaluation of patients should include an erythrocyte sedimentation rate (ESR), complete blood count (CBC) with differential and platelet count, serum ANA, and serum protein electrophoresis. The ESR is elevated in most connective tissue diseases, and it can be used to follow responses to treatment. The CBC is also altered in many of these conditions. Diagnostic criteria for lupus include hemolytic anemia, leukopenia, or thrombocytopenia. Leukopenia can also occur with rheumatoid arthritis (Felty's syndrome), but leukocytosis is a more common finding in JRA. Hypergammaglobulinemia is a nonspecific finding in many of the connective tissue diseases, and ANAs are also positive in a significant proportion of patients. The pattern and titer of ANAs are often of diagnostic value (Table 3-1). The RF is also positive in many of these disorders but the titer is often high in rheumatoid arthritis.

In addition to the aforementioned laboratory tests, LE is characterized by a number of specific and nonspecific abnormalities. There is often a chronic false positive serologic test for syphilis. Proteinuria, hematuria, or cellular casts may signal renal involvement. Depression of complement levels is a sign of disease activity. The LE cell preparation, which has been a criterion for the diagnosis of systemic LE, is still a simple test that yields rapid results. Unclotted blood is allowed to incubate for 30 to 60 minutes and stained with Wright's stain. The LE cell represents a polymorphonuclear leukocyte that has phagocytosed the homogeneous-appearing debris of a damaged cell. With the widespread availability of lupus band tests and tests for a number of ANAs, a positive LE cell preparation is no longer the sole immunologic criterion for the diagnosis of lupus. Perhaps the most specific serologic test for LE is the antibody against double-stranded DNA. This antibody is present in high titer in acute LE but is often negative in subacute cutaneous LE. Antibodies against the Sm antigen are specific for LE and have been associated with a poor prognosis. Subacute cutaneous LE has a better prognosis, and antibodies against the Ro antigen are frequently present.

A recently described test using direct immunofluorescence to examine skin biopsy specimens for deposition of immunoglobulins and complement at the dermoepidermal junction is called the *lupus band test*. Biopsy of lesional skin is very sensitive, with 98 percent positivity in acute LE and 50 percent in subacute cutaneous LE. Unfortunately, biopsy of lesional skin is not specific, and the lupus band test is often positive in lesional skin or sun-exposed nonlesional skin of patients with other conditions. Therefore, the most specific lupus band test is one performed on non-sun-exposed nonlesional skin; this is positive in 75 percent of patients with acute LE. The presence of at least two immunoglobulins on a lupus band test further reinforces the diagnosis of LE. It should not be forgotten, however, that lupus has characteristic features on routine skin biopsy stained with hematoxylin and eosin.

In a patient with symptoms of muscle weakness, laboratory tests can establish or exclude a diagnosis of dermatomyositis. Serum levels of muscle enzymes, including creatine phosphokinase, aldolase, serum glutamic-oxaloacetic transaminase, and lactic dehydrogenase may be so high that alternate diagnoses are unlikely. Characteristic changes also occur on the electromyogram and on muscle biopsy. For patients with symptoms of several of the connective tissue diseases, the presence of antibodies to nRNP may support a diagnosis of MCTD. However, it is the combination of clinical and serologic features that establishes each diagnosis.

ACKNOWLEDGMENT

This study was supported by NIH grants AM 27608 and AM 07376.

REFERENCES

1. Calabro JJ, Marchesano JM: Rash associated with juvenile rheumatoid arthritis. J Pediatr 72:611, 1968
2. Petty RE, Cassidy JT, Sullivan DB: Serologic studies in juvenile rheumatoid arthritis: A review. Arthritis Rheum 20(suppl 2):260, 1977
3. Sibbitt WL, Williams RC Jr: Cutaneous manifestations of rheumatoid arthritis. Int J Dermatol 21:563, 1982
4. Hurd ER: Extraarticular manifestations of rheumatoid arthritis. Semin Arthritis Rheum 8:151, 1979
5. Scott DGI, Bacon PA, Tribe CR: Systemic rheumatoid vasculitis: a clinical and laboratory study of 50 cases. Medicine (Baltimore) 60:288, 1981
6. Theofilopoulos AN, Burtonboy G, LoSpalluto J, et al: IgM rheumatoid factor and low molecular weight IgM. An association with vasculitis. Arthritis Rheum 17:272, 1974
7. Gilliam JN, Sontheimer RD: Clinically and immunologically defined subsets of lupus erythematosus. p. 147. In Fleischmajer R (ed): Progress of Diseases of the Skin. Grune & Stratton, Orlando, FL, 1981
8. Maddison PJ, Provost TT, Reichlin M: Serological findings in patients with "ANA-negative" systemic lupus erythematosus. Medicine (Baltimore) 60:87, 1981
9. Sontheimer RD, Maddison PJ, Reichlin M, et al: Serologic and HLA associations in subacute cutaneous lupus erythematosus, a clinical subset of lupus erythematosus. Ann Intern Med 97:664, 1982
10. Sontheimer RD, Stastny P, Gilliam JN: Human histocompatibility antigen associations in subacute cutaneous lupus erythematosus. J Clin Invest 67:312, 1981
11. Kephart DC, Hood AE, Provost TT: Neonatal lupus erythematosus: new serologic findings. J Invest Dermatol 77:331, 1981
12. Esscher E, Scott JS: Congenital heart block and maternal systemic lupus erythematosus. Br Med J 1:1235, 1979
13. Tuffanelli DL: Lupus erythematosus. Arch Dermatol 106:553, 1972
14. Prystowsky SD, Herndon JH Jr, Gilliam JN: Chronic cutaneous lupus erythematosus (DLE): a clinical and laboratory investigation of 80 patients. Medicine (Baltimore) 55:183, 1977
15. Gilliam JN, Cohen SB, Sontheimer RO, Moschella SL: Connective tissue diseases. p. 1087. In Moschella SL, Hurley HJ (eds): Dermatology. WB Saunders, Philadelphia, 1985
16. Bohan A, Peter JB: Polymyositis and dermatomyositis. N Engl J Med 292:403, 1975
17. Banker BQ, Victor M: Dermatomyositis (systemic angiopathy) of childhood. Medicine (Baltimore) 45:261, 1966
18. Bohan A, Peter JB, Bowman RL, et al: A computer-assisted analysis of 153 patients with polymyositis or dermatomyositis. Medicine (Baltimore) 56:255, 1977
19. Behan WMH, Barkas T, Behan PO: Detection of immune complexes in polymyositis. Acta Neurol Scand 65:320, 1982
20. Sharp GC, Irwin WS, Tan EM, et al: Mixed connective tissue disease—an apparently distinct rheumatic disease syndrome associated with a specific antibody to an extractable nuclear antigen (ENA). Am J Med 52:148, 1972
21. Sharp GC: Association of progressive systemic sclerosis with other connective tissue diseases ("overlap syndromes"). p. 33. In Black CM, Myers RW (eds): Systemic Sclerosis (Scleroderma). Gower Medical Publishing, New York, 1985

4

Raynaud's Phenomenon and Related Forms of Cutaneous Vasospasm

Jonathan L. Halperin

"Asphyxia of the fingers." So it was described in 1862 by Maurice Raynaud, who first set down the clinical phenomena associated with spastic closure of digital blood vessels: pallor, cyanosis, and rubor provoked by cold exposure or emotional stress. The classical sequence of color changes in the fingers or toes is typically well demarcated, beginning with an ischemic phase, often accompanied by numbness of the distal segment, which is followed by a hyperemic phase, associated with throbbing or burning paresthesias as vasospasm subsides. These symptoms bridge the gap between unpleasant coldness of the hands and feet and the extremes of ulceration and gangrene. Raynaud wrote of "local syncope":

> . . . without appreciable cause, one or many fingers become pale and cold all at once. In many cases it is the same finger which is always first attacked; the others become dead successively in the same order. . . . The determining cause is often the impression of cold . . . sometimes even a simple mental emotion is enough. . . . In the more pronounced cases, the pallor of the extremities is replaced by a cyanotic color . . . a vermilion color shows itself at the margin; little by little it gains

ground. . . . Finally, a patch of deep red is formed on the extremities of the fingers. This patch gives place to the normal pink color, and then the skin is found to have entirely returned to the primitive condition.

He also described a more malevolent potential for gangrene:

> . . . I hasten now to the symptoms of symmetrical gangrene properly so called. . . . In the slight cases the ends of the fingers and toes become cold, cyanosed, and livid, and at the same time more or less painful. In grave cases the area affected by cyanosis extends upwards for several centimeters. . . . Finally, if this state is prolonged for a certain time we see gangrenous points appear on the extremities; the gangrene is always dry, and may occupy the superficial layers of the skin from the extent of a pin's head up to the end of a finger, rarely more.[1]

Although excessive spastic vasoconstriction seemed at the root of these digital ischemic syndromes because radial arterial pulses were so often palpable at the wrists, Hutchinson at the turn of the century emphasized that Raynaud's phenomenon also occurred in association with obstructive arterial disease.[2] Recognition that there could be a multiplicity of causes led Allen and Brown in 1932 to propose a system of classification based upon clinical features, which formalized the distinction between primary (idiopathic) and secondary forms of Raynaud's phenomenon.[3] The common denominator is generally thought to be vascular spasm, but understanding of the exact pathophysiologic mechanism has remained elusive for over 100 years.[4]

What distinguishes Raynaud's phenomenon from other cutaneous vasospastic conditions, such as acrocyanosis, livedo reticularis, and cutis marmorata, is the episodic ischemia of well-demarcated segments of the skin caused by reversible closure of small arteries. Women are affected five to eight times more frequently than men, and Raynaud's phenomenon may occur in as many as 10 percent of otherwise healthy females.[5] In most cases the symptoms represent a fairly benign condition, a nuisance paradoxically designated Raynaud's disease. While over 90 percent of cases are idiopathic, Raynaud's phenomenon has also been linked with a variety of disorders of connective tissue, blood vessels, and blood constituents as well as with environmental factors. The principal clinical challenge is to distinguish idiopathic cases of primary Raynaud's disease from Raynaud's phenomenon secondary to underlying disease of connective tissues (e.g., scleroderma or systemic lupus erythematosus), obstructive arterial disease (e.g., thromboangiitis obliterans), blood dyscrasias (e.g., cryoglobulinemia), drug toxicity (e.g., ergotism), or arterial injury, as shown in Table 4-1. A sensible clinical approach to the problem of Raynaud's phenomenon depends upon detailed understanding of each patient's situational characteristics and a firm foundation in cutaneous hemodynamics.

PATHOPHYSIOLOGY

The pathogenesis of vasospasm is poorly understood and multiple factors are probably responsible, but the mechanisms appear to differ from those involved in the physiologic vasoconstriction that modulates skin blood flow as environmental temperature varies. Vasospasm may occur spontaneously in certain individuals and it has long been debated whether this reflects sympathetic nervous system overactivity—what Raynaud termed "a vice of innervation"—or the local vascular fault proposed two generations later by the renowned cardiovascular physiologist Sir Thomas Lewis.[6] On the other hand, while ischemic attacks commonly occur spontaneously in relation to cold or emotional stimuli, they cannot regularly be reproduced in the laboratory, a major hindrance to study. Ischemia may develop as a result of abnormal vasoconstrictor tone, structural disorders of blood vessels, reduced perfusion pressure, or hemorheologic disturbances affecting the flow properties of blood. Normal digital circulation involves balance between the sum of arterial constrictor and extravascular compressive forces, which impede blood flow, and the intraluminal distending forces, which favor patency and flow. Distortion of this equilibrium sufficiently severe to overcome the distal arteriolar reserve leads to temporary ischemia.[7] Capillary perfusion is reduced below that in normal individuals during cold exposure, but the benignity of the idiopathic form of Raynaud's phenomenon may be related both to the meager nutritional perfusion requirements of acral skin and to the reversible nature of the vasomotor disturbance.

The large effective surface area of the digits serves to radiate body heat, and the cutaneous vessels of the hands and feet are essential to regulation of body temperature. Skin vasculature of the hands, feet, elbows, knees, nose, forehead, and earlobes is characterized by relatively large numbers of anastomotic glomus bodies[8] (Fig. 4-1). These arteriovenous shunt networks usually respond to autonomic neural and hormonal stimulation. The sympathetic nervous system clearly plays a major role in regulating the cutaneous circulation and largely accounts for the wide variation in the rate of blood flow through the digital vessels. Cold exposure results in selective constriction of shunt vessels

Table 4-1. Secondary Causes of Raynaud's Phenomenon

Connective tissue diseases
  Scleroderma
  Systemic lupus erythematosus
  Rheumatoid arthritis
  Dermatomyositis
  Polymyositis
  Mixed connective tissue disease
  Sjögren's syndrome
  Necrotizing angiitis

Occlusive arterial disease
  Arteriosclerosis obliterans
  Thromboangiitis obliterans
  Thromboembolism

Drug-induced
  Ergot alkaloids, methysergide
  β-adrenergic antagonists
  Clonidine
  Bleomycin
  Sulfasalazine

Neurologic disorders
  Cerebrovascular accidents
  Poliomyelitis
  Carpal tunnel syndrome
  Intervertebral disc compression
  Thoracic outlet compression syndromes
  Syringomyelia
  Shoulder girdle compression syndrome
  Reflex sympathetic dystrophy

Blood dyscrasias
  Cryoglobulinemia
  Macroglobulinemia
  Cryofibrinogenemia
  Polycythemia vera
  Paroxysmal hemoglobinuria
  Cold hemolysis
  Hepatitis B antigenemia

Neoplastic
  Multiple myeloma
  Leukemia
  Occult carcinoma
  Pheochromocytoma

Occupational or environmental exposure
  Occupational acro-osteolysis
  Pneumatic hammer disease (vibration)
  Sequelae of blunt trauma
  Sequelae of cold injury
  Vinyl-chloride manufacture

Miscellaneous
  Mitral valve prolapse
  Myxedema
  Primary pulmonary hypertension
  Fabry's disease
  Heavy metals (lead, arsenic)

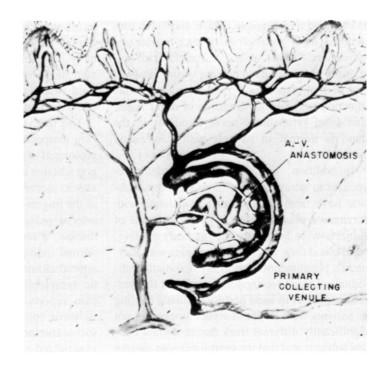

Fig. 4-1. Schematic drawing of main vessels in a digital glomus. (Mescon H, Hurley JH Jr, Moretti G: The anatomy and histochemistry of the arteriovenous anastomosis in human digital skin. J Invest Dermatol 27:133–145, 1956. © by Williams & Wilkins, 1956.)

A.-V. ANASTOMOSIS

PRIMARY COLLECTING VENULE

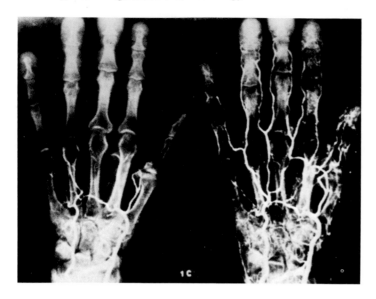

Fig. 4-3. (Right) Baseline hand angiogram showing no organic occlusive disease. **(Left)** Same patient demonstrating severe vasospasm following immersion of hand in ice water. (Holmgren K, Baur GM, Porter JM: Vascular laboratory evaluation of Raynaud's syndrome. Bruit 5:19, 1981.)

Spontaneous attacks of Raynaud's phenomenon typically develop during cold exposure or emotional stress. In normal individuals mental arithmetic stress produces digital vasoconstriction along with a rise in heart rate and blood pressure. This finger hemodynamic response is mediated by the sympathetic nerves since digital nerve block eliminates the vasoconstrictor response.[21] In patients with primary Raynaud's disease, similar stressful stimuli result in digital vasodilation.[22] This paradoxical observation raises the possibility of an active vasodilator mechanism in the digital vessels of patients with a vasospastic disorder. Since nerve blockade fails to alter this vasodilator response, neither sympathetic vasodilator nerves nor withdrawal of sympathetic vasoconstrictor influences can be invoked for explanation. The vasodilation that develops during mental stress in patients with Raynaud's disease is difficult to reconcile with the vasospastic symptoms that accompany periods of emotional stress in these cases, and it is at odds with traditional teaching that sympathetic vasodilation of the cutaneous vascular beds results solely from withdrawal of α-adrenergic vasoconstrictor activity. Nevertheless, the finding of an abnormal relationship between cerebral cortical activity and digital hemodynamics points to a fundamental derangement

of neurovascular physiology even in patients with primary Raynaud's disease.

Digital vasospastic phenomena provoked by β-adrenergic blocking drugs such as propranolol force reconsideration of the possibility of a β-adrenergic vasodilator mechanism in the hands and feet. Intra-arterial isoproterenol has been shown to increase total fingertip blood flow during vasoconstriction induced by norepinephrine, but capillary flow was not changed.[23] This cutaneous vasodilator effect of the β-adrenergic agonist was not observed when vasoconstriction was induced by the reflex sympathetic stimulus of body cooling. Hence, while a β-adrenergic vasodilator mechanism may exist in digital skin, its activity seems to be limited to the arteriovenous shunts and attenuated during neurogenic vasoconstriction. The mechanism by which β blockers induce cold hands and feet or episodes of Raynaud's phenomenon remains an unsettled issue, made all the more mysterious by the observation that total fingertip blood flow is not significantly affected by the agents propranolol or metoprolol when measured in either a warm or a cool environment.[24]

An active mechanism for dilatation of cutaneous arteriovenous anastomoses is vested in the parasympathetic, cholinergic nervous system. Glomus apparatus visualized in the rabbit ear constricts in response to administration of epinephrine and dilates after local application of acetylcholine.[25] Specific histochemical staining of specimens of volar skin of human digits has demonstrated cholinesterases in nerve fibers around the arteriovenous anastomoses just as around the secretory tubules of eccrine sweat glands, while the enzymes were absent around other cutaneous vessels and the ducts of sweat glands, which indicates a cholinergic nerve supply to the arteriovenous anastomoses.[26] These vessels are thus unique in the skin for having dual adrenergic and cholinergic innervation, accounting for both active constriction and dilatation. The cholinergic fibers are thought important in the cold vasodilatation "hunting" reaction[27] and may mediate the spontaneous termination of vasospastic attacks. What is clear is that vasospastic events leading to Raynaud's phenomenon involve a complex interplay of factors that extend beyond the limits of physiological vasoconstriction and involve other mechanisms than the autonomic nervous system alone.

In 1981 Miller et al. reported a statistical correlation of migraine headache and variant angina pectoris with Raynaud's phenomenon, raising the possibility of a systemic factor in some patients with vasospasm.[28] Another disorder possibly linking vasospasm in more than one region of the circulation is pulmonary hypertension, which in either primary or secondary forms is often associated with Raynaud's phenomenon.[29] There are also paradoxical observations about the responses to pharmacologic agents in patients with these vasomotor disorders. Both variant angina pectoris and Raynaud's phenomenon are occasionally aggravated by β-receptor blocking drugs, yet propranolol has been used both as prophylaxis against migraine headaches and to relieve acute attacks.[30,31] Reserpine may be beneficial in the treatment of Raynaud's phenomenon, yet can induce migraine headaches, and ergotamine, effective against migraine, can induce vasospastic angina and digital ischemia. Organic nitrates help relieve variant angina pectoris but provoke headaches and yet produce no proven benefit

in Raynaud's phenomenon. These differing effects support the thesis that there is more than one mechanism for vasospasm.[32] The possibility of a systemic factor cannot be discounted, however, in view of the recent observation that calf vascular reactivity to cold stimulation is increased in patients with variant angina pectoris only in proximity to attacks of myocardial ischemia.[33]

Following the description of a vasoconstrictor substance in blood serum, subsequently identified as serotonin, Halpern and associates reported reduction in the severity and duration of the ischemic response by a serotonin inhibitor in patients with Raynaud's phenomenon induced by immersion of the hands in cold water.[34] These attacks of digital ischemia provoked by local cooling were intensified by injection of synthetic serotonin. As other investigators have generally been unable to induce attacks of Raynaud's phenomenon regularly by these or other means, the experiments have not been confirmed. There have been no convincing reports that antiserotonin agents are effective in the treatment of Raynaud's disease, and the hydroxytryptamine antagonist ketanserin had no effect on blood flow at rest, during cooling, or after recovery from a cold challenge in a controlled trial in patients with Raynaud's phenomenon.[35]

Pickering proposed in 1951 that attacks of ischemia in Raynaud's disease might derive from repeated intravascular coagulation with transient thrombotic occlusion of digital vessels.[36] This concept was explored by Pringle et al., who noted increased intravascular erythrocyte aggregation in the conjunctival vessels, assessed by slit lamp microscopy in a group of patients with Raynaud's disease.[37] The role of prostaglandins in the pathophysiology of vasospastic disorders has been a subject of parallel speculation, although drugs that inhibit the prostaglandin synthetase enzyme system are of no proven value in the management of patients with Raynaud's phenomenon. On the other hand, intermittent infusions of prostacyclin (epoprostenol) have reportedly been helpful in some cases.[38] Inhibition of thromboxane-A2 with dazoxiben does not appear to alter digital vascular resistance in patients with primary Raynaud's disease.[39]

Even measurements of blood viscosity, reported by several investigators using varying methods, have been inconsistent. Whole blood viscosity does not appear to be a fundamental abnormality in patients with the primary disorder but may play a major role in cases of cryoglobulinemia or dysproteinemia. A reduction in blood viscosity did not alter the response to cold stimuli in one investigation, while another (uncontrolled) trial found serial plasmapheresis useful in the attenuation of symptoms in cases of Raynaud's disease.[40,41] As the available data are contradictory, physiologically important variations in hemorheology in Raynaud's disease could be a contributing pathogenetic factor.

The vascular wall itself may appear morphologically normal in patients with mild symptoms, but digital arterial endothelial thickening has been described in patients with more advanced ischemic changes.[17] This may be a particularly important development in patients with vasculitis or immunologically mediated fibrosis, and edema may add substantial compressive forces. Indeed, it is ultimately the imbalance between intraluminal distending forces and extravascular compressive forces, mediated by the components of the vascular wall, which underlies the clinical symptom complex characteristic of the vasospastic response.

APPROACH TO THE PATIENT

Clinical History

The diagnosis of Raynaud's phenomenon depends upon eliciting a history of isolated episodes of well-demarcated color changes in the hands, feet, earlobes, nose, forehead, elbows, or knees, generally provoked by cold exposure or emotional stress. The triphasic color response may be accompanied by pain or numbness during the ischemic phase of pallor and by burning paresthesias during the rubor related to reactive hyperemia. There is no fully diagnostic test for the abnormal cutaneous vasospastic response that seems to be at the root of this condition, but the evaluation of patients must proceed even when attacks cannot be produced by exposure to relatively intense constrictive stimuli at the bedside or in the office or laboratory.

In general, the cutaneous vasospastic syndromes are characterized more by changes in skin color or temperature than they are by intermittent claudication, which represents muscular ischemia. Gangrene occurs occasionally, although this usually signifies more severe or persistent vasospasm, often due to obstructive arterial disease or associated with intraluminal thrombosis. Vasospastic conditions are generally associated with smaller arterial derivatives, and occlusive disorders involve larger arteries, but this is not invariably the case and pulses may evanescently disappear in vasospastic disorders, with or without symptoms and signs of ischemia. When both vasospasm and arterial obstruction occur concurrently, the former is more often caused by the latter. At times, though, vasospasm is the earliest manifestation of a significant but otherwise occult underlying disorder. Fortunately, the differentiation of vasospastic states from obstructive arterial disease is usually clear on clinical grounds. For the most part vasospastic conditions can be fully evaluated and successfully managed on an ambulatory basis.

Although vasospasm may occur in either an episodic or persistent fashion, the distinction is often incomplete. Persistent acrocyanosis in the absence of systemic arterial oxygen desaturation may be punctuated by episodes of ischemic pallor. Livedo reticularis constitutes another form of persistent cutaneous vasospasm in which nonhomogeneous mottled discoloration occurs, which is generally more pronounced over the knees and lower extremities and is also aggravated by exposure to cold. The association of Raynaud's phenomenon and these other cutaneous vasospastic syndromes with sundry disturbances of blood vessels, neural structures, connective tissue, and blood constituents necessitates distinction from the more benign primary vasospastic diseases.

Detailed clinical history should therefore seek to disclose symptoms of possible collagen or rheumatoid disease, large vessel obstructive arterial disease, exposure to digital trauma, positional symptoms in the extremities, hematologic dyscrasias, malignant neoplasms, use of vasoconstrictive medications, embolic disorders, pulmonary hypertension, certain viral antigenemias, metabolic conditions such as myxedema, or humoral disturbances such as pheochromocytoma. A number of medications, such as the ergot derivatives and methysergide employed for migraine headaches, β-adrenergic antagonists used for hypertension or angina pectoris, and bleomycin for chemotherapy of testicular carcinoma, have also been related to secondary Raynaud's phenomenon.

Information about the onset and course of vasospastic episodes may be helpful in differentiating primary from secondary Raynaud's phenomenon. The typical patient with primary Raynaud's disease is a young female who has had symptoms of bilateral cutaneous vasospasm for more than 2 years without fixed ischemic changes or systemic symptoms. Unilateral symptoms, persistent pain, or cutaneous ulceration usually bespeaks a secondary form of the disorder, as does the development of the syndrome beyond the age of 40 years or its occurrence in male patients. Constitutional symptoms are generally absent in the benign forms of Raynaud's phenomenon, and the development of anorexia, bowel disturbances or weight loss should trigger a more intensive search for underlying disorders. Associated skin rash, arthralgias, and edema are also characteristics of complicated cases and are unusual in the idiopathic disease. Raynaud's phenomenon confined to one upper extremity is usually secondary in type, and the underlying disorder is usually present in the same extremity. It is also unusual for primary Raynaud's phenomenon to repeatedly occur in the lower extremities without symptoms in the upper limbs.

Occasionally, patients can be identified as having features of a systemic vasospastic diathesis by virtue of a history of headache syndrome with vasomotor features (in that they are preceded by aura and are unilateral, clustered in time, or familial). Such patients may also complain of anginal chest pain, either related to effort or occurring at rest. Since Raynaud's phenomenon and sympathetic adrenergic hyperresponsiveness may be correlates of the mitral valve prolapse syndrome, however, other mechanisms of chest pain may also occur in patients with otherwise functional syndromes of cutaneous vasospasm. Hyperthyroidism is at times associated with Raynaud's phenomenon, but the mechanism of this relationship is mysterious. Raynaud's phenomenon associated with intervals of neurologic derangements, bleeding, chest pain, or dyspnea should bring to mind intravascular coagulation. Major central hemodynamic derangements such as severe or acute hypertension, congestive heart failure, or pulmonary hypertension may be connected with Raynaud's phenomenon through the action of autonomic reflexes or humoral fluctuations. By far the most important disorder associated with Raynaud's phenomenon, however, is systemic sclerosis (scleroderma), and the occurrence of Raynaud's phenomenon as a new symptom in any patient should lead to the consideration of this connective tissue disease or the syndromes of systemic lupus erythematosus, periarteritis nodosa, or rheumatoid arthritis. The occurrence of constitutional symptoms, skin tightness, Sjögren's syndrome, recent acceleration of dental caries, dysphagia, heartburn related to gastroesophageal reflux, constipation, arthralgias, or hematuria is particularly relevant in such cases.

Physical Examination

The integumentary examination should be directed, in particular, to notation of skin color and temperature, trophic changes of ischemia in the extremities, fissures, ulceration, eschars, subcutaneous thickening, and associated rashes.

Sclerodactyly, calcinosis, petechiae, and telangiectases are important signs of structural organic disease. The general examination should include palpation of the arterial pulses and assessment of joint abnormalities, neurologic deficits, splenomegaly, and signs of pulmonary hypertension (Table 4-2). The ulnar pulses are often absent in cases of thromboangiitis obliterans, and there may be evidence of superficial venous inflammation. When symptoms are confined to the upper extremities, the Adson, hyperabduction, and costoclavicular maneuvers designed to elicit dynamic neurovascular compression at the thoracic outlet should be performed. Most commonly, the thoracic outlet syndromes are associated with unilateral Raynaud's phenomenon, especially when digital ulceration occurs; occasionally there are bilateral symptoms of cold sensitivity and color changes. The basis for necrosis in these cases is generally thromboembolic occlusion of palmar or digital arteries, sometimes associated with poststenotic axillosubclavian arterial dilatation. Elevation and dependency tests of the hands help to determine digital arterial occlusive disease. The Allen and reversed Allen tests may help identify palmar arterial arch occlusion as well as functional insufficiency of the ulnar or radial arterial supply. When Raynaud's phenomenon is limited to the lower extremities, the abdomen, groin, and popliteal fossae should be carefully examined for atherosclerotic arterial aneurysms by palpation as well as by auscultation for bruits (present, however, in only about 40 percent of aneurysm cases). Other sources of microembolism to the feet include Takayasu's aortitis of the distal type and aortoiliac arteriosclerosis obliterans. Petechial microinfarction is a valuable early sign in these cases and may progress to calf muscle tenderness and patchy necrosis of the toes.

Discomfort in the foot provoked by straight leg raising often represents lumbosacral radiculopathy on the basis of spinal canal stenosis, osteophyte formation, vertebral compression, or tumor. Tinel's sign might signify a local neurologic disorder such as median neuropathy related to carpal tunnel compression. Peripheral neuropathy may rarely occur as a consequence of ischemia in persistent vasospastic states, but disorders causing neuropathy (such as amyloidosis, accelerated atherosclerosis in diabetes mellitus, or hyperthyroidism) may be independently associated with Raynaud's phenomenon.

Cutaneous telangiectases in a patient with Raynaud's phenomenon and sclerodactyly with or without calcinosis cutis usually signifies scleroderma, even when there are no other signs of sclerosis. The presence of abdominal organomegaly may be a sign of more advanced

Table 4-2. Differential Diagnosis of Primary and Secondary Raynaud's Phenomenon

Some Useful Features	Raynaud's Disease	Secondary Raynaud's Phenomenon
Sex	Often female	Often male
Age at onset	<40 years	>40 years
Bilateral involvement	+	±
Systemic symptoms	−	±
Asymmetric involvement	−	±
Ischemic changes	−	+
Sclerodactyly	−	±
Telangiectases	−	±
Petechiae	−	±
Diminished pulses	Transient	Fixed
Neurologic deficits	−	±
Pulmonary hypertension	−	±
Splenomegaly	−	±
Blood test abnormalities	−	±

(Modified from Spittell JA, Jr: Vasospastic disorders. p. 280. In Brandenburg RO (ed): Office Cardiology. Cardiovascular Clinics. Vol. 10, No. 3. FA Davis, Philadelphia, 1980.)

systemic involvement in connective tissue disease syndromes associated with Raynaud's phenomenon and other cutaneous vasospastic states. The same is true of fixed pulmonary arterial hypertension associated with restrictive respiratory defects or neuromuscular disturbances of gastrointestinal motility.

Laboratory Evaluation

Testing should include hemogram, erythrocyte sedimentation rate, detection of rheumatoid factor, antinuclear antibodies, cryoglobulins, and serum protein electrophoresis, as well as urinalysis for erythrocyte casts or proteinuria. Chest roentgenography for cervical ribs should also be performed as part of the minimum evaluation (Table 4-3). Nerve conduction studies are abnormal in some but not all cases of thoracic

Table 4-3. Approach to the Patient

History
Cold sensitivity
    Episodic vs. persistent color changes, unilateral vs.
      bilateral involvement
Symptoms of connective tissue disease
    Arthralgias, sun sensitivity, dysphagia
Systemic hematologic or neoplastic disease
Medications
    Bleomycin, β-blocking drugs, ergot alkaloids, methysergide
Positional symptoms
Occupational history
    Vibration, trauma
Migraine

Physical Examination
    Pulses
    Ulcers
    Telangiectases
    Sclerodactyly
    Pulmonary hypertension
    Splenomegaly

Laboratory Investigation
Initial screening
    Hemogram, platelets, erythrocyte sedimentation rate,
      rheumatoid factor, antinuclear antibodies, cryoglobulins, serum protein electrophoresis, urinalysis,
      chest x-ray
In-depth evaluation
    Nerve conduction studies, Doppler ultrasound, digital
      subtraction angiography, vascular imaging, arteriography, digital plethysmography

outlet syndromes and carpal tunnel syndromes. The Doppler ultrasound technique may be employed to identify blood flow through patent vessels when pulses are not palpable or occlusion is suspected at the level of the palmar/plantar arches or digital arteries. Digital subtraction angiography, vascular imaging, and formal arteriography are of value in defining both the level and the morphology of arterial obstruction (fixed or dynamic) in cases of suspected secondary vasospasm.

Intermittent hand ischemia does lend itself to evaluation in the vascular hemodynamic laboratory with a view toward distinguishing fixed arterial obstructive disease from reversible vasomotor disorders. While there is no specific diagnostic test for Raynaud's phenomenon, digital plethysmography may be used to record pulse waveform by volumetric, photoelectric, or laser velocimetric means. Abnormalities may sometimes be detected in a warm environment, but a more pronounced disturbance may develop on cooling of the hand. This may consist of delayed arterial upstroke and crest time; if this pattern persists after warming, obstructive vascular lesions are suggested.[42] Doppler sonography may be used to map the course of patent digital arteries and to evaluate the palmar or plantar arches as adjuncts to the Allen and reversed Allen maneuvers. Perhaps the most reproducible technique is that introduced by Nielsen and Lassen, which involves estimation of systolic digital arterial pressure during the combined stimulus of local cooling and arterial occlusion produced by a miniature sphygmomanometric cuff while pulse volume is recorded from a mercury-in-Silastic strain gauge placed on the fingertip. Pressures from an uncooled digit on the contralateral hand are recorded simultaneously with those of the digit subjected to local cooling while temperatures are measured by thermocouples and brachial pressure is noted. Normally, successive cooling does not result in a fall of more than 5 percent in digital pressure from the control level. Patients with vasospastic disease (and others with "cold sensitivity") display abrupt loss of digital arterial systolic pulsations, perhaps reflecting dynamic arterial closure.[19] The sensitivity and specificity of this critical closing phenomenon as an aid to the diagnosis of the vasospastic disease have not been determined, but it likely underlies the long known clinical phenomenon whereby the rewarming time of digits subjected to local cooling is prolonged in patients with Raynaud's phenomenon.

Treatment

Primary Raynaud's disease is generally benign and patients can usually be managed without vasodilator medication. They should be carefully instructed to avoid cold exposure and to protect their hands from mechanical trauma or excessive dryness. Most patients with progressive ischemic symptoms, cutaneous ulceration, fissures, or infections have secondary vasospasm, which is best managed in conjunction with treatment of the underlying disorder. In such cases the response to pharmacological therapy is frequently less successful and the prognosis is worse than when disorders known to accompany vasospastic symptoms have been excluded.

Drug therapy would ideally counteract the cause of digital vasospasm, dilating specifically only those vessels supplying ischemic zones. Generalized vasodilation might produce "steal" phenomena, diverting blood flow from ischemic areas. Even regional administration by the intra-arterial route may redistribute perfusion to the skeletal muscle of more proximal parts of the limbs and away from skin beds. A variety of vasodilator drugs are available in oral preparations, and attention must be given to their modes of action, onset and duration of action, dosage, effectiveness, and side effects (Table 4-4). Evaluations by controlled studies using objective methods for measuring changes in circulation have seldom been conducted.

Since spontaneous vasospastic attacks cannot readily be reproduced for study in the laboratory, even drugs which dilate digital vessels may be ineffective in preventing ischemic episodes. Conventional therapy employs agents affecting adrenergic receptors, mainly α-adrenergic antagonists rather than β-adrenergic stimulants. Substances that block angiotensin or dilate vascular smooth muscle by direct action have been of limited value, but inhibitors of calcium influx channels and certain prostaglandins hold greater therapeutic promise.

α-ADRENERGIC ANTAGONISTS

Among the α-adrenergic antagonists, perhaps the most extensive experience has been obtained with reserpine, which depletes sympathetic nerves of the neurotransmitter norepinephrine. When injected intra-arterially, reserpine displays additional brief vasodilator activity unrelated to catecholamine depletion. Oral reserpine reduces the vasoconstrictor responses in the hand to infused tyramine, which releases norepinephrine from adrenergic terminals, and to cooling of the face in patients with Raynaud's phenomenon.[11] Oral doses of 0.25 to 0.50 mg daily for a period of 3 weeks increased fingertip capillary blood flow in one series of patients with Raynaud's disease.[15] Painful digital ulcers have been anecdotally reported to respond to intra-arterial administration of reserpine in doses of 0.5 to 1 mg, but a controlled study disclosed no advantage over saline injections.[43] The most frequent side effects include nasal congestion, orthostatic hypotension, reflex tachycardia, flushing, gastrointestinal upset, and psychic depression. Reports that it heightens the incidence of breast carcinoma have not been confirmed.

Guanethidine prevents release of norepinephrine at adrenergic neuroeffector junctions. After 4 to 6 weeks of therapy at doses of 30 to 40 mg daily, guanethidine increased finger capillary blood flow during cooling in patients with Raynaud's phenomenon due to scleroderma, enhancing nutritional perfusion in those patients prone to cutaneous tissue loss.[44] Tolazoline, in comparatively large doses of 75 to 100 mg, acts as an α-adrenergic inhibitor and produces cutaneous vasodilation in the feet in vasoconstricted normal subjects.[45] Oral preparations are

Table 4-4. Drug Therapy of Cutaneous Vasospastic Syndromes

Type of Drug	Uses	Side Effect

α-Adrenergic antagonists
  Reserpine
  Guanethidine
  Tolazoline
  Methyldopa
  Phentolamine
  Phenoxybenzamine
  Prazosin
	Persistent vasospasm—acrocyanosis
	Prevention of gangrene after vasocon-
	  strictor drug infiltration
	Healing ulcers after microembolization
		Nasal congestion
		Orthostatic hypotension
		Depression
		Gastrointestinal disturbances
		Fluid retention
		Flushing
		Reflex tachycardia
		Piloerection
		Exacerbation of angina

β-Adrenergic agonists
  Isoproterenol
  Terbutaline
  Nylidrin
	Reversal of vasoconstriction produced
	  by β-blockers
		Raynaud's phenomenon
		Bradycardia
		Impotence
		Neuropsychological phenomena

Calcium channel blocking agents
  Nifedipine
  Verapamil
  Diltiazem
	Episodic vasospasm
	Raynaud's phenomenon attacks
		Hypotension
		Dizziness
		Flushing
		Headache
		Edema
		Bradycardia
		Atrioventricular block
		Congestive heart failure
		Nausea

Nitrates	Ergotism	Headache Hypotension
Prostacyclin Epoprostenol	Undetermined	Facial flushing Headache

Converting enzyme inhibitors
  Captopril
  Enalapril
	Vasoconstrictor phenomena complicat-
	  ing severe hypertension or con-
	  gestive heart failure
		Fever
		Skin rash
		Leukopenia
		Proteinuria
		Hypotension
		Azotemia
		Dysgeusia

Vascular smooth muscle relaxants
  Hydralazine
  Nicotinic acid
  Isoxuprine
  Cyclandelate
  Papaverine
  Ethaverine
  Griseofulvin
	Little evidence to support their use in
	  peripheral vascular disease
	
	Griseofulvin used for cutaneous vaso-
	  constriction complicated by fundal
	  infection	

no longer available in the United States. The parenteral form in doses of 20 to 50 mg exerts a direct vasodilator effect by an unknown mechanism when injected intra-arterially. The false neurotransmitter methyldopa acts as a competitive antagonist of norepinephrine at peripheral sympathetic effectors, but central neurogenic actions contribute significantly to vasodilatation. In one study a majority of patients with Raynaud's phenomenon reported subjective benefit at doses of 1 to 2 g daily. The rate of surface rewarming of fingers after local cooling increased during this experiment.[46] It has been tolerated somewhat better than reserpine or guanethidine in the long-term treatment of hypertension, but hemolytic anemia and hepatitis have proved problematic in occasional patients treated with this drug. The α-receptor blocking agent phenoxybenzamine induces cutaneous vasodilatation in oral maintenance doses of 10 to 20 mg three or four times daily. Reports of benefit in some patients with Raynaud's disease have not been confirmed.[47] Parenteral phentolamine has been employed for the prevention of dermal necrosis when intravenous therapy with vasopressor substances such as norepinephrine, phenylephrine, or dopamine becomes complicated by extravasation and local accumulation. Regional intra-arterial or dermal injection of 1 to 10 mg results in less systemic hypotension than that produced by intravenous infusion.

Prazosin, an antihypertensive quinazoline, exerts peripheral vasodilator effects through blockade of α-adrenergic receptors. A relative affinity for postsynaptic (vascular) α_1-adrenergic receptors distinguishes it from less selective α blocking agents, which also affect presynaptic (neuronal) α_2 receptors. The usual starting dose is 1 to 2 mg given orally two or three times daily, but clinical tachyphylaxis may develop, requiring increments in dosage up to 10 mg three times daily. This is reminiscent of the experiences of some patients who have moved to areas of warmer climate only to find that vasospastic attacks begin to occur at higher temperatures. Little additional benefit generally accrues from larger doses of prazosin, although amounts as high as 80 mg daily have apparently been tolerated.[48] The dose must be tailored to each patient, and caution must be exercised regarding the development of syncope as therapy is initiated. This first-dose phenomenon results from profound postural hypotension, which can be minimized by starting treatment with prazosin as the patient retires to bed. In most cases, hypotension resolves as therapy is continued, although in occasional patients the agent must be stopped because the side effect

persists. This adverse response, which is related to pharmacological vasodilatation, also poses difficulty when intermittent therapy is desired. Hence, prazosin finds greatest value in the management of patients with persistently cold hands and feet or continuous vasospastic syndromes such as acrocyanosis, although the frequency of attacks of intermittent Raynaud's phenomenon may also be diminished. Clinical effectiveness was reported in a group of patients with Raynaud's phenomenon, but these observations did not include a placebo control.[49] In a single case complicated by digital ulceration, symptomatic improvement was not accompanied by more rapid fingertip rewarming following hand cooling. Prazosin does not increase hand blood flow in patients with coldness of the extremities during treatment with propranolol or atenolol. Fortunately, other than for problematic hypotension at the onset of therapy, prazosin is better tolerated than other α-adrenergic inhibitor agents and we now favor this drug when oral sympatholytic drug therapy is selected for patients with Raynaud's disease whose symptoms are refractory to conservative measures.[50,51]

Adverse reactions to oral maintenance therapy limit dosage and acceptance of most α-adrenergic antagonist medications. Common side effects include orthostatic light-headedness, nasal congestion, reflex tachycardia, flushing, gastrointestinal hypersecretion, renin release, fluid retention, piloerection, exacerbation of angina, and psychiatric reactions. Because of more selective blockade of α_1-adrenergic receptor function, palpitations and central nervous system reactions are relatively infrequent during therapy with prazosin, but first-dose hypotension remains a troublesome side effect.

β-ADRENERGIC AGONISTS

The β-adrenergic agonist isoproterenol has been used for its bronchodilator properties in inhaled, sublingual, and intravenous forms. It exerts limb vasodilator effects largely through activation of β_2 receptors on skeletal muscle vasculature. Intra-arterial isoproterenol displays potent vasodilator activity in the forearm and calf but has little effect on hand or foot blood flow[53]; intra-arterial isoproterenol also increases total fingertip perfusion when vasoconstriction has been established by norepinephrine, but does not affect capillary flow.[23] Terbutaline produces relatively selective β_2 receptor stimulation, which also dilates the limb vasculature. In therapeutic doses terbutaline produces less cardioacceleratory and inotropic effects than does isoproterenol, but this specificity is lost at higher doses. Nylidrin has been available for several decades in oral form as a peripheral vasodilator agent. Its action is not completely blocked by propranolol; hence a direct vasodilator effect of nylidrin is suspected in addition to stimulation of β-adrenergic receptors. Increases in limb blood flow occur largely through dilatation of skeletal muscle beds, and most investigations have found no effect on cutaneous perfusion.

Clinically, β-adrenergic agonists generally provoke vasodilatation in skeletal muscle, and blood flow could theoretically even be diverted from skin beds. At present, there exists no evidence to substantiate the use of these agents in the treatment of patients with cutaneous vasospastic symptoms, except possibly when vasoconstriction is provoked by β-adrenergic blocking drugs.

In patients with cutaneous vasospastic symptoms some care should be taken in the selection of β-adrenergic antagonist drugs if these are needed for therapy of other cardiovascular disorders such as hypertension, angina pectoris, or tachyarrhythmias. Raynaud's phenomenon and even dermal gangrene have been described during therapy with both β_1-selective (e.g., atenolol) and nonselective (e.g., propranolol) antagonists. Whether intrinsic sympathomimetic activity (e.g., pindolol) or combined α-adrenergic antagonist properties (e.g., labetalol) will offer clinical advantages with respect to digital perfusion remains unclear.

CALCIUM CHANNEL BLOCKING AGENTS

The encouraging results of calcium channel antagonist therapy in patients with variant angina pectoris raises the possibility that an abnormality of excitation-contraction coupling depending upon the slow inward flux of calcium ions may be fundamental to the pathophysiology of episodic vasospasm. Nifedipine and verapamil inhibit norepinephrine-induced constriction of isolated blood vessel strips[53] and delay the onset of cutaneous vasospastic symptoms provoked by cold water hand immersion.[54] In short term placebo-controlled trials involving a small number of patients with primary and secondary Raynaud's phenomenon, nifedipine seemed to reduce the frequency and severity of vasospastic phenomena and to accelerate healing of digital ulcers when given in oral doses of 10 to 20 mg qid.[55–56] Creager et al. performed venous occlusion plethysmography in 10 patients with Raynaud's phenomenon (5 of whom had primary Raynaud's disease) in a cool environment and demonstrated fingertip vasodilatation after administration of sublingual nifedipine.[57] During maintenance therapy side effects of edema, nausea, and light-headedness were reported.

Preliminary clinical reports of amelioration of digital vasospastic symptoms with verapamil in patients with scleroderma described more rapid recovery of finger pulse pressure after local cooling.[58] Plethysmographic blood flow studies have not been completed, but the frequency of spastic attacks seemed diminished. Another calcium channel blocking agent, diltiazem (60 mg orally three times daily), was compared with placebo administration in 26 patients with Raynaud's disease, favorably influencing both disability and the frequency of ischemic attacks. The assessment was subjective, however, and again, digital circulation was not measured in this study.[59]

NITRATES

Various nitrate preparations have been beneficial in variant angina, and abrupt nitrate withdrawal is suspected to relate to Raynaud's phenomenon in ammunition workers outside of the factory. Nitroglycerin seems effective in reversing ergonovine-provoked constriction of coronary arteries and could possibly be helpful in the acute management of ergot intoxication. Intravenous nitroprusside, sublingual nitroglycerin, and other preparations have been advocated for acute management of vasospastic states, but nitrates are not of proven value in controlling vasospasm outside the heart.

PROSTAGLANDINS

The role of prostaglandins in the pathophysiology of vasospastic disorders has been a subject of speculation for over a decade. Drugs that inhibit the prostaglandin synthetase enzyme system, commonly given to relieve arthritis, are of no proven value in the management of patients with Raynaud's phenomenon. Their effects could theoretically be disadvantageous in that prostaglandins may mediate the vasodilatation produced by organic nitrates. Intermittent infusions of prostacyclins (epoprostenol) have reportedly been beneficial in patients with Raynaud's phenomenon.[38] Inhibition of thromboxane A_2 does not appear to alter digital vascular resistance in patients with primary Raynaud's disease[39] but may favorably affect the rheology of the blood in other circulatory diseases.

CONVERTING ENZYME INHIBITORS

The angiotensin-converting enzyme inhibitors captopril and enalapril exert peripheral vasodilator activity through several mechanisms, including interference with formation of the pressor substance angiotensin II and with degradation of the intrinsic vasodilator peptide bradykinin. Of 12 patients with Raynaud's phenomenon due to scleroderma, 6 were felt to improve during oral therapy with captopril in doses ranging from 25 to 300 mg daily.[60] Since release of cutaneous vasoconstriction may accompany any measure which effectively controls malignant hypertension in this disorder, therapy with angiotensin inhibitors seems to bring about most dramatic improvement in fingertip perfusion when it corrects severe hypertension in scleroderma renal crisis. Although converting enzyme inhibition has produced skin vasodilatation in animal preparations, preliminary human studies have not demonstrated beneficial changes in digital blood flow in normotensive patients with systemic sclerosis or in those with idiopathic Raynaud's disease. The limb hemodynamic effects of the converting enzyme inhibitors captopril and enalapril are probably comparable. They may differ, however, in pharmacokinetics and in frequency of adverse reactions, including fever, skin rash, leukopenia, proteinuria, hypotension, azotemia, and dysgeusia.

VASCULAR SMOOTH MUSCLE RELAXANTS

The fungistatic agent griseofulvin acts directly to relax vascular smooth muscle and increases finger temperature slightly during body cooling in patients with secondary Raynaud's phenomenon. Satisfactory evidence of clinical effectiveness in peripheral vasospasm has not been provided. Nicotinic acid and its derivatives produce more vasodilatation of the face, scalp, and neck than of the extremities. There is little basis for their use in peripheral vascular disease, particularly when an obstructive component is present, but they could rationally be tried in a patient whose symptoms predominantly involve the face.

Hydralazine is a generalized vasodilator, but there is little evidence to suggest specific usefulness in treating cold sensitivity of the extremities. Similarly, cyclandelate has no demonstrable effect on foot blood flow in single doses up to 800 mg in normal subjects. Claims of benefit in patients with Raynaud's phenomenon are unconfirmed, and there is no evidence to support its use in peripheral vasospastic states. Isoxsuprine exerts vasodilator activity, which is not antagonized by β-adrenergic receptor blocking drugs. Like the β-adrenergic agonists, however, its vasodepressor effects are usually limited to musculature of the limbs. The methylxanthine derivative pentoxifylline lacks major bronchodilator or vasodilator activity but increases erythrocyte deformability in vitro, a property which may be shared by isoxsuprine. While both have been advocated for use in patients with intermittent exertional claudication, there is little evidence that these drugs are of value in treating the cutaneous ischemia that occurs at rest in Raynaud's phenomenon.

Papaverine and ethaverine have peripheral vasodilator actions, but they preferentially affect skeletal muscular rather than cutaneous beds. Oral therapy is not recommended, but when given parenterally they may be of value in reversing the intense constriction of larger proximal limb arteries sometimes encountered during angiographic or surgical procedures.[61]

CONCLUSIONS

Currently, we favor therapy with an α-adrenergic antagonist such as prazosin to relieve symptoms of persistent vasospasm such as coldness, acrocyanosis, and ulceration, particularly when obstructive lesions of proximal large arteries are absent. Generally, α-adrenergic inhibitors seem most effective in attenuating the cutaneous vasoconstriction that results from sympathetic nervous system stimulation. They are less successful in preventing episodic ischemic attacks of Raynaud's phenomenon, which may depend on other vasomotor mechanisms.

Encouraging preliminary reports suggest that calcium channel blocking agents such as nifedipine may prove helpful in reducing the frequency and severity of episodic attacks of spontaneous vasospasm. More extensive controlled studies incorporating measurements of digital blood flow are needed, however, before this form of therapy can be recommended for patients with either primary or secondary vasospastic phenomena. Vasodilator drugs are generally less effective when obstructive arterial lesions are present, although sympathetic blockade sometimes provides dramatic relief in patients with thromboangiitis obliterans. In scleroderma patients drug therapy of cutaneous ischemia seems most beneficial when it reduces severe hypertension. The usefulness of angiotensin inhibition may be limited to such patients

or to those with congestive heart failure. Pharmacologic agents are helpful in little more than half the cases, and side effects limit the acceptance of drug therapy. In nearly all patients with peripheral vasospastic disease, pharmacologic therapy should be accompanied by careful attention to protection of the skin, keeping warm, and avoidance of vasoconstrictor stimuli. The idiopathic forms of peripheral vasospastic disease (coldness, livedo reticularis, Raynaud's disease and primary acrocyanosis) seldom lead to digital ulceration except in severe, longstanding cases. In patients with other forms of cold sensitivity secondary to associated disorders, treatment should be directed mainly to the underlying pathology.

REFERENCES

1. Raynaud M: New research on the nature and treatment of local asphyxia of the extremities. Barlow translation. Selected monographs. New Sydenham Society, London, 1888
2. Hutchinson J: Raynaud's phenomena. Med Press Circular 123:402, 1901
3. Allen EV, Brown GE: Raynaud's disease: a critical review of minimal requisites for diagnosis. Am J Med Sci 183:187, 1932
4. Halperin JL, Coffman JD: Pathophysiology of Raynaud's disease. Arch Intern Med 139:89, 1979
5. Hines EA, Christensen NA: Raynaud's disease among men. JAMA 129:1, 1945
6. Lewis T: Experiments relating to the peripheral mechanism involved in spasmodic arrest of the circulation of the fingers. A variety of Raynaud's disease. Heart 15:7, 1929
7. Cohen RA, Coffman JD: Digital vasospasm—the pathophysiology of Raynaud's phenomenon. Int Angiol 3:47, 1984
8. Greenfield ADM, Shepherd JT: A quantitative study of the response to cold of the circulation through the fingers of normal subjects. Clin Sci 9:323, 1950
9. Peacock JH: Vasodilatation in the human hand. Observations on primary Raynaud's disease: acrocyanosis of the upper extremities. Clin Sci 17:575, 1957
10. Peacock JH: Peripheral venous blood concentration of epinephrine and norepinephrine in pri-

mary Raynaud's disease. Clin Res 7:821, 1959

11. Kontos HA, Wasserman AJ: Effect of reserpine in Raynaud's phenomenon. Circulation 39:259, 1969

12. Mendlowitz M, Naftchi N: The digital circulation in Raynaud's disease. Am J Cardiol 4:580, 1959

13. Downey JA, Frewin DB: The effect of cold on blood flow in the hand of patients with Raynaud's phenomenon. Clin Sci 44:279, 1973

14. Downey JA, LeRoy EC, Miller JM, Darling RC: Thermoregulation and Raynaud's phenomenon. Clin Sci 40:211, 1971

15. Coffman JD, Cohen AS: Total and capillary fingertip blood flow in Raynaud's phenomenon. N Engl J Med 285:259, 1971

16. Coffman JD: Total and nutritional blood flow in the finger. Clin Sci 42:243, 1972

17. Lewis T: The pathological changes in the arteries supplying the fingers in warm handed people and in cases of so called Raynaud's disease. Clin Sci 3:287, 1938

18. Jamieson GG, Ludbrook J, Wilson A: Cold hypersensitivity in Raynaud's phenomenon. Circulation 44:254, 1971

19. Krahenbuhl B, Nielson SL, Lassen NA: Closure of digital arteries in high vascular tone states as demonstrated by measurement of systolic blood pressure in the fingers. Scand J Clin Lab Invest 37:71, 1977

20. Rosch J, Porter JM, Gralino BJ: Cryodynamic hand angiography in the diagnosis and management of Raynaud's syndrome. Circulation 55:807, 1977

21. Nyberg G, Graham RM, Stokes GS: The effect of mental arithmetic in normotensive and hypertensive subjects and its modifications by β-adrenergic receptor blockade. Br J Clin Pharmacol 4:469, 1977

22. Halperin JL, Cohen RA, Coffman JD: Digital vasodilatation during mental stress in patients with Raynaud's disease. Cardiovasc Res 17:671, 1983

23. Cohen RA, Coffman JD: Beta-adrenergic vasodilator mechanism in the finger. Clin Res 28:161A, 1980

24. Coffman JD, Rasmussen HM: Effects of β-adrenoreceptor blocking drugs in patients with Raynaud's phenomenon. Circulation 72:466, 1985

25. Grant RT: Observations on direct communications between arteries and veins in the rabbit ear. Heart 15:281, 1930

26. Hurley HJ, Mescon H: Cholinergic innervation of the digital arteriovenous anastomoses of human skin. A histochemical localization of cholinesterase. J Appl Physiol 9:82, 1956

27. Lewis T: Observations upon reactions of vessels in human skin to cold. Heart 15:177, 1930

28. Miller D, Waters DD, Warnica W, et al: Is variant angina the coronary manifestation of a generalized vasospastic disorder? N Engl J Med 304:763, 1981

29. Winters WL, Joseph RR, Learner N: Primary pulmonary hypertension and Raynaud's phenomenon. Arch Intern Med 114:821, 1964

30. Weber RB, Reinmuth OM: The treatment of migraine with propranolol. Neurology (Minneap) 22:366, 1972

31. Tokola R, Hokkanen E: Propranolol for acute migraine. Br Med J 2:1089, 1978

32. Coffman JD, Cohen RA: Vasospasm, ubiquitous? N Engl J Med 304:780, 1981

33. Serneri GGN, Gensini GF, Masotti G, et al: Enhanced peripheral vasoconstrictor response and increased thromboxane A_2 synthesis after the cold pressor test in patients with angina at rest. Circulation 73:409, 1986

34. Halpern A, Kuhn PH, Shaftel HE, et al: Raynaud's disease, Raynaud's phenomenon and serotonin. Angiology 11:151, 1960

35. Longstaff J, Gush R, Williams EH, et al: Effects of ketanserin on peripheral blood flow, hemorheology and platelet function in patients with Raynaud's phenomenon. J Cardiovasc Pharmacol 7:599, 1985

36. Pickering GW: Vascular spasm. Lancet 2:845, 1951

37. Pringle R, Walder DN, Weaver JPA: Blood viscosity and Raynaud's disease. Lancet 1:1086, 1965

38. Belch JJ, Drury J, Capell H, et al: Intermittent epoprostenol (prostacyclin) infusion in patients with Raynaud's syndrome. Lancet 1:313, 1983

39. Coffman JD, Rasmussen HM: Effect of thromboxane synthetase inhibition in Raynaud's phenomenon. Clin Pharmacol Ther 36:369, 1984

40. Jahnsen T, Nielsen SL, Skovberg F: Blood viscosity and local response to cold in primary Raynaud's phenomenon. Lancet 2:1001, 1977

41. Talpos G, White JM, Horrocks M, et al: Plasmapheresis in Raynaud's disease. Lancet 1:416, 1978

42. Thulesius O: Problems in the evaluation of hand ischemia. p. 404. In Bernstein EF (ed): Noninva-

sive diagnostic techniques in the evaluation of hand ischemia. CV Mosby, St. Louis, 1982

43. McFadyn IJ, Housely E, MacPhersen AIS: Intraarterial reserpine administration in Raynaud's syndrome. Arch Intern Med 132:526, 1973

44. LeRoy EC, Downey JA, Cannon PF: Skin capillary blood flow in scleroderma. J Clin Invest 50:930, 1971

45. Coffman JD: Effect of vasodilator drugs in vasoconstricted normal subjects. J Clin Pharmacol 8:302, 1968

46. Varadi DP, Lawrence AP: Suppression of Raynaud's phenomenon with methyldopa. Arch Intern Med 124:13, 1969

47. Gifford RW: Arteriospastic disorders of the extremities. Circulation 27:970, 1963

48. Graham RP, Pettinger WA: Prazosin. N Engl J Med 300:232, 1979

49. Waldo R: Prazosin relieves Raynaud's phenomenon. JAMA 241:1037, 1979

50. Halperin JL: Peripheral vasospastic syndromes: current pharmacologic therapy. Primary Cardiol 9:110, 1983

51. Halperin JL: Drug therapy for cold sensitivity. Vas Diagn Ther 4:21, 1983

52. Coffman JD: Vasodilator drugs in peripheral vascular disease. N Engl J Med 300:713, 1979

53. Mikkelsen E, Andersson DE, Lederballe Pederson O: Verapamil and nifedipine inhibition of contractions induced by potassium and noradrenaline in human mesenteric arteries and veins. Acta Pharmacol Toxicol (Copenh) 44:110, 1979

54. Kahan A, Weber S, Amos B, et al: Nifedipine and Raynaud's phenomenon. Ann Intern Med 94:546, 1981

55. Smith DC, McKendry RJR: Controlled trial of nifedipine in the treatment of Raynaud's phenomenon. Lancet 2:1299, 1982

56. Rodeheffer RJ, Rommer JA, Wigley F, et al: Controlled double-blind trial of nifedipine in the treatment of Raynaud's phenomenon. N Engl J Med 308:880, 1983

57. Creager MA, Pariser KM, Winston EL, et al: Nifedipine induced fingertip vasodilatation in patients with Raynaud's phenomenon. Am Heart J 108:370, 1984

58. Kinney EL, Nicholas B, Petrokubi R, et al: The treatment of severe Raynaud's phenomenon with verapamil. J Clin Pharmacol 22:74, 1982

59. Vayssairat M, Capron L, Fiessinger SN, et al: Calcium channel blockers and Raynaud's disease. Ann Intern Med 95:243, 1981

60. Whitman HH, Case DB: New developments in the treatment of scleroderma. Drug Ther 5:97, 1981

61. Asby GR Jr, Stein M, Conrad MC, et al: Hemodynamic effects of ethaverine hydrochloride in patients with peripheral vascular disease. Curr Ther Res 16:1096, 1974

5

Immunocompromised Patients with Recurrent Cutaneous Infection

Virginia L. Chen
Bijan Safai

Immunodeficiency disorders can be classified as primary or acquired and can result either from a defect in T lymphocytes or B lymphocytes or from dysfunction of the phagocytic or complement systems. The possibility of a defect in the immune system should be considered in the evaluation of a patient who presents with recurrent or chronic cutaneous infections, since immunodeficiencies can often manifest with a skin eruption and/or infection. Although certain immunodeficiency disorders are not commonly seen, the dermatologist should be familiar with their signs and symptoms and with the approach toward making the correct diagnosis and providing appropriate care, therapy, and in some instances, genetic counseling (Table 5-1).

Recurrent cutaneous infections encountered in immunodeficient patients can present as chronic refractory or extensive viral infections, recurrent bacterial infections, chronic mucocutaneous candidiasis, or opportunistic fungal infections. Other features of immunodeficiency disorders can include recurrent infections of the upper respiratory tract, chronic diarrhea, and failure to thrive.

The type of infection may yield useful infor-mation regarding the corresponding immune defect. For example, recurrent *Neisseria* infections may suggest an underlying complement deficiency, while candidal infections may be suggestive of a cell-mediated immune deficiency or phagocytic disorder.

This chapter is intended to briefly review the clinical presentations of immunodeficiency disorders associated with cutaneous manifestations. These disorders should be considered in the evaluation of a patient susceptible to unexplained, recurrent infections, often of early onset and unresponsive to standard therapy. In addition, work-up essential to establishing the patient's immune status and underlying immune defect is discussed, as well as available therapy.

Secondary or acquired immunodeficiencies can also occur as a result of a number of disease states, which should be considered in evaluation of an immunocompromised patient. These include infections, protein-losing enteropathy, malnutrition, collagen vascular disease, neoplasia, sarcoidosis, histiocytosis, nephrotic syndrome, sickle cell disease, uremia, and iron deficiency as well as surgery, trauma, aging, and immunosuppressive therapy. Secondary

Table 5-1. Clinical Differential Diagnosis of Some Immunodeficiency Disorders

Disease	Mode of Inheritance	Cutaneous Findings	Other Clinical Manifestations
X-linked agammaglobulinemia	X-linked recessive	Pyodermas, furunculosis, atopic dermatitis, dermatomyositis, rheumatoid arthritis, urticaria	Recurrent bacterial infections, pneumonia, bronchiectasis, meningitis, septicemia, lymphoreticular malignancies
Transient hypogammaglobulinemia of infancy	—	Pyodermas, abscesses	Recurrent sinopulmonary infections, failure to thrive, diarrhea, spontaneous recovery by age 3
Selective IgA deficiency	—	Dermatomyositis, systemic lupus erythematosus, rheumatoid arthritis, dermatitis	Chronic pulmonary infections, sinusitis, anemia, thyroiditis, allergic reactions, chronic diarrhea
DiGeorge's syndrome	—	Oral and cutaneous candidiasis, abscesses	Tetany, abnormal facies, cardiovascular abnormalities, diarrhea, failure to thrive, recurrent infections (viral and fungal), *Pneumocystis carinii* pneumonia
Chronic mucocutaneous candidiasis	Sporadic, autosomal recessive	Candidiasis of skin, mucous membranes, and nails; alopecia	Endocrinopathies, thymoma, autoimmune disorders
Severe combined immunodeficiency	Autosomal recessive, X-linked recessive, sporadic	Pyodermas, oral and cutaneous candidiasis, graft vs. host disease, exfoliative dermatitis	Recurrent sinopulmonary infections, diarrhea, septicemia, failure to thrive
Common variable immunodeficiency	Autosomal recessive, autosomal dominant	Oral and cutaneous candidiasis, vitiligo, scleroderma, dermatomyositis, rheumatoid arthritis, purpura, systemic lupus erythematosus	Recurrent sinopulmonary infections, bronchiectasis, malabsorption, increased incidence of malignancy
Immunodeficiency with thymoma	—	Pyoderma, abscesses, oral and cutaneous candidiasis, stomatitis, pemphigus, systemic lupus erythematosus	Autoimmune disorders
Wiskott-Aldrich syndrome	X-linked recessive	Pyoderma, dermatitis, purpura, petechiae, herpes simplex infections	Recurrent sinopulmonary infections, otitis, lymphoreticular malignancy
Ataxia-telangiectasia	Autosomal recessive	Telangiectases, sclerodermoid changes, dermatitis, impetigo, pigmentary changes, candidiasis	Recurrent sinopulmonary infections, cerebellar ataxia, lymphoreticular malignancy
Chronic granulomatous disease	Autosomal recessive	Furunculosis, abscesses, dermatitis, pyodermas	Recurrent otitis, osteomyelitis, failure to thrive, suppurative lymphadenitis, hepatosplenomegaly
Chediak-Higashi syndrome	Autosomal recessive	Pyoderma, pigment dilution	Recurrent pneumonia, partial albinism, hepatosplenomegaly
Hyperimmunoglobulinemia E	—	Furunculosis, abscesses, dermatitis, candidiasis	Recurrent infections, abnormal facies

immunodeficiencies will not be reviewed in detail in this chapter with the exception of the acquired immunodeficiency syndrome (AIDS).

PRIMARY IMMUNODEFICIENCY DISORDERS

The primary immunodeficiency disorders can be classified into five categories: B-cell immunodeficiency, T-cell immunodeficiency, combined B-cell and T-cell immunodeficiency, deficiency of the phagocytic system, and complement-related immunodeficiency.

B-Cell-Associated Primary Immunodeficiency Disorders

Patients with B-cell immunodeficiency disorders are characteristically susceptible to bacterial infections. Recurrent cutaneous infections commonly present as pyodermas and recurrent furunculosis, primarily caused by high-grade, encapsulated pyogenic organisms. Viral and fungal infections are uncommonly encountered. Other dermatologic manifestations have included urticaria, a dermatomyositis-like syndrome, and atopic dermatitis. Defects in humoral immunity may involve one or more classes of immunoglobulins.

Six immunodeficiency disorders in this category merit discussion:

1. Infantile X-linked agammaglobulinemia (Bruton type)
2. Common variable immunodeficiency (or acquired agammaglobulinemia)
3. Selective IgA deficiency
4. Transient hypogammaglobulinemia of infancy
5. Job's syndrome
6. Buckley's syndrome

INFANTILE X-LINKED AGAMMAGLOBULINEMIA (BRUTON TYPE)

Clinical Presentation. Cutaneous infections frequently present as pyodermas and severe furunculosis, usually secondary to *Staphylococcus aureus*. An increased incidence of atopic dermatitis, urticaria, and dermatomyositis-like and rheumatoid arthritis-like manifestations has been documented.[1]

The disorder is transmitted as an X-linked recessive trait. Affected individuals are male infants and children who initially present with repeated bacterial infections, including pneumonia, bronchiectasis, otitis media, sinusitis, meningitis, and septicemia. Chronic diarrhea, usually caused by *Giardia lamblia* or *Bacteroides,* may be present. Upper respiratory tract infections are usually caused by *Hemophilus influenzae* and *S. aureus*. Infections usually occur around 4 to 12 months of age, probably because maternal antibodies provide sufficient protection to the infant during the first few months after birth.[1–5]

Many of these children develop small tonsils and adenoids. There is an increased incidence of malignancy, including leukemias and lymphomas.[6]

Laboratory Tests. Diagnosis is made by the markedly reduced levels or absence of all immunoglobulins, which is due to the absence of B cells from the peripheral blood of most affected individuals; the number of T cells is generally normal. Antibody responses to antigenic stimulation are undetectable. Isohemagglutinin titers are low or absent. Plasma cells are characteristically absent in lymph nodes, spleen, bone marrow, and gastrointestinal tract. The lymph nodes are small and lack germinal centers. Cell-mediated immunity is unaffected.[1,3,4]

Treatment. Early diagnosis and treatment will ameliorate the prognosis. Administration of gamma globulin intramuscularly (25 mg/kg per week) has been effective in preventing pyogenic infections. Appropriate antibiotic therapy is used to treat infections. Infusion of plasma is an alternative treatment but is associated with a risk of hepatitis. Genetic counseling is important, since this disorder is inherited.[3,4]

COMMON VARIABLE IMMUNODEFICIENCY (ACQUIRED AGAMMAGLOBULINEMIA)

Clinical Presentation. In contrast to X-linked agammaglobulinemia, acquired agammaglobulinemia can occur at any age and affects males and females equally. It is inherited in both autosomal recessive and autosomal dominant forms.

Autoimmune diseases, including rheumatoid arthritis, dermatomyositis, scleroderma, systemic lupus erythematosus, vitiligo, and idiopathic thrombocytopenic purpura have been reported in association with common variable immunodeficiency. There is an increased susceptibility to malignancy, including lymphoreticular cancers and gastric carcinomas. Most patients develop respiratory infections and bronchiectasis, usually in the second or third decades of life. Many of these infections are caused by *H. influenzae,* staphylococci and pneumococci. Malabsorption due to *G. lamblia* is frequently found. Lymphadenopathy and hepatosplenomegaly may be present. More commonly, tonsils and lymphoid tissue are absent.[3]

Laboratory Tests. Levels of all classes of serum immunoglobulin are low but usually higher than those of X-linked agammaglobulinemia. The total number of B cells is usually normal, but antibody responses are impaired and B cells do not differentiate in vivo into immunoglobulin-producing cells. Isohemagglutinin titers are decreased and the Schick test is positive. Cell-mediated immunity is usually normal. Declining T-cell function has been observed in association with progression of the disease in some cases. Lymphoid tissues are found to lack both lymphoid cells in B-cell-dependent areas and plasma cells.[3,4,7–9]

Treatment. Prognosis is improved in patients treated with intramuscular injections of gamma globulin (25 mg/kg per week). Chronic pulmonary disease may develop, and treatment of infections with appropriate antibiotics should be instituted.[3,4]

SELECTIVE IgA DEFICIENCY

Clinical Presentation. The dermatologic features of selective IgA deficiency are associated with an increased incidence of autoimmune diseases such as systemic lupus erythematosus. Other autoimmune disorders have been reported, including rheumatoid arthritis, pernicious anemia, and thyroiditis.[10] Most cases are sporadic, while some are autosomal recessive or autosomal dominant. The incidence is estimated to be 1:600. Many affected patients are asymptomatic but others develop recurrent sinopulmonary infection. There is an increased frequency of allergy, and many patients have circulating anti-IgA antibodies. Blood transfusion reactions are common, and gastrointestinal diseases including chronic diarrhea, gluten-sensitive enteropathy, ulcerative colitis, Crohn's disease, and giardiasis have been seen. The IgA deficiency has been found in association with partial deletion of the long arm of chromosome 18.[11] Recently, IgA deficiency has been reported in patients on anticonvulsant drugs, particularly dilantin.[12]

Laboratory Tests. Levels of IgA in serum and respiratory secretions are less than 5 mg/dl in most cases, but serum levels of all other immunoglobulins are unaffected. The total number of B cells is normal, while the total T-cell count is reduced. Cell-mediated immune responses are usually intact, in contrast to the responses of patients affected with ataxia-telangiectasia who have IgA deficiency and impaired cell-mediated immunity. Approximately 40 percent of patients have anti-IgA antibodies circulating in their sera.[4,13]

Treatment. Associated disorders should be managed appropriately. Immunoglobulin replacement or blood transfusion produces no benefit, and no therapy is effective at present.

TRANSIENT HYPOGAMMAGLOBULINEMIA OF INFANCY

Clinical Presentation. Infants affected by transient hypogammaglobulinemia at the age of 3 to 6 months commonly develop recurrent otitis media, bronchitis, pneumonia, recurrent diarrhea, and, rarely, pyodermas of the skin. The disease is self-limited and usually remits spontaneously in 6 to 18 months.[1,14]

Laboratory Tests. Total serum immunoglobulin is low (less than 400 mg/dl), and serum IgG is usually below 250 mg/dl. The total number of B cells is normal, and antibody responses to antigenic stimulation are intact. Cell-mediated immunity is normal. The number of plasma cells in bone marrow and lymph nodes is reduced.[4]

Treatment. Because this disease is self-limited, intramuscular gamma globulin injections are generally not indicated.[14]

JOB'S SYNDROME

Clinical Presentation. Job's syndrome was first described in fair-skinned, red-haired girls who presented with recurrent "cold" staphylococcal abscesses and dermatitis similar to atopic dermatitis.[15] These patients develop pulmonary infections, otitis media, conjunctivitis, and sinusitis. Abscesses can also involve the lung, joints, and other sites.[15,16]

Laboratory Tests. Serum IgE is markedly elevated (greater than 2,000 IU/ml). Antibody and cell-mediated responses to neoantigens are impaired, but T-cell and B-cell numbers are normal. Eosinophilia may be present, and neutrophil chemotactic defects are variable. Strongly positive wheal and flare skin test reactions to multiple allergens are elicited in many of these patients.[15–17]

Treatment. Penicillinase-resistant penicillins are used to treat infections.

BUCKLEY'S SYNDROME

Clinical Presentation. The clinical features of Buckley's syndrome are recurrent furunculosis, which begins in early infancy, recurrent pneumonias, usually caused by *S.*

aureus, and a pruritic dermatitis similar to atopic dermatitis. Patients have a peculiarly coarse facial appearance.[9,18]

Laboratory Tests. Elevated serum IgE and IgD are present, but T-cell and B-cell numbers are normal. In vitro lymphocyte responses to mitogens are intact, while in vitro lymphocyte responses to *Candida albicans* and tetanus toxoid are impaired, and antibody responses to booster immunizations are poor. Chemotactic abnormalities are variable.[9,18]

Treatment. Penicillinase-resistant penicillins are recommended, along with surgical drainage of cutaneous abscesses and pneumatoceles.

T-Cell-Associated Primary Immunodeficiency Disorders

Defects in cell-mediated immunity are characterized by susceptibility to opportunistic infections and a high incidence of malignancy. Recurrent infections are commonly caused by fungi, viruses, *Pneumocystis carinii,* or other infectious agents with low-grade pathogenicity.

Three immunodeficiency disorders in this category will be discussed:

1. DiGeorge's syndrome (congenital thymic aplasia)
2. Nezelof's syndrome (cellular immunodeficiency with immunoglobulins)
3. Chronic mucocutaneous candidiasis

DIGEORGE'S SYNDROME (CONGENITAL THYMIC APLASIA)

Clinical Presentation. Children affected by DiGeorge's syndrome have a peculiar facies characterized by hypertelorism, micrognathia, cleft palate, low-set ear malformations, and nasal clefts.[3] Other dermatologic features include extensive oral and perineal candidiasis, and susceptibility to graft-versus-host disease if any nonirradiated blood product is given. Hypocalcemic tetany may be the initial presenting clinical sign of affected neonates. Cardiovascular anomalies can also be present: absent aortic arch, transposition of the great vessels, tetralogy of Fallot, and other aberrations have been reported. Affected children are susceptible to viral, fungal, bacterial, and parasitic infections. Some develop *Pneumocystis carinii* pneumonia, chronic diarrhea, and failure to thrive.

The absence or hypoplasia of the thymus, often accompanied by the absence of parathyroids, probably results from a defect in the embryogenesis of the third and fourth pharyngeal pouches, from which the thymus and parathyroid glands are derived.[3,19]

Laboratory Tests. Diminished T-cell-mediated immunity is reflected by lack of T cells in the peripheral blood and the absence of in vitro lymphocyte responses to mitogens and antigens. Total blood lymphocyte count and B-cell number and function are usually normal, as are serum immunoglobulin levels. Hypocalcemia and low parathyroid hormone levels may be observed. Thymic shadow is absent on chest X-ray.[20]

Treatment. Hypocalcemia and cardiovascular problems should be managed promptly. Transplantation of human fetal thymus tissue has successfully restored cell-mediated immunity in some cases.[21–23] Less severe forms of DiGeorge's syndrome exist in which cell-mediated immune responses may spontaneously recover.[24]

NEZELOF'S SYNDROME (CELLULAR IMMUNODEFICIENCY WITH IMMUNOGLOBULINS)

Clinical Presentation. Skin manifestations include oral or cutaneous candidiasis refractory to all forms of therapy as well as recurrent bacterial and viral infections. Gram-negative sepsis, urinary tract infections, otitis, severe varicella, or progressive vaccinia may develop.[9,25]

In addition, most affected children have recurrent or chronic pulmonary infections and chronic diarrhea, and fail to thrive.

Laboratory Tests. Common laboratory findings are lymphopenia, neutropenia, eosinophilia, diminished lymphoid tissue, abnormally developed thymus architecture with abnormal cell-mediated immunity, and normal or increased serum levels of immunoglobulins. Total T-cell count is decreased, with a normal T-cell helper to suppressor ratio.[9,25]

Treatment. Antibiotic therapy and immunoglobulin replacement are advocated. Bone marrow transplantation has been beneficial in a few cases.[9,26]

CHRONIC MUCOCUTANEOUS CANDIDIASIS

Clinical Presentation. Chronic mucocutaneous candidiasis may appear as a sporadic or autosomal recessive trait. In early childhood chronic superficial *Candida* infection of the skin, nails, and oral and genital mucosa occurs (Figs. 5-1 and 5-2). Chronic *Candida* infection can manifest with granulomatous lesions of the skin, and alopecia may also be observed. Endocrinopathy may be associated with this disorder, most commonly hypoparathyroidism and adrenal insufficiency.[27]

Laboratory Tests. The characteristic laboratory abnormality is the absence of a delayed hypersensitivity skin test reaction to *Candida* in the presence of a *Candida* infection. In some patients the migration-inhibition factor is absent following lymphocyte stimulation with *Candida* antigen. Total T- and B-cell populations and serum immunoglobulin levels are usually normal, as are B-cell immunity and formation of antibody to *Candida* antigen.[27]

Treatment. Treatment is very difficult. The treatment of choice in cases of *Candida* meningitis or septicemia is intravenous ampho-

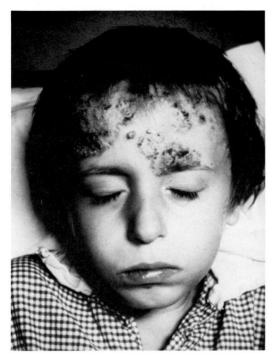

Fig. 5-1. Extensive forehead involvement in a patient with chronic mucocutaneous candidiasis. (Reproduced with permission from Weinberg S, Leider M, Shapiro L: Color Atlas of Pediatric Dermatology. McGraw-Hill, New York, 1975. Print courtesy of Sam Weinberg, M.D., New York University.)

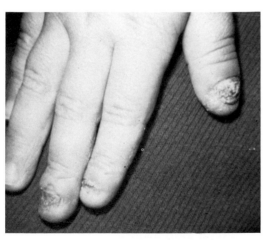

Fig. 5-2. Chronic mucocutaneous candidiasis with characteristic nail involvement. (Reproduced with permission from Weinberg S, Leider M, Shapiro L: Color Atlas of Pediatric Dermatology. McGraw-Hill, New York, 1975. Print courtesy of Sam Weinberg, M.D., New York University.)

tericin B. Alternative effective therapy is ketoconazole.[28]

Combined B-Cell- and T-Cell-Associated Primary Immunodeficiency Disorders

Conditions associated with both B-cell and T-cell defects have dermatologic features found in immunodeficiency disorders that affect either the B-cell or T-cell system primarily and have already been discussed.

The various types of immunodeficiency disorders in this category are as follows:

1. Severe combined immunodeficiency
2. Immunodeficiency with thymoma (Good's syndrome)
3. Wiskott-Aldrich syndrome
4. Ataxia-telangiectasia

SEVERE COMBINED IMMUNODEFICIENCY

Clinical Presentation. Oral candidiasis is commonly the initial finding in severe combined immunodeficiency and progresses to extensive involvement of the skin. Some children have died from complications of common viral infections (varicella, measles, mumps). Immunization against smallpox may lead to progressive vaccinia. Graft-versus-host disease may develop following a transfusion or in utero and is characterized by a skin eruption with a generalized maculopapular, erythrodermic, or morbilliform appearance.[3,29] Affected children are susceptible to bacterial infections of the skin, which may resemble ecthyma gangrenosum or toxic epidermal necrolysis. Some patients develop intractable diarrhea, hepatosplenomegaly, and enlarged lymph nodes, and fail to thrive. Pulmonary infections caused by *Pneumocystis carinii* or *Pseudomonas aeruginosa* can be fatal.

Laboratory Tests. Lymphopenia (usually less than 1,000 lymphocytes/mm³) with a deficiency of T cells and B cells is common. Immunoglobulin levels are low, antibody responses to antigenic stimulation are abnormal, and lymphoid tissue is sparse. A pathognomonic finding is a small, poorly differentiated thymus with complete absence of Hassall's corpuscles. Peripheral lymphocytes are unresponsive to phytohemagglutinin or allogeneic stimulation. Biopsy of a lymph node reveals a depletion of germinal centers, plasma cells, and lymphocytes.[3,29]

Treatment. The treatment of choice is bone marrow transplantation.[30,31] Administration of transfer factor and thymic hormones has limited benefit. Enzyme replacement is advocated in patients with severe combined immunodeficiency associated with adenosine deaminase deficiency.[32,33]

IMMUNODEFICIENCY WITH THYMOMA (GOOD'S SYNDROME)

Clinical Presentation. Good's syndrome is encountered in individuals over 40 years old and affects females and males in a 2:1 ratio. Cutaneous findings include fungal and pyogenic infections and nonspecific dermatitis.[34] Primary benign and malignant thymic tumors have been reported. There is an increased susceptibility to infection, particularly sinopulmonary infections, septicemia, and urinary tract infections. Chronic diarrhea and aplastic anemia may develop.[4]

Laboratory Tests. Progressive lymphopenia develops, with a reduction of total T-cell and B-cell numbers. Cell-mediated immune responses are usually impaired, antibody formation is poor, and panhypogammaglobulinemia is present. Chest X-ray may reveal an anterior mediastinal mass.[4]

Treatment. Prognosis is poor. Removal of the primary tumor and gamma globulin therapy are recommended. The immunodeficient state is not affected by removal of the thymic tumor.[4]

WISKOTT-ALDRICH SYNDROME

Clinical Presentation. Wiskott-Aldrich syndrome, an X-linked recessive disorder, is characterized by a triad of dermatitis, thrombocytopenic purpura, and immunodeficiency, with recurrent infections caused by bacteria, viruses, or fungi. Bleeding episodes, petechiae, and purpura occur in the first few months of life. Within the first year a dermatitis appears, which resembles atopic dermatitis as it usually involves the face and antecubital and popliteal fossae. Patients can develop herpes simplex infection of the skin and eyes. Meningitis, otitis media, pneumonia, and sepsis are frequent. Over 10 percent of patients develop malignancies, particularly lymphoreticular tumors and leukemias.[9,29]

Laboratory Tests. Serum IgM levels are diminished, while serum IgE levels are elevated and serum IgA and IgG levels may be normal or abnormally high. Antibody responses to polysaccharide antigens are poor, isohemagglutinin titers are low or absent, and total T-cell count is normal, but cell-mediated immune responses may be impaired. Cutaneous anergy is common. Platelet count is usually low and platelet size is abnormally small. Anemia, eosinophilia, and progressive lymphopenia may be present.[29]

Treatment. Bleeding can be controlled by platelet transfusion, infections are treated with appropriate antibiotic therapy, and dermatitis responds to topical steroids. About 50 percent of patients given transfer factor have responded with an improved immunologic status and prolonged survival.[3] Bone marrow transplants following total body irradiation or pretreatment with busulfan and cyclophosphamide have been beneficial in a few cases.[35]

ATAXIA-TELANGIECTASIA

Clinical Presentation. Ataxia-telangiectasia, an autosomal recessively transmitted disorder, presents with progressive cerebellar ataxia,

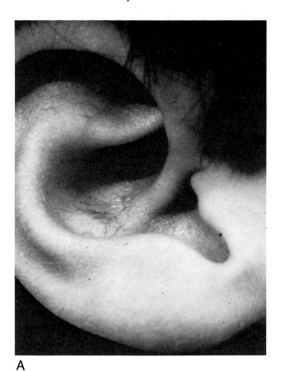

A

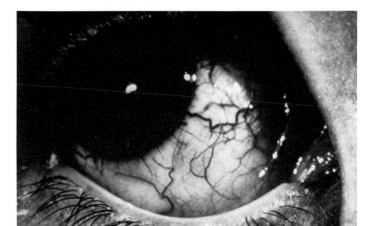

B

Fig. 5-3. Ataxia-telangiectasia. Telangiectases on **(A)** the pinna of the ear and **(B)** the conjunctiva. (Reproduced with permission from Weinberg S, Leider M, Shapiro L: Color Atlas of Pediatric Dermatology. McGraw-Hill, New York, 1975. Print courtesy of Sam Weinberg, M.D., New York University.)

telangiectases (Fig. 5-3), and recurrent infections. Ataxia can begin around the age of 1 year or in early childhood. Choreoathetoid movements, nystagmus, and mental retardation may develop and progress by adolescence. Telangiectases occur on the bulbar conjunctivae and are present later on ear pinnae, eyelids, face, and extremities. Other associated cutaneous manifestations are impetigo, candidiasis, sclerodermoid changes, pigmentary changes, and atopic, nummular, and seborrheic dermatitides.[34,36] Repeated bacterial and viral infections of the lungs and sinuses develop. Associated abnormalities include growth retardation, gonadal hypoplasia, and insulin-dependent diabetes.[37] Over 10 percent of patients develop malignancy, particularly lymphoma and acute lymphocytic leukemia.[3]

Laboratory Tests. Serum IgA is absent in over 50 percent of cases, and IgE is also often absent, whereas T-cell number and function may be normal initially but decline with age, and B-cell number is usually normal. The thymus is hypoplastic and depleted of Hassall's corpuscles and T-cell dependent areas.[9,29] Serum levels of α-fetoprotein are elevated in many cases for unknown reasons.[38] Chromosomal abnormalities, particularly those affecting chromosome 14, have been reported.[39]

Treatment. Little success in treating this fatal disease has been achieved with the use of thymus transplant, thymosin, or transfer factor.[29]

Phagocytic Cell-Associated Immunodeficiency Disorders

Infections in phagocytic disorders are more severe than those encountered in antibody deficiency disorders. Bacterial and fungal infections commonly occur, although other infections can develop as well. Organisms that are not highly virulent in normal hosts can cause severe infection in patients with phagocytic disorders.

The various types of immunodeficiency disorders in this category may be summarized as follows:

1. Chronic granulomatous disease
2. Chediak-Higashi syndrome
3. Lazy leukocyte syndrome

CHRONIC GRANULOMATOUS DISEASE

Clinical Presentation. Chronic granulomatous disease, an X-linked recessive disorder, is characterized by chronic cervical adenitis occurring in the first year of life, followed by

recurrent purulent granulomatous infections of the skin, lungs, intestinal tract, liver, and lymphoreticular organs. The cutaneous manifestations are commonly seen and may resemble seborrheic dermatitis or may appear as granulomatous nodules or pyodermas (Fig. 5-4). Clues to the diagnosis may be found in the type of organisms cultured; *Staphylococcus aureus, Staphylococcus albus, Serratia marcescens, Candida albicans, Escherichia coli, Klebsiella enterobacter,* and *Pseudomonas aeruginosa* are common infectious pathogens in this disease.[40,41] Lymphadenopathy, chronically draining lymph nodes, and hepatosplenomegaly are commonly present; 25 percent of cases develop osteomyelitis.[3]

Laboratory Tests. Failure of leukocytes to reduce a colorless nitroblue tetrazolium dye to a purple formazan dye is indicative of a func-

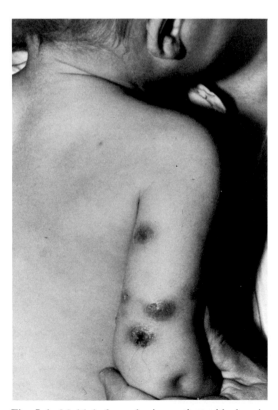

Fig. 5-4. Multiple furuncles in a patient with chronic granulomatous disease.

tional defect of phagocytes and is diagnostic of this disorder.[41,42] The inability of phagocytes to kill catalase-positive bacteria and fungi is believed to be due to a deficiency of NADH or NADPH oxidase,[40,43–45] an enzyme required for hydrogen peroxide production by phagocytes.

Treatment. No specific therapy exists other than appropriate antibiotics and surgical drainage of abscesses. Prognosis is good.

CHEDIAK-HIGASHI SYNDROME

Clinical Presentation. Patients affected with Chediak-Higashi syndrome, an autosomal recessive disorder, present with an increased susceptibility to infection. They develop recurrent pyogenic infections of the skin and may have partial albinism and progressive spinocerebellar degeneration. Pigment dilution of the skin, hair, and eyes is typical and probably results from abnormal melanosome synthesis. There is an increased incidence of malignancy, including lymphomas and reticulum cell sarcomas.[41]

Laboratory Tests. Gigantic lysosomal intracytoplasmic inclusions (2 to 4 μm diameter) are found in leukocytes. It is suggested that autophagocytic activity of leukocytes may be responsible for the formation of giant inclusions, resulting in slow degranulation of lysosomes.[46]

Treatment. There is currently no effective treatment. Bone marrow transplantation has restored the leukocyte defect in a few cases.[47,48]

LAZY LEUKOCYTE SYNDROME

Clinical Presentation. Affected children develop recurrent episodes of gingivitis and stomatitis in addition to recurrent otitis media and mild upper respiratory tract infections.[49]

Laboratory Tests. The major defect is a deficiency in motility of polymorphonuclear leukocytes as assessed by the Rebuck skin window. A decreased number of polymorphonuclear leukocytes in the peripheral blood and poor mobilization of granulocytes from the bone marrow are found. Intracellular killing, cell-mediated immunity, and humoral immunity are not affected.[49]

Treatment. Treatment consists of appropriate antibiotics and local care; there is no therapy available for the underlying defect.

Complement Deficiencies

Deficiency of certain complement components can lead to infections of the skin, lungs, kidneys, and gastrointestinal tract. Table 5-2 lists clinical findings that have been reported in disorders of selective complement deficiencies.[50] In particular, hereditary angioedema is caused by an autosomal dominant deficiency of C1 esterase inhibitor, while collagen vascular diseases and, more commonly, a systemic lupus erythematosus-like syndrome have been reported in association with deficiencies of the

Table 5-2. Complement Deficiencies and Associated Clinical Findings

C1q: SLE-like syndrome, recurrent infection, glomerulonephritis
C1r: SLE-like syndrome, recurrent infections, chronic nephritis
C1s: SLE
C1INH: Hereditary angioedema, SLE, DLE
C2: SLE, DLE, nephritis, vasculitis, dermatomyositis, recurrent infections, glomerulonephritis, Henoch-Schönlein purpura
C3: Pyogenic infections
C3bINA: Pyogenic infections
C4: SLE, glomerulonephritis, Henoch-Schönlein purpura
C5: SLE, *Neisseria* infections
C5 dysfunction: Pyoderma, septicemia, Leiner's disease
C6: *Neisseria* infections
C7: *Neisseria* infections, Raynaud's phenomenon, sclerodactyly and telangiectasia, SLE, nephritis
C8: *Neisseria* infections, SLE
C9: None

SLE = systemic lupus erythematosus; DLE = discoid lupus erythematosus.

early components of the classical pathway, namely, C1q, C1r, C1s, C2, C4, and C5.

Recurrent infections may develop secondary to a defect in the complement system. Deficiency of C3 and C3b inactivator is associated with an increased susceptibility to pyogenic infections. These include pneumonia, meningitis, recurrent otitis media, and septicemia.[50–52] Recurrent *Neisseria* infections are associated with deficiency of the late components C5 to C8. Familial C5 dysfunction occurs in Leiner's disease, which is characterized by gram-negative skin and bowel infection, recalcitrant generalized seborrhea-like dermatitis, sepsis, and failure to thrive. Defective serum opsonization of yeast particles has been reported. Some patients affected with this disorder have shown clinical improvement following fresh plasma transfusions.[53,54]

Laboratory investigation of the complement system should be initiated in a patient who presents with recurrent infections, *Neisseria* infections, or collagen vascular disease. The complement system can be evaluated by assays of total hemolytic complement, such as serum CH50, which measures the ability of complement to lyse sheep erythrocytes sensitized with antierythrocyte antibodies. If the results of this test are normal, there is usually little need to study individual complement components.

ACQUIRED IMMUNODEFICIENCY SYNDROME

Clinical Presentation

The Centers for Disease Control (CDC) define AIDS as the fully developed stage of human immunodeficiency virus (HIV) infection. It is characterized by development of one or more life-threatening opportunistic infections[55] and/or Kaposi's sarcoma of the epidemic form or other unusual neoplastic processes in a patient without an identifiable cause of the underlying immune defect.[56]

As a result of the identification of HIV [also called human T-cell lymphotropic virus type III (HTLV III) and lymphadenopathy-associated virus (LAV)] and the development of reliable blood screening tests, this case definition was revised by the CDC[57] in June, 1985 in response to recommendations by the Conference of State and Territorial Epidemiologists and now includes the following refinements:

1. In the absence of the opportunistic diseases required by the current case definition, any of the following diseases is considered indicative of AIDS if the patient has a positive serologic or virologic test for HIV:

    a. Disseminated histoplasmosis (not confined to lungs or lymph nodes) diagnosed by culture, histology, or antigen detection

    b. Isosporiasis causing chronic diarrhea (more than 1 month), diagnosed by histology or stool microscopy

    c. Bronchial or pulmonary candidiasis, diagnosed by microscopy or by the presence of characteristic white plaques grossly on the bronchial mucosa (not by culture alone)

    d. Non-Hodgkin's lymphoma of high-grade pathologic type (diffuse, undifferentiated) and of B-cell or unknown immunologic phenotype, diagnosed by biopsy

    e. Histologically confirmed Kaposi's sarcoma in patients who are 60 years old or older when diagnosed

2. In the absence of the opportunistic diseases required by the current case definition, a histologically confirmed diagnosis of chronic lymphoid interstitial pneumonitis in a child (under 13 years of age) is considered indicative of AIDS unless test(s) for HIV are negative.

3. Patients who have a lymphoreticular malignancy diagnosed more than 3 months after the diagnosis of an opportunistic disease used as a marker for AIDS will now be included as AIDS cases.

4. To increase the specificity of the case definition, patients are excluded as AIDS cases if they have a negative test result for serum antibody to HIV, have no other type of HIV test with a positive result, and do not have a low number of T-helper lymphocytes or a low ratio of T-helper to T-suppressor lymphocytes. In

the absence of test results, patients satisfying all other criteria in the definition continue to be included.

Classification

The CDC classification of HIV infection reads as follows[58]:

Group 1: Acute infection

Group 2: Asymptomatic infection

Group 3: Persistent generalized lymphadenopathy (PGL): palpable lymph nodes, 1 cm or greater in diameter, at 2 or more extrainguinal sites, lasting for more than 3 months.

Group 4: Other diseases:

    Subgroup A: Constitutional disease: fever for more than 1 month, involuntary weight loss of greater than 10 percent of body weight, or diarrhea of more than 1 month's duration without other underlying disease.

    Subgroup B: Neurologic disease: dementia, myelopathy, or peripheral neuropathy

    Subgroups C: Secondary infectious diseases

    Subgroup C-1: Specific secondary infectious diseases listed in the CDC surveillance definition for AIDS (12 diseases): *Pneumocystis carinii* pneumonia, chronic cryptosporidiosis, toxoplasmosis, extraintestinal strongyloidiasis, isosporiasis, candidiasis (esophageal, bronchial, or pulmonary), cryptococcosis, histoplasmosis, mycobacterial infection (*Mycobacterium avium* or *Mycobacterium kansasii*), cytomegalovirus infections, chronic mucocutaneous or disseminated herpes simplex (Fig. 5-5), progressive multifocal leukoencephalopathy.

    Subgroup C-2: Other specified secondary infectious diseases, specifically, symptomatic or invasive disease due to oral hairy leukoplakia, multidermatomal herpes zoster, recurrent *Salmonella* bacteremia, nocardiosis, tuberculosis, oral candidiasis (thrush)

    Subgroup D: Secondary cancers: Kaposi's sarcoma, non-Hodgkin's lymphoma

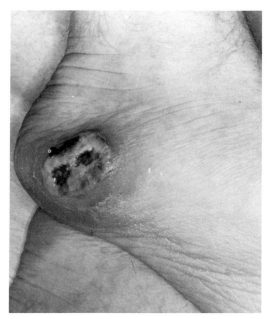

Fig. 5-5. Chronic herpetic ulceration of the heel in a patient with AIDS.

(small, uncleaved lymphoma or immunoblastic sarcoma), primary lymphoma of the brain

    Subgroup E: Other conditions

In accordance with these recommendations, only AIDS—the more severe manifestation of HIV infection—will be reportable nationally. The reportability of milder disease associated with HIV infection [AIDS-related complex (ARC) and persistent generalized lymphadenopathy (PGL)] as well as asymptomatic infections will continue to be determined by individual states.

The AIDS-related complex is a clinical and laboratory syndrome characterized by minor conditions associated with clinical immunosuppression and with laboratory evidence of immunosuppression that is probably associated with HIV infection. Thus, ARC may be diagnosed on the basis of clinical presentation of an unexplained chronic persistent and asymptomatic lymphadenopathy along with laboratory evidence of a quantitative T-cell deficiency. Other clinical symptoms may include an unexplainable chronic fever, night sweats, malaise, weight loss, and diarrhea. Patients with ARC are frequently predisposed to cutaneous infections, such as oral candidiasis, herpes simplex or zoster virus infections, extensive molluscum contagiosum, and fungal infections. Skin testing for delayed hypersensitivity may be negative. Whether or not ARC progresses to AIDS has not been conclusively determined, although it has been estimated that 5 to 20 percent of ARC patients develop AIDS over a 3-year period.[59,60]

In addition, unexplained idiopathic thrombocytopenia is probably associated with HIV infection, as are a variety of non-life-threatening fungal, viral, and bacterial infectious processes that probably represent manifestations of virus-induced immunologic perturbation. These manifestations are sometimes termed *lesser AIDS*.

Also recognized as associated with HIV infection is PGL, a symptom complex characterized by the occurrence of persistent, unexplained lymph node enlargement in several extrainguinal lymph node groups. The relationship of the lymphadenopathy syndrome to progression to overt clinical AIDS is uncertain but probably is as high as 10 percent. (Of course, PGL can be caused by agents other than HIV.)

Immunologic Defect

As already stated, the etiologic agent of AIDS has been identified to be HIV. The virus is transmitted mostly by sexual contact and by blood and blood products, and preferentially infects T_4 helper (inducer) lymphocytes.[61] Progressive destruction of T_4 lymphocytes results not only in defects of the cell-mediated immune system[62] but also in disturbances of the B-cell system, as well as phagocytic and monocytic dysfunctions.[63]

Epidemiology

The disease AIDS was initially recognized in homosexual and bisexual men. Soon after, however, intravenous drug abusers, hemophili-

Table 5-3. Distribution of AIDS Cases by Risk Group (Adults)

Adults/Adolescents	Total Cumulative	
	Number	(%)
Homosexual/bisexual male	26,631	(66)
Intravenous (IV) drug abuser	6,617	(16)
Homosexual male and IV drug abuser	3,052	(8)
Hemophilia/coagulation disorder	369	(1)
Heterosexual cases	1,562	(4)
Transfusion, blood/components	850	(2)
Undetermined	1,201	(3)
Total	40,282	(100)

(Data from AIDS Weekly Surveillance Report, Centers for Disease Control, August 24, 1987.)

acs, children born to mothers with AIDS, and transfusion recipients were recognized as high-risk populations. Recently, the disease has appeared in heterosexuals not in the above categories, and it seems that it has the same pattern of spread in heterosexuals as in homosexuals. Tables 5-3 to 5-7 show the cases of AIDS (not ARC) recently reported to the CDC and the distribution by risk population, location in the United States, and disease manifestation in children and in adults.

In Haiti and Africa the spread of the disease is by hetero- and homosexual contact. It seems that a large proportion of the population is infected by this virus and is dying of what is locally called SLIM disease. In Europe as well as in other parts of the world HIV infection is reaching a pandemic level and constitutes a major world health problem.

Recently, heterosexual transmission has been discovered in female partners of men with AIDS or at high risk for AIDS.[64–66] In addition to sexual and parenteral routes of transmission, prenatal or perinatal infection with HIV from

Table 5-4. Distribution of AIDS Cases by Risk Group (Children)

Children	Total Cumulative	
	Number	(%)
Hemophilia/coagulation disorder	30	(5)
Parent with/at risk of AIDS	440	(78)
Transfusion, blood/components	68	(12)
Undetermined	25	(4)
Total	563	(100)

(Data from AIDS Weekly Surveillance Report, Centers for Disease Control, August 24, 1987.)

Table 5-5. Distribution of AIDS Cases by Location

City	Cumulative Total
New York, NY	10,554
San Francisco, CA	4,009
Los Angeles, CA	3,506
Houston, TX	1,347
Miami, FL	1,184
Washington, DC	1,149
Newark, NJ	989
Chicago, IL	952
Philadelphia, PA	792
Dallas, TX	784
Atlanta, GA	654
Boston, MA	637
Ft. Lauderdale, FL	525
Nassau-Suffolk, NY	516
Jersey City, NJ	508
San Diego, CA	462
Seattle, WA	395
Denver, CO	353
New Orleans, LA	347
Anaheim, CA	333
Rest of US	10,849
Total	40,845

(Data from AIDS Weekly Surveillance Report, Centers for Disease Control, August 24, 1987.)

mothers with AIDS or at risk for AIDS has been reported.[67] Malignancies associated with AIDS include Kaposi's sarcoma, Burkitt's lymphoma, non-Hodgkin's lymphomas, Hodgkin's disease, chronic lymphocytic leukemia, and carcinomas of the oropharynx, liver, and lung.[68]

Laboratory Tests

Diagnosis is made on the basis of clinical findings described above in otherwise healthy individuals with no history of any primary immunodeficiency disorder, cancer, or immunosuppressive therapy. A number of laboratory tests that are not necessarily diagnostic of AIDS help to confirm the immune status of the patient. Screening blood tests should include a complete blood count with differential leukocyte count, platelet count, erythrocyte sedimentation rate, blood chemistry, and antibody test for HIV. Routine blood studies may reveal a mild depression of the total white blood count, hematocrit and hemoglobin values, or total platelet count. Elevated serum thymosin, β_2-microglobulin, and globulins are often seen. Skin testing with common antigens shows variable results in patients with ARC or AIDS.[63]

The presence of the HIV antibodies is identi-

Table 5-6. AIDS Case Fatality Rate

Year	Months	Number of Cases	Number of Known Deaths	Case-Fatality Rate (%)
Before 1981		76	63	83
1981	Jan–June	86	78	91
	July–Dec	180	163	91
1982	Jan–June	363	315	87
	July–Dec	648	561	87
1983	Jan–June	1,221	1,071	88
	July–Dec	1,588	1,353	85
1984	Jan–June	2,444	1,970	81
	July–Dec	3,188	2,539	80
1985	Jan–June	4,366	3,295	75
	July–Dec	5,429	3,753	69
1986	Jan–June	6,516	3,732	57
	July–Dec	7,332	2,872	39
1987	Jan–June	7,060	1,763	25
	July–Aug 24	348	31	9
Total		40,845	23,559	58

(Data from AIDS Weekly Surveillance Report, Centers for Disease Control, August 24, 1987.)

Table 5-7. Reported Cases and Deaths of AIDS by Disease Category

Disease Category Reported	Cumulative Cases/Deaths			
	Reported Cases		Known Deaths	
	Number	(% Total)	Number	(% Cases)
Pneumocystis carinii pneumonia	26,553	(65)	15,350	(58)
Other opportunistic diseases	9,285	(23)	5,890	(63)
Kaposi's sarcoma	5,007	(12)	2,319	(46)
Total	40,845	(100)	23,559	(58)

(Data from AIDS Weekly Surveillance Report, Centers for Disease Control, August 24, 1987.)

fied by an enzyme-linked immunosorbent assay (ELISA). This is a relatively inexpensive and rapid test, which relies upon viral lysates as antigen targets. False positive ELISA results have been seen in a small proportion of patients with autoimmune diseases, as well as alcoholics and patients with lymphoproliferative malignancies. False negative results may be seen in the terminal stage of AIDS, during the incubation period, and in other virus-positive seronegative carriers. A more sensitive and specific test is the Western blot, which is utilized in cases that yield negative or false positive results by the ELISA method. Purified HIV antigens are electrophoresed on sodium dodecyl sulfate gels, and the separated polypeptides are then transferred onto sheets of nitrocellulose paper. After blocking of protein binding sites with suitable nonspecific proteins, the nitrocellulose paper is incubated with the serum specimen in question. Any antibody that binds to the separated polypeptides present on the nitrocellulose paper will be detected by a secondary antihuman antibody that has been conjugated to a suitable enzyme marker and then incubated with the appropriate enzyme substrate. Antibody specificities against known viral components (generally the core component p24 and/or the envelope component gp120) are considered to be true positive results, while antibody specificities against nonviral cellular contaminants are scored as nonspecific, false positive results. A positive ELISA confirmed with a positive Western blot is strongly supportive of an HIV infection. More than 90 percent of all AIDS and ARC patients are seropositive for HIV.[69]

Quantitative studies of T cells, helper T cells, and suppressor T cells are performed in cases suggestive or diagnostic of ARC or AIDS. A deficiency in the helper T-cell count develops progressively as a result of HIV infection, thereby reversing the ratio of helper T cells to suppressor T cells. A persistent finding of a helper T-cell count less than $400/mm^3$ and helper/suppressor ratio less than 1.0 is indicative of impaired immune function.[62,63] The ability of helper T cells to stimulate antibody production by B cells is impaired in several cases.[70] A defect in natural killer cell activity and cell-mediated cytotoxicity against virus-infected targets has been observed in AIDS patients.[71]

Levels of serum immunoglobulins, especially IgG and IgA, are frequently elevated[62] as a result of polyclonal activation of B cells. Proliferative responses to plant lectins, antigens, and allogeneic cells are diminished. Production of γ- and α-interferon by mononuclear cells is reduced.[71,72] Increased levels of acid-labile α-interferon are reported in AIDS and ARC cases. Anti-T-cell antibodies, antisperm antibodies, and antiplatelet antibodies as well as some other autoantibodies are seen in patients with HIV infection.

Special stains and cultures of appropriate specimens from various sites of infection should be made in search of infectious bacteria, fungi, protozoa, and viruses. Biopsies of suspicious skin lesions should be performed and analyzed by acid-fast and fungal staining, as well as obtaining cultures for bacteria, fungi and atypical *Mycobacterium* species.[73]

Evaluation of the patient with AIDS should also include examination of cutaneous and mucosal surfaces for Kaposi's sarcoma. This vascular tumor presents as erythematous, violaceous, or hyperpigmented macules, papules, nodules, or plaques and has been reported to occur in up to 48 percent of all homosexuals with AIDS.[74] Approximately 23 percent of AIDS patients with Kaposi's sarcoma develop visceral or lymph node involvement.[63] Diagnosis is made by biopsy of skin lesions.

Treatment

Patients with AIDS usually die of one or more opportunistic infections. While the treatment of these infections in most instances is possible, the patients remain susceptible to the same or other opportunistic infections because of their immune defect.

Kaposi's sarcoma can be treated by the conventional approach of radiation and chemotherapy. Treatment modalities include recombinant α-interferon, vinblastine, or radiation.[75,76]

Early detection, patient education, and prevention of this devastating disease are important in controlling HIV infection. Recently attempted modalities to help restore the immune system of AIDS patients have included bone marrow transplantation and systemic administration of various drugs, including interleukin-2, interferons, and other antiviral agents, which have all unfortunately resulted in, at best, minimal clinical benefit at present.[77]

As for the treatment of the HIV infection, a recent study by Yarchoan and colleagues[78] indicates that thymidine analogs are most promising. The first of this family of compounds is zidovudine (Retrovir), also known as azidothymidine (AZT). This compound is a derivative of thymidine and has been shown to interfere with the replication of HIV. Several clinical trials are underway to test these agents. Similar compounds are being synthesized and tested in the laboratory and preclinical settings.

While it is difficult to believe that a medication will soon be available to eradicate HIV from all different tissues in a given patient, it is likely that control of this viral infection will become a reality by the use of a combination of several different antiviral agents.

Production of HIV vaccine is also underway, and preliminary work in immunizing animals has already started. The available technology should allow development of such a vaccine in a short time. However, at this time it is unclear whether an effective vaccine could be produced.[79]

APPROACH TO THE PATIENT WITH RECURRENT CUTANEOUS INFECTION

A detailed history and physical examination are of great importance in the diagnosis of immunodeficiency diseases (Table 5-8). History of infection with opportunistic organisms should suggest a defect in cell-mediated immunity. Unusually severe and frequent bacterial infections can occur in disorders of humoral immunity, and *Neisseria* infections suggest complement deficiency. Repeated monilial infections are seen in chronic mucocutaneous candidiasis, but this organism can be pathogenic in patients with defects of cell-mediated immunity or phagocytic disorders.

Family history of severe or recurrent infections or a history of consanguinity may be important, since several of the immunodeficiency diseases are inherited. Wiskott-Aldrich syndrome, chronic granulomatous disease, and Bruton's agammaglobulinemia, for example, are inherited in X-linked recessive fashion. Common variable immunodeficiency can have autosomal dominant or autosomal recessive modes of inheritance, and severe combined immunodeficiency is transmitted in an autosomal or X-linked recessive pattern. A history of age of onset of infections can also be helpful. Many immunodeficiency diseases become apparent in infancy or early childhood, although selective IgA deficiency and common variable immunodeficiency affect adults.

Characteristic physical findings of a particular immunodeficiency syndrome are frequently of diagnostic value; for example, characteristic facial features and cardiac anomalies occur in DiGeorge's syndrome. Nystagmus and telangiectases occur in ataxia-telangiectasia; partial albinism is characteristic of the Chediak-Higashi syndrome; thrombocytopenic purpura oc-

Table 5-8. Approach to the Patient

History
    Type of infections
    Age of onset
    Family history
    Consanguinity

Physical Examination

Laboratory Investigation

Initial screening
    Complete blood count with differential and platelet count
    Peripheral blood smear
    Appropriate bacterial, fungal, and viral cultures
    Gram stain; KOH and Tzanck smears
    Quantitative immunoglobulin levels
    X-rays (chest, soft-tissue of neck for lymphoid tissue)

In-depth examination

Antibodies to human immunodeficiency virus

Assessment of B-cell lymphocyte system
    Total B-cell lymphocyte number
    Isohemagglutinin titers (for IgM antibodies)
    Schick test or poliomyelitis titers in previously immunized individuals (for IgG antibodies)
    Further studies
        In vitro immunoglobulin synthesis
        In vivo antibody responses to antigens: streptolysin O titer, heterophil titer, vaccine antigens (rubella, rubeola, tetanus)
        Lymph node or rectal biopsy

Assessment of T-lymphocyte system
    Total T-lymphocyte number
    Delayed cutaneous tests using purified protein derivative, *Candida albicans, Trichophyton,* mumps, tetanus toxoid, streptokinase-streptodornase (SKSD), dinitrochlorobenzene (DNCB)

Further studies
    Ratio of helper to suppressor cells
    In vitro lymphocyte proliferation to mitogens, phytohemagglutinin, or antigens
    Lymphokine production (lymphocyte mediator assays): migration-inhibition factor
    Cytotoxicity assays
    Enzyme assays for adenosine deaminase and nucleoside phosphorylase
    Thymic hormone assays
    Lymph node biopsy

Assessment of phagocytic system
    Neutrophil count and morphology
    Nitroblue tetrazolium dye reduction test
    IgE level
    Further studies
        Bactericidal assays
        Rebuck skin window (assesses leukocyte mobility)
        Capillary tube migration (assesses random mobility)
        Phagocytic assays (opsonic defects)
        Lysosomal enzymes (glutathione peroxidase, myeloperoxidase)

Assessment of complement system
    CH50 level
    C3 level
    C4 level
    Further studies
        Levels of individual complement components
        Opsonic assays
        Chemotactic factor
        Complement activator assays
        Alternative pathway activity (factor P, factor B, factor D)

---

curs in the Wiskott-Aldrich syndrome; and various dermatitides can occur in several immunodeficiency diseases. Small tonsils and adenoids and the absence of palpable lymph nodes may also be important findings. On the other hand, the presence of lymphadenopathy is often one of the only findings in the early stages of AIDS and can also occur in common variable immunodeficiency.

Laboratory tests are essential to confirm the presence of an immunodeficiency disorder (Table 5-9). Repeated absolute lymphocyte counts of less than 1,500 cells/mm^3 or absolute neutrophil counts of less than 1,800 cells/mm^3 may

indicate significant cellular immunodeficiency. Anemia and thrombocytopenia are occasionally associated findings; thrombocytopenia, for example, is found in the Wiskott-Aldrich syndrome, as mentioned above. Also, X-rays and cultures of suspected sources of infection should be obtained.

If the initial work-up is normal, immunodeficiency is likely to be excluded. If the initial work-up reveals an abnormality or if chronic infections are unexplained, further evaluation should be made in order to determine the presence of a possible defect in the immune system.

Populations of T and B lymphocytes are as-

Table 5-9. Laboratory Findings for Suspected Immunodeficiency Disorders

Suspected Disease	Defect	Diagnostic Laboratory Tests
X-linked agammaglobulinemia	Absent mature B cells in lymphoid tissue	Reduced or absent levels of all serum immunoglobulins Absent circulating B cells in peripheral blood and in antigen-stimulated lymph nodes Low or absent isohemagglutinin titers Absent antibody responses
Common variable immunodeficiency	?Defective differentiation of B cells	Reduced levels of all serum immunoglobulins Low isohemagglutinin titers Inability of B cells to differentiate in vivo into immunoglobulin-producing cells
Transient hypogammaglobulinemia	Delayed synthesis of immunoglobulins	Reduced serum IgG levels Reduced total serum immunoglobulin level
Selective IgA deficiency	Unknown	Markedly reduced serum and secretory IgA levels
DiGeorge's syndrome	Developmental defect of third and fourth pharyngeal pouches	Reduced T-cell number Absent thymic shadow on chest x-ray Hypocalcemia and reduced parathormone levels Absent in vitro lymphocyte responses to mitogens and antigens
Severe combined immunodeficiency	?Defective bone marrow stem cell	Lymphopenia Poor in vitro lymphocyte response to mitogens or allogeneic cells Poor antibody response to antigenic stimulation
Nezelof's syndrome	Unknown	Reduced T-cell number Impaired cell-mediated immune responses Antibody responses often impaired
Wiskott-Aldrich syndrome	Unknown	Thrombocytopenia, reduced platelet size Poor antibody responses to polysaccharide antigens Reduced serum IgM and elevated IgE titers Low isohemagglutinin titers
Ataxia-telangiectasia	Unknown	Serum IgA and IgE often absent Elevated α-fetoprotein Progressive decline in T-cell number and mitogen response
Job's syndrome	Unknown	Markedly elevated serum IgE levels
Buckley's syndrome	Unknown	Markedly elevated serum IgE levels
Chronic granulomatous disease of childhood	Phagocytic killing defect	Decreased nitroblue tetrazolium dye reduction
Chediak-Higashi syndrome	Phagocytic killing defect	Giant inclusions or granules in leukocytes
Leiner's disease	Familial C5 dysfunction	C5 dysfunction
Lazy leukocyte syndrome	Polymorphonuclear leukocyte migration defect	Abnormal Rebuck skin window

sessed as follows. Total B-cell counts can be obtained by immunofluorescence to detect surface membrane immunoglobulins or by EA and EAC rosette formation with sheep erythrocytes coated with antibody and C3 for receptors of B cells. Total T-cell number can also be determined by immunofluorescence with antiserum specific for T cells or by E rosette formation with sheep erythrocytes.

If a defect is suspected in the B lymphocyte system, quantitation of serum immunoglobulins (IgG, IgM, and IgA) should be performed by the radial diffusion technique. Levels of IgG subclasses should also be assessed. Levels of IgE are detected more accurately by radioimmunoassay. Antibody function tests are indicated in the presence of an abnormal serum level of total immunoglobulins (IgG + IgM + IgA) less than 600 mg/dl. Both the Schick test for diphtheria toxin and poliomyelitis titer reflect IgG function and depend on previous immunization. A positive Schick test indicates deficient IgG antitoxin antibody. Except in blood group AB, isohemagglutinin titers reflect the presence of functional IgM antibodies in patients over 6 months of age.

Specific antibody responses are measured by quantitating anti-streptolysin O titers, heterophil titers, and titers to typhoid, inactivated poliomyelitis, and influenza vaccines. In vitro immunoglobulin synthesis should be assessed if hypogammaglobulinemia is detected in the presence of normal B-cell numbers (as occurs in common variable immunodeficiency). Biopsy of lymph nodes (or rectal mucosa) is generally not necessary in most cases and would reveal extraneous information regarding the architecture of the lymph node and assessment of plasma cells.

To measure T-cell-mediated responses, delayed hypersensitivity skin reactions are assessed with commercial antigens (e.g., streptokinase-streptodornase, *Candida*, purified protein derivative (PPD), mumps, *Trichophyton*) placed intradermally. Function of T cells can be further assessed by tests listed in Table 5-8.

Suspected defects of the phagocytic system are evaluated by total white blood count, including a neutrophil count, and peripheral blood smear for morphology. An elevated serum IgE level should alert the clinician to investigate leukocyte mobility. The nitroblue tetrazolium dye reduction test correlates with the ability of phagocytes to generate hydrogen peroxide and is specific for chronic granulomatous disease of childhood. The presence of giant lysosomal granules in leukocytes is characteristic of the Chediak-Higashi syndrome. Further studies of phagocytic function are listed in Table 5-8.

The integrity of the entire complement system is reflected by the serum CH50 level, an assay of total hemolytic complement. A low CH50 level is therefore indicative of a defect in the complement cascade and requires further investigation of individual complement levels and functional ability.

REFERENCES

1. Rosen FS, Janeway CA: The gamma globulins. III. The antibody deficiency syndromes. N Engl J Med 275:709, 1966
2. Ochs HD, Ament ME, Davis SD: Giardiasis with malabsorption in X-linked agammaglobulinemia. N Engl J Med 287:341, 1972
3. Good RA, Pahwa RN, West A: Primary immunodeficiences of man. p. 399. In Safai B, Good RA (eds): Immunodermatology. Plenum, New York, 1981
4. Leung DYM, Rosen FS, Geha RS: Disorders of immunoglobulin-antibody system. p. 44. In Chandia RK (ed): Primary and Secondary Immunodeficiency Disorders. Churchill Livingstone, New York, 1983
5. Rotstein J, Good RA: Significance of the simultaneous occurrence of connective tissue disease and agammaglobulinemia. Ann Rheum Dis 21:202, 1962
6. Page AR, Hansen AE, Good RA: Occurrence of leukemia and lymphoma in patients with agammaglobulinemia. Blood 21:197, 1963
7. Waldmann TA, Durm M, Broder S, et al: Role of suppressor T cells in pathogenesis of common variable hypogammaglobulinemia. Lancet 2:609, 1974

8. Geha RS, Schneeberger E, Merler E, Rosen FS: Heterogeneity of "acquired" or common variable agammaglobulinemia. N Engl J Med 291:1, 1974

9. Buckley RH: Immunodeficiency. J Allergy Clin Immunol 72:627, 1983

10. Ammarin AJ, Hong R: Selective IgA deficiency: presentation of 30 cases and a review of the literature. Medicine (Baltimore) 50:223, 1971

11. Feingold M, Schwartz RS, Atkins L, et al: IgA deficiency associated with partial deletion of chromosome 18. Am J Dis Child 117:129, 1969

12. Kanoh T, Uchino H: Immunodeficiency and epilepsy. Lancet 1:860, 1976

13. Vijas GN, Holmandahl L, Perkins HA, Fudenberg HH: Serologic specificity of human anti-IgA and its significance in transfusion. Blood 34:573, 1969

14. Tiller TL, Buckley RH: Transient hypogammaglobulinemia of infancy: review of the literature, clinical and immunologic features of 11 new cases and long-term follow-up. J Pediatr 92:347, 1978

15. Paslin D, Norman ME: Atopic dermatitis and impaired neutrophil chemotaxis in Job's syndrome. Arch Dermatol 113:801, 1977

16. Davis SS, Schaller J, Wedgwood DRJ: Job syndrome, recurrent cold staphylococcal abscesses. Lancet 1:1013, 1966

17. Hill HR, Quie PG, Pabst HF, et al: Defect in neutrophil granulocyte chemotaxis in Job's syndrome of recurrent "cold" staphylococcal abscesses. Lancet 2:617, 1974

18. Buckley RH, Wray BB, Belmaker EZ: Extreme hyperimmunoglobulinemia E and undue susceptibility to infections. Pediatrics 49:59, 1972

19. Lischner HW, Punnett HH, DiGeorge AM: Lymphocytes in congenital absence of the thymus. Nature 214:580, 1967

20. Kretschmer R, Say B, Brown D, Rosen FS: Congenital aplasia of the thymus gland (DiGeorge's syndrome). N Engl J Med 279:1295, 1968

21. August CS, Rosen FS, Filler RM, et al: Implantation of a foetal thymus restoring immunological competence in a patient with thymic aplasia (DiGeorge's syndrome). Lancet 2:1210, 1968

22. Cleveland WW, Fogel BJ, Brown WT, Kay HEM: Foetal thymic transplant in a case of DiGeorge's syndrome. Lancet 2:1211, 1968

23. Ammann AJ, Wara DW, Doyle NE, Golbus MS: Thymus transplantation in patients with thymic hypoplasia and abnormal immunoglobulin synthesis. Transplantation 20:457, 1975

24. Barrett DJ, Ammann AJ, Wara DW, et al: Clinical and immunologic spectrum of the DiGeorge syndrome. J Clin Lab Immunol 6:1, 1981

25. Lawlor GJ, Ammann AJ, Wright WC Jr, et al: The syndrome of cellular immunodeficiency with immunoglobulins. J Pediatr 84:183, 1974

26. Rubenstein A, Speck B, Jeannet M: Successful bone-marrow transplantation in a lymphopenic immunologic deficiency syndrome. N Engl J Med 285:1399, 1971

27. Kirkpatrick CH, Sohnle PG: Chronic mucocutaneous candidiasis. p. 495. In Safai B, Good RA (eds): Immunodermatology. Plenum, New York, 1981

28. Horsburgh CR Jr, Kirkpatrick CH: Long-term therapy of chronic mucocutaneous candidiasis with ketoconazole: experience with twenty-one patients. Am J Med 74(1B):23, 1983

29. Rosen FS, Cooper MD, Wedgwood RJP: The primary immunodeficiencies. Part 2. N Engl J Med 311:300, 1984

30. O'Reilley RJ, DuPont B, Pahwa S, et al: Reconstitution in severe combined immunodeficiency by transplantation of marrow from an unrelated donor. N Engl J Med 297:1311, 1971

31. Levey RH, Klemperer MR, Gelfand EW, et al: Bone-marrow transplantation in severe combined immunodeficiency syndrome. Lancet 2:571, 1971

32. Hirschhorn R, Vawter GF, Kirkpatrick JA Jr, Rosen FS: Adenosine deaminase deficiency: frequency and comparative pathology in autosomally recessive severe combined immunodeficiency. Clin Immunol Immunopathol 14:107, 1979

33. Palmar SH, Stern RC, Schwartz AL, Hirschhorn R: Enzyme replacement therapy for adenosine deaminase deficiency and severe combined immunodeficiency disease. N Engl J Med 295:1337, 1976

34. Helfer N: Cutaneous symptoms in primary immunodeficiencies. Curr Probl Dermatol 13:50, 1985

35. Parkman R, Rappaport J, Geha R, et al: Complete correction of the Wiskott-Aldrich syndrome by allogeneic bone-marrow transplantation. N Engl J Med 298:921, 1978

36. Reed WB, Epstein WL, Broder E, Sedgwick R: Cutaneous manifestations of ataxia-telangiectasia. JAMA 195:746, 1966

37. Ammann AJ, DuQuesnoy RJ, Good RA: Endocrinological studies in ataxia-telangiectasia and

other immunological deficiency diseases. Clin Exp Immunol 6:587, 1969

38. Waldmann TA, McIntire KR: Serum alphafetoprotein levels in patients with ataxia-telangiectasia. Lancet 2:1112, 1972

39. McCaw BK, Hecht F, Harnden DG, Teplitz RL: Somatic rearrangement of chromosome 14 in human lymphocytes. Proc Natl Acad Sci USA 72:2071, 1975

40. Johnston RB Jr, Newman SL: Chronic granulomatous disease. Pediatr Clin North Am 2:365, 1977

41. Dahl MV, Cates KL, Quie PG: Deficiency of phagocytic function and related disorders. p. 425. In Safai B, Good RA (eds): Immunodermatology. Plenum, New York, 1981

42. Baehner RL, Nathan DG: Quantitative nitroblue tetrazolium test in chronic granulomatous disease. N Engl J Med 278:971, 1968

43. DeChatelet LR, McPhail LC, Mullikin D, McCall CE: An isotopic assay for NADPH oxidase activity and some characteristics of the enzyme from human polymorphonuclear leukocytes. J Clin Invest 55:714, 1975

44. Baehner RL, Karnovsky MS: Deficiency of reduced nicotinamide–adenine dinucleotide oxidase in chronic granulomatous disease. Science 162:1277, 1968.

45. Curmitte JT, Whitten DM, Babior BM: Defective superoxide production by granulocytes from patients with chronic granulomatous disease. N Engl J Med 290:593, 1974

46. Blume RS, Bennett JM, Yankee RA, Wolff SM: Defective granulocyte regulation in the Chediak-Higashi syndrome. N Engl J Med 279:1009, 1968

47. Virclizier JL, Lagrue A, Durandy A, et al: Reversal of natural killer defect in a patient with Chediak-Higashi syndrome after bone-marrow transplantation. N Engl J Med 306:1055, 1982

48. Blume R, Wolff S: The Chediak-Higashi syndrome; studies in four cases and a review of the literature. Medicine (Baltimore) 51:247, 1972

49. Miller ME, Oski FA, Harris MB: Lazy leukocyte syndrome. A new disorder of neutrophil function. Lancet 1:665, 1971

50. Guenther LC: Inherited disorders of complement. J Am Acad Dermatol 9:815, 1983

51. Alper CA, Colten HR, Rosen FS, et al: Homozygous deficiency of C3 in a patient with repeated infections. Lancet 2:1179, 1972

52. Gigli I: The complement system: mechanism of action, biology and participation in dermatological diseases. p. 65. In Safai B, Good RA (eds): Immunodermatology. Plenum, New York, 1981

53. Miller ME, Koblenzer PJ: Leiner's disease and deficiency of C5. J Pediatr 80:879, 1972

54. Jacobs LC, Miller ME: Fatal familial Leiner's disease: a deficiency of the opsonic activity of serum complement. Pediatrics 49:225, 1972

55. Centers for Disease Control. Update on acquired immunodeficiency syndrome (AIDS)—United States. MMWR 31:507, 1982

56. Masur H, Kovacs JA, Ognibene F, et al: Infectious complications of AIDS. p. 161. In DeVita VT Jr, Hellman S, Rosenberg SA, et al (eds): AIDS. Etiology, Diagnosis, Treatment, and Prevention. JB Lippincott, Philadelphia, 1985

57. Centers for Disease Control. Revision of the case definition of acquired immunodeficiency syndrome for national reporting—United States. MMWR 34:373, 1985

58. Centers for Disease Control. Classification system for human T lymphotropic type III/lymphadenopathy associated virus infection. MMWR 35:334, 1986

59. Krause RM: Koch's postulates and the search for the AIDS agent. Rev Infect Dis 6:270, 1984

60. Fischinger PJ, Bolognesi DP: Prospects for diagnostic tests, intervention, and vaccine development in AIDS. p. 275. In DeVita VT Jr, Hellman S, Rosenberg SA, et al (eds): AIDS. Etiology, Diagnosis, Treatment, and Prevention. JB Lippincott, Philadelphia, 1985

61. Gallo RC, Salahuddin SZ, Popovic M, et al: Frequent detection and isolation of cytopathic retroviruses (HTLV-III) from patients with AIDS and at risk for AIDS. Science 224:500, 1984

62. Fauci AS, Macher AM, Longo DL, et al: Acquired immunodeficiency syndrome: epidemiologic, clinical, immunologic, and therapeutic considerations. Ann Intern Med 100:92, 1984

63. Bowen DL, Lane HC, Fauci AS: Immunologic features of AIDS. p. 89. In DeVita VT Jr, Hellman S, Rosenberg SA, et al (eds): AIDS. Etiology, Diagnosis, Treatment, and Prevention. JB Lippincott, Philadelphia, 1985

64. Harris C, Small CB, Klein RS, et al: Immunodeficiency in female sexual partners of men with the acquired immunodeficiency syndrome. N Engl J Med 308:1181, 1983

65. Redfield RR, Markham PD, Salahuddin SZ, et

al: Heterosexually acquired HTLV-III/LAV disease (AIDS-related complex and AIDS). Epidemiologic evidence for female-to-male transmission. JAMA 254:2094, 1985

66. Kreiss JK, Kitchen LW, Prince HE, et al: Antibody to human T-lymphotropic virus type III in wives of hemophiliacs. Evidence for heterosexual transmission. Ann Intern Med 102:623, 1985

67. Centers for Disease Control. Update: Acquired immune deficiency syndrome—United States. MMWR 35:20, 1986

68. Goedert JJ, Blattner WA: The epidemiology of AIDS and related conditions. In DeVita VT Jr, Hellman S, Rosenberg SA, et al (eds): AIDS. Etiology, Diagnosis, Treatment, and Prevention. JB Lippincott, Philadelphia, 1985

69. Safai B, Sarngadharan MG, Groopman JE, et al: Seroepidemiological studies of human T-lymphotropic retrovirus type III in acquired immunodeficiency syndrome. Lancet 1:1438, 1984

70. Lane HC, Masur H, Edgar LC, et al: Abnormalities of B-cell activation and immunoregulation in patients with the acquired immunodeficiency syndrome. N Engl J Med 309:453, 1983

71. Lopez C, Fitzgerald PA, Siegal FP: Severe acquired immunodeficiency syndrome in male homosexuals: diminished capacity to make alpha-interferon in vitro associated with severe opportunistic infections. J Infect Dis 148:962, 1983

72. Murray HW, Rubin BY, Masur H, et al: Impaired production of lymphokines and immune (gamma) interferon in the acquired immunodeficiency syndrome. N Engl J Med 310:883, 1984

73. Freed J, Pervez NK, Chen VL, et al: Cutaneous mycobacteriosis: occurrence and significance in two patients with the acquired immune deficiency syndrome. Arch Dermatol (in press)

74. Gallo RC: The etiology of AIDS. p. 31. In DeVita VT Jr, Hellman S, Rosenberg SA, et al (eds): AIDS. Etiology, Diagnosis, Treatment, and Prevention. JB Lippincott, Philadelphia, 1985

75. Gelmann EP: New concepts in Kaposi's sarcoma. The acquired immunodeficiency syndrome: an update. Ann Intern Med 102:800, 1985

76. Volberding P: Therapy of Kaposi's sarcoma in AIDS. Semin Oncol 11:60, 1984

77. Lane HC, Fauci AS: Immunologic reconstitution in the acquired immunodeficiency syndrome. Ann Intern Med 103:714, 1985

78. Yarchoan R, Klecker RW, Weinhold KJ, et al: Administration of 3'-azido-3'-deoxythymidine, an inhibitor of HTLV-III/LAV replication, to patients with AIDS or AIDS-related complex. Lancet 1:575, 1986

79. Marwick C: Task force formed to coordinate study, testing of AIDS therapies. JAMA 255:1233, 1986

6

Chronic Generalized Erythroderma

Eric Vonderheid

Chronic generalized erythroderma (CGE) is a clinical syndrome characterized by a persistent, seemingly self-perpetuating, universal or nearly universal diffuse erythema of the skin accompanied by a variable degree of exfoliation. *Chronic generalized erythroderma* is considered by the author to be a more appropriate term than the more widely used *exfoliative dermatitis,* because use of the word *dermatitis* may not be appropriate in cases mediated by malignant infiltrates, and because clinically apparent exfoliation is not always present. The use of the term *CGE* also excludes short-lasting diffuse erythrodermas, such as those observed in viral or bacterial exanthems, some drug eruptions, angioimmunoblastic lymphadenopathy, early phases of toxic epidermal necrolysis, staphylococcal scalded skin syndrome, toxic shock syndrome, boric acid or trichloroethylene poisoning, and other toxic or hypersensitivity states of limited duration.

CLINICAL SYMPTOMS

Patients with CGE present with diverse clinical manifestations, and this contributes to the difficulty in establishing the specific underlying cause or diagnosis for the condition. Males are affected two to three times more often than females. In general most patients with CGE complain of pruritus, which varies considerably in severity, but some patients experience a burning sensation or tenderness. Constitutional symptoms associated with CGE often consist of chills accompanied by shivering due to heat loss from the skin surface and fatigue, but low-grade fever may occur in some situations. The clinician should be alert to the possibility of concealed fever caused by the relative hypothermia due to heat loss.

The intensity of skin erythema in CGE varies from bright red in cases with sudden onset to a deeper, dusky red in long-standing cases. The degree of desquamation varies greatly, from virtually absent to quite profuse, resulting in significant loss of protein, vitamins, and other nutrients over time. Secondary bacterial infection may lead to a component of crusting or folliculitis. Postinflammatory hyper- or hypopigmentation also is a common sequela of CGE, especially in dark-skinned peoples, and, rarely, vitiliginous depigmentation may occur.[1]

The physical examination of patients with CGE frequently reveals the nail plates to be thickened (onychauxis) and lusterless, often with transverse depressions (Beau's lines). Keratinaceous material may accumulate beneath the nail plate (subungual hyperkeratosis), which contributes to separation of the nail plate from the nail bed distally (onycholysis). Occasionally, the entire nail plate may be shed (onychomadesis). Similarly, the growth cycle of hair may be disturbed in CGE, resulting in partial or total alopecia of the scalp and body.[2]

In addition, many patients with CGE have moderate enlargement of peripheral lymph nodes bilaterally, particularly when severe pruritus is present. Lymph node specimens in these situations usually show expanded paracortical regions containing histiocytes and dendritic cells (dermatopathic lymphadenitis). The ocular manifestations consist of contractural ectropion of the lower eyelids, which may be accompanied by an exposure keratitis. The skin on involved eyelids may exfoliate into the conjunctival sacs to cause a nonspecific conjunctivitis and/or superficial punctate keratitis. Oral and joint manifestations are not observed in most cases of CGE, but may provide diagnostic clues in occasional patients. Mild hepatomegaly may occur nonspecifically in up to 20 percent of patients, and splenomegaly is not a feature except in patients with malignancy, sarcoidosis, histoplasmosis, or severe hypersensitivity reactions. Nonspecific clinical findings associated with CGE include peripheral edema, gynecomastia, and an increased risk of cardiac failure.

Skin biopsies generally are not helpful in determining the etiology of CGE. In most cases the histopathologic features are those of a subacute or chronic dermatitis, with findings depending on the acuteness of the eruption. Usually there are varying degrees of parakeratosis, spongiosis, acanthosis with elongation of rete ridges, exocytosis of lymphocytes into the epidermis, vasodilation, edema, and a polymorphous inflammatory infiltrate in the upper dermis. As a rule, cases with acute onset tend to show relatively more spongiosis and exocytosis, and chronic cases show more prominent acanthosis and elongation of rete ridges (psoriasiform hyperplasia). Laboratory tests likewise are not helpful as a rule and may show anemia, leukocytosis with eosinophilia or monocytosis, elevated sedimentation rate, hypoalbuminemia, hypergammaglobulinemia (including IgE), increased basal metabolic rate, low serum folate level, hypoferremia, hyperuricemia, and electrolyte abnormalities.

ETIOLOGY

Hypothetically all cases of CGE are manifestations of a specific underlying cause. Consequently, the objective of the physician's evaluation is to establish the appropriate diagnosis whenever possible because specific therapy other than corticosteroids or other anti-inflammatory measures may be required to improve the patient's condition. For example, failure to recognize Norwegian scabies, disseminated histoplasmosis, or a malignant condition as an etiology for CGE will prove to be frustrating to both patient and physician and will result in potentially harmful delays in treatment.

Table 6-1 provides an overview of the major etiologic factors responsible for CGE from 13 reviews available in the literature.[3-15] In approximately half of all cases the etiology of CGE can be attributed to a primary dermatologic condition, and the remaining cases are almost equally divided among systemic drug-induced, malignant, and undetermined etiologies. Rarely, a systemic illness may have CGE as a manifestation. Considerable variation in the relative proportions of each type is found from study to study, reflecting differences in patient populations and diagnostic criteria.

Dermatoses

Of the 451 cases of CGE classified as being secondary to a dermatosis in the composite series, the most frequent causes were various forms of eczema (62.4 percent), and psoriasis (29.5 percent), followed by pemphigus foliaceus (2.3 percent), lichen planus (2.3 percent), pityriasis rubra pilaris (2.0 percent), and congenital ichthyosiform erythroderma (0.9 percent). In addition, the literature contains several reports of CGE attributed to dermatophyte infec-

Table 6-1. Major Etiologic Factors in Adults with Chronic Generalized Erythroderma

Series (Year)	Number of Patients	Dermatoses	Systemic Drug Reactions	Malignancy	Miscellaneous[b]	Undetermined
Montgomery[3] (1933)[a]	72	34	11	18	2	7
Richter[4] (1939)	79	57	18	3	0	1
Wilson[5] (1954)	50	29	4	5	1	11
Gentele et al[6] (1958)	135	89	11	21	0	14
Abrahams et al[7] (1963)	101	35	11	8	0	47
Adam[8] (1968)[a]	23	7	4	5	0	7
Everett[9] (1969)	48	40	1	7	0	0
Anderson & Loeffel[10] (1970)[a]	39	24	0	8	0	7
Singh & Garg[11] (1970)	20	10	5	0	0	5
Nicolis & Helwig[12] (1973)[a]	134	35	54	28	1	16
Ndiaye et al[13] (1979)	77	39	11	3	0	24
Hasan & Jansén[14] (1983)	50	27	5	2	0	16
King et al[15] (1986)	82	25	28	16	0	13
Total	910	451	163	124	4	168
Percentage of total		49.6%	17.9%	13.6%	<0.1%	18.5%

[a] Five cases of staphylococcal scalded skin syndrome (Ritter's disease) were eliminated from these series according to current definition of CGE.

[b] Includes Reiter's disease (1), toxic erythroderma (2), and polyarteritis nodosa (1).

tion,[12,16] actinic reticuloid,[17,18] and Norwegian scabies.[19] Additional citations, which either are not well documented or represent extremely rare causes, include pityriasis rosea,[20] dermatitis herpetiformis,[10] bullous pemphigoid,[21] and hyperthyroidism.[22] This latter group of diseases will not be discussed further.

Most instances of adult onset CGE that are secondary to a dermatosis are preceded by more typical manifestations of the disease, but occasionally CGE may be the initial manifestation (e.g., in atopic dermatitis, psoriasis, or pemphigus foliaceus). In the former circumstance a historical account is of paramount importance in diagnosing the cause correctly while in the latter instance the history is less useful. In the eczemas and psoriasis there is often a history of local irritation prior to the onset of CGE, sometimes from scratching, poorly tolerated medications, or infections. Auto-allergy, the emergence of an autoimmune phenomenon, has been postulated to play a role in some instances.

ECZEMA

Of the causes of CGE attributed to eczema, over half (52.3 percent) of cases in reviews are not classified into a specific subtype. Many cases are examples of adult onset eczema of unknown cause, but some are probably drug-induced systemic types of contact dermatitis. Of the remaining causes of eczematous CGE, the identifiable types include contact or photocontact dermatitis (16.6 percent), atopic dermatitis (13.7 percent), seborrheic dermatitis (11.6 percent), stasis dermatitis (4.7 percent), photosensitive eczematous dermatitis (0.7 percent), and, rarely, nummular eczematous dermatitis (0.4 percent). The frequency of photosensitive eczema probably is higher than indicated because it was recognized to be an entity only in 1973.[23] The histopathologic features of the various eczemas are not specific, but an eczematous etiology should be suspected whenever intraepidermal vesiculation is present.

PSORIASIS

Psoriasis is the particular dermatosis most likely to cause CGE (nearly 30 percent of all cases). Both the vulgaris and pustular variants of psoriasis may gradually or suddenly evolve into the erythrodermic state or, rarely, they may begin as erythroderma.[24] Sudden exacerbations may be precipitated by corticosteroid withdrawal, infection, pregnancy, hypocalcemia, or medications (β-adrenergic blocking agents, tar, chloroquine, lithium). The histopathologic features of erythrodermic psoriasis overlap with those of chronic eczema and therefore are not distinctive enough to establish a diagnosis. However, the finding of neutrophils infiltrating the epidermis (Munro's microabscesses, spongiform pustules of Kogoj) is suggestive of the diagnosis.

PEMPHIGUS FOLIACEUS

Pemphigus foliaceus likewise usually progresses from an eruption localized to the scalp, butterfly regions of the face, and upper trunk (seborrheic distribution) but may appear in a generalized distribution at onset. The diagnosis should be suspected from the moist, erosive, or crusted appearance of the skin and occasional presence of intact bullae. Histopathologic sections show distinctive acantholysis at the stratum granulosum of the epidermis, and direct immunofluorescent studies confirm IgG deposition in the epidermal intercellular spaces.

LICHEN PLANUS

CGE caused by lichen planus may be precipitated by exposure to certain drugs, and such cases probably are better classified as a lichenoid drug eruption. The diagnosis should be suspected clinically from the bluish hue imparted to the skin by deposition of melanin in the upper dermis and the presence of fine, lacy white streaks on lesions (Wickham's striae). Biopsy specimens show a lichenoid tissue reaction pattern, and direct immunofluorescent studies may demonstrate IgM-positive cytoid bodies.

PITYRIASIS RUBRA PILARIS

Pityriasis rubra pilaris beginning in adulthood does not have the strong hereditary factor found in cases beginning in childhood. Like pemphi-gus foliaceus, pityriasis rubra pilaris often resembles seborrheic dermatitis at its onset but then progresses over weeks or years into CGE. Typical cases develop acuminate follicular papules on an erythematous base, which coalesce into plaques. Characteristically, well-demarcated islets of uninvolved skin may remain visible for some time as the disease becomes generalized, but this finding also may be observed in psoriasis, cutaneous T-cell lymphoma, or sarcoidosis. Other helpful clinical findings include a distinctive salmon red coloration caused by the thickened orthokeratotic horny layer and diffuse keratoderma of the palms and soles (keratodermic sandals). The histopathologic features of pityriasis rubra pilaris generally are not helpful unless follicular lesions are biopsied.

CONGENITAL ICHTHYOSIFORM ERYTHRODERMA

Congenital ichthyosiform erythroderma is an inclusive term for several inherited disorders with abnormal keratinization, including lamellar ichthyosis (autosomal recessive trait), epidermolytic hyperkeratosis (autosomal dominant trait), and associated syndromes, which are clinically apparent at birth or shortly thereafter. Thus, in a differential diagnosis of CGE the recognition of congenital ichthyosiform erythroderma is seldom a problem aside from its proper subclassification. Adult patients with lamellar ichthyosis (nonbullous variant of congenital ichthyosiform erythroderma) generally have coarse, platelike scaling with ectropion formation and histopathologic evidence of marked hyperkeratosis with increased thickness of the granular layer. By contrast, patients with epidermolytic hyperkeratosis (bullous variant of congenital ichthyosiform erythroderma) have a more verrucous-appearing skin, with occasional bullae and absence of ectropion, and their diagnostic histopathologic findings consist of massive hyperkeratosis with extensive vacuolization of cells in the midepidermis and granular layer.

OTHER DERMATOSES

The remaining dermatoses that occasionally cause CGE include actinic reticuloid, Norwegian scabies, and certain dermatophyte infections. These often are misdiagnosed as eczema, cutaneous T-cell lymphoma, or idiopathic erythroderma unless the physician maintains an index of suspicion. *Actinic reticuloid* in particular may be confused with erythrodermic forms of cutaneous T-cell lymphoma, since histopathologic findings of skin lesions closely resemble a lymphomatous infiltrate and substantial numbers of atypical lymphocytes resembling Sézary cells may be found in the peripheral blood.[17,18] The diagnosis becomes apparent only when the exquisite sensitivity to ultraviolet radiation is revealed. *Norwegian scabies* likewise may be confused with cutaneous T-cell lymphoma clinically and histopathologically although large numbers of *Sarcoptes* mites usually are evident on skin biopsy specimens (Fig. 6-1). Extensive infection by *Trichophyton violaceum* may cause CGE, but this organism is rarely encountered in the United States.[16] Dermatophyte-induced CGE can be confirmed by biopsy specimens stained with periodic acid–Schiff or by fungal cultures.

Systemic Drug Induced Chronic Generalized Erythroderma

Drugs are implicated as a major cause of CGE (Table 6-2).[25–30] In the author's opinion the reported incidence (17.9 percent of combined series) may be erroneously high for two reasons: (1) many generalized drug eruptions are classified inappropriately as CGE because they have a limited duration; and (2) drug-induced erythema multiforme or toxic epidermal necrolysis may be misdiagnosed as CGE. However, it is clear that about 2 to 4 percent of adverse reactions to systemic drugs will result in CGE.[31,32] The time interval from the beginning of drug ingestion to the onset of the eruption that eventuates in CGE varies greatly but usually ranges between 1 and 4 weeks.

Most reported cases of drug-induced CGE start out as an acute exanthemic type of drug eruption, usually associated with fever and malaise. Other patients may manifest urticaria, purpura, or an erythema multiforme-like eruption that precedes or accompanies the erythrodermic state, and there may be clinical and/or laboratory evidence of stomatitis, hepatitis, nephritis, or arthritis. In addition, certain drugs may cause a generalized eczematous type of CGE in patients who have been sensitized topically to an allergen such as ethylenediamine (aminophylline sensitivity) or paraphenylenediamine (e.g., sensitivity to sulfonamides, sulfonylurea hypoglycemic agents, thiazide diuretics, and related compounds).[33] Histopathologic specimens from patients with systemic drug-induced CGE generally show nonspecific features but may be helpful if the drug causes a lichenoid tissue reaction pattern or, rarely, leukocytoclastic vasculitis.

Malignancy

Of 124 cases of CGE associated with malignant conditions in the combined series, 98 (79.0 percent) were attributed to lymphomas, 19 (15.3 percent) were attributed to leukemias, and 7 (5.6 percent) were linked to an underlying carcinoma. Because the erythroderma frequently is a nonspecific manifestation of the malignancy, the correct diagnosis may be difficult to establish in these patients, and many are considered to have idiopathic CGE.

Erythroderma secondary to lymphomas and leukemias may be caused either by direct infiltration of the skin by malignant cells or by poorly understood nonspecific mechanisms. Therefore, skin biopsies are useful to suggest or confirm a diagnosis in the former circumstance and are of no help in the latter.

CUTANEOUS T-CELL LYMPHOMA

The most frequently identified lymphoma to cause CGE is cutaneous T-cell lymphoma (72.0 percent), followed by Hodgkin's disease (14.7

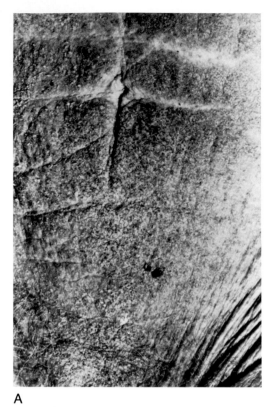

A

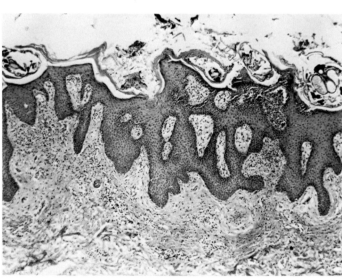

B

Fig. 6-1. (A) This 86-year-old demented man developed chronic generalized erythroderma of 8 months' duration while in a nursing home. He was referred to the author with a presumptive diagnosis of cutaneous T-cell lymphoma. (Photo of lower abdominal skin.) **(B)** Histopathologic examination of the skin shows the presence of several *Sarcoptes* mites in the stratum corneum and a patchy perivascular infiltrate containing lymphocytes and eosinophils. (H&E, original magnification × 25.)

percent) and various non-Hodgkin's lymphomas (13.3 percent). Cutaneous T-cell lymphoma patients include those with erythrodermic mycosis fungoides and Sézary syndrome, the differentiation being based primarily on whether a leukemic component (Sézary cells) is present. The clinical manifestations of cutaneous T-cell lymphoma are quite

Table 6-2. Drugs Reported to Cause Chronic Generalized Erythroderma

Antibacterial agents
    Amithiazone (occasional)
    Cefoxitin (occasional)
    Dapsone (occasional)
    Isoniazid (frequent)
    Nalidixic acid (rare)
    Nitrofurantoin (rare)
    Para-aminosalicylic acid (frequent)
    Penicillins (frequent)
    Streptomycin sulfate (frequent)
    Sulfonamides (frequent)
    Tetracyclines (rare)
Antifungal agents
    Griseofulvin (rare)
    Ketoconazole (rare)
Antiparasitic agents
    Chloroquine salts (rare)
    Hydroxychloroquine sulfate (rare)
    Quinacrine hydrochloride (frequent)
    Tetrachloroethylene (rare)
    Trimethoprim (rare)
Analgesic and anti-inflammatory agents
    Acetaminophen (rare)
    Aminopyrine (occasional)
    Antipyrine (occasional)
    Aspirin (frequent)
    Benoxaprofen (rare)
    Codeine phosphate (occasional)
    Diflunisal (rare)
    Indomethacin (occasional)
    Meclofenamate (rare)
    Oxyphenbutazone (occasional)
    Phenylbutazone (frequent)
    Sulindac (rare)
Heavy metals
    Antimonials (rare)
    Arsenicals (frequent)
    Gold salts (frequent)
    Mercurials (frequent)

Cardiovascular agents
    Captopril (frequent)
    Nifedipine (rare)
    Organic nitrates (occasional)
    Practolol (frequent)
    Quinidine sulfate (rare)
Diuretic agents
    Furosemide (occasional)
    Meralluride (rare)
    Thiazides (occasional)
Anticonvulsant agents
    Barbiturates (frequent)
    Carbamazepine (frequent)
    Hydantoins (frequent)
    Phenacemid (rare)
    Pheneturide (rare)
    Trimethadione (rare)
Psychotropic agents
    Desipramine hydrochloride (rare)
    Imipramine hydrochloride (rare)
    Lithium carbonate (rare)
    Phenothiazines (frequent)
Miscellaneous
    Acetazolamide (rare)
    Allopurinol (frequent)
    Aminophylline (ethylene diamine) (frequent)
    Cimetidine (rare)
    Dactinomycin (rare)
    Diethylstilbesterol (rare)
    Iodides (occasional)
    Lidocaine hydrochloride (rare)
    Phenindione (frequent)
    Phenolphthalein (rare)
    Potassium thiocyanate (rare)
    Sulfonylurea hypoglycemic drugs (occasional)
    Terbutaline sulfate (rare)
    Vitamin A (rare)

varied, but the diagnosis should be suspected whenever there is diffuse or focal infiltration of the skin, markedly enlarged or asymmetrically enlarged lymph nodes, or splenomegaly on physical examination. Histopathologic assessment will help establish the diagnosis in most instances (Fig. 6-2), but many examples of clear-cut cutaneous T-cell lymphoma show only nonspecific changes, particularly in Sézary syndrome. Several studies have found quantitation of Sézary cells on blood smears to be a useful test to distinguish erythrodermic forms of cutaneous T-cell lymphoma from other causes of CGE.[15,34]

HODGKIN'S DISEASE

The erythroderma observed in patients with Hodgkin's disease more often than not preceded documentation of lymph node involvement by several years. For this reason CGE associated with Hodgkin's disease usually shows only a nonspecific chronic inflammatory infiltrate; however, in some instances characteristic Sternberg-Reed giant cells are present, which permit a presumptive diagnosis. Hodgkin's disease should be suspected clinically whenever fever, night sweats, or weight loss accompany CGE, particularly in a young adult, or massive or

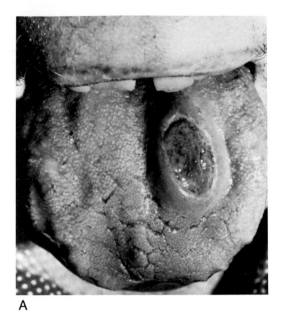

A

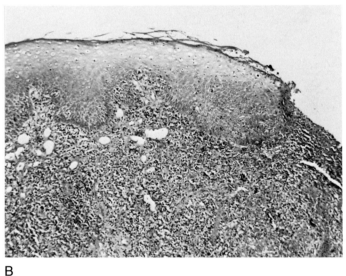

B

Fig. 6-2. (A) This 56-year-old man with Sézary syndrome developed a 1½-cm-diameter ulcerated plaque on the tongue. **(B)** A biopsy taken from the margin of the ulcer showed the histopathologic features of cutaneous T-cell lymphoma. (H&E, original magnification × 25.)

asymmetric lymph node enlargement or splenomegaly is present.

NON-HODGKIN'S LYMPHOMA

The occurrence of CGE as a manifestation of non-Hodgkin's lymphomas other than cutaneous T-cell lymphoma has also been reported.

The author believes the reported frequency of CGE associated with non-Hodgkin's lymphomas may be spuriously high because many such cases are in actuality examples of nonepidermotropic cutaneous T-cell lymphoma. Immunophenotyping of the malignant cellular infiltrate in the skin is useful to distinguish between these two possibilities. CGE also may occur as a nonspecific inflammatory process in patients with non-Hodgkin's lymphomas.

LEUKEMIA

As with lymphoma, CGE may be a specific or nonspecific manifestation of various leukemias. The vast majority of reported cases are associated with chronic lymphocytic leukemia, but the association has been observed with chronic myelogenous leukemia, monocytic leukemia, and acute leukemias. Erythroderma due to infiltration of skin by leukemic cells occurs in 4.5 percent of patients with chronic lymphatic leukemia[35]; most of these cases are presumably of T-cell origin rather than the more usual B-cell origin. The clinical diagnosis should be suspected whenever the erythroderma is accompanied by diffuse or focal infiltration of the skin, often with a distinctive orange coloration, or there is marked lymphadenopathy or splenomegaly. The histopathology generally shows sharply demarcated patches of normal-appearing lymphocytes around blood vessels in the dermis. Clear-cut differentiation from Sézary syndrome may require electron microscopy to characterize the shape of the nucleus and bone marrow biopsy. CGE also may occur as a nonspecific manifestation of chronic lymphocytic leukemia, in which case the histopathology is nonspecific. Of interest, cell marker studies performed on the cutaneous infiltrate in some cases of erythroderma associated with B-cell chronic lymphocytic leukemia have demonstrated predominantly T cells, which indicates that the erythroderma is not caused by a specific leukemic infiltrate.[36]

CARCINOMA

Infrequently, CGE may occur in patients with an underlying, often occult carcinoma.[1,37] Of cases reported in the literature, five patients had pulmonary carcinoma (three squamous cell, one oat cell, one undefined type), three patients had prostatic carcinoma, two patients had rectosigmoid carcinoma, and individual patients had carcinomas of the pancreas, liver, thyroid, stomach, tongue, and cervix. Removal of the tumor may cause the erythroderma to disappear.

The clinical and histopathologic features of CGE in this circumstance are entirely nonspecific, so diagnosis requires a high index of suspicion and adequate evaluation when looking for the tumor.

Miscellaneous Systemic Diseases

GRAFT-VERSUS-HOST DISEASE

With the advent of bone marrow transplantation for treatment of leukemia, aplastic anemia, and primary immunodeficiency states, CGE is recognized to be a frequent consequence of graft-versus-host disease. The history and histopathologic evidence of a lichenoid reaction pattern with satellite cell necrosis of keratinocytes[39] should establish the diagnosis.

REITER'S DISEASE, SARCOIDOSIS, AND DISSEMINATED HISTOPLASMOSIS

In addition, the literature contains a few well-documented reports of CGE associated with Reiter's disease,[12,40,41] sarcoidosis,[42–44] and disseminated histoplasmosis.[45,46] CGE caused by Reiter's disease, which in effect is generalized keratoderma blennorrhagicum, may easily be confused with erythrodermic pustular psoriasis, particularly since each condition commonly has significant seronegative arthropathy as a clinical feature. The diagnosis should be considered in young male adults whose eruption begins insidiously within a few weeks after an episode of dysentery or sexual indiscretion and is accompanied by nonspecific urethritis, mouth ulcers, or iridocyclitis. The histopathology may reveal psoriasiform features with spongiform pustules of Kogoj. Likewise, multisystemic sarcoidosis rarely may cause erythroderma, with associated joint and eye manifestations. The cutaneous infiltrate may be relatively diffuse in such cases, but the presence of granulomatous inflammation (clusters of epithelioid cells) will suggest the histopathologic diagnosis. Finally, CGE may occur in progressive disseminated infection with *Histoplasma capsulatum,* an organism that in the United States is endemic to the Mississippi–Ohio–St. Lawrence river valleys. These cases may closely resemble cutaneous T-cell lymphoma, but the diagnosis should be suspected whenever chronic ulcers with an indurated base are present on the skin or oral mucosa or characteristic chorioretinal lesions are found in the eyes. The diagnosis can be established by demonstrating the organism on fungal cultures or on skin sections prepared with special stains.

APPROACH TO THE PATIENT WITH CHRONIC GENERALIZED ERYTHRODERMA

The appendix summarizes the clinical clues that may suggest a specific etiology for CGE. A careful history should be taken, with emphasis on antecedent manifestations. Was the eruption provoked by sunlight, topical exposure to a potential allergen, or a drug systemically administered before the onset of the eruption?

The coloration of the skin may implicate atopic dermatitis (pallor), pityriasis rubra pilaris (salmon red hue), chronic lymphocytic leukemia (orange hue), or conditions associated with lichenoid injury patterns (bluish hue). The presence of ichthyosiform scaling is a characteristic feature of congenital ichthyosiform erythroderma but may be seen in some cases of atopic dermatitis, sarcoidosis, lymphoma, or leukemia. Vesicles or bullae are seen in acute eczema but also in pemphigus foliaceus, drug eruptions, epidermolytic hyperkeratosis, and graft-versus-host reaction. Ulceration of the skin suggests the possibility of lymphoma, leukemia, or histoplasmosis. Significant nail plate pitting (more than 20 fingernail pits) is suggestive of psoriasis but may occur in Reiter's disease, pemphigus foliaceus, and atopic dermatitis, or the nails may be completely normal in dermatoses of recent onset, epidermolytic hyperkeratosis, or systemic illnesses. The eruption may be accompanied by diagnostically important oral manifestations (lichen planus, drug eruption, histoplasmosis, Reiter's disease), ocular manifestations (atopic dermatitis, Reiter's disease, sarcoidosis, histoplasmosis), or joint manifestations (psoriasis, drug eruption, Reiter's disease, sarcoidosis). The physical examination also may reveal massive or asymmetric lymph node enlargement suggestive of lymphoma, leukemia, drug reaction, or sarcoidosis. Splenomegaly most often occurs from lymphoma or leukemia but may be a feature of drug reaction, sarcoidosis, histoplasmosis, Reiter's disease, and graft-versus-host disease.

Laboratory studies are of limited help in establishing the cause of CGE. They may provide some information in the diagnosis of pityriasis rubra pilaris (decreased vitamin A levels), sarcoidosis (hypercalcemia or hypercalcuria), Sézary syndrome and actinic reticuloid (15 or more Sézary cells per 100 lymphocytes), and leukemias (leukemic cells). A chest radiograph may be abnormal in sarcoidosis, histoplasmosis, or malignant conditions.

Several skin biopsies from representative areas should be obtained on all patients with CGE because the histopathologic findings may be suggestive of a diagnosis of Reiter's disease, pustular psoriasis, and lamellar ichthyosis or may be almost diagnostic in pemphigus foliaceus, epidermolytic hyperkeratosis, Norwegian scabies, sarcoidosis, and histoplasmosis. Moreover, a lichenoid tissue reaction is characteristic for lichen planus, lichenoid types of systemic drug eruptions, and graft-versus-host disease. Direct immunfluorescent studies would be of benefit in these conditions as well as in pemphigus foliaceus.

Finally, it should be recalled that a lymphoma of the skin can evolve over a period of many months or years. Repeating skin biopsies after intervals of time have passed may eventually yield the correct diagnosis.

REFERENCES

1. Schwartz RA, Trotter MG: Generalized vitiligo after erythroderma. Dermatologica 167:42, 1983
2. Kostanecki W, Kwiatkowska E, Gawkowska M:

The effect of inflammatory conditions of the scalp upon hair growth and hair melanogenesis in man. Dermatologica 136:95, 1968

3. Montgomery H: Exfoliative dermatosis and malignant erythroderma. Arch Dermatol 27:253, 1933
4. Richter R: Zur Klinik der generalisierten exfolierenden Erythrodermien (mit besonderer Berücksichtigung der sekundären Erythrodermien). Arch Dermatol Syphilis 179:611, 1939
5. Wilson HTH: Exfoliative dermatitis: its etiology and prognosis. Arch Dermatol 69:577, 1954
6. Gentele H, Lodin A, Skog E: Dermatitis exfoliativa. Acta Derm Venereol (Stockh) 38:296, 1958
7. Abrahams I, McCarthy JT, Sanders SL: 101 cases of exfoliative dermatitis. Arch Dermatol 87:96, 1963
8. Adam JE: Exfoliative dermatitis. Can Med Assoc J 99:661, 1968
9. Everett MA: Exfoliative dermatitis and generalized erythroderma. J Okla State Med Assoc 62:461, 1969
10. Anderson PC, Loeffel ED: Erythrodermatitis: a review of 40 cases. Mo Med 67:252, 1970
11. Singh R, Garg BR: A clinical study of exfoliative dermatitis. Indian J Dermatol 16:11, 1970
12. Nicolis GD, Helwig EB: Exfoliative dermatitis. Arch Dermatol 108:788, 1973
13. Ndiaye B, Sissoko F, Stroebel M, et al: Les érythrodermies de l'adulte (à propos de 77 cas à Dakar). Dakar Med 24:65, 1979
14. Hasan T, Jansén CT: Erythroderma: a follow-up of fifty cases. J Am Acad Dermatol 8:836, 1983
15. King LE Jr, Dufresne RG Jr, Lovett GL, et al: Erythroderma: Review of 82 cases. South Med J 79:1210, 1986
16. Levi L, della Torre B, Cozza G: Un caso clinico di dermatofizia chronica granulomatosa ed eritrodermica da *Trichophyton violaceum*. Giorn Ital Dermatol 106:81, 1965
17. Ive FA, Magnus IA, Warin RP, et al: "Actinic reticuloid": a chronic dermatosis associated with severe photosensitivity and the histological resemblance to lymphoma. Br J Dermatol 81:36, 1969
18. Neild VS, Hawk JLM, Eady RAJ, et al: Actinic reticuloid with Sézary cells. Clin Exp Dermatol 7:143, 1982
19. Maguire HC Jr, Kligman AM: Norwegian scabies. Arch Dermatol 82:62, 1960
20. Kierland RR: Exfoliative dermatitis: classifica-

tion, diagnosis, and treatment. Med Clin North Am 31:962, 1947
21. Tappeiner G, Konrad K, Holubar K: Erythrodermic bullous pemphigoid. J Am Acad Dermatol 6:489, 1982
22. Pegum JS, Grice K: Unusual skin eruption with eosinophilia associated with hyperthyroidism. Br J Dermatol 88:295, 1973
23. Ramsey CA, Kobza Black A: Photosensitive eczema. Trans St Johns Hosp Dermatol Soc 59:152, 1973
24. Baker H, Ryan TJ: Generalized pustular psoriasis: a clinical and epidemiological study of 104 cases. Br J Dermatol 80:771, 1968
25. Baer RL: Cutaneous aspects of drug toxicity. Ann NY Acad Sci 123:354, 1965
26. Cram DL: Life-threatening drug eruptions. Drug Ther 3:31, 1973
27. Bruinsma W: A Guide to Drug Eruptions. Excerpta Medica, Amsterdam, 1973
28. AMA Drug Evaluations. 5th Ed. WB Saunders, Philadelphia, 1983
29. Dukes MNG: Meyler's Side Effects of Drugs. 10th Ed. Elsevier, New York, 1984
30. Stern RS, Bigby M: An expanded profile of cutaneous reactions to nonsteroidal anti-inflammatory drugs. JAMA 252:1433, 1984
31. Kauppinen K: Cutaneous reactions to drugs with special reference to severe bullous mucocutaneous eruptions and sulphonamides. Acta Derm Venereol (Stockh) 52(suppl. 68):1, 1972
32. Kuokkanen K: Drug eruptions. Acta Allerg 27:407, 1972
33. Fisher AA: Contact Dermatitis. 2nd Ed. Lea & Febiger, Philadelphia, 1973
34. Vonderheid EC, Sobel EL, Nowell PC, et al: Diagnostic and prognostic significance of Sézary cells in peripheral blood smears from patients with cutaneous T-cell lymphoma. Blood 66:358, 1985
35. Bonvalet D, Foldes C, Civatte J: Cutaneous manifestations in chronic lymphocytic leukemia. J Dermatol Surg Oncol 10:278, 1984
36. Greenwood R, Barker DJ, Tring FC, et al: Clinical and immunohistological characterization of cutaneous lesions in chronic lymphocytic leukaemia. Br J Dermatol 113:447, 1985
37. Harper TG, Latuska RF, Sperling HV: An unusual association between erythroderma and an occult gastric carcinoma. Am J Gastroenterol 79:921, 1984
38. Glucksberg H, Storb R, Fefer A, et al: Clinical

manifestations of graft-versus-host disease in human recipients of marrow from HLA-matched sibling donors. Transplantation 18:295, 1974

39. Grogan TM, Odom RB, Burgess JH: Graft-versus-host reaction. Arch Dermatol 113:806, 1977
40. Carr JL, Friedman M: Keratoderma blennorrhagicum, report of a case with autopsy. Am J Pathol 20:709, 1944
41. Hancock JAH: Surface manifestations of Reiter's disease in the male. Br J Vener Dis 36:36, 1960
42. Wigley JEM, Musso LA: A case of sarcoidosis with erythrodermic lesions. Treatment with calciferol. Br J Dermatol 63:398, 1951
43. Simpson JR: Sarcoidosis with erythrodermia and ulceration. Br J Dermatol 75:193, 1963
44. Greer KE, Harman LE Jr, Kayne AL: Unusual clinical manifestations of sarcoidosis. South Med J 70:666, 1977
45. Fox H: Exfoliative dermatitis complicated by fatal acute disseminated histoplasmosis. Arch Dermatol 68:734, 1953
46. Samovitz M, Dillon TK: Disseminated histoplasmosis presenting as exfoliative erythroderma. Arch Dermatol 101:216, 1970

APPENDIX:
APPROACH TO THE PATIENT—USEFUL CLUES IN THE DIFFERENTIAL DIAGNOSIS OF CHRONIC GENERALIZED ERYTHRODERMA

Differential Diagnosis of CGE

	Contact or Photocontact Dermatitis	Atopic Dermatitis
Age Predilection	Any	Younger adults
History	Exposure to allergen	Pre-existing lichenified rash on face, neck, antecubital or popliteal fossae Positive family history
Associated Disorders		Asthma Hayfever Cholinergic urticaria Ichthyosis vulgaris
Symptoms	Pruritus relatively intense	Pruritus relatively intense
Coloration		Relative pallor (frequent)
General Findings	Vesicles or oozing (frequent)	Prominant lichenification (frequent) Xerosis or keratosis pilaris (frequent)
Nail Findings Hair Findings		Coarse pitting (frequent)
Oral Findings		
Ocular Findings		Epicanthal fold of lower eyelid (frequent) Allergic conjunctivitis (frequent) Interstitial keratitis (rare) Keratoconus (rare) Subcapsular cataracts (occasional)
Joint Findings		
Visceral Findings		
Skin Histopathology	Relatively more spongiosis (frequent)	
Laboratory		Normal IgE level mitigates against diagnosis
Other Useful Tests	Positive patch or photopatch tests (frequent)	White dermatographism (frequent)

Differential Diagnosis of CGE

	Seborrheic Dermatitis	Stasis Dermatitis
Age Predilection	Any	Older adults
History	Pre-existing dermatitis on scalp, face, ears, or presternal areas Otitis externa	Pre-existing dermatitis on lower leg(s) Varicose veins or phlebitis
Associated Disorders	Acne vulgaris Parkinsonism Epilepsy	
Symptoms	Pruritus relatively mild	Pruritus relatively intense
Coloration		Hemosiderin deposits at ankles (frequent)
General Findings	Greasy scale on face and scalp (frequent)	Ulcers or scars at ankles (frequent)
Nail Findings		
Hair Findings		
Oral Findings		
Ocular Findings	Erythema with greasy scale along lid margin (frequent)	
Joint Findings		
Visceral Findings		
Skin Histopathology		
Laboratory		
Other Useful Tests		

Differential Diagnosis of CGE

	Photosensitive Eczema	Nummular Dermatitis
Age Predilection	Older adults	Older adults
History	Pre-existing dermatitis that flares after sun exposure	Pre-existing exudative coin-like patches on extensor aspects of extremities, buttocks, and posterior trunk
Associated Disorders		
Symptoms	Pruritus relatively intense	Pruritus relatively intense
Coloration		
General Findings	Relatively worse on sun-exposed skin (frequent)	Vesicles or oozing (occasional)
Nail Findings		
Hair Findings		
Oral Findings		
Ocular Findings		
Joint Findings		
Visceral Findings		
Skin Histopathology		Relatively more spongiosis (occasional)
Laboratory		
Other Useful Tests	Positive patch tests to Compositae plant oleoresin or fragrances (frequent) Abnormal phototest responses to UVB (frequent)	

Differential Diagnosis of CGE

	Psoriasis	Pityriasis Rubra Pilaris
Age Predilection	Any	Any
History	Pre-existing scaly plaques on knees, elbows, lumbosacrum, or scalp Positive family history	Resembles seborrheic dermatitis at onset Positive family history in childhood forms
Associated Disorders	Ankylosing spondylitis (HLA-B27)	
Symptoms	Pruritus relatively mild Skin tenderness and fever in pustular variant (frequent)	Pruritus relatively mild
Coloration		Salmon-red color (frequent) Islets of normal skin (frequent)
General Findings	Micaceous scale (occasional) Pustules in pustular variant (frequent)	Exfoliation relatively mild (frequent) Prominent keratoderma of palms and soles (frequent)
Nail Findings	Prominent pitting (frequent) Paronychia or subungual pus in pustular variant (frequent)	
Hair Findings	Alopecia relatively mild	Acuminate horny plugs in follicles (frequent) Alopecia relatively mild
Oral Findings	Localized grayish-white or pink patches on buccal mucosa or palate (rare) Geographic tongue (rare)	Diffuse hyperkeratosis with grayish white streaks on buccal mucosa and palate (rare)
Ocular Findings	Small yellowish-red scaly papules on bulbar conjunctiva (rare)	Mother-of-pearl papules on bulbar conjunctiva (rare) Interstitial keratitis (rare)
Joint Findings	Chronic asymmetric mono- or oligoarthritis predominantly of upper limbs, often including distal interphalangeal joints (frequent)	
Visceral Findings		
Skin Histopathology	Munro's microabscesses or spongiform pustules of Kogoj (occasional)	Hyperkeratotic follicular plugs (frequent)
Laboratory		Decreased serum vitamin A levels (occasional)
Other Useful Tests		

Differential Diagnosis of CGE

	Pemphigus Foliaceus	Lichen Planus
Age Predilection	Any	Young adults
History	Resembles seborrheic dermatitis or dermatitis herpetiformis at onset Penicillamine may induce	Certain drugs may induce
Associated Disorders	Thymoma Myasthenia gravis	
Symptoms	Pruritus relatively mild Burning (rare)	Pruritus relatively intense
Coloration		Bluish hue (frequent)
General Findings	Superficial bullae or erosions (occasional) Scaling or crusting in gyrate patterns (frequent) Malodor (frequent)	Coalescent angulated papules with Wickham's striae (frequent) Fine reticulate scale (frequent)
Nail Findings	Prominent pitting (frequent) Lamination of nailplate (occasional) Pterygium formation (occasional)	Longitudinal grooves or fissures (frequent) Papular paronychia (frequent) Pterygium formation (occasional)
Hair Findings		Cicatricial alopecia (occasional)
Oral Findings	Trivial superficial erosions on buccal mucosa (rare)	Bilateral lace-like bluish-white streaks on buccal mucosa or tongue (frequent) Erosions (occasional) White papules or plaques (occasional)
Ocular Findings	Interstitial keratitis (rare) Cataracts (rare)	
Joint Findings		
Visceral Findings		
Skin Histopathology	Acantholysis at stratum granulosum (frequent) IgG in epidermal intercellular spaces by direct immuno-fluorescence (frequent)	Lichenoid injury pattern (frequent) IgM positive cytoid bodies by direct immuno-fluorescence (frequent)
Laboratory	Serum IgG pemphigus antibody (frequent)	
Other Useful Tests	Positive Nikolsky's sign (frequent)	

Differential Diagnosis of CGE

	Lamellar Ichthyosis	Epidermolytic Hyperkeratosis
Age Predilection	Newborn Infants	Newborn Infants
History	Collodion baby followed by chronic ichthyosiform eruption Positive family history	Erythema and blisters at birth followed by verrucous eruption Positive family history
Associated Disorders	Intellectual impairment Decreased fertility Dwarfism in associated syndromes	
Symptoms	Pruritus relatively mild	Pruritus relatively mild
Coloration	Bright red (frequent)	Dark red (frequent)
General Findings	Coarse yellowish-brown scales (frequent) Malodor (frequent)	Verrucous hyperplasia (frequent) Flaccid bullae (occasional) Malodor (frequent)
Nail Findings		Usually normal
Hair Findings	Hair shaft abnormalities in associated syndromes (rare)	Usually normal
Oral Findings		
Ocular Findings	Ectropion	Usually normal
Joint Findings		
Visceral Findings		
Skin Histopathology	Marked hyperkeratosis with thickened granular layer (frequent)	Massive hyperkeratosis with vacuolization in midepidermis and granular layer (frequent)
Laboratory		
Other Useful Tests		

Differential Diagnosis of CGE

	Norwegian Scabies	Systemic Drug Reactions
Age Predilection	Any	Any
History	Preceding eruption typical for scabies Outbreaks in close contacts	Pre-existing drug ingestion May resemble erythema multiforme at onset
Associated Disorders	Mental retardation	
Symptoms	Pruritus relatively mild	High fever (occasional)
Coloration		Bright red (frequent) Purpuric component (occasional) Bluish hue in lichenoid type (occasional)
General Findings	Crusting prominent, especially elbows, intergluteal area (frequent)	Vesicles or oozing (occasional)
Nail Findings		Normal in acute phase
Hair Findings		
Oral Findings		Bullous stomatitis (occasional)
Ocular Findings		
Joint Findings		Transient arthritis (occasional)
Visceral Findings		Massive lymphadenopathy (occasional) Splenomegaly (rare) Interstitial nephritis (occasional) Hepatocellular injury (occasional) Pulmonary infiltrate (rare)
Skin Histopathology	Sarcoptes mites in stratum corneum (frequent)	Lichenoid injury pattern (occasional) Leukocytoclastic vasculitis (rare)
Laboratory		Increased hepatic transaminases, alkaline phosphatase, or direct bilirubin (occasional)
Other Useful Tests	Sarcoptes mites on microscopic examination of crusts (frequent)	Positive patch or provocative test (occasional)

Differential Diagnosis of CGE

	Cutaneous T-Cell Lymphoma	Hodgkin's Disease
Age Predilection	Older adults	Younger adults
History	Pre-existing widespread patches that coalesce slowly over time Pruritus may precede eruption	Pruritus often precedes eruption
Associated Disorders		
Symptoms	High fever (rare) Weight loss (rare)	Pruritus relatively severe (frequent) High fever (occasional) Weight loss (frequent) Night sweats (frequent)
Coloration	Islets of normal skin (rare)	
General Findings	Ichthyosiform scaling (rare) Coexisting plaques or tumors (occasional)	Ichthyosiform scaling (frequent)
Nail Findings		
Hair Findings	Follicular mucinosis (occasional) Follicular papules resembling pityriasis rubra pilaris (rare)	Follicular mucinosis (rare)
Oral Findings	Indurated ulcers on palate, tongue, or buccal mucosa (rare)	Indurated ulcers at any location (occasional) Gingival hyperplasia (rare)
Ocular Findings		
Joint Findings		
Visceral Findings	Massive or asymmetrical lymphadenopathy (frequent) Splenomegaly (occasional) Multiorgan involvement (rare)	Massive or asymmetrical lymphadenopathy (frequent) Splenomegaly (frequent) Multiorgan involvement (frequent)
Skin Histopathology	Pautrier microabscesses (frequent) Atypical lymphocytes in infiltrate (frequent)	Sternberg-Reed cells in infiltrate (occasional)
Laboratory	Leukemic T cells (Sézary cells) in peripheral blood (frequent)	
Other Useful Tests	Abnormal chromosome studies (frequent)	Skin test anergy

	Differential Diagnosis CGE	
	Miscellaneous Lymphomas/Leukemias	Carcinoma
Age Predilection	Any	Older adults
History	Pruritus may precede eruption	
Associated Disorders		
Symptoms	High fever (occasional) Weight loss (occasional) Night sweats (occasional)	Weight loss (occasional)
Coloration	Purpuric component (occasional)	
General Findings	Coexisting plaques or tumors (occasional) Ichthyosiform scaling (rare)	
Nail Findings		
Hair Findings		
Oral Findings	Gingival hyperplasia (occasional) Indurated ulcers at any location (rare)	
Ocular Findings	Keratoconjunctivitis sicca (occasional)	
Joint Findings	Symmetric migratory polyarthritis (occasional)	
Visceral Findings	Massive or asymmetric lymphadenopathy (frequent) Splenomegaly (frequent) Multiorgan involvement (frequent)	Primary involvement of lung, prostate, or gastrointestinal tract (frequent)
Skin Histopathology	Atypical lymphocytes in infiltrate (occasional)	
Laboratory	Leukemic B cells in peripheral blood (frequent)	Chorioembryonic antigen (occasional)
Other Useful Tests	Abnormal bone marrow (frequent)	

Differential Diagnosis of CGE

	Graft-Versus-Host Disease	Reiter's Disease
Age Predilection	Younger adults	Younger adults
History	Preceding bone marrow or blood transfusion Resembles toxic epidermal necrolysis or lichen planus at onset	Pre-existing urethritis or diarrhea
Associated Disorders	Primary or secondary immunodeficiency states	Ankylosing spondylitis (HLA-B27)
Symptoms	Nausea, vomiting, diarrhea, high fever in acute phase (frequent)	Pruritus relatively mild High fever (rare)
Coloration	Bluish hue (occasional) Poikilodermatous hyperpigmentation (occasional)	
General Findings	Bullae or epidermal sloughing in acute phase (frequent) Ichthyosiform scaling (occasional)	Keratoderma blennorrhagicum (occasional) Circinate balanitis (frequent)
Nail Findings		Prominent pitting (occasional) Paronychia (occasional)
Hair Findings		
Oral Findings	Lichen planus-like white patches with reticulation (occasional)	Painless erosions with white circinate border on buccal mucosa, palate, or tongue (occasional)
Ocular Findings	Keratoconjunctivitis sicca (frequent)	Mucopurulent discharge (frequent) Anterior uveitis (frequent) Interstitial keratitis (occasional)
Joint Findings	Transient arthritis (occasional)	Acute and transient asymmetric polyarthritis predominantly of lower limbs, often with plantar fasciitis (frequent)
Visceral Findings	Hepatocellular injury (frequent) Gastrointestinal tract injury (frequent) Splenomegaly (occasional) Multiorgan involvement (occasional)	Multiorgan involvement (rare)
Skin Histopathology	Lichenoid injury pattern ± satellite cell necrosis (frequent) IgM deposition at dermoepidermal junction (frequent)	Spongiform pustules of Kogoj (frequent)
Laboratory	Increased hepatic transaminases, alkaline phosphatase, or direct bilirubin (frequent)	
Other Useful Tests		

Differential Diagnosis of CGE

	Sarcoidosis	Histoplasmosis
Age Predilection	Younger adults	Older adults
History	Pre-existing widespread patches that coalesce slowly over time	Exposure in endemic area Immunosuppressive disease or treatment
Associated Disorders	Erythema nodosum	Erythema multiforme or nodosum
Symptoms	Pruritus relatively mild High fever (rare)	Cough, weight loss, night sweats, or high fever (frequent)
Coloration	Islets of normal skin (frequent)	
General Findings	Ichthyosiform scaling (occasional) Ulceration (rare)	Ulceration (occasional)
Nail Findings	May appear normal (frequent)	May appear normal (frequent)
Hair Findings	Follicular papules resembling pityriasis rubra pilaris (frequent) Cicatricial alopecia (rare)	
Oral Findings	Painless parotid gland enlargement (frequent) Single or multiple papules with or without ulceration at any location (rare)	Indurated ulcers on tongue and buccal mucosa (frequent)
Ocular Findings	Keratoconjunctivitis sicca (occasional) Conjunctival follicles (occasional) Acute or chronic anterior uveitis (frequent) Posterior uveitis or chorioretinitis (occasional)	Chorioretinitis (frequent)
Joint Findings	Symmetric migratory arthritis of knees, ankles, elbows, wrists, and proximal interphalangeal joints (occasional)	
Visceral Findings	Bilateral hilar adenopathy with or without parenchymal disease on chest x-ray (frequent) Massive lymphadenopathy (occasional) Splenomegaly (occasional) Multiorgan involvement (frequent)	Apical infiltrates or fibrosis on chest x-ray (frequent) Massive lymphadenopathy (occasional) Splenomegaly (occasional) Multiorgan involvement (occasional)
Skin Histopathology	Epithelioid cell granulomas (frequent)	Histiocytes containing organisms (frequent)
Laboratory	Hypercalcemia (occasional) Increased serum angiotensin-converting enzyme (frequent)	Complement fixation titers >1:32 (frequent)
Other Useful Tests	Skin test anergy	Positive fungal cultures (frequent)

7

The Immunobullous Skin Diseases

Robert E. Jordon

The immunobullous skin diseases comprise most of the nonhereditary blistering diseases of man. Included are the pemphigus group (pemphigus vulgaris, pemphigus vegetans, pemphigus foliaceus, Brazilian pemphigus foliaceus, pemphigus erythematosus, and drug-induced pemphigus), the pemphigoid group (bullous pemphigoid, cicatricial pemphigoid, localized scarring pemphigoid, and herpes gestationis), the IgA bullous disease group (dermatitis herpetiformis, linear IgA bullous dermatosis, chronic bullous disease of childhood), erythema multiforme, epidermolysis bullosa acquisita, and bullous lupus erythematosus. All the above blistering skin diseases have specific immunopathologic features, which allow us to better classify and diagnose them. This chapter presents a brief review of the important clinical, histopathologic, and immunopathologic findings of this group of diseases. We have attempted to classify the diseases based upon their specific immunopathologic findings, including those based upon routine immunofluorescence (IF) and immuno-electron microscopy.

THE PEMPHIGUS GROUP

Pemphigus Vulgaris

Although different clinical variants exist, diseases of the pemphigus group share similar histopathologic and immunopathologic findings. The most common and unfortunately the most severe form of the disease is pemphigus vulgaris, which accounts for roughly 75 percent of all diagnosed cases of pemphigus.[1] Oral lesions in this form of the disease are common, may precede skin lesions by 4 to 5 months, and are often the earliest presenting symptom of the disease.[1,2] In rare instances pemphigus may remain entirely confined to the oral cavity.[2] The nasal, vaginal, anal, and laryngeal mucosa, the ocular membranes, and the vermilion border of the lips may also be involved. Cutaneous sites of involvement include the scalp, face, back, and chest. Any area of the body may be involved when the disease process is generalized.

Pemphigus Vegetans

Pemphigus vegetans represents a rare variant of pemphigus vulgaris.[3] Although two types of this variant have been recognized in the past, only the Neumann type is considered a true member of the pemphigus group. Lesions of pemphigus vegetans in the early stages are identical to those of pemphigus vulgaris. Later in the course, however, lesions become hypertrophic and papillomatous, particularly in the intertriginous areas.

Lesions of both pemphigus vulgaris and pemphigus vegetans share common histopathologic findings. Both demonstrate suprabasalar or deep intraepidermal blister formation and acantholysis. In pemphigus vulgaris, the cellular infiltrate may be sparse, although eosinophils, often in clusters (eosinophilic spongiosis), may be apparent in early lesions.[4] In pemphigus vegetans, these infiltrates may be heavy, especially in verrucoid lesions. Dissolution of the desmosomes is the earliest pathologic event observed by electron microscopy.[5]

Pemphigus Foliaceus

Pemphigus foliaceus is a less severe, superficial member of the pemphigus group.[6] Blistering skin lesions are rarely seen because of the superficial nature of the disease. Shallow erosions with scaling and crusting are common. Oral lesions are extremely rare in this form of the disease. The scalp, face and chest are common areas of involvement. An interesting variant of pemphigus foliaceus, which is endemic to certain areas of South America, is called *fogo selvagem* ("wild fire"). This disease is clinically, histopathologically and immunopathologically identical to true pemphigus foliaceus.[7] Although no absolute proof exists, an arthropod vector has been implicated in this form of the disease process.

Pemphigus Erythematosus

Another superficial member of the pemphigus disease group is pemphigus erythematosus. First recognized by Senear and Usher,[8] this condition combines clinical and serologic features of pemphigus and lupus erythematosus. Immunopathologically these patients may have deposition of immunoglobulins and complement at the dermal-epidermal junction in skin lesions and measurable antinuclear antibodies in their serum in addition to the more typical immunopathologic features of pemphigus.[9] Concurrent myasthenia gravis and thymoma have also been associated with this unique form of the disease.[10,11] By routine histopathology, pemphigus foliaceus and pemphigus erythematosus are characterized by intraepidermal bulla formation occurring high in the epidermis. Clefting in these two forms of pemphigus occurs in or near the granular layer.[3,6] A moderate infiltrate, mostly eosinophils, again may be present.

Drug-Induced Pemphigus

Drug-induced pemphigus was first recognized by Degos et al.[12] in a patient treated with D-penicillamine (β,β-dimethylcysteine) for hepatolenticular degeneration (Wilson's disease). Approximately 40 additional cases have been documented thus far in the world literature.[13] Clinically most of these patients manifest pemphigus foliaceus; a few, however, have presented clinically with either pemphigus vulgaris or pemphigus erythematosus. Almost all these cases have been associated with the administration of D-penicillamine. In most instances the eruption resolves spontaneously with cessation of therapy.

Immunopathology

Pemphigus is an autoimmune disease of the skin. Indirect IF staining has been used in numerous studies to confirm the presence of serum autoantibodies reactive with antigens localized to the intercellular substance (ICS) of epidermis or the surface of epidermal cells.[1,7,14,15] These antibodies are of the IgG type, reside in all subclasses of IgG, and are present in all types of pemphigus, an additional feature that unifies members of this disease group (Table 7-1). Levels of pemphigus antibodies often fluctuate with disease activity; they may be absent during peri-

Table 7-1. Approach to Patient: Diagnostic Features of the Pemphigus Group of Bullous Diseases

	Clinical Features	Histology	Immunopathology
Pemphigus vulgaris	Oral lesions often precede cutaneous bullae Nikolsky sign	Suprabasalar clefts extending along adnexa Acantholytic keratinocytes	Normal or perilesional skin: IgG and C3 at intercellular spaces of epidermis Serum anti-intercellular substance antibodies correlate with disease activity
Pemphigus vegetans	Bullae are followed by hypertrophic, papillomatous lesions in intertriginous sites	Suprabasalar clefts Acantholytic cells Eosinophilic abscesses Epidermal hyperplasia	Resembles pemphigus vulgaris
Pemphigus foliaceus	Oral lesions rare Rapid crusting of bullae	Subcorneal or granular layer cleft Acantholytic cells Dyskeratotic cells in granular layer Eosinophilic pustules	Resembles pemphigus vulgaris, immune deposits more superficial
Pemphigus erythematosus	Bullae, crusts, and impetiginous lesions Prominent facial involvement	Identical to pemphigus foliaceus	Immunoglobulins and complement at dermal-epidermal junction, intercellular IgG and C3 Positive antinuclear antibody
Penicillamine-induced pemphigus	Often resembles pemphigus foliaceus	Identical to pemphigus foliaceus or pemphigus vulgaris	IgG and C3 at intercellular spaces

ods of clinical remission. Considerable investigative effort has been focused upon the antigens reactive with pemphigus antibodies in recent years. Stanley and co-workers have recently shown that the antigens reactive with pemphigus vulgaris and pemphigus foliaceus sera differ.[16] Whatever their composition, these antigens are clearly produced by and expressed on the surface of epidermal cells and appear to be important in cell-cell adhesion.[17,18]

By direct IF staining both IgG and complement deposits are found in ICS areas of early acantholytic lesions of both deep and superficial forms of pemphigus.[7,19] If performed properly, this test is positive in virtually all cases of pemphigus, including early pemphigus vulgaris confined to the oral cavity. In pemphigus vulgaris these immune deposits are most intense in deep acantholytic areas (Fig. 7-1A), while in pemphigus foliaceus the deposits are more superficial in location (Fig. 7-1B). These tests are particularly valuable in the diagnosis of all cases of pemphigus. Early lesions should be chosen for biopsy.

The mechanism by which epidermal cells detach in pemphigus (acantholysis) has also received considerable investigative attention in recent years. The first convincing evidence that the antibodies found in sera of patients with pemphigus are responsible for acantholysis was presented several years ago by Michel, Schultz, and co-workers.[20] In their studies histologic evidence of acantholysis occurred when explants of normal human skin were placed in organ culture in the presence of pemphigus IgG. Later, others showed that by adding pemphigus IgG to monolayers of epidermal cells in culture, detachment of epidermal cells occurred.[18,21] Further studies suggested that pemphigus IgG would stimulate the release of proteases in culture systems, implicating proteinases in the detachment of epidermal cells.[21,22] Hashimoto et al.[23] subsequently reported that the protease released by epidermal cells when treated by pemphigus antibodies is a plasminogen activator. Thus, the plasminogen-plasmin system has been implicated as a possible mechanism for acantholysis.

Studies performed in our laboratories suggest that pemphigus antibodies will fix complement components to the surface of epidermal cells.[24] We have further demonstrated that complement will enhance the detachment of epidermal cells mediated by pemphigus antibody.[25] This mechanism of epidermal cell detachment appears to be independent of the plasminogen-plasmin sys-

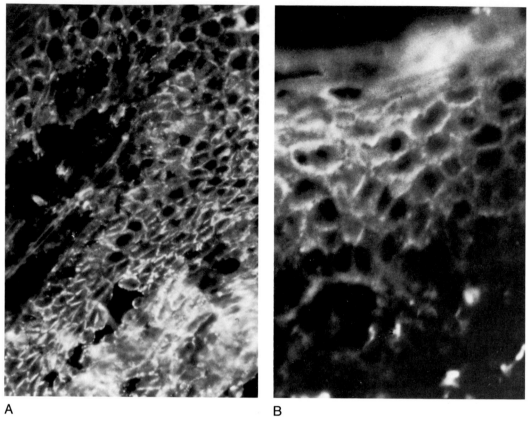

A   B

Fig. 7-1. Direct IF staining of lesions of patients with pemphigus using labeled antiserum to human IgG. (**A**) Pemphigus vulgaris. (**B**) Pemphigus foliaceus. (Original magnifications: A, × 400; B, × 500.)

tem. Further studies have shown that when complement is fixed to the surface of epidermal cells in culture by pemphigus antibody, the membranes of these cells are damaged.[26] Thus, at the present time there is no question that the antibody found in the serum of patients with pemphigus is responsible for the acantholytic changes seen in skin lesions. The elegant passive transfer studies reported by Anhalt et al.[27] also support this contention.

THE PEMPHIGOID GROUP

Bullous pemphigoid, herpes gestationis, cicatricial pemphigoid, and localized scarring pemphigoid (Brunsting-Perry) are diseases of the pemphigoid group. These diseases all share similar histopathologic and immunopathologic features despite different clinical presentations (Table 7-2).

Bullous Pemphigoid

For years bullous pemphigoid was confused with other blistering diseases of the skin, such as pemphigus, dermatitis herpetiformis, and erythema multiforme. Lever,[3] who first recognized this disease as a distinct clinical entity, chose the term *bullous pemphigoid* because clinically it has a close similarity to pemphigus vulgaris but histopathologically is without acantholysis.

Clinically the major feature of bullous pemphigoid is the presence of large, tense bullae,

Table 7-2. Approach to the Patient: Diagnostic Features of the Pemphigoid Group of Bullous Diseases

	Clinical Features	Histology	Immunopathology
Bullous pemphigoid	Large tense bullae Oral lesions rarely the initial manifestation	Subepidermal bullae Infiltrate with eosinophils can be present	Perilesional skin: C3, IgG, and other immunoglobulins in linear pattern at basement membrane zone (BMZ) (lamina lucida) Serum anti-BMZ antibodies
Herpes gestationis	Urticarial, vesicular, and bullous lesions in pregnancy	Subepidermal blisters Spongiosis Papillary edema Infiltrate with eosinophils	Perilesional skin: C3 and occasionally IgG in linear patterns at BMZ Serum HG factor
Cicatricial pemphigoid	Scarring blisters of mucous membranes	Subepithelial blisters	Linear deposition of immunoglobulins and complement in BMZ
Localized scarring pemphigoid (Brunsting-Perry)	Localized patches of recurrent scarring blisters on head and neck	Subepidermal blisters	Resembles cicatricial pemphigoid

arising either on clinically normal or erythematous skin. Urticaria-like lesions are not uncommon early in the disease process. Common sites of involvement include the flexural surfaces of the forearms, the groin, the axillae, and the lower abdomen. Unlike the lesions of pemphigus vulgaris, these lesions usually show a good tendency to heal and only rarely extend peripherally. Mucous membrane lesions are also less common in this disease and are rarely the initial manifestation. When present, they appear as intact blisters.

The disease is self-limited, with a course characterized by periodic remissions and exacerbations; recurrences are usually less severe than the initial episode. Well-documented spontaneous remissions occur in bullous pemphigoid.[3]

Bullous pemphigoid occurs predominantly in the sixth, seventh, and eighth decades of life, but well-documented cases have been reported in children.[28] Age-matched studies reported by Stone and Schroeter[29] have failed to substantiate the previous notion of an increased incidence of malignancy. Although the mortality rate is thought to be low for bullous pemphigoid, death from unrelated causes may intervene before the disease has run its course because of the age of many of the patients. Bullous pemphigoid may affect all ethnic groups; there is no genetic predisposition for this disease process.

IMMUNOPATHOLOGY

Bullous pemphigoid is also an autoimmune disease that affects the skin. Autoantibodies reactive with the basement membrane zone (BMZ) of skin and mucosa are present in serum samples from about 75 percent of patients with this disease.[7,15,30] Like pemphigus antibodies, these antibodies are of the IgG type and are found in all subclasses of IgG. Many studies have demonstrated that they avidly fix a variety of complement components.[31,32]

By direct IF staining, IgG may be detected bound in vivo to the BMZ of skin lesions.[30] Other immunoglobulins, including IgM, IgA, IgD, and IgE, have also been detected in the BMZ, but much less frequently. C3 deposition occurs in virtually all bullous pemphigoid lesions (Fig. 7-2A) and at times in the absence of immunoglobulins. Other complement components, including classical and alternative pathway and terminal sequence components, are also present in perilesional skin bound to the BMZ.[33,34] By immuno-electron microscopy the immunoreactants in bullous pemphigoid have been localized to the lamina lucida region of the BMZ.[35,36]

Attempts to isolate and purify antigens reactive with bullous pemphigoid antibodies have led to controversial findings. Molecular weights of these isolated proteins vary from 20,000 kD

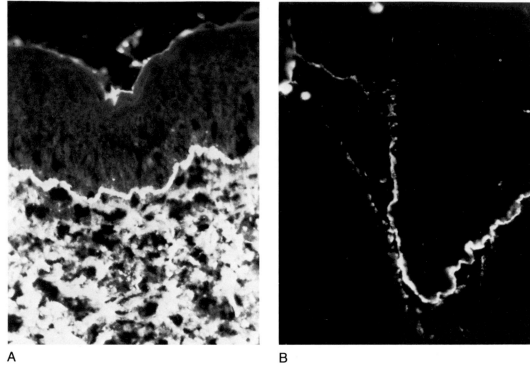

A   B

Fig. 7-2. Direct IF staining of perilesional skin and oral mucosa from patients with pemphigoid using labeled antiserum to human C3. **(A)** Bullous pemphigoid (perilesional skin). **(B)** Cicatricial pemphigoid (oral mucosa). (Original magnifications × 400.)

to 200,000 kD.[37,38] It has now been clearly demonstrated, however, that the antigen(s) are produced by basal cells and deposited in the BMZ. Further, Zhu and Bystryn[39] have demonstrated different reactivities for bullous pemphigoid antibodies using indirect IF on multiple substrates. Mutasin et al.[40] recently demonstrated that bullous pemphigoid antigen appears to be in close proximity to the hemidesmosomes of the basal cells. The true nature of bullous pemphigoid antigen, however, needs further clarification.

The mechanism of blister formation in bullous pemphigoid is thought to be due to the interaction of anti-BMZ antibody with lamina lucida antigen, activation of complement, subsequent attraction of neutrophils and eosinophils, and release of their proteolytic enzymes.[15] Examination of blister fluids helps substantiate this theory of pathogenesis. Low levels of complement and individual comple-

ment components, activated complement components, and C5-related chemotactic activity have been identified.[41,42] Gammon and coworkers[43] have demonstrated that BMZ antibody in the presence of complement will fix neutrophils in vitro to normal skin BMZ. Immune complexes, both in serum and in blister fluids, form and may contribute to further activation of the complement cascade.[44]

Complement activation may also account for the attraction of eosinophils in this disease process. With complement activation, anaphylatoxins (C4a, C3a, and C5a) are elaborated. Anaphylatoxins could activate mast cells to release histamine, eosinophilic chemotactic factor of anaphylaxis (ECF-A), and eosinophil colony-stimulating material (ESM).[15] Bullous pemphigoid antibodies of the IgG$_4$ subclass could also activate mast cells.[45] All these factors could be involved in the subepidermal separation that occurs in this disease process.

Immunologic mechanisms other than IgG, autoantibody, and complement may also participate in the pathogenesis of bullous pemphigoid. Two groups of investigators have identified low levels of serum IgE anti-BMZ antibodies.[33,46] In addition, Arbesman et al.[47] reported increased serum IgE levels in many bullous pemphigoid patients. Baba et al.[46] and Wintroub et al.[48] have isolated and identified the eosinophilic chemotactic factor of anaphylaxis in bullous pemphigoid blister fluids. Evidence has also been presented to suggest activation of both mast cells and eosinophils in bullous pemphigoid skin lesions. Mast cell enzymes, including arginine esterase and a Hageman factor cleaver, have also been identified in bullous pemphigoid blisters.[49] Thus, the IgE system may also participate in the pathogenesis of bullous pemphigoid.

Herpes Gestationis

Herpes gestationis is an uncommon, intensely pruritic, blistering disease of pregnancy and the immediate postpartum period. The disease occurs once in every 10,000 deliveries, although herpes gestationis may be more common than the reported incidence. The onset usually occurs in the second trimester of pregnancy, but cases in the first trimester and the immediate postpartum period have been well documented.[50,51] The disease is usually self-limited, but with subsequent pregnancies bullous lesions may occur earlier and be more severe. Estrogen- and/or progesterone-containing medications are contraindicated, as these may initiate an episode of herpes gestationis. A high frequency of the HLA antigens DR3 and DR4, suggesting a genetic predisposition, has been reported.[52]

The clinical presentation of herpes gestationis varies. Erythematous and urticaria-like lesions, vesicles (sometimes in an annular configuration), and large, tense bullae may be present. The disease process and accompanying pruritus may be mild or severe. The abdomen, extremities, and flexural areas are common sites of involvement. Other sites, however, may also be involved.

Although transient urticarial and vesicular lesions have been reported in some infants born of affected mothers, most infants are not affected. An increased mortality in infants born of affected mothers, however, has been well documented. The relationship between disease severity (as judged by the necessity for more aggressive therapy) and fetal complications has been reported. Although not diagnostic, the histopathologic features of herpes gestationis are somewhat characteristic.[50] As in other members of the pemphigoid group, bullous lesions are subepidermal. Necrosis of the tips of the basal cells may be a characteristic feature, but the same phenomenon may occur in selected cases of bullous pemphigoid. Ultrastructurally, the earliest change appears to be vacuolar degeneration of the endoplasmic reticulum in basal cells, with destruction of the plasma membranes.[53] Blister formation in herpes gestationis therefore may result from basal cell degeneration with fluid accumulation in the lamina lucida area of the BMZ.

Immunopathologically, herpes gestationis is strikingly similar to bullous pemphigoid. Heavy BMZ deposition of C3, often in the absence of IgG, occurs in herpes gestationis skin lesions.[54–56] Alternative pathway complement components, in particular properdin and factor B, are frequently present, while classical pathway components (C1q and C4) may again be absent. Linear C3 deposition at the BMZ has also been reported in infants born of mothers with herpes gestationis.[57] Again, these deposits usually occur in the absence of concomitant immunoglobulin deposition.

By immuno-electron microscopy C3 deposition has been shown to occur in the area of the lamina lucida of the cutaneous BMZ, as with other members of the pemphigoid group.[58] Less frequently, IgG deposition has also been noted in a similar distribution pattern; these studies also suggest that herpes gestationis may be related to bullous pemphigoid. On the basis of these similar clinical and immunopathologic findings, some investigators have proposed that we change the name of herpes gestationis to *pemphigoid gestationis*.

Circulating anti-BMZ antibodies are detectable by indirect IF in only 10 to 20 percent of herpes gestationis patients. When present, titers of these IgG autoantibodies are usually low, in contrast to bullous pemphigoid. In the vast majority of herpes gestationis sera, however, a C3-fixing factor is present, which also reacts with the BMZ.[54–56] In vitro complement-staining techniques are necessary to demonstrate this C3-fixing factor. This factor, also called HG factor, was initially thought to activate complement via the alternative pathway. Studies performed in several laboratories, however, suggest that HG factor is an avid complement-fixing IgG autoantibody but that it is present in such low levels that it escapes detection by routine indirect IF methods. The factor has also been shown to activate complement via the classical pathway in the same fashion as bullous pemphigoid antibodies.[54–56] Thus, the immunopathogenesis of this interesting blistering skin disease of pregnancy is thought to be similar to that of bullous pemphigoid.

Cicatricial and Localized Pemphigoid

Cicatricial pemphigoid (ocular pemphigus, benign mucous membrane pemphigoid) is a rare, well-defined clinical entity characterized by scarring, erosive subepidermal blistering lesions of the mucous membranes.[59,60] In this condition the oral mucosa and ocular membranes are most commonly involved. A variant of this condition, localized pemphigoid (Brunsting-Perry), is characterized by cutaneous vesiculobullous lesions, which are localized usually to the head and neck areas.[61] Often in this condition only one anatomic site is involved. Both these members of the pemphigoid group are characterized clinically by scarring lesions, which is distinctly different from the presentation of bullous pemphigoid and herpes gestationis. Conjunctival scarring occurs in approximately 60 percent of patients with cicatricial pemphigoid, a process that may lead to total blindness. Oral lesions are common and are often the presenting symptomatology. As in bullous pemphigoid and herpes gestationis, cicatricial and localized pemphigoid are characterized by subepidermal bulla formation.[60] By immuno-electron microscopy, however, blister formation is shown to occur at the level of the lamina lucida but below the areas associated with bullous pemphigoid and herpes gestationis.[62] This lower anatomic site in the BMZ may be the cause of scarring in both these conditions.

By direct IF staining (Fig. 7-2B), immunoglobulins, particularly IgG and IgA, and a variety of complement components (C1q, C4, C3, factor B, and properdin) are demonstrable along the BMZ of oral and ocular lesions.[63–65] Similar deposition is seen in skin lesions of the localized Brunsting-Perry pemphigoid. With the exception of a few sera, most patients with cicatricial pemphigoid do not possess circulating anti-BMZ antibodies. Sera from most of the rare cicatricial pemphigoid patients who possess such antibodies usually exhibit restricted specificity, reacting only with certain substrates.[63] Although histopathologic and immunopathologic findings relate these diseases to the other members of the pemphigoid group, both cicatricial and localized pemphigoid are dissimilar to the other members. The recent observations by Fine and co-workers[62] suggest, in fact, that these two diseases may be distinct from other members of the pemphigoid group.

THE IGA BULLOUS DISEASE GROUP

Dermatitis Herpetiformis

Dermatitis herpetiformis is a chronic, blistering skin disease characterized clinically by symmetrical, pleomorphic, intensely pruritic, grouped vesicles arising on erythematous bases. The disease usually begins in the late teens or early twenties but may affect any age group. Well-documented childhood cases have been described. Common sites of involvement include the extensor surfaces, the buttocks, the lower back, and the scapular areas. Pruritus, which is always present and often severe, may be the presenting symptom of the disease process.

By routine histopathology dermatitis herpetiformis is also a subepidermal blistering dermatosis. Early lesions may be somewhat characteristic, demonstrating neutrophilic microabscesses at the tips of the dermal papillae with fibrin deposition.[66] These same findings, however, have been noted in a few cases of early herpes gestationis and bullous pemphigoid, and identical histologic features have been described in bullous lupus erythematosus.[67]

In addition to vesicular skin lesions, systemic manifestations may also be present. Small intestinal biopsies of dermatitis herpetiformis patients reveal patchy duodenal and jejunal atrophy, a pattern associated with adult celiac disease.[68,69] Signs and symptoms of malabsorption, however, are usually not present. The duodenal-jejunal atrophy, and in some cases the cutaneous lesions, are responsive to a diet free of gluten.

Dermatitis herpetiformis, like the other immunobullous skin diseases, has specific immunopathologic findings (Table 7-3). First reported by van der Meer,[70] IgA deposition in the tips of the dermal papillae (Fig. 7-3A) is a characteristic finding in this disease.[69] The deposits are usually granular or fibrillar and on occasion may be found along the dermal-epidermal junction. These IgA findings are now thought to be distinctive for dermatitis herpetiformis and different from the IgA deposits observed in linear IgA bullous dermatosis and chronic bullous disease of childhood. IgA deposition in the dermal papillae, as depicted in Figure 7-3A, has now become a diagnostic hallmark of true dermatitis herpetiformis. More recently these IgA deposits have been shown to be of the IgA_1 subclass[71] and appear to be dimers, which is characteristic of IgA produced in the gastrointestinal tract.[72.]

Dermatitis herpetiformis may in some fashion be mediated immunopathologically by immune complex formation and deposition. Immune complexes containing IgA have been identified in patients with this disease process.[73,74] IgG- and/or IgM-containing immune complexes may be present at very low levels and are most likely of no pathologic significance.[75] In addition to containing IgA, these immune complexes may also contain gluten.[76,77] Zone et al.[77] have further shown that gluten- and IgA-containing immune complexes arise in these patients following the ingestion of gluten. They do not contain secretory piece, however. The relationship between the IgA deposits in normal skin and the IgA- and gluten-containing immune complexes has not yet been clearly defined. Defective removal of immune complexes from the circulation, however, has also been documented.[78]

Dermatitis herpetiformis also appears to be a disease with immunogenetic linkage. Approximately 90 percent of patients have the surface antigen HLA-B8, compared with 20 to 30 percent of the general population.[69] In addition, these patients also have a very high incidence of HLA-DR3.[69] These same immunogenetic findings are also found in patients with gluten-sensitive enteropathy. These HLA associations are only seen in patients with the typical granu-

Table 7-3. Approach to the Patient: Diagnostic Features of the IgA Bullous Disease Group

	Clinical Features	Histology	Immunopathology
Dermatitis herpetiformis	Severe pruritus Symmetrical grouped vesicles, associated with gluten-sensitive enteropathy	Subepidermal blisters Papillary microabscesses with neutrophils	Uninvolved skin: IgA deposition in dermal papillae
Linear IgA bullous disease	Vesicles and bullae, not associated with enteropathy	Subepidermal blisters Features of dermatitis herpetiformis and bullous pemphigoid	Linear deposits of IgA at dermal-epidermal junction
Chronic bullous disease of childhood	Vesicles or bullae in young children	Subepidermal blisters Infiltrate with neutrophils	Perilesional skin: linear deposits of IgA at basement membrane zone

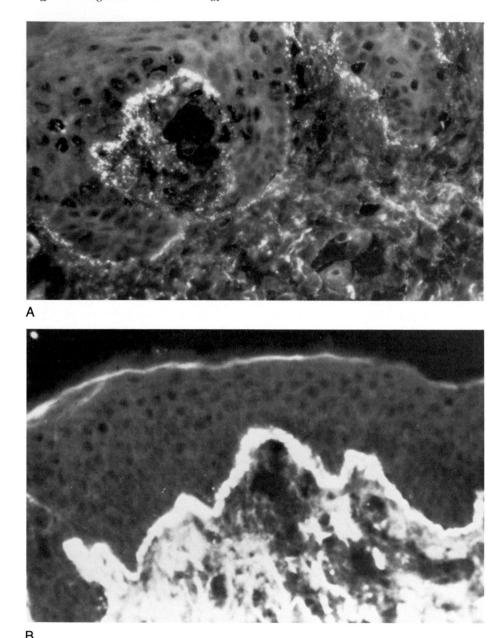

Fig. 7-3. Direct IF staining of perilesional skin from patients with dermatitis herpetiformis and linear IgA bullous disease using labeled antiserum to human IgA. (**A**) Dermatitis herpetiformis. (**B**) Linear IgA bullous disease. (Original magnifications × 400.)

lar IgA deposits in the tips of the dermal papillae and only in those patients who histologically manifest evidence of duodenal-jejunal atrophy.[79]

A variety of antibodies have been described in these patients, including antithyroid[80] and anti-wheat protein antibodies.[81] These latter antibodies have been implicated in the pathogenesis of both dermatitis herpetiformis and gluten-sensitive enteropathy. More recently, Chorzelski and co-workers[82] have described IgA antiendomysium antibodies in approximately 80 percent of patients with dermatitis herpetiformis. These antibodies are also found in patients with adult celiac disease but not in patients with linear IgA bullous disease.

Linear IgA Bullous Disease

Although recent evidence suggests that IgA bullous disease is a distinct, separate entity, the condition remains controversial. It has been previously reported as mixed bullous disease, polymorphic pemphigoid, dermatitis herpetiformis linear IgA type, etc. The reason for the confusion is that it combines clinical features of both bullous pemphigoid and dermatitis herpetiformis. In addition, many patients with this disease will respond to dapsone therapy. Histopathologically this is a subepidermal blistering disease, which again may show features of both bullous pemphigoid and dermatitis herpetiformis, many of the patients having neutrophilic microabscesses in the tips of the dermal papillae.[82] By direct IF staining the major feature of this disease process is shown to be a linear deposit of IgA (Fig. 7-3B) at the BMZ and/or dermal-epidermal junction; C3 deposits may also be apparent. In contrast to bullous pemphigoid, IgG deposits are not usually seen in this disease process, and in contrast to true dermatitis herpetiformis, in which the IgA deposits are in the tips of the dermal papillae, these deposits are linear and along the BMZ.

In addition, these patients do not have the HLA associations of true dermatitis herpetiformis nor do they have the histologic findings seen in patients with duodenal-jejunal atrophy.[82,83] By immuno-electron microscopy many of these patients demonstrate their IgA deposits at the lamina densa or below. Recent evidence suggests that these linear IgA deposits lack J chains and thus do not represent dimeric IgA as seen in true dermatitis herpetiformis.[84] Chorzelski et al.[82] have also shown that these patients do not have antiendomysium antibodies. Because of these differences, linear IgA bullous disease should be considered a distinct, separate bullous skin disease.

Chronic Bullous Disease of Childhood

Chronic bullous disease of childhood is an uncommon blistering dermatosis that affects primarily children of preschool age.[85] Of all the nonhereditary blistering diseases of childhood, this disease is probably one of the most common but is often misdiagnosed.[86] It has long been confused with other nonhereditary bullous skin diseases of children such as bullous pemphigoid, dermatitis herpetiformis, and erythema multiforme,[87] but IF data now allow us to consider chronic bullous disease of childhood as a distinct, separate clinical entity.

Three distinct clinical lesions characterize this disease process: large, tense bullae, as seen in bullous pemphigoid; grouped vesicles, as seen in dermatitis herpetiformis; or annular bullous lesions, as seen in erythema multiforme. One lesion type may predominate, or combinations of the three may occur in the same patient. Bullae may arise on normal-appearing skin or on erythematous bases. The mucous membranes are usually not involved.

Common areas that are involved include the inner thighs, the groin and pelvic areas, and the central facial areas, especially around the mouth. Lesions, however, may be widespread. Itching may be severe, leading to numerous excoriations, or it may be entirely absent. The course of chronic bullous disease of childhood is marked by periodic remissions, with decreasingly severe exacerbations. The disease does not persist into the teens or adult life, a feature that separates this condition from true bullous pemphigoid, dermatitis herpetiformis, and the linear IgA bullous disease of adults.

By routine histopathology blistering skin lesions in this disease process show subepidermal bulla formation, with an inflammatory infiltrate of eosinophils and/or neutrophils. Microabscesses, as seen in dermatitis herpetiformis, may occasionally be present. Most lesions, however, are histologically similar to those present in bullous pemphigoid.

Early studies using IF methods were inconclusive. Negative IF findings in chronic bullous dermatosis of childhood, however, differed from positive IF findings in true bullous pemphigoid and dermatitis herpetiformis of childhood.[85,87] Linear BMZ deposits of IgA and C3 have been found in perilesional skin of children affected with this condition in recent years.[86,88,89] This IgA pattern is dissimilar to that of the IgA deposits noted in dermatitis herpetiformis but similar to those of the adult IgA linear bullous disease. By immuno-electron microscopy most of these IgA deposits appear in the lamina lucida region of the BMZ.[90,91] Circulating autoantibodies have yet to be identified in this condition. The etiology of chronic bullous disease of childhood remains obscure.

OTHER IMMUNOBULLOUS DISEASES

Erythema Multiforme

Erythema multiforme is an acute, erythematous inflammatory process with a variety of clinical presentations. Erythematous papules, plaques, macular erythema, bullous lesions, and the typical target lesions may be apparent. Extreme malaise may accompany the cutaneous manifestations. A severe variant of this disease process, called Stevens-Johnson syndrome, can occur, and affected patients often have extensive involvement of mucous membranes.

Erythema multiforme is thought to represent a reaction pattern in the skin rather than a specific disease per se. Thus, it may be associated with a wide variety of underlying causes. Infections, drugs, malignancies, and exposure to chemicals and a variety of other noxious substances have all been implicated.[92] Infections are perhaps the most common associations and include those caused by bacteria, fungi, mycoplasma, and a variety of viruses. The most common viral illness associated with erythema multiforme and the major cause of recurrent episodes is preceding herpes simplex infection.[93] In a small prospective study of such patients, an increased incidence of HLA-B15 was found when compared with controls.[94] Thus, a genetic predisposition to recurrent episodes of herpes simplex infection associated with erythema multiforme seems to be present. Interestingly, it has been recently shown that oral acyclovir is helpful in patients with recurring episodes of herpes-associated erythema multiforme.[95] Milker's nodules, infectious mononucleosis, and infections with enteroviruses such as coxsackie and echo are other virus-associated illnesses that can result in erythema multiforme.

Histopathologically, subepidermal bulla formation may also be apparent in lesions of erythema multiforme (Tabel 7-4). Vacuolar and necrotic degeneration of the cells, leading to epidermal necrosis, are distinctive histopathologic features.[96] An infiltrate composed of lymphocytes may also be present.

The cause of erythema multiforme is not known. Evidence suggesting that the condition is at least in part mediated by immune complex

---

Table 7-4. Approach to the Patient: Diagnostic Features of Other Immunobullous Diseases

	Clinical Features	Histology	Immunopathology
Erythema multiforme	Target lesions	Subepidermal blister Necrotic keratinocytes	Deposits of IgM and C3 in walls of superficial vessels
Epidermolysis bullosa acquisita	Scarring vesiculobullous lesions Milia and skin fragility Acral distribution	Subepidermal blister	Perilesional skin: linear IgG and C3 in basement membrane zone (BMZ) (below lamina densa) Serum anti-BMZ antibodies
Bullous lupus erythematosus	Patients with systemic lupus erythematosus More common in blacks	Subepidermal blister Mucin in upper dermis Mixed infiltrate with neutrophils	Granular deposits of IgG and IgM at dermal-epidermal junction

formation and subsequent deposition has been presented by several investigators. Deposition of IgM, C3, and fibrin in the superficial microvasculature of skin lesions of erythema multiforme has been demonstrated.[97–99] In addition to the IF studies, circulating immune complexes have been detected in a high percentage of erythema multiforme patients by a variety of detection methods.[97–99] Blister fluids of these patients also appear to contain immune complex-like materials.[100] In a study performed by us at least some of the immune complexes were of rather large size.[98] Although one study has suggested that these circulating immune complexes might contain herpes simplex antigens,[101] these studies have never been confirmed or extended.

Evidence presented by Orton et al.,[102] however, suggests that herpes simplex viral antigen is present in skin lesions of erythema multiforme. Fritz et al.[103] have shown that erythema multiforme serum will support herpes simplex-specific cellular cytotoxicity reactions. It is possible that herpes simplex-containing epidermal cells may become targets for antibody-dependent cellular cytotoxicity, resulting in lesions of erythema multiforme.

Epidermolysis Bullosa Acquisita

Epidermolysis bullosa acquisita is a nonhereditary subepidermal blistering dermatosis with distinctive clinical, histopathologic, and immunopathologic findings.[104] The disease clinically may mimic bullous pemphigoid, but milia, scarring, and skin fragility, particularly in an acral distribution, appear to be distinctive features. Unlike the hereditary forms of epidermolysis bullosa, this disease has its onset during adulthood. Other blistering dermatoses and porphyria cutanea tarda must be excluded before a diagnosis of epidermolysis bullosa acquisita can be entertained.

By routine histopathology, lesions of epidermolysis bullosa acquisita demonstrate subepidermal blister formation with or without mild inflammation. When inflammation is apparent, it usually consists of an infiltrate of neutrophils.[105] By direct IF staining, linear IgG (Fig. 7-4) and C3 deposits are shown to be present in the BMZ of perilesional skin, as in bullous pemphigoid. Unlike the situation in bullous pemphigoid, however, these immune deposits are found within the BMZ immediately below the lamina densa. In addition, these pa-

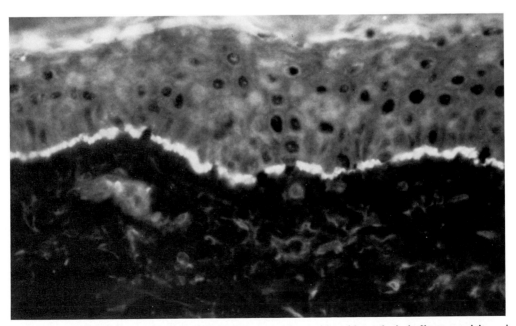

Fig. 7-4. Direct IF staining of perilesional skin from a patient with epidermolysis bullosa acquisita using labeled antiserum to human IgG. (Original magnification × 400.)

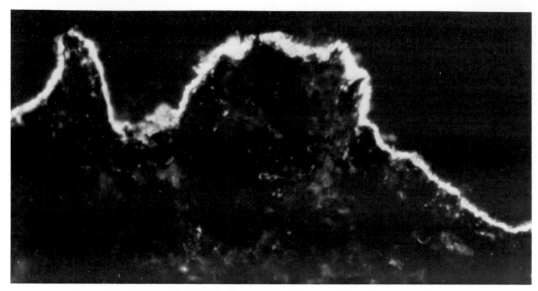

Fig. 7-5. Direct IF staining of perilesional skin from a patient with the bullous eruption of systemic lupus erythematosus using labeled antiserum to human IgM. (Original magnification × 400.)

tients have circulating antibodies reactive with the BMZ, which also react with antigens located below the lamina densa.[106,107] These antibodies have been shown to be capable of complement fixation and will attract neutrophils to this anatomic area.[108] Thus, epidermolysis bullosa acquisita is clearly a distinct, separate subepidermal blistering disease with characteristic immunologic features.

On the basis of these findings Woodley and Gammon[104] have recently proposed specific criteria for the diagnosis of epidermolysis bullosa acquisita. These include (1) separation of the blister below the lamina densa; (2) the presence of IgG antibodies directed against a sublamina densa antigen; (3) IgG and C3 deposits immediately below the lamina densa; (4) milia formation; (5) scar formation; (6) lack of family history for blistering diseases; and (7) adult onset of the disease process.

Bullous Lupus Erythematosus

Bullous lesions are an uncommon cutaneous manifestation of systemic lupus erythematosus (SLE). When present, they are often misdiag-

nosed as another blistering skin disease such as bullous pemphigoid, erythema multiforme, or dermatitis herpetiformis. To add to the confusion, concurrences of some of these bullous diseases with SLE have been well documented. Recent reports, however, have documented patients who, while undergoing an exacerbation of their SLE, developed vesiculobullous lesions.[67,109] This author has recently seen two patients at our institution who developed similar lesions with a severe flare of their SLE.

Several features of this form of SLE are worthy of note. When blistering lesions develop, they often appear in a herpetiform configuration. They tend to be more common in blacks and most often are associated with a severe flare of SLE. By routine histopathology lesions of bullous SLE bear striking resemblance to lesions of dermatitis herpetiformis. By direct IF, however, granular deposits of IgG and IgM (Fig. 7-5), rather than IgA, are present at the dermal-epidermal junction.[67] Interestingly, some of these patients respond to dapsone therapy. In our experience, however, these lesions usually clear with the administration of systemic corticosteroids needed to treat the severe exacerbation of the SLE. Recently, some of these patients have been shown to have anti-sublamina densa antibodies, which suggests a relationship to patients with epidermolysis bullosa acquisita.[110]

REFERENCES

1. Ahmed AR, Graham J, Jordon RE, Provost TT: Pemphigus: current concepts. Ann Intern Med 92:396, 1980
2. Meurer M, Millns JL, Rogers RS III, Jordon RE: Oral pemphigus vulgaris: a report of ten cases. Arch Dermatol 113:1520, 1977
3. Lever WF: Pemphigus and Bullous Pemphigoid. Charles C. Thomas, Springfield, IL., 1965
4. Emmerson RW, Wilson-Jones E: Eosinophilic spongiosis in pemphigus: a report of an unusual histologic change in pemphigus. Arch Dermatol 97:252, 1968
5. Hashimoto K, Lever WF: An electron microscopic study of pemphigus vulgaris of the mouth and skin with special reference to the intercellular cement. J Invest Dermatol 48:540, 1967
6. Perry HO, Brunsting LA: Pemphigus foliaceus: further observations. Arch Dermatol 91:10, 1965
7. Beutner EH, Chorzelski TP, Jordon RE: Autosensitization in Pemphigus and Bullous Pemphigoid. Charles C Thomas, Springfield, IL., 1970
8. Senear FE, Usher B: An unusual type of pemphigus combining features of lupus erythematosus. Arch Dermatol 13:761, 1926
9. Chorzelski TP, Jablonska S, Blaczcyzk M: Immunopathologic investigations in the Senear-Usher syndrome (coexistence of pemphigus and lupus erythematosus). Br J Dermatol 80:211, 1968
10. Beutner EH, Chorzelski TP, Hale WL, Hausmanowa-Petruzewiez L: Autoimmunity in concurrent myasthenia gravis and pemphigus erythematosus. JAMA 203:845, 1968
11. Maize JC, Dobson RL, Provost TT: Pemphigus and myasthenia gravis. Arch Dermatol 111:1334, 1975
12. Degos R, Tourraine R, Beliach S, Revus J: Pemphigus chez un malade traité pour maladie de Wilson. Bull Soc Fr Dermatol Syphilis 76:751, 1969
13. Santa Cruz DJ, Marcus MD, Prioleau PG, Uitto J: Pemphigus-like lesions induced by D-penicillamine: analysis of clinical, histopathologic and immunofluorescence features of 34 cases. Am J Dermatopathol 3:85, 1981
14. Beutner EH, Jordon RE: Demonstration of skin antibodies in sera of pemphigus vulgaris patients by indirect immunofluorescence staining. Proc Soc Exp Biol Med 117:505, 1964
15. Jordon RE, Kawana S, Fritz KA: Immunopathologic mechanisms in pemphigus and bullous pemphigoid. J Invest Dermatol 85:72s, 1985
16. Stanley JR, Kowler L, Thivolet L: Distinction between epidermal antigens binding pemphigus vulgaris and pemphigus foliaceus autoantibodies. J Clin Invest 74:313, 1984
17. Diaz LA, Marcelo CL: Pemphigoid and pemphigus antigens in cultured epidermal cells. Br J Dermatol 98:631, 1978
18. Woo TY, Hogan VA, Patel H, et al: Specificity and inhibition of the epidermal cell detachment induced by pemphigus IgG in vitro. J Invest Dermatol 81:115s, 1983
19. Jordon RE, Schroeter AL, Rogers RS III, Perry HO: Classical and alternate pathway activation of complement in pemphigus vulgaris lesions. J Invest Dermatol 63:256, 1974
20. Schiltz JR, Michel B, Papay R: Pemphigus antibody interaction with human epidermal cells in culture: a proposed mechanism for pemphigus acantholysis. J Clin Invest 62:778, 1978
21. Farb RM, Dykes R, Lazarus GS: Antiepidermal cell surface pemphigus antibody detaches viable epidermal cells from culture plates by activation of proteinase. Proc Natl Acad Sci USA 75:459, 1978
22. Singer KH, Sawka NJ, Samowitz HR, Lazarus GS: Proteinase activation: a mechanism for cellular dyshesion in pemphigus. J Invest Dermatol 81:115s, 1980
23. Hashimoto K, Shafran KM, Webber PS, Singer KH: Anti-cell surface pemphigus autoantibody stimulates plasminogen activator activity of human epidermal cells. A mechanism for loss of cohesion and blister formation. J Exp Med 157:259, 1983
24. Kawana S, Janson M, Jordon RE: Complement fixation by pemphigus antibody. I. In vitro fixation to organ and tissue culture skin. J Invest Dermatol 82:506, 1984
25. Kawana S, Geoghegan WD, Jordon RE: Com-

plement fixation by pemphigus antibody. II. Complement enhanced detachment of epidermal cells. Clin Exp Immunol 61:517, 1985

26. Kawana S, Geoghegan WD, Jordon RE: Complement fixation by pemphigus antibody. III. Altered epidermal cell membrane integrity mediated by pemphigus antibody and complement. J Invest Dermatol 86:29, 1986

27. Anhalt GJ, Labib RS, Voorhees JJ, et al: Induction of pemphigus in neonatal mice by passive transfer of IgG from patients with the disease. N Engl J Med 306:1189, 1982

28. Bean SF, Jordon RE: Chronic nonhereditary blistering disease in children. Arch Dermatol 110:941, 1974

29. Stone SP, Schroeter AL: Bullous pemphigoid and associated malignant neoplasms. Arch Dermatol 111:991, 1975

30. Jordon RE, Beutner EH, Witebsky E, et al: Basement membrane zone antibodies in bullous pemphigoid. JAMA 200:751, 1967

31. Jordon RE, Nordby JM, Milstein H: The complement system in bullous pemphigoid. III. Fixation of C1q and C4 by pemphigus antibody. J Lab Clin Med 86:733, 1975

32. Jordon RE, Nordby-MacFarland JM, Tappeiner G: The complement system in bullous pemphigoid. V. In vitro fixation of properdin by pemphigoid antibody. J Clin Lab Immunol 1:59, 1978

33. Provost TT, Tomasi TB Jr: Immunopathology of bullous pemphigoid: basement membrane deposition of IgE, alternate pathway components and fibrin. Clin Exp Immunol 18:193, 1974

34. Jordon RE, Schroeter AL, Good RA, Day NK: The complement system in bullous pemphigoid. II. Immunofluorescent evidence for both classic and alternate pathway activation. Clin Immunol Immunopathol 3:307, 1975

35. Holubar K, Wolff K, Konrad K, Beutner EH: Ultrastructure localization of immunoglobulins in bullous pemphigoid skin. J Invest Dermatol 64:220, 1975

36. Schmidt-Ulrich B, Rule A, Schamberg-Lever G, Lablac C: Ultrastructural localization of in vivo bound complement in bullous pemphigoid. J Invest Dermatol 65:217, 1976

37. Diaz LA, Calvanico NJ, Tomasi TB Jr, Jordon RE: Bullous pemphigoid antigen: isolation from normal human skin. J Immunol 118:455, 1977

38. Stanley JR, Woodley DT, Katz SI: Identification and partial characterization of pemphigoid antigen extracted from normal human skin. J Invest Dermatol 82:108, 1984

39. Zhu XJ, Bystryn JC: Heterogeneity of pemphigoid antigens. J Invest Dermatol 80:16, 1983

40. Mutasim DF, Takahashi Y, Labib RS, et al: A pool of bullous pemphigoid antigen(s) is intracellular and associated with the basal cell cytoskeleton-hemidesmosome complex. J Invest Dermatol 84:47, 1985

41. Jordon RE, Day NK, Sams WM Jr, Good RA: The complement system in bullous pemphigoid. I. Complement and component levels in sera and blister fluids. J Clin Invest 52:1207, 1973

42. Diaz-Perez JL, Jordon RE: The complement system in bullous pemphigoid. IV. Chemotactic activity in blister fluid. Clin Immunol Immunopathol 5:360, 1976

43. Gammon WR, Merritt CC, Lewis DM, et al: An in vitro model of immune complex mediated basement membrane zone separation caused by antibodies, leukocytes and complement. J Invest Dermatol 78:285, 1982

44. Jordon RE, Struve MF, Bushkell LL: Serum and blister fluid immuno complexes in bullous pemphigoid: detection with C1q and monoclonal rheumatoid factor. Clin Exp Immunol 45:129, 1981

45. Bird P, Friedmann PS, Ling N, et al: Subclass distribution of IgG autoantibodies in bullous pemphigoid. J Invest Dermatol 86:21, 1986

46. Baba T, Sonozaki H, Seki K, et al: An eosinophilic chemotactic factor present in blister fluids of bullous pemphigoid patients. J Immunol 116:112, 1976

47. Arbesman CE, Wypych JI, Reisman RE, Beutner EH: IgE levels in sera of patients with pemphigus and bullous pemphigoid. Arch Dermatol 110:378, 1974

48. Wintroub BU, Mihm MC Jr, Geotzl EJ, et al: Morphologic and functional evidence for release of mast-cell products in bullous pemphigoid. N Engl J Med 298:417, 1978

49. Mogavero HS Jr, Meier HS, Newball HH: Enzymatic activity in bullous pemphigoid blister fluid. Clin Res 30:598A, 1982

50. Hertz KC, Katz SI, Maize J, Ackerman AB: Herpes gestationis: a clinicopathologic study. Arch Dermatol 112:1543, 1976

51. Lawley TJ, Stingl G, Katz SI: Fetal and mater-

nal risk factors in herpes gestationis. Arch Dermatol 114:552, 1978

52. Shornick JK, Stastny P, Gilliam JN: High frequency of histocompatability antigens HLA-DR3 and DR4 in herpes gestationis. J Clin Invest 68:553, 1981

53. Schamberg-Lever G, Saffold OE, Orfanos CE, Lever WF: Herpes gestationis: histology and ultrastructure. Arch Dermatol 107:888, 1973

54. Jordon RE, Heine KG, Tappeiner G, et al: The immunopathology of herpes gestationis: immunofluorescence studies and characterization of HG factor. J Clin Invest 57:1426, 1976

55. Katz SI, Hertz KC, Yaoita H: Herpes gestationis. Immunopathology and characterization of HG factor. J Clin Invest 57:1434, 1976

56. Carruthers JA, Ewins AR: Herpes gestationis: studies on the binding characteristics, activity and pathogenetic significance of the complement-fixing factor. Clin Exp Immunol 31:38, 1978

57. Chorzelski TP, Jablonska S, Beutner EH, et al: Herpes gestationis with identical lesions in the newborn. Arch Dermatol 112:1129, 1976

58. Honigsman J, Stingl G, Holubar K, Wolff K: Herpes gestationis: fine structural pattern of immunoglobulin deposits in the skin in vivo. J Invest Dermatol 66:389, 1976

59. Hardy KM, Perry HO, Pingree GC, Kirby TJ Jr: Benign mucous membrane pemphigoid. Arch Dermatol 104:467, 1971

60. Shklar G, McCarthy P: Oral lesions of mucous membrane pemphigoid. Otolaryngology 93:354, 1971

61. Michel B, Bean SF, Chorzelski TP, Fedele CF: Cicatricial pemphigoid of Brunsting-Perry. Arch Dermatol 113:1403, 1977

62. Fine JD, Neises GR, Katz SI: Immunofluorescence and immunoelectron microscopic studies in cicatricial pemphigoid. J Invest Dermatol 82:39, 1984

63. Bean SF: Cicatricial pemphigoid. Immunofluorescent studies. Arch Dermatol 110:552, 1974

64. Holubar K, Honigsmann H, Wolff K: Cicatricial pemphigoid: immunofluorescence investigations. Arch Dermatol 108:50, 1973

65. Rogers RS III, Perry HO, Bean SF, Jordon RE: Immunopathology of cicatricial pemphigoid: studies of complement deposition. J Invest Dermatol 68:39, 1977

66. Pierard J, Whimster I: The histological diagnosis of dermatitis herpetiformis, erythema multi-forme and bullous pemphigoid. Br J Dermatol 73:253, 1961

67. Hall RP, Lawley TJ, Smith HR, Katz SI: Bullous eruption of systemic lupus erythematosus: dramatic response to dapsone therapy. Ann Intern Med 97:165, 1982

68. Marks J, Shuster S, Watson A: Small bowel changes in dermatitis herpetiformis. Lancet 2:1280, 1966

69. Katz SI, Strober W: The pathogenesis of dermatitis herpetiformis. J Invest Dermatol 70:63, 1978

70. van der Meer JB: Granular deposits of immunoglobulins in the skin of patients with dermatitis herpetiformis: an immunofluorescent study. Br J Dermatol 81:493, 1969

71. Hall RP, Lawley TJ: Characterization of circulating and cutaneous IgA immune complexes in patients with dermatitis herpetiformis. J Immunol 135:1760, 1985

72. Egelrud T, Back O: Dermatitis herpetiformis. Biochemical properties of the granular deposits of IgA in papillary dermis. Characterization of SDS-soluble IgA-like material and potentially antigen-binding IgA fragments. J Invest Dermatol 84:239, 1985

73. Hall RP, Lawley TJ, Jeck JA, Katz SI: IgA-containing circulating immune complexes in dermatitis herpetiformis, Henoch-Schönlein purpura, systemic lupus erythematosus and other diseases. Clin Exp Immunol 40:431, 1980

74. Zone JJ, LaSalle BA, Provost TT: Circulating immune complexes of IgA type in dermatitis herpetiformis. J Invest Dermatol 75:152, 1980

75. Jordon RE, Tappeiner G, Kohl JC, Wolff K: Dermatitis herpetiformis: immune complex detection with C1q and monoclonal rheumatoid factor. Br J Dermatol 105:159, 1981

76. Huff JC, Weston WL, Sirkes DK: Wheat protein antibodies in dermatitis herpetiformis. J Invest Dermatol 73:570, 1979

77. Zone JJ, LaSalle BA, Provost TT: Induction of IgA circulating immune complexes after wheat feeding in dermatitis herpetiformis. J Invest Dermatol 78:375, 1982

78. Lawley TJ, Hall RP, Fauci AS, et al: Defective Fc-receptor functions associated with the HLA-DRW3 haplotype: studies in patients with dermatitis herpetiformis and normal subjects. N Engl J Med 304:185, 1981

79. Lawley TJ, Strober W, Yaoita H, Katz SI: Small intestinal biopsies and HLA types in der-

matitis herpetiformis patients with granular and linear IgA skin deposits. J Invest Dermatol 74:9, 1980

80. Seah PP, Fry L, Hoffbraud AV, Holborow EJ: Tissue antibodies in dermatitis herpetiformis and adult celiac disease. Lancet 1:834, 1971

81. Lane AT, Huff JC, Zone JJ, Weston WL: Class-specific antibodies to gluten in dermatitis herpetiformis. J Invest Dermatol 80:402, 1983

82. Chorzelski TP, Beutner EH, Sulej J, et al: IgA anti-endomysium antibody. A new immunologic marker of dermatitis herpetiformis and celiac disease. Br J Dermatol 111:395, 1984

83. Smith SB, Harrist TJ, Murphy GF, et al: Linear IgA bullous dermatosis v dermatitis herpetiformis. Arch Dermatol 120:324, 1984

84. Leonard JN, Haffenden GP, Unsworth DJ, et al: Evidence that the IgA in patients with linear IgA disease is qualitatively different from that of patients with dermatitis herpetiformis. Br J Dermatol 110:315, 1984

85. Jordon RE, Bean SF, Triftshauser CT, Winkelmann RK: Childhood bullous dermatitis herpetiformis: negative immunofluorescent tests. Arch Dermatol 101:629, 1970

86. Esterly NB, Furey NL, Kirschner BS, et al: Chronic bullous dermatosis of childhood. Arch Dermatol 13:42, 1977

87. Bean SF, Jordon RE: Chronic non-hereditary blistering diseases in children. Arch Dermatol 110:941, 1974

88. McGuire J, Norlund J: Bullous disease of childhood. Arch Dermatol 108:284, 1973

89. Prystowsky S, Gillian JN: Benign chronic bullous dermatosis of childhood: linear IgA and C3 deposition on the basement membrane. Arch Dermatol 112:837, 1976

90. Dabrowski J, Chorzelski TP, Jablonska S, et al: The ultrastructural localization of IgA deposits in chronic bullous disease of childhood. J Invest Dermatol 72:291, 1979

91. Ahmed AR, Moy R: Chronic bullous dermatosis of childhood. Am J Dis Child 136:214, 1982

92. Tonnesen MG, Soter NA: Erythema multiforme. J Am Acad Dermatol 1:357, 1979

93. Howland WW, Golitz LE, Weston WL, Huff JC: Erythema multiforme: clinical, histopathologic and immunologic study. J Am Acad Dermatol 10:438, 1984

94. Duvic M, Reisner EG, Dawson DV, Ciftan E: HLA-B15 association with erythema multiforme. J Am Acad Dermatol 8:493, 1983

95. Lemak MA, Duvic M, Bean SF: Oral acyclovir for the prevention of herpes-associated erythema multiforme. J Am Acad Dermatol 15:50, 1986

96. Ackerman AB, Penneys NS, Clark WS: Erythema multiforme exudativum. Br J Dermatol 84:554, 1971

97. Wuepper KD, Watson PA, Kazmierowski JA: Immune complexes in erythema multiforme and the Stevens-Johnson syndrome. J Invest Dermatol 74:368, 1980

98. Bushkell LL, Mackel SE, Jordon RE: Erythema multiforme: direct immunofluorescent studies and detection of circulating immune complexes. J Invest Dermatol 74:372, 1980

99. Huff JC, Weston WL, Carr RI: Mixed cryoglobulinemia: I^{125}-C1q binding and skin immunofluorescence in erythema multiforme. J Invest Dermatol 74:375, 1980

100. Safai B, Good RA, Day NK: Erythema multiforme: report of two cases and speculation of immune mechanisms involved in the pathogenesis. Clin Immunol Immunopathol 7:379, 1977

101. Kazmierowski JA, Peizner DS, Wuepper KD: Herpes simplex antigen in immune complexes of patients with erythema multiforme. Presence following recurrent herpes simplex infection. JAMA 2457, 1982

102. Orton PW, Huff JC, Tonnesen MG, Weston WL: Detection of a herpes simplex viral antigen in skin lesions of erythema multiforme. Ann Intern Med 101:48, 1984

103. Fritz KA, Norris DA, Ryan SR, et al: Herpes specific cellular cytotoxicity induced by erythema multiforme serum. (Abstract) J Invest Dermatol 78:343, 1982

104. Woodley DT, Gammon WR: Epidermolysis bullosa acquisita: an autoimmune disease with distinctive immunoultrastructural features. Cutis 32:521

105. Gammon WR, Briggaman RA, Wheeler CE: Epidermolysis bullosa acquisita presenting as an inflammatory bullous disease. J Am Acad Dermatol 7:382, 1982

106. Neibor C, Boorsma DM, Woerdman MJ, Kalsbeek GL: Epidermolysis bullosa acquisita: immunofluorescence, electron microscopic and immunoelectron microscopic studies in four patients. Br J Dermatol 102:383, 1980

107. Yaoita H, Briggaman RA, Lawley TJ, et al: Epidermolysis bullosa acquisita: ultrastructural

and immunologic studies. J Invest Dermatol 76:288, 1981

108. Gammon WR, Inman AO III, Wheeler CE: Differences in complement-dependent chemotactic activity generated by bullous pemphigoid and epidermolysis bullosa acquisita immune complexes: demonstration by leukocyte attachment and organ culture methods. J Invest Dermatol 83:57, 1984

109. Pennys NS, Wiley HE III: Herpetiform blisters in systemic lupus erythematosus. Arch Dermatol 115:1427, 1979

110. Gammon WR, Woodley DR, Dole KC, Briggaman RA: Anti-basement membrane zone antibodies in bullous eruption of systemic lupus erythematosus recognize epidermolysis bullosa acquisita autoantigen. (Abstract). J Invest Dermatol 84:288, 1985

8

Fever and Rash

Michael Fisher
Susan Katz

In the febrile patient with a rash, the physician is liable to consider a multiplicity of possible diseases, and a methodical approach to diagnosis may be elusive. As the dilemma is a clinical one and bedside scrutiny is the first, and sometimes the only, diagnostic tool employed, we have proposed a simple plan of organization based primarily on the morphology of the rash, i.e., on erythematous, purpuric, and vesicopustular reaction patterns. Each category may be further divided into infectious and noninfectious etiologies, with emphasis again laid upon the distinctive appearance of the rash as well as the mode of presentation and outstanding laboratory features of each specific entity.

The overall scheme is as it appears in Table 8-1. It is our hope that such a basic analysis will enable the clinician to weigh the differential diagnosis with greater confidence.[1-7]

ERYTHEMATOUS ERUPTIONS (TABLE 8-2)

Infectious Disorders

VIRAL INFECTIONS

Erythema Infectiosum

Erythema infectiosum (fifth disease) is an acute viral infection characterized initially by a ''slapped cheek'' appearance and later by a reticulate erythema of the extremities and trunk; there is usually no associated morbidity.

Etiology. Recently, a parvovirus (single-stranded DNA) was implicated in an epidemic of an erythema infectiosum-like illness. However, the associated slapped cheek and reticulate erythema were less pronounced; palms and

Table 8-1. Approach to the Patient: Differential Diagnosis of Fever and Rash

Erythematous eruptions
  Infectious disorders
    Viral infections
      Erythema infectiosum
      Measles (rubeola)
      Rubella
      Roseola infantum
      Enteroviruses
      Infectious mononucleosis
      Hepatitis B
    Bacterial infections
      Scarlet fever
      Toxic shock syndrome
      Secondary syphilis
      Lyme disease
  Noninfectious disorders
    Kawasaki's disease
    Erythema multiforme
    Erythema marginatum
    Juvenile rheumatoid arthritis
    Systemic lupus erythematosus
    Drug reactions

Purpuric eruptions
  Infectious disorders
    Viral infections
      Atypical measles
      Echovirus 9
      TORCHS
    Rickettsial infections
      Rocky Mountain spotted fever
      Epidemic typhus
    Bacterial infections
      Meningococcemia
      Gonococcemia
      Staphylococcal sepsis
      Pseudomonas sepsis
      Subacute bacterial endocarditis
  Noninfectious disorders
    Allergic vasculitis—Henoch-Schönlein purpura
    Drug reactions

Vesicopustular eruptions
  Infectious disorders
    Viral infections
      Herpes simplex
      Varicella and herpes zoster
      Kaposi's varicelliform eruption
      Variola
      Hand-foot-and-mouth disease
      Enterovirus
    Rickettsial infections
      Rickettsialpox
    Bacterial infections
      Staphylococcal scalded skin syndrome
      Congenital syphilis
  Noninfectious disorders
    Drug reactions

soles were often involved, and upper respiratory symptoms were more pronounced. Thus, the definitive cause of erythema infectiosum has yet to be shown but is presumably viral.

Epidemiology. In 80 percent of cases the patients are below age 15; most are 2 to 12 years old. The disease is mildly contagious, with clusters of cases mostly within households; there is an increased incidence in winter and early spring.

Course. The incubation period is 7 to 28 days, with an average of 16 days. Occasionally there is a mild 1- to 2-day prodrome with low-grade fever (up to 100°F), malaise, and occasionally nausea, vomiting, and diarrhea.

The initial major sign is the acute onset of marked malar erythema with or without circumoral pallor, mimicking sunburn or slapped cheeks. This erythema begins as 3- to 5-mm blanching, pinpoint, red papules, which rapidly coalesce to form asymptomatic warm, red, often edematous plaques with palpable borders. Other discrete erythematous macules or papules may be found on the chin or forehead or behind the ears. Fading of the facial erythema usually occurs in 4 to 5 days.

The secondary eruption presents in 1 to 4 days with blanching, occasionally pruritic, erythematous macules and/or papules on the extensor arms and thighs; it then spreads to the flexural and distal extremities and at times to the buttocks and trunk. The initial lesions fade in their centers and coalesce to form a characteristic reticulate network. On the average, total fading occurs in 10 to 11 days. Importantly, the rash may be reactivated by sunlight, heat, cold, friction, and exertion. There is no enanthem.

During the rash, the child is classically asymptomatic but there may be mild fever or malaise; arthralgias and arthritis are more common in adults. The course is very rarely complicated by pneumonitis, encephalopathy, or hemolytic anemia. No congenital defects due to infection during pregnancy have been reported.

Table 8-2. Approach to the Patient: Clinical and Laboratory Features of Generalized Erythematous Eruptions Associated with Fever

Disorder	Clinical Features	Laboratory
Erythema infectiosum	Children; "slapped cheeks"	
Measles	Cough, coryza, conjunctivitis, Koplik's spots	Sputum smears (Warthin-Finkeldey cells); acute and convalescent titers
Rubella	Tender lymphadenopathy, Forschheimer spots	Acute and convalescent titers
Roseola	Children; rash follows fever	
Viral exanthems	Occasional enanthem; associated symptoms variable	Stool and oropharyngeal cultures; acute and convalescent titers
Infectious mononucleosis	Pharyngitis, adenopathy, splenomegaly, supraorbital edema	Lymphocytosis with atypical lymphocytes; heterophil/monospot
Hepatitis B	Jaundice, urticaria, erythema multiforme, palpable purpura, and papular acrodermatitis can occur	Hepatitis B surface antigen; elevated liver function tests; rising anti-HBc and anti-HBs antibody titers
Scarlet fever	Pharyngitis, strawberry tongue, Pastia's lines, desquamation of palms and soles	Culture of nose or throat; elevated antistreptolysin O (ASLO), streptozyme hemagglutination
Toxic shock syndrome	Tampon use or bacterial infection, hypotension, desquamation of palms and soles, gastrointestinal symptoms, neurologic symptoms	Elevated liver function tests, creatine phosphokinase, blood urea nitrogen, and creatinine; abnormal urinalysis; *Staphylococcus aureus* cultured from vagina or other source
Kawasaki's disease	Children; conjunctivitis, chapped lips, strawberry tongue, desquamation of palms and soles, cervical adenopathy; neurologic, gastrointestinal, and cardiovascular symptoms	Elevated platelets, white blood cells, and erythrocyte sedimentation rate; electrocardiographic abnormalities; infiltrates on chest x-ray
Drug reaction	History of drug ingestion	
Connective tissue diseases	Malar rash, discoid lesions, photosensitivity, mucosal ulcers, arthritis, muscle weakness, alopecia, Raynaud's phenomenon	Antinuclear antibodies, creatine phosphokinase, aldolase, blood urea nitrogen, creatinine, complement, rheumatoid factor, LE cell preparation, erythrocyte sedimentation rate, VDRL, urinalysis, skin biopsy, and immunofluorescence
Erythema multiforme (toxic epidermal necrolysis, Stevens-Johnson syndrome)	Preceding infection or drug; target lesions, mucosal lesions; diffuse erythema and erosions (TEN)	Skin biopsy; skin peel and Tzanck prep for toxic epidermal necrolysis
Secondary syphilis	Preceding chancre; condylomata lata, symptoms variable	VDRL, FTA; dark-field exam of non-intraoral lesions
Lyme disease	Endemic areas; preceding tick bite; annular lesions, arthritis, meningoencephalitis, myocarditis, neuropathy	Lyme disease serology; spirochetes on silver stain of skin biopsy

Diagnosis. Erythema infectiosum is distinguished by its clinical features from the other toxic erythemas, such as scarlet fever, rubella, enterovirus infections, systemic lupus erythematosus (SLE), and drug rashes. The diagnosis is strongly suggested by a slapped cheek appearance, which is followed by a reticulate erythema of the extremities and at times also the trunk and is exacerbated or recalled by sunlight, heat, and trauma, with minimal or nonexistent constitutional signs and symptoms. Routine laboratory examinations and skin biopsy are nondiagnostic; serologic and DNA hybridization examinations for parvovirus are not routinely available.

Treatment. Therapy is usually not needed except for occasional pruritus (antihistamines, shake lotions, colloidal baths). Isolation is not necessary.[8,9]

Measles

Measles (rubeola or first disease) is an acute, highly contagious disease (attack rate exceeds 90 percent) with a significant prodrome of fever, coryza, conjunctivitis, enanthem (Koplik's spots), and a characteristically progressive morbilliform rash. Morbidity due to viral involvement and/or secondary bacterial involvement is frequent and under conditions of poor nutrition and sanitation may lead to death (2 to 500 deaths per 100,000 cases). Significantly, this disease was thought to have been eradicated, but failure to completely vaccinate all populations has led to recent epidemics (e.g., in New Jersey, 800 cases reported in 1983 and more than 900 cases reported in 1986).

Etiology. The disease is due to a paramyxovirus (RNA).

Epidemiology. Droplet or fomite spread leads to the initial invasion of the respiratory or conjunctival epithelium. There is no known carrier state. The disease is endemic throughout the year, but the peak incidence is in the dry early spring. (Increased virion survival is associated with low humidity.) Crowded urban or primitive environments favor earlier exposure, usually by the age of 3 years; infection is rare under age 6 months owing to protective maternal antibody. Infectivity extends from the onset of the prodrome until 4 to 5 days after the appearance of the rash.

Course. The prodrome usually begins about 11 days after infection. The rash usually follows in 3 to 5 days, average 14 days, and viremia ends and constitutional symptoms begin to decrease 1 to 2 days after the onset of rash. Uncommonly, there may be transient mild malaise and faint rash before the prodrome.

The prodrome is marked by coryza, incessant barking cough (tracheobronchitis), keratoconjunctivitis, photophobia, prostration, chills, and high fever up to 104 to 105°F. The fever may be present for 1 to 2 days and then decrease for 1 day, to return with the onset of the rash. Frequently, there is generalized lymphadenopathy and splenomegaly. Nonspecific erythema or petechiae may be found on the soft palate. Later, Koplik's spots begin on the mucosa of the inner lip or the cheek opposite the lower molars as small, bright red erythematous macules with pinpoint bluish white centers. They can spread quickly throughout the mouth to give an appearance of grains of sand surmounting widespread erythema. Koplik's spots can sometimes be found on other mucosal surfaces, such as those of the conjunctiva, labia, and gastrointestinal tract. (Similar findings have been noted in echovirus 9 and coxsackievirus A16 infections.) The enanthem usually appears 1 to 2 days before the exanthem and fades by the latter's peak.

The rash proper begins with faint pink macules at the frontal hairline, in the scalp, and behind the ears. It then becomes morbilliform, extending in 3 days sequentially over the face, neck, and upper trunk and then the remainder of the trunk and extremities. As it progresses, the discrete lesions, particularly on the face, may coalesce. The color intensifies to a deep reddish blanching purple, which can be edematous. As the rash peaks, constitutional signs and symptoms, which are pronounced on days 2 and 3 of the rash, diminish. Fading occurs in the same progression as the onset of the rash, starting on the face. Some residual nonblanching reddish brown pigment may temporarily remain; this represents hemosiderin due to capillary hemorrhage. Fine branny desquamation may occur in conjunction with fading, sparing the distal extremities.

Unusual presentations of the rash include hemorrhagic ("black") measles, a rare and potentially fatal form of the disease characterized by hemorrhage into the skin and mucous membranes. Atypical measles, particularly that associated with previous administration of inactivated vaccine, is discussed separately below in connection with purpuric eruptions. Modified measles, marked by prolonged incubation (2 to 3 weeks), mild prodrome, and faint or absent rash, is seen in infants still partly protected by maternal antibodies or in naive persons receiving pooled globulin after exposure.

Complications can arise from viral infection, secondary bacterial infection, and hypersensitivity phenomena. Respiratory involvement is frequent, with 20 to 60 percent of patients' x-rays showing interstitial infiltrates and hilar node enlargement. Infants frequently suffer from viral bronchiolitis and croup. Bacterial pneumonia due to pneumococcus, hemophilus, streptococcus (group A hemolytic), and staphylococcus is the leading cause of death. Giant cell (Hecht's) pneumonitis is a fatal complication seen especially in the immunosuppressed (leukemics); it is difficult to distinguish from routine measles interstitial pneumonitis. Tuberculous disease is classically exacerbated; the purified protein derivative (PPD) reaction may be inhibited for 2 to 3 weeks. The central nervous system (CNS) may be involved in 1 or 2 per 1,000 cases, with encephalitis occurring even before the rash, during the rash, or days to weeks after the rash fades; it is unclear if this is an infectious or hypersensitivity condition. The encephalitis may be symptomatic or subclinical, with transient electroencephalographic changes and pleiocytosis of the cerebrospinal fluid (CSF). Of those affected, 5 to 10 percent die (particularly those under age 4 years); up to 35 percent have residual brain damage. Subacute measles encephalopathy, a fatal condition, is seen in some patients with depressed cellular immunity weeks to months after the initial infection. Subacute sclerosing panencephalopathy (SSPE) is a late complication especially associated with contraction of measles before age 2. Bacterial otitis media (hemophilus) is seen in up to 10 percent of cases. A viral punctate keratoconjunctivitis may persist for months. Viral myocarditis or pericarditis, often subclinical, may occur; up to one-third of patients may have transient electrocardiographic changes. Enteritis, if it occurs, is usually mild. Thrombocytopenic purpura due to peripheral platelet destruction, possibly on an immune basis, has been noted with live virus vaccination and rarely after natural infection; hemorrhage of mucous membrane surfaces usually ends after 1 to 2 weeks, but CNS bleeds may occur. Infection during pregnancy is not associated with birth defects but can cause fetal death or premature birth.

Pneumonia and encephalitis, particularly in the very young, lead to 1.2 deaths per 10,000 cases. Prognosis is poor for the immunosuppressed and the malnourished; otherwise the prognosis is good.

Diagnosis. The severity of the prodrome, the presence of Koplik's spots, and the distinctive intensity, progression, and time course of the rash help to distinguish measles from rubella, enterovirus infections, roseola, infectious mononucleosis, scarlet fever, and other diseases. The ameliorated course of modified measles may make diagnosis more difficult. Nasopharyngeal, sputum, and even urinary sediment smears stained with Giemsa or methylene blue reveal epithelial giant cells and multinucleated reticuloendothelial giant cells (Warthin-Finkeldey cells). Direct immunofluorescence of nasopharyngeal smears reveals viral antigen. Skin biopsy of the rash (Koplik's spots) can also show giant cells, as well as nonspecific focal parakeratosis, epidermal hyperplasia, focal spongiosis and intracellular edema, and occasional necrotic keratinocytes. The diagnosis is most specifically substantiated by serologic testing (neutralizing antibodies, complement fixation, hemagglutination, or enzyme-linked immunoabsorbent assay (ELISA)) of acute and convalescent (2 to 3 weeks) sera; a fourfold rise in titer is confirmational. Viral cultures of body fluids, secretions, and blood are not routinely available.

Treatment. In uncomplicated cases supportive therapy such as humidification of inspired air and room darkening suffice. Bacterial infections are treated as indicated by smears and cultures. The role of steroids in treating thrombocytopenic purpura and CNS complications is unclear. Active cases should be isolated until 5 days after the onset of the rash. Prevention is most important. Vaccination with live attenuated virus (but not before 15 months of age) should be almost universal, even for those previously immunized with killed vaccine; exceptions should be made, however, for the immunocompromised (candidates for killed, inactivated vaccine), pregnant women, and persons with untreated tuberculosis or severe febrile illness or who have received blood products within the previous 12 weeks. To ameliorate the course and prevent complications, exposed naive hosts should be given gamma globulin (0.05 ml/kg up to 6 days after exposure; 0.1 ml/kg 6 to 9 days after exposure.)[10]

Rubella

Rubella (also known as German measles, three-day measles, and third disease) is a mild, moderately contagious disease with minimal prodromal illness, a morbilliform rash characteristically milder and briefer than that of measles, and tender posterior auricular and suboccipital nodes. Of the greatest significance is the congenital rubella syndrome, in which many defects may arise following infection in pregnancy.

Etiology. The infection is due to a togavirus (RNA). Although the clinical and epidemio-

logical aspects of rubella resemble paramyxovirus infections, the togavirus is antigenically distinct.

Epidemiology. Infection is by droplet spread; prolonged close contact is usually required (unlike the highly contagious measles). The period of greatest infectivity ranges from 5 days before to 5 days after the appearance of the rash, although virus can be found in secretions from as early as 13 days before to 21 days after the rash. (Subclinical disease is also contagious.) Since it is not markedly contagious, the majority of people susceptible are over age 15 years, with clusters in college, military, and hospital settings. More cases are seen in the spring. The incidence since the introduction of the vaccine in 1969 is 0.4 per 100,000; 10 to 15 percent of women of childbearing age are susceptible.

Course. The incubation period averages 18 (12 to 23) days; a prodrome lasting 1 to 5 days is marked by conjunctivitis with eye pain, mild sore throat, headache, low-grade fever, chills, aches, cough, anorexia, and nausea. Characteristic tender lymphadenopathy (posterior auricular, posterior cervical, and suboccipital; occasionally generalized) may precede the rash by as much as 10 days, peak with the rash, and recede in 1 week (rarely, months). Forschheimer spots (petechiae on the soft palate) are seen just before or with the rash in up to 20 percent of cases; a similar enanthem may be seen in scarlet fever, roseola, infectious mononucleosis, and other infections. As the rash appears, symptoms abate, although mild fever may persist. Discrete, even pinpoint, occasionally pruritic blanching pink papules and macules first appear on the face and then extend over the trunk and extremities in a day, sometimes in hours. By the end of day 2 the rash may be confluent on the trunk and already fading from the face. By day 3 fading has usually proceeded downwards, leaving a fine desquamation, mainly centrally. Many cases are atypical in the presentation of the prodrome, rash, or adenopathy; the entire course may be subclinical, or one or more features, e.g., rash, may be very muted.

Complications include neurologic findings such as acute encephalitis (1 in 6000 cases; 20 percent mortality), ascending polyneuritis, and the rare progressive rubella parencephalitis seen in chronic rubella infections originally acquired in the fetal or neonatal period. Joint involvement, more commonly seen in adult females (up to one-third), includes arthralgia or arthritis of fingers, wrists, or knees; it may resemble rheumatic fever, and an elevated erythrocyte sedimentation rate (ESR) and positive rheumatoid factor may be found. However, no neutrophils are present in the joint fluid, and joint symptoms resolve in 2 to 30 days. Rarely, particularly in children, a transient thrombocytopenia may result in hemorrhage of the skin and mucous membranes, beginning a few days after the onset of rash and persisting for up to 2 weeks. Rarely, myocarditis and pericarditis may occur.

The greatest complication is the congenital rubella syndrome, usually noted for the triad of cataracts, deafness, and heart disease, but also including low birth weight, microcephaly, mental retardation, microphthalmia, buphthalmos, hypospadias, club foot, and many other multisystemic defects. Of particular dermatologic concern is the "blueberry muffin" appearance of the newborn caused by dermal (extramedullary) hematopoiesis or thrombocytopenia (see discussion of the TORCHS syndrome below). Infection incurred in the first 12 weeks results in defects in 90 percent of surviving infants; 50 percent are at risk during the second trimester, and the risk diminishes greatly in the third trimester. Viral shedding in the affected infant may persist for more than 2 years, with potential infectivity lasting up to 18 months.

With the exception of the congenital rubella syndrome and rare CNS complications, the prognosis is excellent.

Diagnosis. Diagnosis may be difficult, except during epidemics, owing to the prevalence of mild, atypical, and subclinical cases. Clinically, rubella is milder and more rapid in its course and resolution than measles. The pronounced adenopathy may at times help to distinguish rubella from more common viral infections (e.g., enterovirus). With respect to the adenopathy and even occasionally palpable spleen tip, it may resemble mononucleosis, but the hematologic changes are absent, with only leukopenia and plasma (Turk) cells seen on the complete blood count. Skin biopsy findings are nonspecific, showing a mild superficial mononuclear cell infiltrate. Although techniques such as direct immunofluorescent detection of viral antigen in throat swabs and even viral culture of amniocentesis fluid have been used, the mainstay of diagnosis is serologic. The hemagglutination inhibition (HI) test is most popular, although neutralization, fluorescent complement fixation, immunodiffusion, and ELISA tests may also be applied. An acute specimen, obtained preferably at the start of the rash, and a delayed specimen (2 to 4 weeks later) should be run simultaneously: a fourfold rise in titer of HI antibodies is confirmatory. A high initial titer alone is not sufficient; a low convalescent titer (not higher than 1:16) alone suggests no infection. The HI antibodies will return to low titer at 4 to 12 months and persist indefinitely. If early specimens cannot be obtained for HI testing, the complement fixation test may be used, as those antibodies do not peak until 4 to 8 weeks after infection. (Some immune patients may have antibodies too low to detect by routine HI; enhanced HI, ELISA, or gel diffusion studies may be used.) Rubella-specific IgM is present in amniocentesis fluid only at 21 or more weeks' gestation.

Treatment. Therapy for routine acute complaints is symptomatic; the occasional arthropathy responds to aspirin. The main concern is that of prevention. Since 1969 live attenuated vaccine has been recommended for children 15 months or older, all naive adult males, and all nonimmune adult females who will not be pregnant for at least 3 months. Vaccination should not be given to those with acute febrile illness or depressed host immunity or to those who have received blood products in the preceding

12 weeks. A mild illness and/or rash may be seen with vaccination; there is a very low risk of transmission for up to 3 weeks after immunization. Abortion should be considered for all first trimester infections; administration of human serum immune globulin may be of some help to prevent fetal disease if abortion is refused. Reinfection may occur in up to 3 to 10 percent of those with natural immunity and up to 18 percent of those vaccinated (strain RA27/3); most reinfection is subclinical, and fetal infection from maternal reinfection is very rare. Nonetheless, all pregnant women should avoid exposure.[11,12]

Roseola Infantum

Roseola infantum (also known as exanthem subitum, sixth disease, and Zahorsky's disease) is a common acute illness of infants and young children marked by 3 to 5 days of high fever followed by a morbilliform rash during or after defervescence; it is classically benign in its course.

Etiology. The disease is transmittable to infants and monkeys by blood, serum, and throat washings. Several viruses have been identified including echovirus 16, coxsackie virus B5, other enteroviruses, and several adenoviruses; Hurwitz suggests that roseola represents a host response to multiple viral infections.[4]

Epidemiology. Roseola is seen throughout the year, with some increase in fall and spring. This is the most common febrile exanthem seen under 2 years of age, but it is rarely seen before 6 months. Up to 30 percent of all children contract roseola; it is exceeded only by varicella in its prevalence in childhood.

Course. In the unusual instance in which a contact is known, incubation averages 12 days (range 5 to 15 days) and is followed by a sudden onset of fever (103 to 106°F) with malaise, mild coryza, and sometimes irritability and mild gastrointestinal upset. Importantly, the severity of the fever is markedly disproportionate to the innocuousness of the other signs and symptoms. The fever is usually sustained in nature. Slight injection of the tympanic membranes or the pharynx may be found, with or without pink specks (lymphoid hyperplasia) on the uvula, soft palate, and tonsillar pillars. Eyelid swelling may be prominent. On day 2 or 3, mild occipital, posterior auricular, or cervical adenopathy (milder than in rubella) may be seen, lasting up to 1 week. In 3 to 5 days the fever falls, usually by crisis; the fever and symptoms are succeeded usually within a day by the rash. Blanching pink 2- to 5-mm papules and/or macules, sometimes with a light halo, appear principally on the neck, trunk and arms, and are rarely disseminated. The rash fades without a trace in hours to 1 to 2 days.

Complications are unusual; they include convulsions (presumably febrile) and, very rarely, encephalitis and thrombocytopenic purpura. Outlook is generally excellent.

Diagnosis. The key to diagnosis is the clinical presentation of an abrupt high fever without obvious cause, followed by a sudden fall in temperature with the onset of a pink morbilliform rash, most pronounced on the trunk. The most distinctive laboratory finding is leukopenia with a relative lymphocytosis and granulocytopenia. Skin biopsy is not diagnostic.

Treatment. Antipyretic medications and cooling baths are indicated during high fever. Isolation is not recommended.[13,14]

Enteroviruses

At least 30 distinct enteroviruses (echo and coxsackie) are responsible for febrile illness, occasionally with exanthem that is often morbilliform in nature. Rash is more frequently seen in children. The symptoms may include malaise and mild upper respiratory and gastrointestinal complaints. The most significant complication sometimes encountered is aseptic meningitis.

Epidemiology. Infections are most common during July to September. Spread is by contact, especially the fecal-oral route; viral shedding in feces may persist for 1 month. Incubation is 2 to 7 days in duration. A clustering of cases amongst close associates and in the community at large is diagnostically helpful. Symptomatic infection with exanthem and sometimes enanthem is most common in young children and infants; asymptomatic infection is frequent. Although in an older population the sexes are equally affected, young males are more susceptible than females.

Diagnostic Features. The enterovirus exanthems themselves are variable in form; they are often morbilliform but may in some cases be urticarial, petechial, or vesicular (Fig. 8-1). They are usually nonpruritic. They often begin centrally but vary in extent and involvement of palms and soles. Variable enanthems, including herpangina, may or may not occur. The illness itself is usually relatively mild, with low-grade to moderately high fever (101 to 102°F), headache, anorexia, occasional rhinopharyngitis, and mild gastroenteritis. Fever may be bi- or triphasic, and rash may recur with each return of fever. Adenopathy (usually cervical, occipital, and postauricular) may be present but is not marked. Significant complications include aseptic meningitis (permanent sequelae are most often seen in those under 12 months of age) and pericarditis/myocarditis (enterovirus is the leading cause); pneumonitis, hepatitis, and pancreatitis may also occur. Laboratory diagnosis is best made by culture of feces and the oropharynx, where virus may persist for one or more weeks after infection. Blood cultures are negative once symptoms are present. Peripheral blood studies may show a leukocytosis and moderately elevated ESR (up to 50 mm/hour). In aseptic meningitis, up to 1,000 cells/mm^3 may be seen (first neutrophils, then mononuclear cells) but CSF protein is usually normal. Skin biopsy is not diagnostic.

With regard to differential diagnosis, adenovirus may, rarely, cause morbilliform or even scarlatiniform or roseola-like rashes. However, symptoms usually include conjunctivitis and more prominent rhinopharyngitis. Reovirus exanthems, while rare, may be hard to distinguish from enteroviral disease, as both may share morbilliform rash and generally mild illness. Respiratory syncytial virus may, rarely, cause a severe toxic erythema in the very young.

Treatment is symptomatic. Prevention depends upon good hygiene, as transmission is by the fecal-oral route. Prognosis is excellent, with the exception of possible sequelae in aseptic meningitis and perimyocarditis.

Significant features of specific enteroviral rashes follow:

The *echoviruses* usually encountered are 2, 4, 5, 6, 9, 11, 16, 17, 18, and 25. The highlights are as follows:

Echo 2: This causes an asymptomatic morbilliform rash, starting on the abdomen and back and then extending. The rash, often copper-colored, lasts 2 to 7 days. Severe neurologic complications are rarely seen.

Echo 4: An asymptomatic blotchy erythema spreads in centrifugal fashion over 1 to 2 days; occasional petechiae or vesicles are reported. Rare CNS complications are seen.

Echo 5: Faint generalized erythema, particularly over the extremities, appears after the onset of fever.

Echo 6: Neurological symptoms are infrequently accompanied by morbilliform rash.

Echo 9: This is the most common enterovirus infection associated with rash. A minority of patients (one in three) experience mild prodrome (fever, anorexia/nausea, sore throat) followed by a brief asymptomatic rest and then the sudden onset of illness with fever, headache, photophobia, upper respiratory complaints, nausea, vomiting, abdominal pain, and sometimes symptoms attributable to aseptic meningitis. Rash is seen in up to one-third of cases (about half under age 3 years); it usually begins as an asymptomatic blanching pink morbilliform eruption on the cheeks, spreading in hours to the trunk, extremities, palms, and soles. The face is the last area to clear (3 to 5 days). A grayish

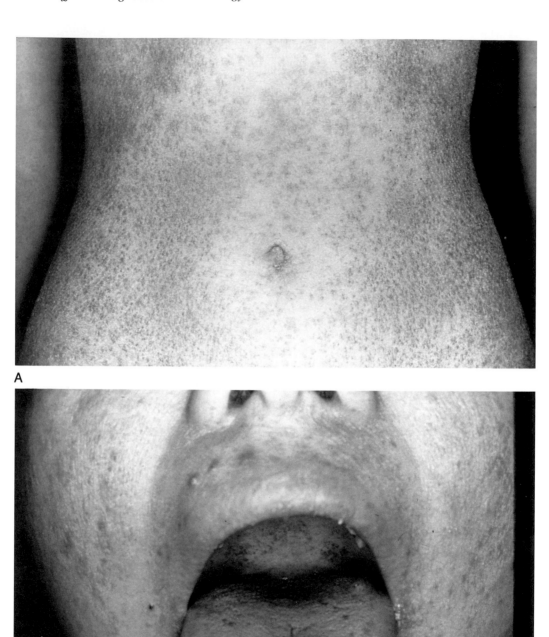

Fig. 8–1. Viral infection. **(A)** Generalized erythematous maculopapular rash. **(B)** Petechiae on the palate.

or red enanthem may be present in some patients. Occasionally the rash may be urticarial or at times petechial, suggesting meningococcemia with neurologic signs and symptoms. Echo 9 disease is most often considered in the differential of purpuric eruptions and is thus classified in that section of this chapter as well.

Echo 11: A morbilliform, sometimes urticarial, rash of the trunk and extremities is sometimes, but not usually, seen; rarely, vesicles have been noted.

Echo 16 (Boston exanthem): Rash is present in approximately one-third of cases and about one-fourth of patients suffer a herpangina-like enanthem. Rash is more common in children; malaise is more common in adults. The rash is usually seen after fever of 1 to 2 days' duration (101 to 102°) subsides. (The appearance of rash with defervescence may suggest a roseola-like syndrome.) There may be headache, gastrointestinal illness, mild pharyngitis, and adenopathy (occipital, cervical, or postauricular, especially with oral ulcerations). The rash begins as small nonpruritic pink to salmon-colored papules on the face and thorax, extending centrifugally even to palms and soles; it may last up to 5 days.

Echo 17: About one-third of patients have a morbilliform, rarely vesicular, rash.

Echo 18: A morbilliform exanthem, at times with enanthem, may be seen; aseptic meningitis is rarely encountered.

Echo 25: A mainly truncal morbilliform rash, rarely vesicular, may be seen after 3 days of fever and pharyngitis. Herpangina-like enanthem is seen occasionally.

The *coxsackievirus* infections often seen with rash are A4, 5, 6, 9, 10, 16, B2, 3, 4, and 5. Noteworthy features include the following:

Coxsackie A4: Illness with fever, pharyngitis, coryza, and anorexia is followed by small pink macules or papules, beginning on the face and trunk and extending peripherally but sparing palms and soles. Vesicles may be present, as may herpangina-like lesions in the mouth.

Coxsackie A5: This virus is one of the causes of the vesicular eruption of hand-foot-and-mouth disease (discussed below under vesicular diseases).

Coxsackie A9: Fever and occipital and/or cervical adenopathy may be accompanied by 1 to 7 days of morbilliform rash, beginning on the face and extending to the trunk and extremities. The rash may sometimes be urticarial, petechial, or even vesicular in nature. (A single-crop varicella-like eruption has been described.)

Coxsackie A10: This virus is associated with hand-foot-and-mouth disease (see discussion of vesicular eruptions below), primarily in children.

Coxsackie A16: This virus is discussed below under vesicular eruptions.

Coxsackie B1: Rarely, a morbilliform rash has been seen, sometimes resembling that of rubella or roseola. Hand-foot-and-mouth disease has been described, as has herpangina.

Coxsackie B3: Children, unlike adults, frequently have a rash, which is usually morbilliform but occasionally petechial like that of echo 9. Hand-foot-and-mouth disease has been reported. Of note is occasional hepatosplenomegaly.

Coxsackie B4: A vesicular exanthem has been seen.

Coxsackie B5: In a small number of cases (particularly in infants under 18 months), a fine morbilliform rash, occasionally urticarial or petechial, starts on the face and neck and spreads in hours to the trunk and extremities, sparing palms and soles. Like the rash of roseola and echovirus 16 infection, this may occur as (or after) fever subsides. There is no enanthem and usually no adenopathy.[15–17]

Infectious Mononucleosis

Infectious mononucleosis is an acute, mildly infectious viral illness which causes fever, pharyngitis, malaise, adenopathy, splenomegaly, and, often, a morbilliform rash. This illness is commonly seen in children and young adults. Characteristically, a transient lymphoproliferation is noted, as are specific serologic markers.

Etiology. The disease is due to Epstein-Barr virus, a herpesvirus (DNA); this virus is also associated with Burkitt's lymphoma in Africa.

Epidemiology. Infection occurs by direct contact and is known worldwide, with a peak incidence in the 15- to 25-year age group. The majority of these cases are subclinical. In children, infection is also common, but symptoms are often mild.

Course. Infection rates are higher in early fall and early spring. Incubation periods range from as low as 10 to 14 days (in children) to 30 to 50 days; a prodrome of headache, fatigue, and malaise lasts 4 to 5 days. The illness proper begins with pharyngitis and even frankly exudative tonsillitis, fever sometimes as high as 104°F in the afternoon (but not so high in childhood), myalgia, headache, and cervical adenopathy. These signs and symptoms may persist for a week or more. Rash begins in the latter half of the first week in anywhere from 3 to 25 percent of cases. Typically, it is morbilliform and most pronounced over the trunk and proximal arms, although it may generalize. It is limited occasionally to palms and soles. Rarely, it is purpuric, scarlatiniform, or urticarial. The rash clears in a few days; erythema multiforme or urticaria sometimes follows. Bilateral supraorbital edema is more common than rash (50 percent) and may even be the presenting sign in children. By the second week one-fourth of patients exhibit transient petechiae at the border of the hard and soft palates; pronounced firm, tender cervical or even generalized adenopathy may persist for weeks. Splenomegaly is found in over one-half of patients in the second and third weeks of illness; rare splenic rupture may cause death. Hepatomegaly occurs in only 10 percent, but an anicteric hepatitis affects the majority. Pneumonitis, pleuritis, and hilar ade-

nopathy may occur. Disease of the CNS is rare (less than 1 percent) and usually is seen in adults; a variety of neurological ailments, including aseptic meningitis, Bell's palsy, meningoencephalitis, and Guillain-Barré syndrome, usually resolve fully. Pericarditis, myocarditis, hemolytic anemia, and thrombocytopenic purpura are other unusual complications. Prognosis is otherwise excellent. Symptoms usually begin to abate by the end of the third week and patients can usually resume activities at 4 to 6 weeks.

A common, almost diagnostic feature is a generalized copper-colored rash seen in up to 90 percent of patients 5 to 8 days after receiving ampicillin; a similar phenomenon occurs in patients receiving allopurinol and in those with lymphatic leukemias, cytomegalovirus (CMV) infection, and viral respiratory infections. This apparent sensitivity to ampicillin is temporary and thus probably does not represent true allergy.

Diagnosis. The clinical presentation of sore throat, morbilliform rash, fever and adenopathy may be confused with nonspecific viral illness, scarlet fever, rubella, and even toxoplasmosis and cytomegalovirus infections (although the last two are not associated with severe pharyngitis). The following specific laboratory findings substantiate the diagnosis:

1. An absolute and relative lymphocytosis (total white blood count 20,000 or even higher) is present by weeks 2 and 3.
2. At least 10 percent atypical lymphocytes with lobulated or indented nuclei and vacuolated basophilic cytoplasm are seen on peripheral smear.
3. Heterophil antibody titer is quantified at 1:40 or higher (based on assay of agglutinins for sheep red blood cells). In adults 38 percent of cases are positive by week 1 and 80 percent are positive by week 3; the test is less sensitive in children. Assay for horse red cell agglutinins is most sensitive and thus is best used in testing children. The monospot test, which assays for antibodies to formalized horse red blood cells

affixed to the slide, provides a rapid diagnosis. Heterophil antibodies are mainly IgM and persist up to 6 months.

4. Specific Epstein-Barr virus antibodies can be assayed by immunofluorescence (most common method; titers of 1:40 to 1:160 are seen early), complement fixation, immunodiffusion, ELISA, or neutralization techniques. The titer does not correlate with severity of illness and may remain qualitatively positive for life.

Treatment. Therapy is generally supportive, with rest and avoidance of trauma to the spleen. Tapering doses of prednisone may be given for severe pharyngitis or hematologic, CNS, or cardiac complications.[18,19]

Hepatitis B

Hepatitis B is a bloodborne infection distinguished by a long incubation period and a prodrome of malaise and often rash preceding an acute icteric phase. Chronic liver disease may sometimes follow apparent convalescence.

Etiology. The disease is due to the distinctive hepatitis B "hepadna" virus (double-stranded DNA).

Epidemiology. The disease is contracted by direct contact with infected blood, blood products, bile, and body fluids. Infection in childhood often arises in conditions of crowding and institutionalization or when the mother is infected. Intrauterine infection is rare. Peak infection is in young adults and among intravenous drug abusers, homosexuals, dialysis patients, laboratory personnel, and transfusion recipients.

Course. After a 40- to 180-day incubation, 10 to 20 percent of patients experience a prodrome of anorexia, nausea, vomiting, fever, headache, malaise, or alterations in olfactory and gustatory senses. Additionally, 20 to 30 percent of patients may experience a serum sickness syndrome with fever, arthralgia, arthri-

tis, proteinuria, or hematuria. The most common sign of this serum sickness is cutaneous, often urticarial. Angioedema, erythema multiforme, toxic erythema, petechiae, and frank palpable purpura (vasculitis) may be associated. The serum sickness may antedate the actual hepatitis by days to weeks and usually resolves within 1 week. If it overlaps the onset of liver disease, yellow hives may be the first manifestation of icterus. A scarlatiniform exanthem of the trunk and proximal extremities has also been described at the start of illness. Other findings include papular acrodermatitis of childhood (Gianotti-Crosti) (Fig. 8-2), periarteritis nodosa, and "essential" mixed cryoglobulinemia. Active hepatitis of variable severity and duration is followed by convalescence and sometimes persistent or chronic active hepatitis. Less than 1 percent of patients may die from fulminant hepatitis. Up to 10 percent of patients may go on to be chronic carriers and be positive for hepatitis B surface antigen (HBsAg). In children, this is especially true of anicteric neonatal infections. Chronic carriers stand an increased risk of chronic active hepatitis and hepatocellular carcinoma.

Diagnosis. The clinical picture of prodromal illness with serum sickness-like signs and symptoms followed by icterus is strongly suggestive of hepatitis B, but serologic confirmation is required to distinguish the disease from other viral illnesses such as infectious mononucleosis. Hepatitis A rarely has cutaneous findings; non-A, non-B hepatitis may, like hepatitis B, occur with a serum sickness syndrome, as well as cryoglobulinemia. The most important marker of activity is HBsAg, which appears 2 to 8 weeks before clinical illness and may last until convalescence. Surface antibody antiHBs is detected after HBsAg is cleared and only indicates previous infection. AntiHBc (core antibody) is seen with the onset of clinical disease and may persist for life; in occasional cases in which HBsAg cannot be found, rising antiHBc and antiHBs titers may be used to confirm the diagnosis. Where there is extreme intensity and prolonged duration of infectivity, hepatitis B e

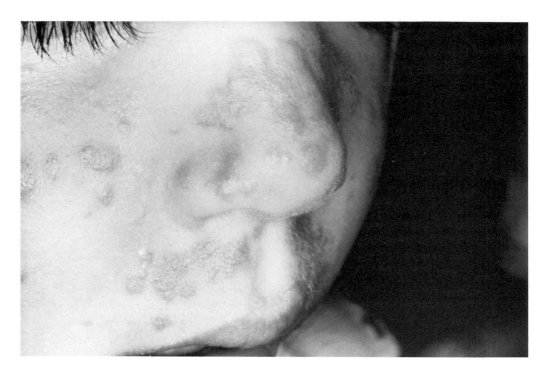

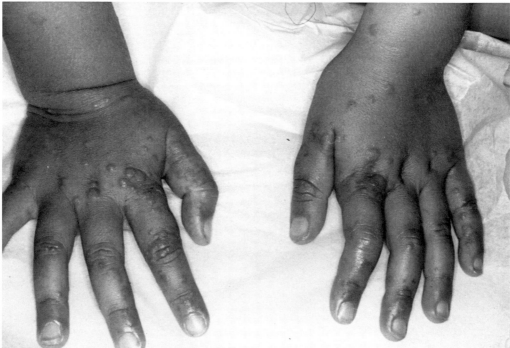

Fig. 8–2. Papular acrodermatitis of childhood (Gianotti-Crosti syndrome). Nonpruritic papules on the face and hands.

antigen (HBeAg), may be seen along with HBsAg.

Treatment. Supportive care and antihistamines for pruritus are employed. Systemic steroids and immunosuppressive drugs may be contraindicated as they may increase the number of circulating virions and thus possibly the risk of chronic active hepatitis. Prevention is important; administration of hepatitis B immune globulin (HBIg) is indicated after an acute intense exposure to (e.g., needle stick) or intimate contact with (e.g., sexual) a person with known or suspected disease. Similarly, newborns should be immunized if their mothers had acute infection in the second or third trimesters or up to 2 months postpartum or are chronic carriers. Infants should receive 0.5 ml intramuscularly within 12 hours of birth and at 3 and 6 months; those percutaneously infected should receive 0.06 ml/kg intramuscularly within 24 hours and possibly again at 1 month. Sexual partners should be immunized within 14 days and possibly again at 1 month. Additionally, infants and percutaneous contacts, but not sexual partners, should receive hepatitis B vaccine; children (up to age 10) receive 0.5 ml intramuscularly within 7 days and again at 1 month and 6 months; percutaneous contacts receive 1 ml within 7 days and again at 1 and 6 months. A dose of 2 ml is recommended for the immunocompromised.[20–22]

BACTERIAL INFECTIONS

Scarlet Fever

Scarlet fever (scarlatina or second disease) is an acute infection arising from streptococcal pharyngitis or occasionally from a streptococcal wound infection and is associated with fever, malaise, and a characteristic diffuse toxic erythema and enanthem. The rash is due to erythrogenic toxin (three types) related to a lysogenic bacteriophage found in some group A β-hemolytic streptococci. (Toxin may also be made by some group C and G streptococci.)

Epidemiology. Infection is due to droplet spread, particularly during the cold months. School children aged 2 to 12 years are most susceptible, as are military recruits. Infants rarely contract scarlet fever, possibly owing to maternal antibody protection as well as seeming insensitivity to erythrogenic toxin. By age 10 most children (80 percent) have immunity, usually due to subclinical infection. As there is more than one distinct toxin, 25 percent of patients may experience a recurrence of scarlet fever. In recent decades it has generally been acknowledged that scarlet fever has evolved into a milder disease.

Course. Incubation averages 36 to 72 hours (but may last up to 7 days), during which time bacterial cultures are negative. There follows a sudden onset of pharyngitis, often with exudate (more severe in older children), fever (102 to 105°F), chills, headache, malaise, and occasional gastrointestinal upset. Anterior cervical, submandibular, and even general adenopathy may be present. On examination the whole pharynx is hyperemic with posterior pharyngeal edema; by day 3 or 4, there may be nonadherent exudate of the tonsils and posterior pharynx. Petechiae may be present. In 50 percent of cases there is a strawberry tongue, which begins as a white tongue with red papillae on the tip and sides; by days 4 to 5, the entire tongue is red with prominent papillae.

The rash, a diffuse blanching toxic erythema, appears in the first 2 days, often after defervescence. It begins on the neck, chest, and axillae, and spreads within 36 hours to the trunk and extremities, sparing palms and soles. Circumoral pallor with erythema of the cheeks and forehead is common. The rash may feel like sandpaper to the touch owing to the presence of 1- to 2-mm papules. Miliaria crystallina may be present. In addition to pressure areas, erythema may be marked in the antecubital and axillary folds; the characteristic linear arrays of petechiae termed *Pastia's lines* may also be found in the folds. The rash persists up to 5 days; branny desquamation begins on the face as early as day 7 and then appears on the abdomen and extremities. Large sheets of skin may peel off the hands and feet, especially at the tips of the digits and periungual areas. Beau's lines of the nails may occur.

In the prepenicillin era mortality approached 1 to 3 percent owing to local spread and bacteremia with subsequent infection in soft tissue, bone, CNS, and other sites. Current complications include glomerulonephritis seen about 10 days after infection with specific M-type (1, 4, 12, 18, 25, 49) or T-type (3, 6) antigens, and rheumatic fever, which may occur in 2 to 3 percent of untreated cases of scarlet fever approximately 19 days after infection with any M type. Rarely, acute arthritis or myocarditis is seen.

Diagnosis. Scarlet fever must be distinguished from Kawasaki's disease, toxic shock syndrome, drug rash, and viral illnesses such as rubella, roseola, or rubeola. Staphylococcal scarlet fever is a mild form of staphylococcal scalded skin syndrome due to infection with phage group II, types 3A, 3C, 55, 71, and 85; it may give a similar picture without pharyngitis and strawberry tongue. Definitive diagnosis rests with identification of the streptococcus on culture of nose or throat. An antistreptolysin O (ASLO) titer of 1:128 or more suggests recent infection and may persist up to 6 months. The streptozyme hemagglutination test can detect early antibody response. General laboratory tests show a granulocytosis and later eosinophilia (5 to 10 percent) and occasional transient microscopic hematuria. Skin biopsy shows dilated capillaries, with perivascular collections of polymorphonuclear granulocytes and occasional hemorrhage. The Dick test, in which intradermally injected erythrogenic toxin produces erythema in a nonimmune host, and the Schultz-Charlton test, in which intradermally injected antitoxin locally blanches the scarlet fever rash, are no longer used.

Treatment. Penicillin is the drug of choice and may be given intramuscularly (benzathine penicillin 600,000 units up to age 8 to 10 years, 900,000 to 1,200,000 units if older) or orally (penicillin VK 25 to 50 mg/kg per day up to 1,000 mg in four divided doses every 6 hours for 10 days). Erythromycin 40 mg/kg per day up to 1,000 mg in four divided doses every 6 hours PO for 10 days or cephalexin/cephteridine 25 to 50 mg/kg per day up to 1,000 mg in four divided doses every 6 hours PO for 10 days may be substituted. Throat cultures should be repeated in 7 to 10 days after oral therapy or 4 to 5 weeks after intramuscular therapy; if cultures are still positive, carriers should be identified by the absence of elevated antibody titers. Persistent infections, reinfections, or new infections (with a different M type antigen) should be retreated. Even after 10 days of infection, rheumatic fever can be prevented by appropriate antibiotic therapy.[23]

Toxic Shock Syndrome

Toxic shock syndrome is an acute, life-threatening illness due to exotoxin-producing staphylococci. This disorder is characterized by fever, hypotension, a toxic erythema with marked desquamation of the distal extremities, and multisystem involvement.

Epidemiology. Most patients have been menstruating females who use tampons, but the illness has been seen with a variety of staphylococcal soft tissue infections. The identity of the specific toxin responsible for the disease remains unknown; toxic shock syndrome toxin-1 (TSST-1), pyrogenic exotoxin C, enterotoxin F, and others still unidentified have been suggested.

Course. A prodrome of myalgias, nausea, vomiting, and diarrhea is followed by fever (greater than 102°F) and rash (a diffuse toxic erythema resembling a sunburn). Erythema and edema of the distal extremities may be present, and petechiae and even subepidermal bullae may be found. In 1 to 2 weeks desquamation, especially of the palms and soles, occurs, and Beau's lines may form. Mucous membrane injection, even with petechiae or frank strawberry tongue, may be found. Hypotension (systolic pressure below 90 mmHg) is characteristically seen. Complications include gangrene, renal failure, cardiac disease, adult respiratory distress syndrome, pancreatitis, thrombocytopenia, and frank disseminated intravascular coagulation. Death (in up to 5 percent of cases) or severe morbidity may result. The disease may recur with menses.

Diagnosis. Strict diagnostic criteria have been presented:

1. Fever
2. Rash
3. Desquamation
4. Hypotension
5. Three or more of the following:
    a. Symptoms of gastrointestinal upset at onset
    b. Myalgia or myositis (creatine phosphokinase twice normal)
    c. Mucous membrane hyperemia
    d. Renal disease (blood urea nitrogen or creatinine twice normal or more than five white blood cells per high-power field on urinalysis)
    e. Liver disease
    f. Nonfocal CNS disease
6. Negative blood, throat, and CSF cultures (though later cases have been seen with positive blood cultures for *Staphylococcus aureus*) and negative serologies for Rocky Mountain spotted fever (RMSF), leptospirosis, and rubeola.

Overly strict adherence to the criteria may result in underdiagnosis. *Staphylococcus aureus* may be cultured from the vagina in affected women (normally 5 to 15 percent of women harbor staphylococci and only a small percent of these produce exotoxin C).

Treatment. Maintenance of blood pressure and perfusion with volume expansion and pharmacologic support is key. β-Lactamase-resistant penicillins do not affect the acute course but may prevent or ameliorate recurrences. The

use of tampons, especially the superabsorbent kind, should be discouraged.[24,25]

Secondary Syphilis

Syphilis (lues) is a sexually transmitted disease, which has several distinctive stages. These are primary, distinguished by the presence of a chancre; secondary, in which flu-like illness and a disseminated papulosquamous or dermal rash is often seen; latent; tertiary, in which complications, particularly neurologic or cardiovascular, may arise; and congenital, in which a variety of musculoskeletal, neurologic, cardiovascular, and ophthalmic abnormalities may be found, at times with a rash, which may be vesicular or hemorrhagic (see discussion of the TORCHS syndrome below).

Epidemiology. Syphilis is seen most commonly in the third decade but may occur at any age, with males predominating by 2:1 to 4:1. The disease can be contracted by contact with the spirochete *Treponema pallidum* in skin lesions, blood, or body fluids. In skin, transmission may occur via intact mucous membranes or damaged cornified skin. Infection may also occur transplacentally and by transfusion.

Course. The secondary stage of syphilis is usually seen about 6 to 8 weeks after the appearance of the primary chancre; as the chancre appears 10 to 90 days after inoculation, secondary disease may occur at any time from 2 to 6 months after exposure. At times the chancriform and secondary stages may overlap. Secondary disease usually clears spontaneously in 4 to 12 weeks; one-fourth of untreated cases relapse. The cutaneous and systemic manifestations of secondary syphilis arise from a spirochetemia.

The patient often presents with a flu-like illness, with low-grade fever, malaise, anorexia, headache, weight loss, and muscle and joint pains. At times there may be sore throat with hoarseness. Nontender, rubbery adenopathy may be generalized; epitrochlear nodes, as well as suboccipital, cervical, axillary, and inguinal nodes, may be especially prominent. It is almost a cliché to note that the manifestations of secondary syphilis are protean; macular erythema, papular, papulosquamous, follicular, pustular, dermal plaque, and nodular forms are described. Vesiculobullous disease is confined to congenital syphilis (see discussion of TORCHS). Erythematous oval macules ("roseola syphilitica") are an early sign of secondary disease and may last only a few days; they often start on the torso but may localize anywhere. Papular syphilids are most common; erythematous follicular papules, acneiform pustules, annular plaques (especially on the face of dark-skinned patients), and papulosquamous round to oval plaques (resembling pityriasis rosea) may be found. The rash may be localized to the head and neck or trunk or may be generalized. Pruritus may be present, especially in dark-skinned patients. Copper-colored macules or scaly plaques may affect palms and soles; diffuse palmoplantar keratoderma ("syphilis cornée") may occur. Condylomata lata, moist pink to gray plaques, may be seen over genitalia and in the folds. Other papular lesions include "split papules" in areas where two surfaces interface, such as the angle of the mouth and intertriginous zones; "frambesiform" eroded hypertrophic nodules and "corymbiform" (bombshell) lesions composed of large central papules with smaller satellite papules. All these lesions usually heal without scarring but at times with dyschromia. Hypopigmentation around the neck ("necklace of Venus") is a classic sign.

A special variant of secondary disease is "malignant syphilis," with prodromal fever, headache, and myalgia followed by widespread necrotic papules and pustules which form dirty, ostraceous (rupioid) scales. The patient may appear toxic; hepatitis may be present.

Mucous patches, round eroded gray patches with surrounding erythema, may be found on oropharyngeal or genital surfaces. Frank oral ulceration may occur in malignant syphilis. As with condylomata lata, the mucous membrane lesions are highly infectious, with large numbers of spirochetes present and the protection of a thick stratum corneum absent. Other clinical findings may include anemia, lymphocytosis, elevation of the ESR, transient proteinuria, acute membranous glomerulonephritis with nephrotic syndrome, anicteric hepatitis, gastritis, myalgias, arthritis mimicking rheumatic disease, osteolysis of the skull, periostitis (tibia, sternum, skull, ribs), osteomyelitis, uveitis, iridocyclitis, and chorioretinitis. Cardiac conduction defects and pulmonary involvement are seen. Between 5 and 15 percent of patients develop an asymptomatic pleiocytosis or elevation of protein in the CSF, but symptoms of acute syphilitic meningitis or transverse myelitis are rare. Eighth nerve damage has also been reported.

If untreated, 25 percent of cases may eventually progress to later (tertiary) disease, with cardiovascular or neurologic sequelae.

Diagnosis. The history of a preceding chancre, known exposure, and certain specifics of presentation, e.g., "copper pennies" of the palms, may be highly suggestive, but confusion with other entities, such as pityriasis rosea, and the need to accurately diagnose and treat demand laboratory confirmation. In secondary syphilis serologic assay is usually the diagnostic test of choice; nontreponemal tests, such as the Venereal Disease Research Laboratories (VDRL) or rapid plasma reagin (RPR) will usually be positive at titers of 1:16 or higher. Titers may be so high, in fact, that in up to 1 percent of cases the slide flocculation tests performed with undiluted serum may be falsely negative (prozone phenomenon); thus, a qualitatively negative nontreponemal test should be repeated with serially diluted screen to ensure that it is quantitatively negative as well. Positive nontreponemal tests should be confirmed by the fluorescent treponemal antibody (FTA) test to rule out the possibility of a false biologic positive. Dark field examination, the mainstay of diagnosis of primary disease, can be performed serially for three days on mucous membrane lesions of secondary disease (preferably nonoral, where nonpathogenic spirochetes are found) and on "dry" lesions, where the stratum corneum has been removed by cellophane tape stripping. Skin biopsy may suggest the diagnosis by the presence of significant numbers of plasma cells in cufflike superficial and deep perivascular infiltrates or in a bandlike infiltrate obliterating the dermal-epidermal junction; endothelial cell swelling may be prominent. Nonspecific spongiotic and/or psoriasiform changes of the epidermis are often present. Silver stains may confirm the presence of spirochetes in the epidermis and dermis and around the vessels.

Treatment. The current recommendation of the American Academy of Dermatology for treatment of secondary syphilis is a single intramuscular dose of benzathine penicillin, 2.4 million units (preferably fractionated into 1.2 million units in each buttock). In over three-quarters of cases, treatment will provoke a Jarisch-Herxheimer reaction, with fevers, chills, flu-like symptoms, and a flare of skin lesions in the first 24 hours. The reaction is self-limited, and bed rest and aspirin are useful. Additionally, patients given parenteral penicillin should be monitored for anaphylaxis for 30 minutes after the dose is given. In penicillin-allergic patients, oral erythromycin or tetracycline, 2 g (fractionated into four doses) daily for 15 days can be given. Nontreponemal serologies are to be repeated at 3, 6, and 12 months; if a sustained fourfold rise in titer or the failure of an initially high titer to decrease fourfold is observed or if clinical signs and symptoms persist or recur, retreatment is warranted. (*Note:* secondary syphilis patients treated by the above regimen normally will revert to negative nontreponemal serologies by 24 months; the FTA test may remain positive for life.) Case reporting to the appropriate local health departments, with appropriate epidemiologic follow-up, is vital.[26]

Lyme Disease

Lyme disease is a spirochetal infection characterized at its onset by acute signs such as fever and headache and a distinctive gyrate erythema, erythema chronicum migrans (ECM), and later by recurrent arthritis, meningoencephalitis, and myocarditis.

Epidemiology. The responsible treponeme, *Borrelia burgdorferi*, is transmitted by the bite of the hard-bodied tick *Ixodes dammini* (variants *Ixodes pacificus, Amblyomma americanum*). There are three major endemic areas in the United States: (1) the East (Connecticut, Massachusetts, Rhode Island, New York, New Jersey, Delaware, Pennsylvania, Maryland, and Georgia); (2) the Great Lakes (Minnesota and Wisconsin) and (3) the West (California, Nevada, and Oregon). The disease has been reported elsewhere in the U.S., and ECM has long been described in northern Europe.

Course. Within 4 to 20 days after a tick bite, a round to oval erythematous macule forms and continues to expand, forming rings with diameters of 20 to 40 or even 70 cm with central clearing (Fig. 8-3). At times, the center or edge may be elevated; there may be bluish discoloration, papule or pustule formation, crust, or even frank ulceration centrally. Scale may be present, the lesion may itch or burn, and in one-fourth of cases multiple lesions may be present (sparing mucous membranes and palms and soles). Accompanying urticaria and generalized erythema have been cited. The ECM usually clears in 3 to 8 weeks. Symptoms of fever, headache, fatigue and arthralgia may occur before, after, or during the rash of ECM. Myalgias, gastrointestinal upset, pharyngitis, conjunctivitis, and regional adenopathy are seen less frequently.

Late sequelae occur weeks to months later; patients with HLA-DR2 B-cell alloantigen may be at increased risk. Major disease, a risk in about 10 percent of untreated cases, includes meningoencephalitis, myocarditis, and recurrent arthritis, usually in the large joints. Minor disease includes peripheral neuropathy (e.g., Bell's palsy), supraventricular tachycardia, headache, arthralgia, and brief arthritis. Even with treatment almost half the patients will have some minor sequelae.

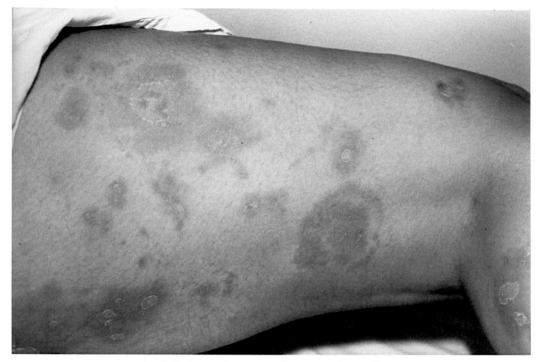

Fig. 8–3. Lyme disease: erythema chronicum migrans.

Diagnosis.   A history of a tick bite followed by an expanding figurate erythema strongly suggests the diagnosis and need for treatment. Differential diagnosis may include insect or spider bites, erythema multiforme, fixed drug eruption, and cellulitis. Serologic confirmation by indirect immunofluorescent techniques indicating titers of 1:256 or higher is available through the Centers for Disease Control and local health departments. Skin biopsy reveals a superficial and deep perivascular infiltrate, with lymphocytes and often plasma cells and eosinophils, which is consistent with an arthropod bite. Spirochetes will be seen on 40 percent of biopsies with silver stain. Other laboratory findings may include an elevated ESR, elevations of IgM and IgG, depressed complement levels, and cryoglobulinemia.

Treatment.   Oral tetracycline, 250 mg four times daily for 10 to 20 days, is the treatment of choice, as it alone apparently prevents late major disease. When tetracycline must be avoided, penicillin VK 50 mg/kg per day (total 1 to 2 g per day) in divided doses for 10 to 20 days, may be given. Erythromycin stearate 30 mg/kg per day in divided doses for 15 to 20 days is less desirable owing to the greater reported incidence of late major disease. Intravenous aqueous penicillin is recommended for treatment of late major disease.[27–29]

Noninfectious Disorders

Kawasaki's Disease

Kawasaki's disease (mucocutaneous lymph node syndrome) is an acute disease of young children, earmarked by high persistent fever, inflammation of the oral and conjunctival mucosae, scarlatiniform changes of the hands and feet, rash, and cervical adenopathy. Later cardiac complications may be fatal. The origin of the disease, first reported by Kawasaki in Japan in 1967, remains unknown despite various infectious and toxic hypotheses.

Epidemiology. The disease is endemic and without seasonal variation, although occasional community epidemics have been reported. It is not highly communicable. In 85 percent of cases the patient is under the age of 5 years, and the majority of patients are under 2½; the disease is very rare in children older than 8. Males outnumber females by 1.6 to 1. Orientals in both hemispheres seem most susceptible, which may be related to the increased prevalence of HLA antigen types BW22 and BW22J2.

Course. High fever, up to 104° F, appears abruptly without a prodrome and lasts a minimum of 5 days and often up to 3 weeks (11 days average); it is unresponsive to antibiotics and only variably responsive to antipyretics. In addition to fever as described, four of the following five features must be present:

1. *Conjunctivitis:* Almost 90 percent of patients have nonprurulent injection, appearing on the first through the third day and lasting up to 3 weeks.
2. *Enanthem:* Red, swollen, chapped lips are seen in 90 percent, while 77 percent have a strawberry tongue within 3 to 5 days of the onset of fever. Simple oropharyngeal hyperemia may be present.
3. *Rash:* In 92 percent of cases there is some exanthem, often starting on the third to fifth day of fever as palmoplantar erythema and then extending to the trunk. It may peel in about 2 weeks. The rash may be papular, morbilliform, or urticarial or may even resemble erythema multiforme; it is often scarlatiniform.
4. *Peripheral edema:* Three-quarters of patients show hand and foot edema followed by desquamation beginning on the fingertips and around the nails.
5. *Cervical adenopathy:* Approximately 50 to 80 percent of patients have cervical adenopathy, which is usually unilateral and often limited to a solitary, nontender, firm node at least 1.5 cm in diameter.

Thrombocytosis, seen after day 10, is apparently responsible for the major cardiac complications of ischemic heart disease and coronary aneurysms, which lead to sudden death in 1 to 5 percent of cases, usually within 1 to 2 months but occasionally even up to years later. Those at particular risk are males under 1 year, with ESR greater than 101, white blood cell count over 30,000, and fever exceeding 16 days. Death may also result from myocarditis, pericarditis, and cardiac conduction defects. Large vessel occlusion and hypertension may be seen. Up to 20 percent of patients may have some cardiovascular involvement. Pulmonary infiltrates and pyuria may be seen acutely, and arthralgia and even arthritis may be seen late in the disease. About one-fourth of patients have nausea, vomiting, and abdominal pain; 10 percent have hepatitis; and a small number have a hydropic gallbladder. Nearly all have CNS involvement, and irritability and sleep disturbances are common. Almost a third may be lethargic or frankly comatose during the acute illness, and 25 percent have aseptic meningitis and may suffer ataxia or cranial nerve palsies.

Diagnosis. The cornerstone of diagnosis remains the clinical diagnostic criteria outlined above. In particular, Kawasaki's disease must be distinguished from scarlet fever and the toxic shock syndrome. Laboratory tests may show a leukocytosis greater than 18,000, mild anemia, and an elevated ESR. Thrombocytosis is seen universally after day 10, ranging from 600,000 to 1,800,000 and normalizing by day 30. Liver function tests may show elevations of bilirubin and transaminases. Urinalysis may reveal white blood cells, and the CSF may have mononuclear cells and some increased protein. In 70 percent of cases EKGs show increased PR and QT intervals or nonspecific ST and T wave changes.

Biopsy of affected tissues show dermal edema, dilated vessels with endothelial swelling, and surrounding mononuclear cell infiltrate. Patchy necrosis may be present. The arteritis of small and medium-size vessels resembles that seen in infantile periarteritis nodosa.

Treatment. Aspirin in doses of 80 to 100 mg/kg daily in four divided doses is given during the acute phase (target serum level at 18 to 25 mg/dl); once the patient is afebrile, aspirin is continued at 10 mg/kg per day divided into two doses until the ESR normalizes (about 6 to 10 weeks after the onset of disease). Patients should be followed with echocardiography. If aneurysms are evident at 4 weeks (up to 20 percent of cases), aspirin should be continued indefinitely and the EKG and echocardiography should be repeated every 3 months. Aneurysms can resolve; two-thirds are no longer seen on angiography after 1 year. Steroids are contraindicated as they may increase the incidence of coronary aneurysms. Recently, intravenous immunoglobulin has been employed in acute treatment.[30-32]

Erythema Multiforme

Erythema multiforme (EM) is an acute, self-limited erythematous rash with distinctive targetoid lesions, mucous membrane involvement, and often mild constitutional complaints; a variety of agents may provoke this dermal vascular reaction. The more common minor variant of EM may be distinguished from the major forms, namely, Stevens-Johnson syndrome and toxic epidermal necrolysis (TEN), by the absence of significant morbidity and mortality.

Epidemiology. Erythema multiforme is fairly common, with a peak incidence in the teens and twenties; although up to 20 percent of those affected are children, they are usually more than 3 years of age. More severe cases are often seen in male children and young adults. Seasonal epidemics may occur when EM is associated with various infectious agents. Recurrences may be expected in 25 percent of cases, especially those associated with herpesvirus infections.

Etiology. The apparent etiologies of EM include (1) infections; (2) drugs (penicillins, sulfas, seizure medications, immunizations); (3) immune complex diseases (collagen vascular disease); (4) neoplasia (leukemias, lympho-

mas, paraproteinemias, carcinomas); (5) metabolic/endocrine disorders; (6) other known sources (contactants, physical agents, inoculations, irradiation of tumors); and (7) unknown sources (50 percent.) The infections include those due to: viruses such as herpes-, adeno-, and enteroviruses and Epstein-Barr virus (infectious mononucleosis); mycoplasmas; chlamydia (lymphogranuloma venereum); bacteria, such as streptococci and *Yersinia;* myobacteria; and fungi and parasites. Additionally, TEN may arise in acute graft-versus-host disease.

Although immune complexes have been detected in lesional tissue, the abundance of T lymphocytes and lymphokines and the absence of vasculitis suggest the effect of cell-mediated immunity; an antibody-dependent cell-mediated cytotoxicity mechanism has been proposed.

Course. Within days to 2 weeks of exposure to a probable inciting cause, a prodrome resembling a mild upper respiratory infection with low-grade fever, muscle aches, and malaise may be seen in one-third of cases. The rash, which may burn or itch, appears acrally and symmetrically, favoring extensor surfaces; palms, soles, trunk, face, and neck may also be involved. Classically, erythematous macules, 1 to 2 cm in size with central duskiness or frank necrosis or blistering, are seen, inspiring the descriptive terms "targetoid," "iris," and "bullseye." Polycyclic and concentric configurations may appear. Swelling, particularly distally, may be marked. Fixed urticarial plaques may also be seen. At least 25 percent of patients with EM minor will have painful blisters, erosions, and crusts of the mucosae (especially oral); although the gums, tongue, and buccal mucosae are often involved, a characteristic finding is hemorrhagic crusting of the lips. Some cases may be limited entirely to the mouth. The acute attack usually resolves within 4 weeks, often with postinflammatory hyperpigmentation.

In EM major the prodrome is more severe and protracted; cough, coryza, and sore throat may be prominent, simulating an upper respiratory infection. Vomiting, diarrhea, and muscle and joint pains may also be present. Usually more than one mucosal surface is affected (conjunctivae, oropharynx, nasopharynx, larynx, esophagus, trachea, bronchi, genitalia); nephritis, hepatitis, and pneumonitis may occur. Early in the course it may be impossible to distinguish Stevens-Johnson syndrome from TEN as both display severe mucosal disease and may involve erythema with blistering limited to the head, neck, upper trunk, and distal extremities. In TEN the erythema may progress to involve the entire skin surface, with sheets of skin eroding without discrete vesicles or bullae being visible; the Nikolsky sign is positive. Thus it would appear that the distinction between the Stevens-Johnson syndrome and TEN is merely one of degree. In both forms of EM major, the principal finding distinguishing them from routine EM is ultimately the severe toxicity present. Fluid and electrolyte imbalances may also be present. Death results in up to 50 percent of cases, usually following sepsis, often staphylococcal in nature. In survivors ocular sequelae may be severe.

Diagnosis. Clinically, the diagnosis of EM may be immediately provided by the acute onset of classic targetoid lesions on distal extremities and prominent erosion and crusting of the lips with relatively minimal involvement more posteriorly in the oropharynx. Although the distinctive morphology of the lesions may be very suggestive, it is often necessary to confirm the diagnosis by biopsy, immunofluorescence, viral cultures, and pertinent laboratory studies to eliminate other possible diagnoses such as primary blistering disease, herpesvirus and other viral infections, lichen planus, lupus erythematosus, Behçet's syndrome, Reiter's syndrome, and Kawasaki's disease. On skin biopsy spongiosis is present, with necrotic keratinocytes and mononuclear cell exocytosis. Subepidermal blistering may be present. Papillary edema with endothelial cell swelling and a mononuclear superficial, perivascular, and at times bandlike infiltrate are also seen. Epidermal necrosis is much more prominent in the severe bullous forms of EM; the pathologic changes may be fully confluent in TEN. Direct immunofluorescence serves to rule out other diseases; occasionally, scarce superficial perivascular and junctional granular deposits of C3 and IgM are seen, as is the binding of immunoreactants to Civatte bodies, but this is nondiagnostic.

In EM major extensive fibrinoid necrosis may be seen in the tracheobronchial tree, spleen, and stomach.

Particularly in TEN, it is vital to rule out staphylococcal scalded skin syndrome (SSSS). Although both may occur in children and adults, SSSS is more commonly seen in infants. The patient with TEN may appear more acutely ill, and, importantly, mucous membrane disease is absent in SSSS. Rapid diagnosis may be achieved with a frozen section of a skin peel, or even with a Tzanck preparation or Papanicolaou test; TEN-involved skin will yield necrotic keratinocytes, neutrophils, and much debris, whereas SSSS skin should show only acantholytic cells with no evidence of inflammation. Similar changes may be documented on fixed tissue, but more time is required. With regard to routine laboratory examinations, prolonged neutropenia may be associated with poorer prognosis in drug-induced TEN.

Efforts should be made by careful history taking, physical examination, and appropriate laboratory studies to identify the inciting agent, if possible.

Treatment. Symptomatic treatment with antihistamines and topical drying agents (for blisters) is often all that is required. Oral lesions may require topical anesthetics or even erythromycin or penicillin for secondary infection. A liquid diet or, rarely, parenteral feedings may be needed. As EM minor is a self-limited disease and may often be due to an (occult) herpesvirus infection, the role of systemic steroids grows increasingly controversial. Suppressive therapy with acyclovir may prove beneficial in cases of recurrent EM due to herpesvirus.

The management required by EM major is best afforded by burn units, with strict attention to wet dressings, topical antibiotics, and fluid management. Systemic antibiotics are employed as dictated by Gram stains and cultures. Continuous monitoring for infection at multiple sites, including skin, eyes, urinary tract, pharynx, and lung, is needed, as is early ophthalmologic consultation. Retrospective studies would seem to indicate that prolonged courses of systemic steroids may increase mortality due to sepsis. The role of early short intervention with steroids by conventional or pulse therapy dosage remains unclear. Plasmapheresis early in the course may also be of use.[33–35]

Erythema Marginatum

Erythema marginatum (erythema annulare, erythema circinatum) is a figurate erythema with characteristically rapid spread seen in 10 to 15 percent of children with rheumatic fever; it is considered a major sign of rheumatic fever by the Jones criteria (Table 8-3).

Etiology. A *Streptococcus pyogenes* infection antedates the rheumatic fever by several days to 5 weeks. The role played by antibodies to cell wall, extracellular products, and heart tissue is unclear regarding erythema marginatum.

Course. In children over 6 rheumatic fever begins suddenly, with high fever and painful, often migratory, swelling of the joints. Usually within days of the onset of arthritis, especially in children, asymptomatic pink papules may appear, often on the abdomen, in the axilla, or elsewhere on the trunk. As the papules rapidly enlarge, they fade centrally to form arcuate, geographic plaques. The spread may be as rapid as 10 mm in half a day. ''Rheumatoid'' nodules may also be present on the extremities, as may erythema papulatum. Erythema marginatum, shown in Figure 8-4 in a patient with a new heart murmur and polyarthritis, is often a hallmark of active carditis but may be seen months later. Usually it is self-limited and abates within several weeks, but in some cases it recurs periodically for years even without other rheumatic activity.

Diagnosis. Review of the Jones criteria is helpful in making the diagnosis. The differential diagnosis is extensive, including many diseases presenting with fever, arthritis, and rash. Of major note are juvenile rheumatoid arthritis, in which carditis is absent and the rash is stationary, and systemic lupus erythematosus, in which specific clinical and serologic criteria prevail. Henoch-Schönlein purpura, with demonstrable leukocytoclastic vasculitis, presents similarly, as may bacterial endocarditis, but acral vasculitic lesions (palpable purpura) constitute the distinctive cutaneous finding. Viral illnesses such as rubella should be ruled out. Other figurate erythemas, such as ECM, EM, and even urticaria, should be excluded by careful clinical evaluation and by laboratory analysis where applicable. Skin biopsy may be corroborative by showing superficial perivascular polymorphonuclear leukocytes.

Table 8-3. Jones Criteria for the Diagnosis of Rheumatic Fever

Major	Minor
Carditis	
Murmurs: prolonged apical systolic, apical mid-diastolic, basal diastolic	Arthralgia (without arthritis)
Cardiomegaly	Previous rheumatic fever or rheumatic heart disease
Pericarditis	Elevated erythrocyte sedimentation rate
Congestive heart failure	Positive C-reactive protein
Polyarthritis	Leukocytosis
Chorea (Sydenham's)	Prolonged PR interval (without carditis)
Erythema marginatum	
Subcutaneous (rheumatoid) nodules	

Diagnosis of rheumatic fever: Evidence of previous streptococcal infection plus two major signs or one major and two minor signs

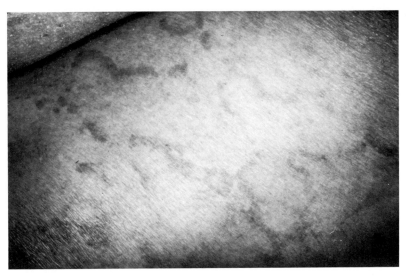

Fig. 8–4. Erythema marginatum on the thigh of a patient with a new heart murmur and polyarthritis.

Treatment. Although appropriate antibiotics and anti-inflammatory therapy, including steroids and salicylates, remedy the infection and the rheumatic complaints of rheumatic fever, the course of erythema marginatum appears to be independent of therapy. Once the diagnosis is made, prophylaxis with 1.2 million units of benzathine penicillin intramuscularly (or 1 g sulfonamide orally) monthly for at least 5 years is recommended.[36–38]

Juvenile Rheumatoid Arthritis

Juvenile rheumatoid arthritis (JRA), also known as Still's disease and chronic juvenile polyarthritis, may present either acutely or insidiously with arthropathy, fever, macular or papular erythematous rash, and a variable extent of systemic illness. The course is often unpredictable, as is the morbidity, especially with respect to the joint symptoms.

Etiology and Epidemiology. The cause is unknown. As the presence of rheumatoid factor is not a consistent finding, especially in children, the immunologic basis is not completely known. The peak incidence is between 2 and 4 years of age, although adolescents and young adults may also be affected. Females outnumber males 2 to 1 in the articular forms of the disease; systemic JRA affects both sexes equally.

Course. Three patterns of disease are seen:

1. *Polyarticular (Still's disease):* This pattern is marked by sudden onset of high fever, adenopathy, splenomegaly, and symmetric polyarthritis of the knees, wrists, ankles, fingers, hips, and cervical spine. Fusiform changes (''spindling'') of the proximal interphalangeal joints are characteristic. In 10 percent of cases severe crippling may result.

2. *Pauciarticular:* This form, accounting for 35 percent of cases, is marked by insidious onset of arthropathy, usually one joint at a time (knee, ankle, elbow) over weeks to months; iridocyclitis may occur.

3. *Systemic (Wessler-Fanconi syndrome):* Features of this pattern (25 percent of cases) are acute onset of high intermittent fever, usually in the afternoon and evening, lymphadenopathy, hepatosplenomegaly, and prominent rheumatoid rash. Complications such as pericarditis, pleuritis, leukemoid reaction, and anemia are common. Joint disease may be delayed in

onset by months or even years and may ultimately resemble that in the polyarticular form. Even when present early, systemic toxicity may overshadow the arthritis. As with polyarticular disease, the major morbidity is seen with crippling arthritis; growth retardation, while common during systemic illness, is rectified during remission.

The rash of JRA is seen in at least half of all patients younger than 2 years and becomes less common with increasing age. It usually occurs with or after the arthritis and less often before. It may be seen with the various forms of JRA but is classically associated with fever (polyarticular and systemic forms), attaining prominence in the afternoon and evening and fading with the morning defervescence. The rash itself consists of occasionally pruritic, light to deep pink macules or papules (about 2 to 5 mm) with surrounding pallor on the extremities, palms, soles, trunk, and face. These lesions rarely coalesce. Unlike the rash of erythema marginatum, this rash does not move. It may be accentuated by fever, as noted above, and by heat, activity, and other sources of flushing; it may also koebnerize. Other skin findings may include rheumatoid nodules, atrophic changes over involved joints, and even periungual telangiectasia.

The rash may persist for weeks or even as long as years, and JRA itself may resolve in months or recur over years, even into adulthood. In addition to joint deformity and growth retardation, secondary amyloidosis is an infrequent but major sequela.

Diagnosis. As with erythema marginatum in rheumatic fever, the rheumatoid rash of JRA must be distinguished from that of a variety of illnesses. The nonmotility of the rash and its accentuation with diurnal variation in fever are helpful features; the relatively long duration of the rash contrasts with the transient nature of the exanthems of viral illnesses such as rubella, adenovirus, and coxsackie virus infections, in which fever, arthropathy, and even splenomegaly may be found. There is no single

laboratory test that is diagnostic. The ESR is usually elevated and anemia is common; the white count may be as high as 75,000 in systemic disease. The antinuclear antibody (ANA) test is positive in 25 percent of polyarticular and pauciarticular disease and correlates significantly with iridocyclitis in the latter. Importantly, the rheumatoid factor is present in only about 25 percent of childhood disease cases compared with 80 percent in adults. Early x-ray changes are fairly nonspecific, with soft tissue swelling and periostitis; late changes may show classic fusiform deformities of hands and wrists. Synovial fluid reveals neutrophils and elevated levels of protein.

Skin biopsy may show a nonspecific mononuclear superficial perivascular infiltrate or polymorphonuclear leukocytes; in JRA, unlike erythema marginatum, mononuclear and plasma cells may be present in addition to neutrophils. Biopsy of a subcutaneous nodule reveals a palisading granuloma with fibrinoid degeneration of collagen, as in rheumatic fever.

Treatment. Aspirin is the mainstay of treatment of systemic illness and arthropathy, with systemic corticosteroids reserved for extreme illness. Intralesional steroids and gold may be used for joint disease; steroid drops are used for iridocyclitis. The rheumatoid rash does not respond to therapy other than antihistamines for the pruritus.[39,40]

Systemic Lupus Erythematosus

Systemic lupus erythematosus (SLE) is an autoimmune disorder that presents with a spectrum of inflammatory vascular changes in the skin and many other organ systems. In addition to characteristic clinical features, a variety of serologic markers are associated with the disease.

Epidemiology. The disease has a predilection for adolescents and young adults, and nearly one-fourth of all cases occur before the age of 20. Females outnumber males by more than 4 to 1. Although a genetic predilection is implicated by the clustering of cases among first-degree relatives and the preponderance of HLA antigen types B8, A11, B35, DR2, and DR3, the exact mode of transmission is not known.

Course. The initial presentation is often one of acute toxicity, with fever, fatigue, weight loss, muscle aches, and joint pain occurring in about half of the cases. Generalized lymphadenopathy and hepatosplenomegaly are often found. Initially 36 percent of patients will have a rash; eventually, about 80 percent will have some cutaneous manifestation.

The skin lesions may be of many types. Malar rash, morbilliform eruptions, photosensitivity, mucosal erosions, discoid plaques, and nonscarring alopecia can occur. Other possible cutaneous findings include: subcutaneous lupus erythematosus (LE) (lupus profundus or lupus panniculitis), characterized by hard plaques of the face, trunk, or extremities with overlying hyperpigmentation or ulceration; livedo reticularis; and leukocytoclastic vasculitis causing a variety of lesions, including purpuric papules and nodules, hemorrhagic bullae, ulcerations, and urticarial vasculitis. Thrombophlebitis, periungual telangiectases, pterygia, Raynaud's phenomenon, and erythromelalgia may also be seen.

Systemic symptoms can be quite variable in their type and severity. Kidney disease, pleuritis, pericarditis, peritonitis, psychosis, and seizures can occur. Patients generally have chronic disease activity marked by exacerbations and remissions, with kidney, CNS, and cardiopulmonary complications clouding their course. Death may be due to sepsis, particularly in patients on steroid or immunosuppressive therapy, or to renal failure.

Diagnosis. Definitive diagnosis rests on the finding of 4 of 11 of the American Rheumatism Association's criteria (see Table 3-5, p. 36). The acute onset of fever, malaise, and rash may initially suggest a wide variety of illnesses, including viral disease. Arthralgias may enhance the possibility of a rheumatoid or collagen vascular disease, and more specific clinical markers, such as malar erythema, may particularly indicate SLE. Mixed connective tissue disease, with its lower incidence of renal disease and its serologic marker of high anti-ribonucleoprotein (RNP) antibody titers, should be ruled out. Similar care should be taken to exclude JRA on the basis of clinical signs (true arthritis) and absent serological markers. Serologic studies in SLE will reveal a positive fluorescent ANA in the vast majority of patients. The ANA test often shows a homogeneous pattern, although a peripheral pattern is more specific for SLE. Anti-DNA antibodies and extractable nuclear antigen (ENA) antibodies, including anti-Sm, anti-RNP, and cytoplasmic (Ro, La) antibodies, should be investigated. The LE preparation is a more specific test than the ANA and is positive in 70 to 85 percent of cases, but instead it is best to use a panel of antibody tests, yielding a multiple antibody profile with titers, in making the specific collagen vascular diagnosis. A false biologic positive nontreponemal test for syphilis, e.g., VDRL, RPR, or ART, should also be sought.

Drug-induced LE usually produces serositis and only rarely cutaneous erythema. In children, the most common agents are anticonvulsants. Serologically, significant titers of antihistone antibodies may help to distinguish this state.

Other laboratory tests of diagnostic importance include a complete blood count (50 percent of patients may have anemia, leukopenia, or thrombocytopenia) and a urinalysis, which may reveal cells, cell casts, or protein. Less specifically, an elevated ESR, hypergammaglobulinemia, and hypocomplementemia (C4, C3, C1q, and CH50) may mark disease activity. Although not included in the American Rheumatism Association's criteria, biopsy of lesional skin for routine hematoxylin-eosin staining may be diagnostic with features of hyperkeratosis, follicular plugging, epidermal atrophy, liquefaction degeneration of the basal layer, thickened basement membrane zone (periodic acid–Schiff (PAS)-positive), and periappendageal and superficial and deep perivascular mononuclear cell infiltrates. Direct immunofluorescence (lupus band test) will demonstrate granular deposition of C3, IgG, IgM, or the complement membrane attack complex in about 90 percent or more of lesional biopsies. Similar findings may be found in over half of nonlesional sun-exposed skin samples in SLE (but not in chronic cutaneous LE). A smaller percentage of nonlesional, non-sun-exposed samples will be positive; this may correlate with more severe renal disease. However, the diagnostic and prognostic value of the lupus band test remains controversial.

Efforts should always be made to rule out coexistent infection, especially in patients with known SLE who are on steroids or other immunosuppressive therapy and are experiencing an apparent flare.

Treatment. Sunlight exposure should be extremely limited, as ultraviolet radiation may not only aggravate or engender skin lesions but also exacerbate underlying systemic disease. Bed rest and salicylates are routinely employed. Systemic steroids (prednisone 1 to 2 mg/kg per 24 hours) are routinely prescribed for severe general toxicity and for renal, neurologic, serosal, or other complications. (Care must be taken that steroids do not mask the signs of intestinal rupture.) As soon as possible, steroids should be given on an alternate-day regimen to minimize potential side effects. Severe bouts of vasculitis particularly may require the addition of cytotoxic or immunosuppressive agents, such as cyclophosphamide and azathioprine.

Antimalarial therapy may play a role in the management of selected patients, but this should be done in conjunction with ophthalmologic consultation because of potential retinal toxicity. Simple cutaneous activity can often be treated by topical or intralesional corticosteroids alone.[41–44]

Drug Reactions

Most drugs are associated with possible rash and fever though with widely varying frequencies. It is the rare drug that has never been known to provoke an untoward cutaneous response. Parenteral administration is associated with a higher rate of reactions than the oral route. In contrast to the overwhelming multiplicity of possible offending agents, the variety of rashes produced is relatively limited. Though there are some distinctive eruptions associated with a comparatively small number of agents, such as lichenoid, pityriasiform, and lupus-like rashes, usually the characteristics of a given drug rash are insufficiently unique to immediately implicate a specific drug or group of drugs. Most of these rashes fall into the vascular reaction pattern, embracing a spectrum that includes toxic erythema (morbilliform), urticaria, EM (minor and major), and allergic vasculitis. The morbilliform drug eruptions are most apt to be confused with the infectious exanthems and are indeed the most common drug rashes encountered; thus they are the prime focus of this discussion.

Etiology. Morbilliform drug rashes usually are presumably immunologic in origin, as repeated exposure to even minute quantities often produces a similar host response. Although cell-mediated immunity is suspected, the exact mechanism remains unknown. The basis for one of the most common drug rashes, the ampicillin rash, is particularly puzzling. When ampicillin is given in the setting of infectious mononucleosis, CMV infection, viral respiratory infections, lymphocytic leukemias, and allopurinol ingestion, rash is very frequent, but it is not usually seen upon reexposure to the drug and hence often is not classified as true allergy. Whether the rash produced under these conditions is due to some toxic mechanism or whether these states somehow affect immunologic memory or other immune function is not known. (Similar questions have been raised with regard to trimethoprim-sulfamethoxazole reactions in AIDS patients.)

Certainly, urticarial drug rashes are morphologically indistinguishable from their counterparts associated with infectious diseases. The features of angioedema and bronchospasm would tend, however, to implicate a drug reaction rather than an infectious cause. Urticarial drug rashes are usually due to an immediate-type hypersensitivity (IgE) response, although some agents (e.g., salicyclates), may cause urticaria by direct mast cell degranulation. Erythema multiforme reactions are thought to be mediated by antibody-dependent cell-mediated cytotoxicity (see discussion of erythema multiforme above). (Purpuric vasculitic drug rashes will be discussed in their entirety below.)

Course. Typically, the morbilliform drug rash begins like other toxic erythemas with blanching erythematous macules and/or papules over the face, upper chest, and back. Pruritus is usual and prominent. In the bedbound patient, the rash may appear over pressure points such as the back and buttocks. There may be accentuation in the folds and in areas of dependency, even to the point of purpura. Individual lesions rapidly coalesce and spread and may even produce frank erythroderma. Injection of mucosal surfaces is sometimes seen. Accompanying fever and lymphadenopathy may further obscure the noninfectious origins of the rash.

The rash typically begins within 1 to 2 weeks of initiation of the drug but, rarely, may be seen even after several months, especially when therapy has been intermittent. Furthermore, rash may be seen as late as 2 weeks after discontinuation of therapy.

Complete resolution of the rash usually occurs within 1 to 2 weeks after the drug is stopped. Rarely, the rash persists and may even worsen; conversely, the rash may resolve even while the drug is continued (possibly by the action of blocking antibodies). The rash may also change character and at times may progress into exfoliative erythroderma or even TEN. Furthermore, repeat exposure to the drug usually produces a similar morbilliform rash but at times may cause a different eruption, e.g., erythema multiforme, or even no reaction.

Diagnosis. History is the main key to diagnosis. Laboratory studies are usually not diagnostic; peripheral eosinophilia, for example, is usually not encountered and may also be seen

with infectious diseases. Skin biopsy of a typical drug exanthem is also usually nondiagnostic in the presence of vasodilatation and a sparse mononuclear superficial perivascular infiltrate; sometimes the presence of eosinophils is suggestive of drug rash. As already stated, nearly all drugs, including over-the-counter agents, are potential offenders, but statistically the most likely drugs include the penicillins, sulfonamides, cephalosporins, barbiturates, hydantoin and other CNS depressants, phenothiazines, antipyretics/nonsteroidal anti-inflammatory drugs, thiazides, and blood products.

Although sometimes an array of associated findings, such as massive facial edema, prominent lymphadenopathy, and renal or liver abnormalities, may indicate fairly specifically the cause of a morbilliform drug rash, as in the dilantin hypersensitivity syndrome, detailed history taking and detective work are usually required. A complete account of all agents given (including over-the-counter drugs) and the time course of ingestion vis à vis the onset of rash is crucial in making the diagnosis. This is particularly true in the setting of a patient with an apparent viral illness and rash who was additionally treated with a variety of agents, including antibiotics and antipyretics; careful scrutiny of the data may relieve the patient of the label of antibiotic-allergic. By analyzing the timing of events and the statistical likelihood of any given agent producing rash, one can reasonably judge if the eruption is drug-related and, if so, which drug is most likely responsible.

The most reliable means of verifying the diagnosis is by rechallenge with the putative offender; however, this is not possible without discomfort, if not hazard, to the patient, and is impracticable under most circumstances. Assays for drug-specific IgG and IgM antibodies, intradermal skin testing for cell-mediated immunity, and in vitro lymphocytic proliferation and stimulation tests have not correlated sufficiently with clinical reactivity to be of use.

Treatment. If suspected, a given drug should be discontinued if at all possible and, additionally, it and related compounds should be avoided in the future. Unlike more dangerous reactions, such as urticaria/anaphylaxis, bullous disease (EM/Stevens-Johnson syndrome/TEN), and vasculitis, the morbilliform drug rash itself probably does not pose an absolute contraindication to continued therapy if the agent in question is needed to treat a potentially life-threatening condition and cannot be readily replaced by a supposedly antigenically unrelated drug. However, the patient should be vigilantly observed for progression of the eruption and ominous alteration in its character.

Supportive therapy includes antihistamines, topical menthol/phenol preparations (not advisable in the very young), oatmeal baths, and other conservative treatment. Topical corticosteroids are usually of little help. The rash is rarely sufficiently severe or prolonged to require systemic steroids.[45,46]

PURPURIC ERUPTIONS (TABLE 8–4)

Infectious Disorders

VIRAL INFECTIONS

Atypical Measles

Atypical measles is an unusual form of measles seen in children and adults exposed to wild virus after vaccination with killed vaccine (used 1963 to 1967) or after live virus vaccine administered before 15 months of age. It is chiefly memorable for its hemorrhagic features, in which it may be likened to Rocky Mountain spotted fever (RMSF) or meningococcemia, requiring swift evaluation and decision.

Etiology. Perhaps a delayed-type hypersensitivity reaction to antigens common to wild and attenuated or killed measles virus is responsible. This may be related to the severe inflammatory changes seen with or without fever at the site of vaccination with live attenuated virus after previous immunization with killed vaccine.

Course. A prodrome lasting 2 to 3 days with high fever, headache, myalgia, abdominal pain, and severe prostration is followed by the exanthem. Erythematous macules and papules with petechiae and sometimes vesicles, urticarial plaques, or even EM first appear on the wrists and ankles, then progress inward onto the more proximal extremities and trunk. The rash remains densest peripherally, and edema of hands and feet may be present. Pruritus and hyperesthesia may accompany the rash. Systemically, severe pneumonitis with or without hilar adenopathy or pleural changes is commonly found; solitary pulmonary nodules up to 5 cm in size may persist on x-ray for 2½ years.

Despite acute toxicity, the disease is self-limited, and prognosis for full recovery is excellent.

Diagnosis. Clinically, the acral hemorrhagic exanthem with systemic toxicity will be most readily confused with Rocky Mountain spotted fever, although bacterial sepsis, such as meningococcemia, and hypersensitivity vasculitis, such as Henoch-Schönlein purpura, should also be considered. The prominent pulmonary involvement here may serve to distinguish atypical measles from RMSF. While demonstration of giant cells in nasopharyngeal scrapings may be attempted to substantiate a diagnosis of measles, detailed history taking is the sine qua non in establishing the possibility of atypical measles in an improperly immunized host. Routine laboratory work, including cultures and Gram stain (buffy coat), should be done to rule out bacterial sepsis. Skin biopsy may disclose multinucleated giant cells and exclude the presence of rickettsia or leukocytoclastic vasculitis.

Specific serologic tests for measles as well as RMSF should be made, but as diagnosis rests upon acute and convalescent titers, all cases not readily identifiable as atypical measles should be presumed on an emergency basis to be RMSF and treated as such, as rapid treatment of that entity is mandatory.

Table 8-4. Approach to the Patient: Clinical and Laboratory Features of Purpuric Eruptions Associated with Fever

Disorder	Clinical Features	Laboratory
Atypical measles	History of killed vaccine (1963–1967); pneumonitis; erythematous macules and papules and petechiae begin on wrists and ankles	Acute and convalescent titers; giant cells in nasopharyngeal scrapings; chest x-ray
Echovirus 9	Upper respiratory, gastrointestinal, and neurologic symptoms	Acute and convalescent titers
Rocky Mountain spotted fever	Endemic areas; rash starts few days after fever; pink macules start on wrists and ankles and become purpuric	Direct immunofluorescence of skin biopsy; Weil-Felix, complement fixation tests
Epidemic typhus	Pink macules start in axillae and become purpuric	Weil-Felix, complement fixation tests
Meningococcemia	Purpuric lesions occur on trunk and legs	Blood, spinal and nasopharyngeal cultures; Gram stain of purpuric lesions; counterimmunoelectrophoresis of CSF
Allergic vasculitis	Purpuric lesions most prominent on lower extremities; arthritis	Urinalysis; stool guaiac; elevated erythrocyte sedimentation rate; skin biopsy and immunofluorescence
TORCHS	Neonatal purpura, "blueberry muffin baby"	*Toxoplasma* antibodies; rubella antibodies; IgM immunofluorescent test for cytomegalovirus; maternal and fetal VDRL; Tzanck prep; Gram stain; dark-field exam; viral and bacterial cultures; CBC
Gonococcemia	Arthritis; 5–20 lesions	Genitourinary, rectal, throat, blood, and synovial cultures
Staphylococcal sepsis	Intravenous drug abusers, other source of infection	Blood and skin cultures; Gram stain of skin lesions
Pseudomonas sepsis	Burn patients, immunosuppressed patients; ecthyma gangrenosum, vesiculobullous lesions, gangrenous cellulitis and rose spot-like lesions	Blood and skin cultures; Gram stain of skin lesions
Subacute bacterial endocarditis	Heart murmur, petechiae, splinter hemorrhages, Osler's nodes, Janeway lesions	Blood cultures; Gram stain of skin lesions sometimes helpful

Treatment. Once the diagnosis of RMSF has been definitely excluded, treatment is chiefly supportive.[47]

TORCHS Syndrome

TORCHS is an acronym (*t*oxoplasmosis, *o*ther, *r*ubella, *c*ytomegalovirus, *h*erpes simplex, and, in our approach, *s*yphilis) applied to a syndrome, or a constellation of clinical findings, in affected infants at birth or shortly thereafter. The common cutaneous link that relates the majority of these congenital conditions, mostly infectious, is the "blueberry muffin" appearance arising from dermal erythropoiesis, as well as the presence of less specific purpuric lesions. Noncutaneous commonality may be found in jaundice, organomegaly, fever, and overall toxicity. Other clinical features and laboratory findings allow for the distinction of one entity from another.

Toxoplasmosis. Toxoplasmosis is a parasitic infection, which may be acquired or congenital; it is often clinically silent. Only 10 to 20 percent of acutely infected pregnant women will be symptomatic, with transient morbilliform rash, lymphadenopathy, and an illness generally suggestive of infectious mononucleosis; their offspring nonetheless remain at risk for infection and possible developmental defects, including chorioretinitis, cerebral calcifications, psychomotor retardation, hydrocephaly, microcephaly, and seizures. Congenital toxoplasmosis follows parasitemia during acute infection; hence, for all intents and purposes, subsequent pregnancies should be risk-free. Cell-mediated immunity prevents reinfection in the mother.

Etiology. The causative organism is *Toxoplasma gondii,* an obligate intracellular protozoan whose definitive host is the cat. The cat acquires infection by ingesting infected small animals; parasite reproduction takes place in the feline intestine, and infective oocysts are shed via the stool. The intestinal oocysts, as well as the trophozoite and cyst forms found in infected tissues, can be killed by freezing, heating, and drying; salting and smoking of foods may also accomplish inactivation.

Epidemiology. Infection in humans is commonly acquired by ingestion of oocysts present in soil contaminated by feline feces. Oocysts from soil or feces may be indirectly introduced into food by insects. Another important source of infection is ingestion of undercooked infected meat. These sources may account for prevalence rates approaching 50 percent in selected populations. Infection may also be acquired from infected blood products and organs as well as in utero. Approximately 14 percent of Americans have antibodies to *T. gondii.* The risk of acquiring toxoplasmosis during pregnancy is approximately 0.1 to 0.2 percent. Once acquired, the risk of fetal infection is about 40

percent. In general, less than one-third of those infected will manifest stigmata of congenital toxoplasmosis. However, first-trimester infections may yield congenital defect rates of about 16 percent.

Course. Congenitally infected infants may be born prematurely or stillborn. Acute illness may include fever, vomiting, diarrhea, icterus, hepatosplenomegaly, lymphadenopathy, pneumonitis, and myocarditis. Chorioretinitis, which is usually bilateral (unlike the unilateral disease seen in relapsing acquired disease), may be present at birth or be delayed. Glaucoma, strabismus, cataracts, and optic atrophy may be found, as well as CNS effects, including deafness, retardation, seizures, and hydro- and microcephaly, although CNS manifestations may be delayed by months or years.

Cutaneous manifestations include blue-red macules and plaques scattered on the skin, apparent at or near birth and lasting up to 6 weeks; these loci of extramedullary hematopoiesis constitute the blueberry muffin lesions. Few or many lesions may be present; they may measure almost 1 cm in diameter and are often clustered about the head or trunk. Petechiae may be seen, as may scarlatiniform eruptions, annular erythema-like lesions, and even vesicles.

Diagnosis. The prevalence of chorioretinitis (80 to 90 percent in affected children) and of nodular calcifications of the subcortex and curvilinear calcifications of the basal ganglia on x-ray may be helpful in diagnosing toxoplasmosis. Routine laboratory tests will show nonspecific anemia, thrombocytopenia, eosinophilia, and monocytosis. The CSF may show xanthochromia, pleiocytosis, and elevated protein. Specific serologic diagnosis may be made by measuring neonatal IgM anti-*Toxoplasma* antibody by dye (Sabin-Feldman), fluorescent, complement fixation, and hemagglutination inhibition techniques; some of the IgM-dependent examinations are frequently falsely negative in up to 7 percent of newborns in the first few days of life (often owing to the presence of maternal IgG-blocking antibodies). Antibody titers do not correlate with severity of disease. The most useful test for diagnosis of acute infection in the neonate may be the IgM-ELISA. (*Note:* The presence of ANAs or rheumatoid factor may lead to a false positive IgM–indirect immunofluorescence antibody test.)

Diagnosis may also be confirmed by inoculating tissue cultures or mice with acutely infected body fluids or tissue and checking for the presence of organisms in 6 to 10 days. Biopsy of infected tissues, e.g., skeletal muscle, may reveal PAS-positive cysts or trophozoites (especially with immunofluorescence or immunoperoxidase techniques).

Treatment. Infected neonates are usually treated with pyrimethamine, sulfonamides, and folinic acid in the hope of preventing sequelae; sometimes clindamycin is employed. Ophthalmic disease may additionally be specifically treated with steroids. Infected pregnant women are not usually treated, especially during first trimester, owing to the teratogenicity of the drugs. As at least 80 percent of infants exposed to *T. gondii* in utero will be either uninfected or without significant disease, therapeutic abortion is not routinely recommended. Prevention is of prime importance; pregnant women should avoid contact with cat feces, cook meat to above 60° C or freeze it at −20° C for more than 24 hours, and exercise extreme care in handling raw meat and unwashed fruits and vegetables.[48]

Other Conditions Producing TORCHS Syndrome. *Congenital listeriosis* may produce a TORCHS syndrome picture, resulting in spontaneous abortion, stillbirth, prematurity, or neonatal death. The organism *Listeria monocytogenes,* a flagellate gram-positive bacillus, is found worldwide in human and animal carriers. In its acquired form the disease is usually seen in the immunosuppressed. Usually, asymptomatic genital tract infection in the mother during the third trimester produces disease in the child. Male infants are more commonly infected than females. Fever may be absent, but organomegaly, vomiting, diarrhea,

cardiopulmonary distress, and meningitis may be present. Skin lesions may include blueberry muffin lesions and nonspecific exanthem. Diagnosis may be difficult, as cultures of the maternal genital tract, placenta, or neonatal body fluids and tissues may not grow the organism; refrigeration of specimens favors recovery of the organism by facilitating release from the intracellular space. Serodiagnosis is also difficult because of cross-reaction with antistaphylococcal antibodies; specific agglutination tests may peak in 2 to 4 weeks. Histopathology of tissues, especially the liver, reveals miliary granulomatosis. Therapy is with intravenous penicillin and tobramycin for 2 weeks during pregnancy or the neonatal period.

Bacterial sepsis may mimic the TORCHS syndrome by producing systemic toxicity as well as the palpable purpura of septic embolic vasculitis, which may in some ways suggest blueberry muffin lesions. (Biopsy of these should show thrombosis of the dermal vessels and not the islands of nucleated and nonnucleated erythrocytes of dermal hematopoiesis.) Petechiae due to thrombocytopenia and ecchymoses due to coagulopathy may be seen here as well as in the TORCHS syndrome. Appropriate cultures should lead to correct identification of the causative agent.

Leukemias may provoke extramedullary hematopoiesis with blueberry muffin lesions. Lymphoproliferation and metastatic disease may produce "purple plumlike" lesions in skin, simulating the plaques of dermal erythropoiesis.[49,50]

Rubella. Congenital rubella infection is specifically associated with the triad of congenital heart disease, deafness, and cataracts, in addition to a long list of other abnormalities. Approximately 15 percent of women of childbearing age are immunologically naive; hence, in the absence of adequate screening and immunization, epidemics of congenital rubella may be expected to follow those of acquired rubella, occurring every 9 to 10 years. The 1964–1965 epidemic produced more than 20,000 cases of congenital rubella and more than 13,000 deaths due to spontaneous or voluntary abortion or neonatal demise.

Etiology. See discussion of rubella in connection with erythematous eruptions.

Epidemiology. Maternal infection produces viremia, which in turn infects the placenta and causes fetal viremia, with potential dissemination to every organ. At least 90 percent of fetuses exposed in the first trimester will be infected; the risk of a major defect ranges from 50 percent in the first month to 20 percent in the third month and 5 percent in the fourth. Viewing infection during gestation as a whole, less than 15 percent of exposed infants may be expected to be completely disease-free.

Infected infants may shed virus for 2 years or more, though they usually do not spread the disease after 18 months. Virus may persist in the eye, ear, or brain even into adulthood and thus, at least theoretically, may cause late-onset disease.

Course. Intrauterine growth retardation, failure to thrive, and microcephaly may be seen in addition to specific defects. The triad of deafness, cataracts, and congenital heart disease is characteristic, but many lesions can be seen. Sensorineural hearing loss, central auditory disease, otitis media, and vestibular abnormalities may be present. (Sensorineural deafness, the most common defect, may be delayed by years.) Retinopathy, microphthalmia, glaucoma, iridocyclitis, and corneal clouding are other ocular defects seen. Multiple cardiovascular anatomic defects, as well as myocarditis and myocardial necrosis, may be present. Interstitial pneumonitis may be seen as late as 1 year. Meningoencephalitis, psychomotor retardation, spasticity, and progressive panencephalitis may occur. More subtle behavioral and cognitive changes may be noted later. Generalized lymphadenopathy, thrombocytopenia, hemolytic or hypoplastic anemia, thymic aplasia, and depressed cell-mediated and humoral immunity have been reported as well as hepatosplenomegaly and gastrointestinal, musculoskeletal,

dental, and genitourinary defects. Metabolic disease, including diabetes mellitus, growth hormone deficiency, and lymphocytic thyroiditis, may be seen at various stages in life.

Skin lesions classically include the blueberry muffin appearance of dermal erythropoiesis, as well as thrombocytopenic petechiae. An exanthem resembling that seen in acquired rubella but persisting much longer has been reported.

As many as 20 to 30 percent of affected newborns may die in the first year.

Diagnosis. The presence of the classic triad of defects may immediately suggest congenital rubella in a TORCHS syndrome baby. The diagnosis may be suggested by careful review of the maternal history, particularly of the first trimester; it may be made in utero by isolation of rubella virus obtained by amniocentesis. After birth cultures of nasopharyngeal secretions, urine, or other body fluids should be obtained to confirm the diagnosis. Detection of IgM-neutralizing antibodies or, after 6 months, IgG hemagglutination antibodies is also helpful. Multiple laboratory abnormalities may be found, as suggested by the plethora of possible defects, but they are not specific except perhaps for findings related to the metabolic abnormalities.

Treatment. Therapeutic abortion should be recommended to women infected at least during the first 18 weeks of pregnancy owing to the considerable risk to the fetus. If abortion is refused, immune globulin may be offered, but this has no proven efficacy in preventing viremia. Symptomatic care, including indicated surgery and ophthalmologic and otologic follow-up, is paramount. Steroids may be beneficial in treatment of interstitial pneumonitis, which is potentially fatal. (Steroids should not be used to treat the causes underlying purpura.)

Prevention is key. Infected infants should be sequestered from pregnant women until viral shedding has ceased, at anywhere from 6 months to 2 years. Vaccination with attenuated virus should be performed in children by 15 months; vaccination should not be administered to women within the 12 months preceding conception. Pregnant women with baseline antibody titers of 1:16 or greater should be considered immune. If titers are insufficient or absent, repeat titers should be checked 2 to 3 weeks following possible infection.[50]

Generalized Cytomegalic Inclusion Disease. Cytomegalovirus (CMV), the cause of generalized cytomegalic inclusion disease, is found worldwide, with antibodies present in 50 percent of the population of industrialized nations and in up to 100 percent of third world peoples. It is a common cause of congenital or perinatal infection though infection is asymptomatic about 90 percent of the time. Active disease prominently involves brain, liver, and bone marrow and often leads to death or mental deficiency. In contradistinction to the other entities comprising TORCHS syndrome, congenital CMV infection may arise not only from primary infection but also from reactivation of latent disease in the mother.

Etiology. The agent is a member of the DNA herpesvirus group.

Epidemiology. The virus may be transmitted transplacentally, by blood products, and by transplanted organs. Presumably, the major damage occurs during first trimester infections; additionally, the baby may be infected in the birth canal during labor. Although virus has been found in the cervix, semen, and milk, transmission by sexual contact and by nursing is still uncertain.

The incidence of viral shedding in pregnant women is unclear, as up to one-fifth of women in the third trimester may have positive cervical cultures, whereas the yield earlier in pregnancy may be as low as 2 percent. Among newborns, 1 to three percent have CMV in the urine at birth; about 10 percent of these have symptomatic illness. Viral shedding by infected infants may persist up to 1 year or longer.

Course. Even apparently asymptomatic newborns may suffer delayed-onset CNS dis-

ease. At birth organomegaly with or without icterus may be present. Microcephaly, retardation, sensorineural deafness, and chorioretinitis are the more frequent defects, but multiple ophthalmic, cardiopulmonary, musculoskeletal, and gastrointestinal defects similar to those of congenital rubella may occur. Depressed markers of CMV-specific cell-mediated immunity may be seen. Death may occur perinatally, and institutionalization for mental deficiency is not infrequent.

In the skin blueberry muffin lesions may be prominent, reflecting the widespread extramedullary hematopoiesis associated with CMV. Petechiae due to thrombocytopenia and, rarely, vesicles are also seen.

Diagnosis. There are no specific clinical markers of congenital CMV infection. Helpful laboratory examinations include skull x-rays and CAT scan, which may reveal the periventricular or subependymal calcifications associated with significant neurologic deficits. Abnormal lucencies of the metaphyses, similar to those in congenital rubella, may also be seen on x-ray. Routine laboratory findings are nonspecific and may show thrombocytopenia, CSF pleiocytosis and elevated protein, and hyperbilirubinemia.

The serologic test of choice is the IgM-immunofluorescent test on cord blood, which is positive in 95 percent of clinically affected neonates. Other techniques, such as complement fixation, may depend upon the presence of IgG; multiple determinations to detect the onset of neonatal IgG (at minimally four times the maternal titer) plus persistence of the IgG (as opposed to the transience of passively acquired maternal antibody) are less practical. Additionally, cultures of body fluids, buffy coat, or tissue should be obtained as soon as possible. In a minority of patients cytologic examination of urine will show the classic 8-μm intranuclear and small intracytoplasmic inclusions; electron microscopic examination increases the yield. Histopathology of infected tissues yields similar findings.

Treatment. Therapy is at best supportive, as currently available antiviral agents such as vidarabine and cytarabine have been found ineffective in eradicating infection. Experimental agents such as dihydroxypropoxymethylguanine (DHPG), an inhibitor of viral DNA polymerase, may prove effective. Long-term follow-up is necessary as sequelae may be delayed in onset. Isolation of infected children with active viral shedding may be warranted.[51]

Herpes simplex. Congenital herpes simplex infection is apparently uncommon but may be associated with 50 percent mortality and up to 50 percent severe morbidity in survivors. With increasing rates of genital herpes infections in recent years, congenital infection is a timely concern.

Etiology. *Herpesvirus hominis,* a double-stranded DNA virus, is the infectious agent. Most congenital infections occur with type 2, as this is the prevalent organism in genital infections.

Epidemiology. An incidence of congenital herpes simplex ranging from 1 in 30,000 to 1 in 2,000 births has been reported, yet active maternal infection during pregnancy has been estimated at about 2.5 percent. The risk of transmission is as great as 10 percent if there is active maternal infection during the final 2 months of pregnancy. The risk approaches 40 percent if there is primary infection at term, but this probably results in acquired neonatal infections rather than in the congenital syndrome. The acquired cases present after the first 2 days of life with evidence of systemic infection, and patients may have localized or disseminated cutaneous herpetiform lesions. Although these cases may be severe and associated with significant morbidity and mortality, they are not associated with congenital defects of the TORCHS complex.

Course. At birth the baby may be small for gestational age. Few, many, or no herpetiform lesions may be present, and systemic con-

genital defects may not always be apparent yet. The CNS findings include microcephaly, hydrocephaly, retardation, seizures, and abnormal muscular tone. A variety of ophthalmic abnormalities, including keratoconjunctivitis, chorioretinitis, and microphthalmia are found. As with other TORCHS diseases, multisystem involvement may be evident, with hepatosplenomegaly, cardipulmonary disease, and musculoskeletal abnormalities. Thrombocytopenia and even disseminated intravascular coagulopathy may occur, as in related conditions.

In herpes simplex, unlike the other TORCHS diseases, grouped umbilicated vesicles or vesicopustules on the skin or mucous membranes are highly distinctive; however, less than 50 percent of infected infants manifest vesicles, ulcers, or keratitis. Again, in contrast to other TORCHS entities, dermal erythropoietic "blueberry muffin" lesions are not seen but petechiae (thrombocytopenia) and ecchymoses (coagulopathy) are.

As stated earlier, mortality and morbidity rates are high. As with other TORCHS entities, sequelae, particularly neurologic effects, may be delayed.

Diagnosis. The presence of herpetiform vesicles is very helpful; as in other herpesvirus group infections, Tzanck preparations (Wright, Giemsa, or Papanicolaou stains) of the base of an unroofed vesicle reveal multinucleated epithelial giant cells and balloon cells with nucleoplasmic margination. Antiherpesvirus immunofluorescent antibody staining of infected skin or other tissue is also of use, as is viral culture of infected tissues and body fluids, such as CSF; cytopathic changes in tissue culture can be seen as early as 1 day. Biopsy of herpetiform skin lesions will show an intraepidermal vesicle, with ballooning of epidermal cells, acantholysis and necrosis of keratinocytes, margination of nucleoplasm, multinucleated epithelial giant cells, dermal edema, and variably dense, round cell perivascular infiltration. Again, as with the Tzanck preparation, other herpesvirus infections will show similar findings. These studies will exclude other causes of vesiculopustules in the newborn, including syphilis, impetigo, epidermolysis bullosa, mastocytosis, and erythema toxicum neonatorum. Serologic diagnosis may provide additional confirmation, but the diagnosis is best made by viral culture.

As with other TORCHS infections, routine laboratory examinations may show thrombocytopenia, anemia, coagulopathy, and pleiocytosis and elevated protein in CSF. Cerebral calcifications and radiographic abnormalities of bone similar to those found in congenital rubella or CMV infection may also be seen.

Treatment. Acyclovir and vidarabine are both employed; the former is less toxic and may prove more effective. Cesarean delivery is indicated when obvious maternal infection is present or when viral cultures (routinely performed near term in known asymptomatic carriers) are positive. At this time, however, there are no recommendations for treatment of active maternal infections earlier in pregnancy when presumably the congenital syndrome may be initiated.[49,50]

Congenital Syphilis. Congenital (prenatal) syphilis is a highly variable syndrome, its manifestations and severity depending on the timing of infection during gestation. Fetal wastage may be as high as 25 percent and perinatal mortality 25 to 30 percent; of the survivors, about 40 percent are estimated to be symptomatic, and the remainder are apparently well and may or may not be serologically positive.

(Syphilis may be acquired by contact with infectious active maternal lesions during birth; such a neonatal infection will begin with a primary chancre and may be expected to manifest the signs of secondary syphilis, discussed earlier in this chapter.)

Etiology. The agent is *T. pallidum* (see the discussion of secondary syphilis).

Epidemiology. Duration of infection in the mother is of prime importance. Although the disease may be transmitted in utero in women with late latent disease and even congenital disease (although acute reinfection may have also occurred), generally maternal infection for more than 4 years poses little risk to the fetus. In other words, the more recent the maternal infection, the greater the danger to the fetus. Additionally, the severity of disease in the child depends upon when in the pregnancy the mother acquires infection. Acute maternal infection early in pregnancy, by about weeks 12 through 16, can cause fetal death as well as severe abnormalities, while maternal infection late in the pregnancy may produce an apparently normal child at birth, who may not show evidence of disease, including seropositivity, for months or even years. (Interestingly, evidence of fetal infection is rare before 16 weeks although spirochetal transplacental passage is documented as early as 8 or 9 weeks. The explanation remains moot; electron microscopic evidence indicates that there is no anatomic change in the Langhans' layer of the chorion, which was previously thought to atrophy and thus allow infection only after the third month. It has been suggested that the early fetus is insufficiently immunocompetent to produce the reactive changes in tissue and resultant damage associated with treponemal infection. Therapeutically, this is of prime importance, as early detection and treatment before 12 to 16 weeks should ensure delivery of a completely normal child.)

Congenital or, more correctly, prenatal, syphilis is customarily divided into two groups, early disease and late disease. Early congenital syphilis presents within the first 2 years of life and is analogous to secondary syphilis; logically, it is associated with more acute maternal infection. Late congenital syphilis is evident after 2 years and is similar to late adult disease. The clinical picture of late congenital syphilis does not resemble TORCHS.

Course of Early Congenital Syphilis. The earlier the presentation, the greater the severity of disease. Babies presenting at or near birth, and thus most reminiscent of other TORCHS victims, are acutely ill and risk nearly a 50 percent chance of death. These infants show signs of intrauterine growth retardation, and the placentas may be abnormally large. Features of hydrops fetalis or, conversely, a "withered old man" appearance are distinctive. Hepatosplenomegaly, jaundice, lymphadenopathy, periostitis and osteomyelitis, hemolytic anemia, thrombocytopenia, leukocytosis, erythroblastosis, and coagulopathy may all be seen. In this early severe form the skin may show purpura mimicking the blueberry muffin appearance of congenital CMV infection and rubella; erosions of the ears and extremities may also be present.

Fortunately, most early-disease babies do not present until the second to sixth week and are much less severely affected. These children may have organomegaly and jaundice. Cutaneously, they develop lesions of secondary syphilis, with copper-colored macules and papules on the head, palms, soles, and anogenital areas; mucous patches and condylomata lata may also be present. They may present with the distinctive vesicopustules of early syphilis, particularly on palms and soles, as well as syphilitic rhinitis ("snuffles"), productive of an often hemorrhagic nasal discharge. This may leave a saddle nose deformity and rhagades. Paronychia may be seen. Periostitis and osteochondritis may cause sufficiently severe pain to inhibit motion (pseudoparalysis of Parrot). Acute glomerulonephritis and nephrotic syndrome may be present, and CNS disease, which may be asymptomatic or evince meningitis, convulsions, and hydrocephalus, occurs in up to one-half of cases.

Course of Late Congenital Syphilis. The onset of signs and symptoms in late congenital syphilis often resembles that of late acquired syphilis at the age of 2 years through the third decade; this phase of congenital syphilis thus does not properly constitute TORCHS syndrome. Findings often include interstitial keratitis, eighth nerve deafness and Hutchinson's teeth (Hutchinson's triad); neurosyphilis; Clutton's joints (syphilitic synovitis of the knees); periostitis and gummata of bone; and paroxysmal cold hemoglobinuria. Skin lesions are the

gummata of late acquired disease. Other stigmata (which may result from early congenital syphilis and from other unrelated causes) include saddle nose, frontal bossing, shortened maxilla and high arched palate, saber shin, sternoclavicular enlargement (Higouménakis' sign) and mulberry molars. Cardiovascular disease is less frequent than in the adult late form. As much as 60 percent of late congenital syphilis may be latent, with positive serology being the only sign of disease.

Diagnosis. In the extremely early form of early congenital syphilis there may be no specific clinical sign distinguishing it from the rest of TORCHS. In the less acute form of that disease the presence of snuffles and localized vesiculopustules, as well as cutaneous manifestations of secondary lues, may readily indicate the diagnosis. Dark-field microscopic examination of the umbilical vein, skin lesions, and nasal discharge will demonstrate treponemes and is the diagnostic examination of choice. Biopsy of skin lesions will demonstrate endothelial cell swelling and perivascular cuffing with mononuclear cells, including plasma cells; silver stains may demonstrate the presence of the spirochete. Radiographic and other laboratory examinations reflect the clinical changes described above.

Serologic examination does not provide the same definitive diagnosis as does dark-field. Owing to passive transplacental passage of maternal IgG, nontreponemal tests may be positive at birth in the offspring of a seropositive mother even if she has been adequately treated. Unfortunately, the FTA-ABS-IgM test is insufficiently sensitive to serve as a definitive screening test.

Treatment. The major treatment is preventive, with adequate maternal care. Routine nontreponemal serologic screening in the first 3 months and at or near delivery would ensure identification and treatment of nearly all mothers and children at risk. Recall that treatment before weeks 12 to 16 virtually guarantees a normal child, while therapy after 18 weeks eradicates infection but may not prevent the stigmata, e.g., bony malformations, arising from the already established inflammation. Treatment of infected mothers is as outlined in standard texts. In penicillin-allergic pregnant women, erythromycin but not tetracycline may be substituted. However, erythromycin treatment failures in the child have been reported, so routine treatment with penicillin is recommended at birth. Similarly, all infants born to mothers given no or unknown treatment should be treated at birth. Even if the mother has been adequately treated, the infant, asymptomatic or not, should be treated if (1) the neonatal nontreponemal antibody titer (e.g., VDRL) of the cord blood exceeds the maternal titer by two or more dilutions or (2) an initial neonatal titer less than or equal to the maternal titer fails to convert to negative by 3 months. (Infants born to mothers treated for syphilis during pregnancy should be examined at birth, 1 month, then every 3 months for 15 months, and then every 6 months until nontreponemal antibody titers are negative or stable.) Examination of CSF should be performed on all patients with congenital syphilis prior to treatment. All patients with congenital syphilis with abnormal CSF should receive aqueous crystalline penicillin G 50,000 units/ kg intravenously or intramuscularly (divided into two daily doses) for 10 days or more; aqueous procaine penicillin G 50,000 units/kg given intramuscularly daily for 10 days or more may be substituted. Congenital syphilis without evidence of neurosyphilis may be treated with benzathine penicillin G 50,000 units/kg intramuscularly once.

Older children may be treated by similar guidelines, with dosages not to exceed those recommended for adults. As in acquired syphilis, Jarisch-Herxheimer reactions may occur. In the case of penicillin allergy erythromycin may be substituted, but tetracycline must not be used before age 8; all patients treated without penicillin should be closely followed.

Early congenital syphilis patients without neurosyphilis should be followed after treatment with quantitative nontreponemal tests at least every 3 months for 1 year. Patients treated for congenital syphilis lasting more than 1 year should be checked again 24 months after treatment. Patients with early congenital syphilis should show negative or low serum titers on quantitative nontreponemal antibody testing within 1 year; cases of longer duration may require more time.

Patients treated with drugs other than penicillin require careful follow-up, and repeat CSF examination at the last follow-up visit is recommended. Patients with neurosyphilis require repeat serologic testing, semiannual clinical examination, and repeat CSF studies for at least 3 years.

Retreatment is recommended if there is new, persistent, or recurrent clinical evidence of disease; if the nontreponemal titer increases fourfold; or if the initial high titer fails to fall fourfold in a year. Unless a diagnosis of early acquired syphilis (reinfection) can be substantiated, a CSF examination should be performed before retreatment. Retreatment is as outlined for standard therapy of acquired syphilis of more than 1 year's duration. As stable low titers may persist, more than one retreatment course is usually not indicated.[48–53]

RICKETTSIAL INFECTIONS

Rocky Mountain Spotted Fever

Rocky Mountain spotted fever (RMSF) is an acute rickettsial illness characterized by fever and a purpuric eruption and transmitted to humans by the bite of an infected tick.

Etiology. The causative organism of RMSF is *Rickettsia rickettsii*.

Epidemiology. The disease is seen in all parts of the United States, with the highest incidence in the southeast and Rocky Mountain regions, and affects all ages, the majority of victims being children between 5 and 9 years of age. It is primarily a disease of spring and summer, corresponding to the increased activity of the tick vectors, *Dermacentor andersoni* (wood tick), *Dermacentor variabilis* (dog tick), and *Amblyomma americanum* (Lone Star tick).

Course. The incubation period varies from 2 to 12 days, with a mean of about 6 days. There is an abrupt onset of high fever, associated with headache, chills, malaise, and myalgias. The rash appears 3 to 4 days after the onset of fever and is characterized by blanchable pink macules on the wrists, ankles, and forearms, which progress to involve the palms, soles, extremities, trunk, and face within 6 to 18 hours. After 2 to 4 days the eruption becomes papular and purpuric (Fig. 8-5) and may lead to gangrene of digits, earlobes, nose, scrotum, or vulva. Bilaterally symmetric purpura of the palms and soles is a characteristic clinical feature. Major complications include CNS involvement, myocarditis, and disseminated intravascular coagulation. The overall mortality rate is 5 to 10 percent but may be up to 80 percent in untreated cases.

Diagnosis. The diagnosis is often based on historic, epidemiologic, and clinical features. Weil-Felix serologic tests using Proteus OX-19 and OX-2 become positive in the second and third weeks and are followed by specific complement fixation tests. The most rapid and efficient diagnosis is made by direct immunofluorescence of a skin biopsy demonstrating fluorescent organisms in the walls of blood vessels.

The major differential diagnostic possibilities include meningococcemia, atypical measles, typhus, echo 9 disease, allergic vasculitis, and drug reactions.

Treatment. Therapy must be instituted immediately in a suspected case. Tetracycline and chloramphenicol are the drugs of choice. Tetracycline may be given orally in a dose of 25 to 50 mg/kg daily up to 2 g/day for 7 to 10 days, or intravenously in a dose of 20 mg/kg daily. Chloramphenicol is administered intravenously

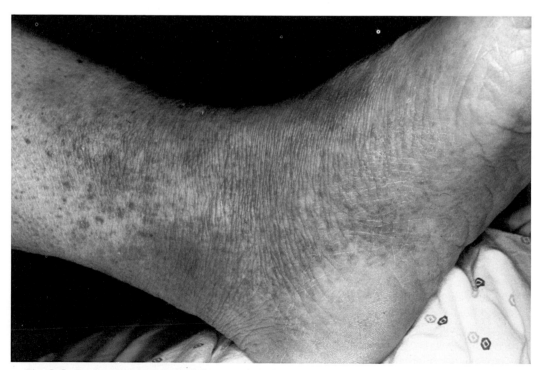

Fig. 8–5. Rocky Mountain spotted fever: rash begins over wrists and ankles and becomes purpuric.

in a dose of 50 to 75 mg/kg daily with a maximum of 2 to 4 g/day. Treatment should be continued for 2 to 4 days after the patient has been afebrile.

The best method of prevention is to protect against tick bites by use of repellants and tight clothing.[54,55]

Epidemic Typhus

Epidemic typhus is an acute rickettsial illness characterized by fever, severe prostration, and a purpuric eruption and transmitted from human to human by the bite of an infected louse.

Etiology. The causative organism is *Rickettsia prowazekii*.

Epidemiology. Epidemic typhus is still endemic in certain parts of the world but has been absent from the United States since the 1920s. It may be seen in all age groups and may recur with holocaust, war, and famine. Man is the predominant reservoir and the major vector is the body louse, followed by the head louse.

Course. The incubation period varies from 7 to 14 days. There is an abrupt onset of high fever associated with headache, chills, malaise, and general myalgias. The rash appears between the fourth and seventh febrile day and is characterized by erythematous, blanching macules occurring initially in the axillae and spreading to the trunk and extremities. The eruption becomes purpuric during the second week, does not become papular, and does not involve the palms and soles. Gangrene may occur over bony prominences. Major complications include CNS involvement, myocarditis, and hypotension. The mortality rate is 10 to 40 percent in untreated cases.

Diagnosis. The diagnosis is often based on the clinical picture, a positive Weil-Felix reaction with Proteus OX-19, and a less positive reaction with OX-2. Specific complement fixation tests are positive during convalescence.

Diseases to be considered in the differential diagnosis include typhoid fever, atypical and typical measles, meningococcemia, RMSF, echo virus 9 disease, and drug reactions.

Treatment. A single oral dose of 100 mg of doxycycline cures most adults and 50 mg cures most children below 10 years of age. Tetracycline and chloramphenicol are also effective but must be continued until the patient is afebrile for 2 to 3 days.[54]

BACTERIAL INFECTIONS

Meningococcemia

Meningococcemia is an acute bacterial illness, which may vary from a mild respiratory illness to fulminant septicemia associated with a purpuric eruption.

Etiology. The causative organism is *Neisseria meningitidis* (meningococcus).

Epidemiology. Meningococcemia is seen worldwide, with a peak incidence in late winter and spring. The attack rate is greatest in males less than 15 years of age. It is spread from person to person by droplet infection.

Course. The incubation period varies from 2 to 10 days. The onset may be mild, with a flu-like illness, or more severe, with an abrupt onset of fever, chills, myalgias, signs of meningitis, hypotension, and shock. Cutaneous manifestations characterized by purpura occur in approximately 50 percent of patients, usually within the first 3 days of illness. Purpuric lesions vary in size from petechiae to ecchymoses, occur most frequently on the trunk and lower extremities, and are often palpable and irregular in shape with gun-metal gray centers. Extensive purpura and gangrene may occur, with disseminated intravascular coagulation. Other complications include septic foci in other organs and rapid death. The mortality rate of untreated meningococcemia is approximately

70 percent, with a rate of 10 to 15 percent for treated cases, death being most frequent in those less than 2 years of age.

Diagnosis. Diagnosis can be made by culturing the meningococcus from blood, CSF, or the nasopharynx. Counterimmunoelectrophoresis (CIE) of CSF is also available. Gram stain of material from purpuric lesions less than 24 hours old may reveal gram-negative diplococci.

The differential diagnosis includes other bacterial septicemias, RMSF, typhus, atypical measles, echo 9 disease and hypersensitivity vasculitis.

Treatment. Penicillin G is the treatment of choice and should be administered intravenously in doses of 80,000 to 240,000 units/kg per day. Chloramphenicol in doses of 25 to 100 mg/kg daily is a good alternative. Therapy should be continued for 7 to 10 days.[56]

Gonococcemia

Gonococcemia is a disseminated gonococcal infection characterized by fever, polyarthritis, and palpable purpura.

Etiology. The causative organism is *Neisseria gonorrhoeae* (gonococcus).

Epidemiology. Gonococcemia may be seen in 1 to 3 percent of all patients with gonorrhea. The disease is more common in females than males and frequently follows menstruation. Transmission is usually venereal.

Course. The incubation period is variable, from a few days to a few weeks postcontact. The dermatitis-arthritis form usually begins with fever, tenosynovitis, a migratory polyarthritis, which usually affects a large joint, and slightly tender, palpable purpuric skin lesions. These lesions are usually distal and asymmetric, number about 5 to 20, and heal in 3 to 5 days without scarring. Complications include septic arthritis, meningitis, and endocarditis.

Diagnosis. Diagnosis can be made by culturing the gonococcus from the genitourinary tract, rectum, throat, synovial fluid, or blood. Gram stain of material from skin lesions rarely demonstrates organisms, although direct immunofluorescence may be positive.

The major differential diagnostic possibilities include other bacterial septicemias, collagen vascular disease, and hypersensitivity vasculitis.

Treatment. Penicillin G is the treatment of choice and should be given intravenously in doses of 10 million units per day until improvement occurs, followed by oral ampicillin 500 mg four times a day for 7 days. Penicillin-sensitive patients may be treated with tetracycline or erythromycin.[57,58]

Staphylococcal Sepsis

Staphylococcal sepsis is an acute bacterial illness characterized by fever and palpable purpuric lesions.

Etiology. The causative organism is *Staphylococcus aureus*.

Epidemiology. Staphylococcal sepsis may be seen at all ages and results from direct inoculation of organisms into the circulation, as in intravenous drug abuse, or from hematogenous spread from other staphylococcal foci, such as deep folliculitis or endocarditis.

Course. The incubation period is variable. The clinical picture consists of fever and chills associated with distal, asymmetric palpable purpuric lesions, from few to several in number, usually with purulent centers. Rarely, firm, tender subcutaneous nodules of the trunk may also be present. Major complications include metastatic spread to various organs leading to suppurative abscesses and disseminated intravascular coagulation. The mortality rate may be up to 50 percent, even with appropriate treatment.

Diagnosis. The diagnosis can be made by culturing organisms from blood or skin lesions. Gram stain of material from purpuric pustular lesions may reveal gram-positive cocci in clusters, both intra- and extracellularly. Differential diagnosis includes other bacterial septicemias, collagen vascular disease, and hypersensitivity vasculitis.

Treatment. Prolonged parenteral therapy is required, with 150 to 200 mg/kg per day of nafcillin, methicillin, or oxacillin for penicillinase-producing organisms. The major alternative drugs are vancomycin, cephalosporins, and gentamicin.[59]

Pseudomonas Sepsis

Pseudomonas sepsis is usually seen in patients with an underlying disease and is characterized by fever and palpable purpuric lesions.

Etiology. The causative organism is *Pseudomonas aeruginosa.*

Epidemiology. Pseudomonas sepsis may be seen in all ages and depends mostly on impaired host defenses rather than on direct transmission of organisms or on their increased pathogenicity. Predisposing risk factors may include malignancy, antibiotic and immunosuppressive therapy, extensive burns, and gastrointestinal or genitourinary infections.

Course. The incubation period is variable. Clinically, the patients frequently demonstrate worsening signs and symptoms of the underlying disease, associated with fever and characteristic cutaneous lesions. These lesions include painful, opalescent vesicles and bullae, which become purpuric and may occur anywhere on the body. Ecthyma gangrenosum is characterized by painless ulcerations with a black eschar and erythematous borders following purpuric bullae; it is often seen in the anogenital or axillary areas. Gangrenous cellulitis and rose spotlike truncal lesions may also be seen. Major complications include septic embolization to other organs, disseminated intravascular coagulation, and death.

Diagnosis. The diagnosis is often based on the characteristic cutaneous lesion of ecthyma gangrenosum and the demonstration of gram-negative rods from skin lesions. The differential diagnosis includes other bacterial septicemias and spider bites.

Treatment. The parenteral treatment of choice is the combination of an aminoglycoside, such as 5 to 6 mg/kg per day of gentamicin, tobramycin, or amikacin, with 400 to 500 mg/kg per day of carbenicillin.[60]

Subacute Bacterial Endocarditis

Subacute bacterial endocarditis is a bacterial infection of the heart associated with *Streptococcus* spp. and characterized by fever and palpable purpuric lesions.

Etiology. The majority of cases are due to *Streptococcus viridans* and group D streptococci.

Epidemiology. The incidence of endocarditis may be related to the frequency of predisposing cardiac disease. Bacteremia secondary to oropharyngeal, gastrointestinal, and genitourinary manipulation leads to the formation of vegetations on damaged valves by relatively avirulent microorganisms.

Course. The incubation period is variable. The clinical picture consists of fever, chills, malaise, anemia, and heart murmur, associated with a variety of purpuric lesions. These include petechiae of the extremities, chest, and mucous membranes, splinter hemorrhages of the nails, painful Osler's nodes of the pads of the fingers and toes, and painless Janeway lesions of the palms and soles. The pathogenesis of the purpuric lesions is unclear, as they may represent examples of microembolization or local immune reactions. The major complications are those of embolization from vegetations to various organs and cardiac failure. Prognosis is variable and depends on the infecting organism, severity of the condition, and time of initiation of therapy.

Diagnosis. The diagnosis is usually made by culturing organisms from the blood. Gram stain of material from skin lesions may reveal gram-positive cocci. Differential diagnosis includes other bacterial septicemias, collagen vascular disease, hypersensitivity vasculitis, and trichinosis.

Treatment. Prolonged parenteral antibiotic therapy is necessary to effect a cure. For the viridans group, 65 to 70 mg/kg per day of penicillin G plus streptomycin 20 mg/kg per day is the treatment of choice, with vancomycin and cefazolin being good alternative drugs. For group D streptococci, the suggested treatment is 200 to 300 mg/kg per day of ampicillin plus 5 to 6 mg/kg per day of gentamicin or tobramycin. Vancomycin plus streptomycin is a good alternative.[61,62]

Noninfectious Disorders

Allergic Vasculitis

Allergic vasculitis is characterized by bilaterally symmetric palpable purpura, often occurring with fever. It is associated with multiple etiologies, which are discussed in detail in Chapter 1.

Etiology. Etiologic factors include infections such as hepatitis B, group A β-hemolytic streptococcal infection, and many others; drugs, including sulfonamides and penicillin; connective tissue diseases, particularly lupus and rheumatoid arthritis; serum sickness; Henoch-Schönlein purpura; and others. Many cases are idiopathic, but deposition of circulating immune complexes in blood vessels appears to play a central pathogenetic role regardless of etiology.

Course. The eruption usually begins over the legs, may involve the buttocks and arms, and is most often characterized by symmetric purpuric papules. Vesicles, necrotic ulcers, and urticarial papules and plaques can also occur. Lesions may appear in crops over days to weeks and usually resolve within 1 week to 1 month. Skin lesions may be accompanied by fever, malaise, and systemic manifestations, including arthralgias and arthritis, hematuria, and proteinuria. Complications are associated with systemic involvement, and in addition to those already mentioned may include pneumonitis and CNS vasculitis. Chronic renal disease is the most serious complication.

Some symptoms suggest specific etiologies or syndromes. Serum sickness, for example, follows administration of antitoxin or drug within 2 weeks and is characterized by fever, arthralgias, lymphadenopathy, and an urticarial rash. Henoch-Schönlein purpura typically affects children and young adults, and the symmetric purpuric lesions of the lower legs are often associated with abdominal pain, gastrointestinal bleeding, and evidence of renal involvement.

Diagnosis. The diagnosis is based on the clinical finding of bilaterally symmetric palpable purpura of the lower extremities and confirmed by the histologic finding of leukocytoclastic vasculitis. Deposits of IgA in dermal blood vessels and in glomeruli are also characteristic of Henoch-Schönlein purpura.

The major differential diagnoses include RMSF, meningococcemia, echovirus 9 disease, collagen vascular disease, and purpura fulminans.

Treatment. Rest, antihistamines, and supportive care are beneficial. Treatment of specific etiologic factors, if found, is warranted. The efficacy of systemic corticosteroid therapy is questionable, although this modality is often used, especially for systemic or severe skin involvement.[63,64]

VESICOPUSTULAR ERUPTIONS (TABLE 8-5)

Infectious Disorders

VIRAL INFECTIONS

Herpes Simplex

Herpes simplex is a viral infection primarily affecting the skin and mucous membranes and characterized by grouped vesicles on an erythematous base.

Etiology. The causative organism is *Herpesvirus hominis.*

Epidemiology. Herpes simplex is seen worldwide and in all age groups, and transmission is usually by person-to-person contact. Humans are the major hosts for the virus, and there are two antigenic types, one associated primarily with nongenital disease and one associated with genital disease. Infection may be primary or recurrent, recurrent infection being associated with the presence of antibodies. Trigger factors implicated in recurrences include stress, fever, sunlight, menses, and infections.

Course. The incubation period of primary herpetic infection is 2 to 12 days, with an average of 6 days. Primary infections include gingivostomatitis, vulvovaginitis, genital infection in the male, herpetic whitlow, keratoconjuncti-

Table 8-5. Approach to the Patient: Clinical and Laboratory Features of Vesicopustular Eruptions Associated with Fever

Disorder	Clinical Features	Laboratory
Herpes simplex	Vesicles on erythematous base become pustules, erosions and crusts; prodromal pain	Viral culture; Tzanck and Pap smears
Varicella	Vesicles on red base, lesions in different stages begin on trunk and spread to face and extremities	Tzanck prep; viral culture
Herpes zoster	Grouped vesicles on erythematous base in a unilateral dermatomal distribution; prodromal pain	Tzanck prep; viral culture
Kaposi's varicelliform eruption	Follows vaccination or herpes simplex infection in a patient with atopic dermatitis, Darier's disease, or other dermatosis	Tzanck prep; viral culture
Variola	Eradicated; started on face and extremities; all lesions in same stage	Tzanck prep with Giemsa stain; electron microscopy; immunofluorescence; viral culture
Hand-foot-and-mouth disease	Children; oral vesicles; oval vesicles on hands, feet and buttocks; 1 day prodrome of fever and abdominal pain	Viral culture; acute serum-neutralizing antibody titers (usually unnecessary)
Enterovirus infection	Occasional exanthem; associated symptoms variable	Viral culture; acute and convalescent titers
Rickettsial pox	Eschar at site of mite bite, erythematous papulovesicles, lymphadenopathy	Negative Weil-Felix; acute and convalescent complement-fixing antibody titers
Staphylococcal scalded skin syndrome	Staphylococcal infection; erythema followed by bulla formation; Nikolsky sign; desquamation of large sheets of skin	Bacterial cultures from primary site of infection (not skin); skin biopsy or peel

vitis, eczema herpeticum, and neonatal infection. Recurrent infections include herpes labialis, herpes progenitalis, herpes cervicitis, herpetic whitlow, lumbosacral infection, keratoconjunctivitis, and eczema herpeticum. In general, primary infection is characterized by painful and more widespread umbilicated vesicles on erythematous bases, affecting the skin and mucous membranes. The lesions become pustular, erosive, and crusted and may last up to 2 to 6 weeks. Recurrent infections are often preceded by paresthesias or pain; the lesions are smaller and less painful than in primary infection and last for 5 to 7 days.

Gingivostomatitis is the most common primary infection with herpes type 1 and has its peak incidence in the 1- to 5-year age group. Dehydration is the most common complication and may require intravenous fluids. The major complications of primary genital herpes are urinary retention and aseptic meningitis. Herpetic keratoconjunctivitis may result in blindness. Disseminated disease, both cutaneous and visceral, may occur in immunocompromised hosts.

Diagnosis. The diagnosis is confirmed by the finding of multinucleated giant cells on a Tzanck preparation from the base of a vesicle and culture of virus from lesions. The differential diagnosis is extensive and varies according to location of the infection. The major considerations include herpangina, EM, aphthous stomatitis, varicella, impetigo, herpes zoster, cellulitis, contact dermatitis, and bullous disease.

Treatment. All types of herpetic infection require supportive and local care. Although there has been no specific treatment available that can consistently promote healing of an existing infection and prevent future recurrence, the use of acyclovir is most promising. It may be used parenterally for severe disease and orally for recurrent infection.[65–67]

Varicella and Herpes Zoster

Varicella, or chickenpox, is a contagious viral infection characterized by disseminated vesicopustular lesions. Herpes zoster, or shingles, is a dermatomal vesicobullous disease caused by reactivation of the virus that causes chickenpox.

Etiology. The causative organism of both disorders is the varicella-zoster virus (herpesvirus varicellae).

Epidemiology. Varicella and herpes zoster are worldwide in distribution and seen only in humans. Varicella occurs most commonly in winter and spring, primarily in children younger than 10 years, with the majority between 2 and 6 years. Herpes zoster occurs throughout the year in all ages, with the majority in the 50- to 80-year age group. Varicella is usually transmitted by direct contact or droplet spread, and crusts are not infectious. Zoster represents reactivation of latent varicella-zoster virus infection, although contact with a zoster patient can produce varicella in a susceptible host, usually by direct contact spread. Possible trigger factors associated with reactivation of virus include reexposure to varicella and local irritation of the dorsal root ganglion secondary to x-ray therapy, malignancy, and Pott's disease.

Course. In varicella the incubation period is 14 to 21 days, with a 1-day prodrome characterized by fever, malaise, myalgias, and headache. The rash begins on the trunk, spreads to the face and extremities, and is characterized by pruritic erythematous macules, which progress to vesicles on a red base ("dew drops on a rose petal"), pustules, and crusts over a 12- to 24-hour period. Lesions usually appear in three crops over a few days, which results in lesions in different stages of development. Vesicles and erosions are also present in the mouth. Other manifestations include pneumonia (rare in children), encephalitis, and orchitis. Major complications include secondary bacterial infection of the skin, neurologic defects, and disseminated intravascular coagulation. The mortality rate is 10 to 20 percent in neonatal varicella.

The incubation period of herpes zoster is unknown. Paresthesias and pain may precede the eruption by 4 to 5 days. The rash is characterized by grouped, umbilicated vesicles on erythematous bases in a dermatomal distribution, which begin as erythematous, edematous plaques and progress to pustules and crusts over a 1- to 3-day period. Crops of lesions may appear for 1 week and may be associated with fever, headache, malaise, and regional lymphadenopathy. The eruption is usually unilateral, most commonly occurring in the thoracic area, and heals within 2 to 4 weeks. The major complications include ocular damage associated with trigeminal involvement, disseminated zoster, usually seen in immunocompromised patients, postherpetic neuralgia which is unusual in children, the Ramsay-Hunt syndrome, and motor paralysis.

Diagnosis. The diagnosis of both varicella and herpes zoster is usually based on clinical presentation. Confirmatory findings include the presence of multinucleated giant cells in a Tzanck preparation of tissue fluid from skin lesions and culture of the virus from lesions.

The major differential diagnoses of varicella include erythema toxicum neonatorum, pustular miliaria, coxsackievirus infection, rickettsial pox, variola, and pityriasis lichenoides et varioliformis acuta (PLEVA). Differential diagnoses of herpes zoster include zosteriform herpes simplex and contact dermatitis.

Treatment. There is no specific therapy for varicella other than supportive measures and local care. In immunocompromised patients antiviral therapy in the form of ara-A and acyclovir has been used.

In herpes zoster local care and analgesics are used for symptomatic relief. Acyclovir has been used for ophthalmic infection, disseminated disease, and, recently, for uncomplicated zoster. Postherpetic neuralgia may possibly be prevented in patients 60 years and older by the use of systemic corticosteroids.[68–70]

Kaposi's Varicelliform Eruption

Kaposi's varicelliform eruption, also referred to as eczema vaccinatum or eczema herpeticum, is a viral infection superimposed on abnormal skin and characterized by umbilicated vesicles on an erythematous base.

Etiology. The causative organism of eczema vaccinatum is the vaccinia virus, and that of eczema herpeticum is herpes simplex virus types 1 and 2.

Epidemiology. Eczema vaccinatum is now rare since routine smallpox vaccination is no longer performed except in the military. It may occur secondary to direct vaccination or contact with a recently vaccinated person. Eczema herpeticum may occur as a primary inoculation or as recurrent disease. Both viruses infect diseased skin such as that affected by atopic dermatitis, Darier's disease, or potentially any chronic dermatosis.

Course. The clinical picture produced by either virus is the same. There is an acute onset characterized by the appearance of umbilicated vesicles on abnormal skin (Fig. 8-6), accompanied by fever, malaise, and lymphadenopathy. Lesions become pustular and crusted over 1 to 2 weeks and may spread to normal skin. Complications include dissemination to internal organs, secondary bacterial infection, and fluid and electrolyte imbalance. The mortality rate may be up to 10 percent.

Diagnosis. A Tzanck preparation differentiates eczema herpeticum (multinucleated giant cells) from eczema vaccinatum (intracytoplasmic inclusions). The major differential diagnosis is pyoderma.

Treatment. For eczema vaccinatum, methisazone and vaccinia immune globin may be effective; for eczema herpeticum, acyclovir is the treatment of choice. Supportive and local care may be required, as well as antibiotics for secondary infection.[71,72]

Variola

Variola, or smallpox, is a highly contagious viral infection characterized by fever and a vesicopustular eruption.

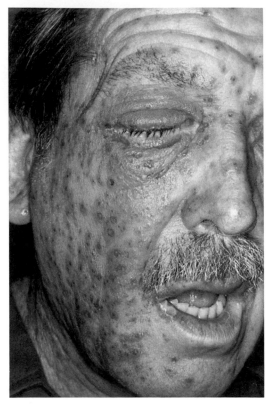

Fig. 8–6. Eczema herpeticum in a patient with atopic dermatitis.

Etiology. The causative organism is the smallpox virus (poxvirus variolae).

Epidemiology. Smallpox has essentially been eradicated worldwide through mass vaccination with the vaccinia virus. It occurred only in humans and was transmitted from person to person via droplet infection from the oropharynx, upper respiratory tract, or skin lesions (including crusts).

Course. The incubation period was 12 to 14 days, with a 2-day prodrome characterized by fever and malaise. The rash was characterized by erythematous papules on the extremities and face, which progressed through umbilicated vesicular, pustular, and crusted stages over 10 days to 2 weeks, all lesions being in the same stage of development. Vesicles and erosions were often seen in the oropharynx, and skin lesions usually healed with scarring. Many clinical variants were seen, and complications included pneumonitis, encephalitis, eye damage, and death in up to 50 percent of patients.

Diagnosis. Typical smallpox in endemic areas was diagnosed clinically. Laboratory diagnosis included a Tzanck preparation with Giemsa stain to find intracytoplasmic inclusion bodies, electron microscopy, immunofluorescence, and viral culture. The major differential diagnostic possibility was chickenpox.

Treatment. There were no effective antiviral agents for treatment, including methisazone and vaccinia immune globulin.[73]

Hand-Foot-and-Mouth Disease

Hand-foot-and-mouth disease is a coxsackievirus infection characterized by a vesicular eruption on the extremities and an enanthem.

Etiology. The causative organism is usually coxsackievirus A16 although coxsackieviruses A5, A7, A9, A10, B2, and B5 can produce the disease.

Epidemiology. Hand-foot-and-mouth disease has been reported from around the world. It is primarily seen in children under 10 years of age and has a peak incidence in the summer and fall. It is transmitted by direct contact via the fecal-oral route or by droplet spread and may occur in epidemics.

Course. The incubation period is 3 to 5 days and may be followed by a 1-day prodrome characterized by fever, malaise, and abdominal pain. The enanthem usually precedes or occurs concomitantly with the exanthem. The oral lesions, found primarily on the anterior oropharynx, are painful vesicles and erosions with erythematous halos. The exanthem is characterized by oval and somewhat linear vesicles on erythematous bases, usually on the hands, feet, and buttocks, with less common involvement of the elbows and knees (Fig. 8-7). The vesicular lesions may be asymptomatic or tender and last for about 1 week. Complications are rare but may include aseptic meningitis, myocarditis, paralysis, and eczema coxsackium in patients with atopic dermatitis.

Diagnosis. The diagnosis is usually based on clinical and epidemiologic findings. A more definitive diagnosis can be made on the basis of virus isolation and serologic tests during the acute illness. The differential diagnoses include herpetic infections, varicella, EM, gonococcemia, and herpangina.

Treatment. There is no specific treatment other than supportive and symptomatic measures.[74]

RICKETTSIAL INFECTIONS

Rickettsialpox

Rickettsialpox is an acute rickettsial disease characterized by a benign course and a vesicular eruption, and is transmitted to man by the house mouse mite.

Etiology. The causative organism is *Rickettsia akari.*

Epidemiology. Rickettsialpox is seen most commonly in the eastern United States especially around New York City. It is seen in all age groups and is spread by the house mouse mite, *Allodermanyssus sanguineus.*

Course. The incubation period varies from 1 to 2 weeks. A primary lesion occurs at the site of the mite bite and is characterized by an erythematous papule, which becomes vesicular after 2 days, develops an eschar, and then sloughs and heals with a scar after 3 weeks (Fig. 8-8). Tender regional lymphadenopathy may be associated. Within 4 to 7 days after the primary lesion, systemic manifestations occur, including fever, chills, headache, and malaise associated with a variable number of erythematous papules surmounted by a vesicle. The rash heals in 1 week without scarring, and there are no complications.

Diagnosis. The diagnosis is usually made on the basis of the clinical picture, a negative Weil-Felix reaction, and specific complement-fixing antibodies, which show a fourfold in-

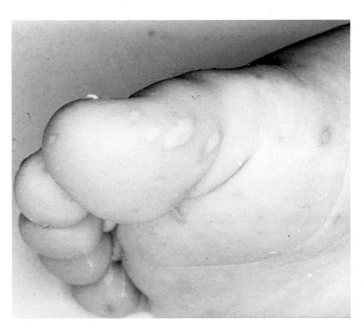

Fig. 8–7. Hand-foot-and-mouth disease: oblong vesicles on a child's foot.

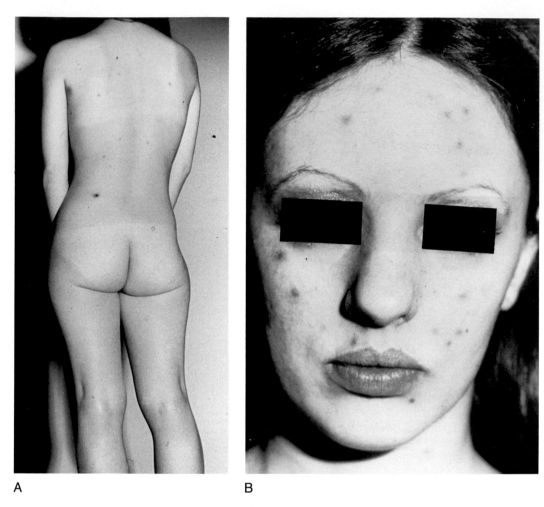

A   B

Fig. 8–8. Rickettsialpox. (**A**) Eschar on lower back at site of mite bite. (**B**) erythematous papulovesicular lesions develop 4 to 7 days after primary lesion. (Photographs courtesy of Bronx VA Medical Center.)

crease in titer 4 to 6 weeks later. The major differential diagnostic possibilities include chickenpox and insect bites.

Treatment. Tetracycline and chloramphenicol are effective in treatment.[75]

BACTERIAL INFECTIONS

Staphylococcal Scalded Skin Syndrome

Staphylococcal scalded skin syndrome, known as *Ritter's disease* in the neonate, is caused by the activity of a staphylococcal exo-toxin on the skin and is characterized by gener-alized redness, blistering, and peeling.

Etiology. The causative organism is *S. aureus,* usually group II, phage types 71 or 55, which elaborates an exotoxin called *exfoliatin.*

Epidemiology. The syndrome is primarily a disease of the neonatal period and infancy, with a peak incidence in the first 3 months of life and a predominance in males, but is also seen in older children and occasionally in adults with renal insufficiency and immunologic ab-normalities. It follows staphylococcal infection at a local site such as the conjunctiva, middle ear, nasopharynx, or umbilical stump. Exotoxin released from organisms at the site then produces changes in the upper epidermis.

Course. The incubation period is variable. A prodromal stage of fever, malaise, and irritability is followed within 1 to 2 days by erythema and cutaneous tenderness. The erythema is initially in the periorificial and intertriginous areas and then generalizes, resembling scarlet fever. Flaccid bullae with a positive Nikolsky sign develop and then rupture, leaving moist erosions and crusts. Desquamation or peeling of the skin in large sheets follows, with healing completed in 5 to 7 days. Complications such as sepsis, pneumonia, cellulitis, and death are rare.

Diagnosis. *S. aureus* cannot be recovered from the skin but may be cultured from the original site of infection or the blood. The diagnosis is made by a skin biopsy or skin peel, which reveals upper epidermal necrosis with separation below the granular layer.

The major differential diagnosis is TEN, which shows complete epidermal necrosis on biopsy or skin peel. Other differential diagnostic possibilities include scarlet fever, graft-versus-host disease, Leiner's disease, and toxic shock syndrome.

Treatment. The treatment of choice is a semisynthetic penicillinase-resistant penicillin such as nafcillin, administered parenterally in doses of 150 to 200 mg/kg daily. Cephalosporins may be used as an alternative in penicillin-sensitive patients. Supportive measures may be necessary for fluid, electrolyte, and protein balance.[76]

REFERENCES

1. Demis DJ (ed): Clinical Dermatology. 13th Revised Ed. Harper & Row, Philadelphia, 1986
2. Fitzpatrick TB, Eisen AZ, Wolff K, et al: (eds): Dermatology in General Medicine. 3rd Ed. McGraw-Hill, New York, 1987
3. Hoeprich PD (ed): Infectious Diseases. 3rd Ed. Harper & Row, Philadelphia, 1983
4. Hurwitz S: Clinical Pediatric Dermatology. W.B. Saunders, Philadelphia, 1981
5. Krugman S, Katz SL: Infectious Diseases of Children. CV Mosby, St. Louis, 1981
6. Moschella SL, Hurley HJ: Dermatology. 2nd Ed. WB Saunders, Philadelphia, 1985
7. Nelson WE, Behrman RE, Vaughan VC (eds): Nelson Textbook of Pediatrics. 12th Ed. WB Saunders, Philadelphia, 1983
8. Balfour HH: Fifth disease: full-fathom five. Am J Dis Child 130:239, 1976
9. Plummer FA, Hammond GW, Forward K, et al: An erythema infectiosum-like illness caused by human parvovirus infection. N Engl J Med 313:74, 1985
10. Morgan EM, Rapp F: Measles virus and its associated diseases. Bacteriol Rev 41:636, 1977
11. Green RH, Balsamo MR, Giles JP, et al: Studies of the natural history and prevention of rubella. Am J Dis Child 110:348, 1965
12. McCarthy K, Taylor-Robinson CH: Rubella. Br Med Bull 23:185, 1967
13. Berenberg W, Wright S, Janeway CA: Roseola infantum (exanthem subitum). N Engl J Med 241:253, 1949
14. Clemens HH: Exanthem subitum (roseola infantum): report of eighty cases. J Pediatr 26:66, 1945
15. Lerner AM, Klein JP, Cherry JD, Finland M: New viral exanthems. N Engl J Med 269:678, 1963
16. Lerner AM, Klein JP, Cherry JD, Finland M: New viral exanthems (concluded). N Engl J Med 269:736, 1963
17. Sanford JP, Sulkin SE: The clinical spectrum of echo-virus infections. N Engl J Med 261:1113, 1959
18. Lund BMA, Bergan T: Temporary skin reactions to penicillins during acute stage of infectious mononucleosis. Scand J Infect Dis 7:21, 1975
19. Patel BM: Skin rash with infectious mononucleosis and ampicillin. Pediatrics 40:910, 1967
20. Findlay GM, Martin NH, Mitchell JB: Hepatitis after yellow fever inoculation. Lancet 247(2):301, 1944
21. Lockshin NA, Hurley H: Urticaria as a sign of viral hepatitis. Arch Dermatol 105:570, 1972
22. Prestia AE, Lynfield YL: Scarlatiniform eruption in viral hepatitis. Arch Dermatol 101:352, 1970

23. McCloskey RV: Scarlet fever and necrotizing fasciitis caused by coagulase-positive hemolytic *Staphylococcus aureus* phage type 85. Ann Intern Med 78:85, 1973

24. Davis JP, Chesney PJ, Wand PJ, LaVenture M: Toxic shock syndrome. N Engl J Med 303:1429, 1980

25. Tofte RW, Williams DW: Toxic shock syndrome. Postgrad Med 73:275, 1983

26. Silber TJ, Niland NF: The clinical spectrum of syphilis in adolescence. J Adolesc Health Care 5:112, April 1984

27. Berger BW: Erythema chronicum migrans of Lyme disease. Arch Dermatol 120:1017, 1984

28. Burgdorfer W, Barbour AG, Hayes SF, et al: Lyme disease: a tick-borne spirochetosis? Science 216:1317, 1982

29. Steere AC, Malawista SE, Hardin JA, et al: Erythema chronicum migrans and Lyme arthritis. Ann Intern Med 86:685,1977

30. Furusho K, Hiroyuki N, Shinomiya K, et al: High-dose intravenous gammaglobulin for Kawasaki disease. Lancet 2:1055, 1984

31. Kawasaki T, Kosaki F, Okawa J, et al: A new infantile febrile mucocutaneous LN syndrome (MLNS) prevailing in Japan. Pediatrics 54:271, 1974

32. Morens DM, Nahmias AJ: Kawasaki disease: a new pediatric enigma. Hosp Pract 13(9):109, 1978

33. Lernak MA, Duvic M, Bean SF: Oral acyclovir for the prevention of herpes-associated erythema multiforme. J Am Acad Dermatol 15:50, 1986

34. Howland WW, Golitz LE, Weston WL, Huff JC: Erythema multiforme: clinical, histopathologic, and immunologic study. J Am Acad Dermatol 10:438, 1984

35. Tonnesen MG, Soter NA: Erythema multiforme. J Am Acad Dermatol 1:357, 1979

36. Burke JB: Erythema marginatum. Arch Dis Child 30:359, 1955

37. Keil H: The rheumatic erythema: a clinical survey. Ann Intern Med 11:2223, 1938

38. Toyer G, Grossman ME, Silvers DN: Erythema marginatum in rheumatic fever. Early diagnosis by skin biopsy. J Am Acad Dermatol 8:724, 1983

39. Calabro JJ: Juvenile rheumatoid arthritis. Mode of onset as key to early diagnosis and management. Postgrad Med 70(3):120, 1981

40. Calabro JJ, Marchesano JM: Rash associated with juvenile rheumatoid activity. J Pediatr 72:611, 1968

41. Fish AJ, Blau EB, Westberg G, et al: Systemic lupus erythematosus within the first two decades of life. Am J Med 62:99, 1977

42. Callen JP (ed): Lupus Erythematosus. Clinics in Dermatology 3(3). Lippincott, Philadelphia, 1985

43. Epstein A, Barland P: The diagnostic value of antihistone antibodies in drug-induced lupus erythematosus. Arthritis Rheum 28:158, 1985

44. Smith CD, Marino C, Rothfield NF: The clinical utility of the lupus band test. Arthritis Rheum 27:382, 1984

45. Kauppinen K, Stubbs S: Drug eruptions: causative agents and clinical types; series of patients during a 10 year period. Acta Derm Venereol (Stockh) 64:320, 1984

46. Wintroub BU, Stern R: Cutaneous drug reaction: pathogenesis and clinical classification. J Am Acad Dermatol 13:167, 1985

47. Rauh LW, Schmidt R: Measles immunization with killed virus vaccine: serum antibody titers and experience with exposure to measles epidemic. Am J Dis Child 109:232, 1965

48. Stagnos S: Congenital toxoplasmosis. Am J Dis Child 134:635, 1980

49. Nahmias AJ: The TORCH complex. Hosp Pract 9:65, May 1974

50. Brough AJ, Jones D, Page RH, Mizukarni I: Dermal erythropoiesis in neonatal infants. A manifestation of intrauterine viral disease. Pediatrics 40:627, 1967

51. Panjavi ZFK, Hanshaw JB: Cytomegalovirus in the perinatal period. Am J Dis Child 135:56, 1981

52. Strabstein JC, Morris N, Larke RPB, et al: Is there a congenital varicella syndrome? J Pediatr 84:239, 1974

53. Breasette M: The laboratory diagnosis of congenital syphilis. A review. Am J Med Technol 45:645, 1979

54. Burnett JW: Rickettsioses: a review for the dermatologist. J Am Acad Dermatol 2:359, 1980

55. Bradford WD, Hawkins HK: Rocky Mountain spotted fever in childhood. Am J Dis Child 131:1228, 1977

56. Dalldorf FG, Jennette SC: Fatal meningococcal septicemia. Arch Pathol Lab Med 101:6, 1977

57. Ackerman AB, Miller RC, Shapiro L: Gonococcemia and its cutaneous manifestations. Arch Dermatol 91:227, 1965

58. Holmes KK, Counts GW, Beaty HN: Disseminated gonococcal infection. Ann Intern Med 74:979, 1971

59. Plaut ME: Staphylococcal septicemia and pustular purpura. Report of cases. Arch Dermatol 99:82, 1969

60. Hall JH, Callaway JL, Tindall JP, Smith JG Jr: *Pseudomonas aeruginosa* in dermatology. Arch Dermatol 97:312, 1968

61. Von Gemmingen GR, Winkelmann RK: Osler's node of subacute bacterial endocarditis. Arch Dermatol 95:91, 1967

62. Alpert JS, Krous HF, Dalen JE, et al: Pathogenesis of Osler's nodes. Ann Intern Med 85:471, 1976

63. Allen DM, Diamond LK, Howell DA: Anaphylactoid purpura in children (Schönlein-Henoch syndrome). Review with a follow-up of renal complications. Am J Dis Child 99:833, 1960

64. Fauci AS, Haynes BF, Katz P: The spectrum of vasculitis. Clinical, pathologic, immunologic and therapeutic considerations. Ann Intern Med 89:660, 1978

65. Nahmias AJ, Roizman B: Infection with herpes-simplex viruses 1 and 2. N Engl J Med 289:667, 1973

66. Nahmias AJ, Roizman B: Infection with herpes-simplex viruses 1 and 2. N Engl J Med 289:719, 1973

67. Nahmias AJ, Roizman B: Infection with herpes-simplex viruses 1 and 2. N Engl J Med 289:781, 1973

68. Rogers RS III, Tindall JP: Herpes zoster in children. Arch Dermatol 106:204, 1972

69. Weller TH: Varicella and herpes zoster. Changing concepts of the natural history, control and importance of a not-so-benign virus. Part I. N Engl J Med 309:1362, 1983

70. Weller TH: Varicella and herpes zoster. Changing concepts of the natural history, control and importance of a not-so-benign virus. Part II. N Engl J Med 309:1434, 1983

71. Swart RNJ, Vermeer BJ, van der Meer JWM, et al: Treatment of eczema herpeticum with acyclovir. Arch Dermatol 119:13, 1983

72. Wheeler CE Jr, Abele DC: Eczema herpeticum, primary and recurrent. Arch Dermatol 93:162, 1966

73. Brennan JG, Arita I: The confirmation and maintenance of small pox eradication. N Engl J Med 303:1263, 1980

74. Miller GD, Tindall JP: Hand-foot-and-mouth disease. JAMA 203:827, 1968

75. Wong B, Singer C, Armstrong D, Millian SJ: Rickettsial pox. Case report and epidemiologic review. JAMA 242:1998, 1979

76. Elias PM, Fritsch P, Epstein EH Jr: Staphylococcal scalded skin syndrome. Clinical features, pathogenesis and recent microbiological and biochemical developments. Arch Dermatol 113:207, 1977

9

Rash and Eosinophilia

Dominick J. Ligresti

The eosinophil was first described by Paul Ehrlich in 1879 as a polymorphonuclear leukocyte containing acidophilic granules found in human blood and tissues. *Eosinophilia* is a term used to describe an increase in the quantity or percentage of eosinophils in peripheral blood. Diverse immunogenetic mechanisms have been proposed and numerous chemotactic factors identified that attract and immobilize eosinophils in peripheral circulation, resulting in eosinophilia. Many diseases are associated with eosinophilia and many of these involve cutaneous eruptions. It is known that blood eosinophilia does not necessarily correlate with tissue eosinophilia. What is not known, however, is whether eosinophilia is an integral part of disease or merely a "reactive" physiologic phenomenon to the disease process. The presence of eosinophilia may suggest active disease, and its recognition may aid in early diagnosis and treatment. Infection with helminthic parasites and drug eruptions are most important in generating blood eosinophilia as well as other immune responses associated with IgE production.

In this chapter the morphology, structure, and function of the eosinophil, drug reactions and diseases associated with blood eosinophilia, and clinical evaluation of the patient with rash and eosinophilia will be reviewed.

MORPHOLOGY AND STRUCTURE OF EOSINOPHILS

The eosinophil is a polymorphonuclear leukocyte 12 to 17 μm in diameter, which has the capacity for phagocytizing and destroying invading organisms through its numerous enzymes.

The nucleus of the eosinophil is bilobed, compared with the multilobed nuclei of neutrophilic and basophilic polymorphonuclear leukocytes. Two types of granules are found in the eosinophil cytoplasm, the *major granule* and the *minor granule*. The major granules number from 25 to 400 and stain acidophilic with eosin dyes; they contain a *core* and *matrix*. The core contains *major basic protein* (MBP), a 10,800-molecular-weight arginine- and lysine-rich protein responsible for the staining properties of the major granule.[1] More than 50 percent of the core consists of MBP,[2] which has activity against parasites[3] and against skin in patients with atopic dermatitis[4]; it adsorbs to cell membranes, precipitates DNA, and neutralizes heparin.[5] Eosinophilia is associated with an increase in serum MBP.[6] *Eosinophil cationic protein* is also found in the core of the major granule—its function remains unknown. The matrix of the major granule contains a unique peroxidase, along with hydrolytic enzymes capable of destroying tissue and invading parasites.[7] Similar enzymes are found in neutrophils and in eosinophils, but they differ quantitatively and morphologically. For example, arylsulfatase is found at higher concentrations and has different substrate specificity in eosinophils than in neutrophils.[7] The minor granule contains arylsulfatase, an enzyme capable of degrading leukotrienes, which are substances with a wide array of biologic activities.[8]

Eosinophil cell membranes contain Fc receptors for IgE, which increase in density upon cell activation.[5] There are also surface receptors for complement components C4, C3b, and C3a and for IgE.[9,10,11]

In patients with eosinophilia resulting from the hypereosinophilic syndrome and parasitic infections, the percentage of surface IgE and C3b receptors increases to the density found in neutrophils.[8] Activation of eosinophilic membranes enhances their capacity to modulate inflammation.[8] The eosinophil also contains surface receptors for estrogens,[12] glucocorticoids,[13] and H_1 and H_2 receptors.[14]

FUNCTIONS OF EOSINOPHILS

The functions of eosinophils include phagocytosis, modulation of inflammation, and host defense against invading helminthic parasites.

Phagocytosis

Eosinophils, with their numerous hydrolytic lysosomal enzymes, are capable of phagocytizing immune complexes, immunoglobulins, mast cell granules, yeast, bacteria, mycoplasmas, and protozoa.[8] The potential of the eosinophil for phagocytosis and intracellular destruction is less than that of the neutrophil.[15] Its bactericidal capacity is dependent on an intact peroxidase-halide-hydrogen peroxide system.

Modulation of Inflammation

The eosinophil, through its numerous enzymes, modulates immediate hypersensitivity reactions of mast cells and basophils by inhibiting release of mast cell and basophil granules containing eosinophil chemotactic factor of anaphylaxis (ECF-A), histamine, heparin, and slow-reacting substance of anaphylaxis (SRS-A). Eosinophil histaminase inactivates histamine[16] and arylsulfatase inactivates SRS-A or leukotrienes.[17] Eosinophil MBP inactivates heparin,[18] and ECF-A is destroyed by cell membrane-bound esterase.[19] Eosinophils are capable of phagocytizing whole mast cell and basophil granules. Activated eosinophils of sensitized individuals produce prostaglandins E_1 and E_2, which inhibit basophil and mast cell granule release. Zinc, found in the eosinophil, may have a similar function.[9] Eosinophil phospholipase D degrades neutrophil-derived platelet-activating factor (PAF),[21] and lysophospholipase lyses cell membranes and degrades cell membrane-active lysophosphatides.[22] The eosinophils also decrease inflammation by phagocytizing immune complexes, thereby preventing complement activation and release of chemotactic factors C3a and C5a.

Host Defense Against Helminthic Parasites

The eosinophil plays a major role against invading parasites through its cytotoxicity and capacity for "frustrated phagocytosis." This has been demonstrated against schistosomes when they are initially sensitized by IgG antibody, which activates complement by both classical and alternative pathways. Mast cells adhere to complement-coated parasites by their surface complement receptors and release their granules, which include ECF-A and histamine. Eosinophils are recruited in the area by ECF-A, complement-derived chemotactic factors, and lymphokines such as eosinophil stimulation promoter (ESP), elaborated by sensitized T lymphocytes.[23] Mast cell mediators enhance eosinophil cytotoxicity by increasing the number of eosinophil complement receptors that serve to bridge the eosinophil with the complement-coated parasite. Eosinophils release their granules, including MBP, eosinophil basic granule protein, peroxidase, and phosopholipase on the parasite surface, which results in parasite destruction. Complement components C3b and IgG are most important in bridging the eosinophil and target cell or parasite, but lecithin and IgE have also been shown to have similar function.[8] Mast cell mediators also enhance eosinophil peroxidase activity.[8]

Factors Affecting Eosinophil Function

EOSINOPHIL CHEMOTAXIS

Eosinophils are influenced by factors secreted from mast cells, lymphocytes, and other cell types. The most important mast cell mediator for eosinophil chemotaxis is ECF-A. Histamine and its major metabolites 5-hydroxyimidazole-acetic acid also have eosinophil chemotactic activity, as do other mast cell products including acidic oligopeptide, a high-molecular weight chemotactic factor, and a lipid chemotactic factor (LCF).[24] This explains the presence of eosinophils in immediate hypersensitivity reactions.

Antigen deposition in tissue can induce eosinophilia through T lymphocyte-dependent mechanisms. Sensitized lymphocytes produce lymphokines with chemotactic properties for eosinophils.[24,25,26]

Serum-derived mediators of eosinophilia include kallikrein, plasminogen activator, and neutrophil proteases.[24] Complement-derived components C3a, C5a, and C567 are potent neutrophilic as well as eosinophilic chemotactic agents, C5a having the most eosinotactic capacity. These serum-derived proteins are liberated through activation of both the classical and alternate pathways.

Neutrophils also generate an antigen-induced

ECF.[27] Hydroxyheptadecatrienoic acid and hydroxyicosatetraenoic acid are arachidonic acid-derived products produced by platelets that are chemotactic for eosinophils and all other leukocytes. Eosinophil chemoattractant substances have been isolated from tumors such as squamous cell carcinoma of the lung[28] and histiocytic lymphoma[29] and from lymph nodes of patients with Hodgkin's disease.[30]

EOSINOPHIL PRODUCTION

A T lymphocyte-dependent substance known as eosinophilopoeitin (EPP) which regulates bone marrow eosinopoiesis, has been demonstrated in mice with parasitic infestations.[24] Its presence in humans has not been determined.

EOSINOPHIL QUANTITATION

The life span of the eosinophil in circulation ranges from ½ to 12 hours, with only 1 percent of the eosinophils circulating under normal conditions. There exists a diurnal variation in circulating levels of eosinophils, the lowest level occurring in the morning and the highest level at night. Studies vary with respect to normal total eosinophil counts, 1 to $600/mm^3$ representing the lower and upper limits of the normal adult range. Other biologic sources of variation include exercise, which results in transient elevation, and menstruation, stress, and β-adrenergic agents, all of which have lowering effect.[8]

BLOOD EOSINOPHILIA WITH SKIN RASH—ETIOLOGY

Drugs

Drug hypersensitivity is the most common cause of eosinophilia and rash (Table 9-1). Eosinophilia may develop 1 or more weeks after a drug is initiated; however, it may occur as

Table 9-1. Disorders Causing Skin Rash and Eosinophilia

Allergic disorders
    Drug hypersensitivity
Inflammatory dermatoses
    Atopic dermatitis
    Exfoliative dermatitis
    Urticaria and angioedema
    Erythema nodosum
    Erythema toxicum neonatorum
    Eosinophilic papulovesicular dermatitis of infancy
    Eosinophilic pustular folliculitis
    Urticaria of serum sickness reactions
    Well's disease
    Granuloma faciale
    Sarcoidosis

Bullous diseases
    Bullous pemphigoid
    Herpes gestationis
    Pemphigus
    Dermatitis herpetiformis

Collagen-vascular diseases
    Rheumatoid arthritis
    Allergic granulomatosis
    Periarteritis nodosa
    Eosinophilic fasciitis

Infections
    Bacterial
        Scarlet fever
        Secondary syphilis
        Leprosy
    Viral
        Erythema infectiosum
    Fungal
        Coccidiomycosis
        Chronic mucocutaneous candidiasis
    Parasitic
        Trematoda
            Schistosomiasis

Infections, parasitic (continued)
    Cestoda
        Taenia solium
        Echinococcus granulosus
    Nematoda
        Necator americanus
        Ancylostoma duodenale
        Ancylostoma caninum
        Toxocara canis
        Strongyloides stercoralis
        Trichinella spiralis
        Wuchereria bancrofti
        Brugia malayi
        Loa loa
        Onchocerca volvulus
    Scabies

Immunodeficiency diseases
    Selective IgA deficiency
    Combined immunodeficiency
        X-linked
        Autosomal recessive (Swiss type)
    Wiskott-Aldrich syndrome
    Nezelof syndrome
    Job's syndrome
    Graft-versus-host disease

Neoplastic and myeloproliferative diseases
    Lymphomatoid papulosis
    Mycosis fungoides
    Sézary syndrome
    Angioimmunoblastic lymphadenopathy
    Heavy chain disease
    Waldenström's primary macroglobulin-
        emia
Other
    Kimura's disease
    Systemic mastocytosis
    Hypereosinophilic syndrome

---

early as 1 day later if prior sensitization has occurred. Drugs associated with skin rash and eosinophilia are listed in Table 9-2. The most common drugs include gold, ampicillin, penicillin, streptomycin, para-aminosalicylic acid, phenytoin, arsenicals, phenothiazines, and sulfonamides. Drug-induced eosinophilia and skin rash are secondary to IgE-mediated immediate hypersensitivity mechanisms, but IgG-mediated serum sickness reactions can also occur.[34] Some drugs induce eosinophilia through direct mast cell-degranulating mechanisms; these drugs include codeine, morphine, polymyxin, stilbamidine, *d*-tubocurarine, dextran, protamine, and viomycin.[35] The mechanism of eosinophilia of aspirin intolerance involves β-adrenergic blockade.[24]

Immediate hypersensitivity or IgE-mediated reactions bring about greater eosinophil counts than immune complex- or IgG-mediated mechanisms. Acute allergic reactions may elicit leukemoid eosinophil responses of greater than 20,000/mm^3 while chronic allergy is rarely associated with counts greater than 2,000/mm^3. Eosinophilia often disappears by 1 week after a drug is discontinued.

Inflammatory Dermatoses

ATOPIC DERMATITIS

In atopic dermatitis decreased suppressor T lymphocytes may result in increased circulating IgE serum levels and peripheral eosinophilia.

Table 9-2. Drugs Causing Rash and Eosinophilia

Acetylsalicylic acid[8]	Para-aminosalicylic acid[8]
Allopurinol[8]	Penicillamine[33]
Arsenicals[8]	Penicillins[8]
Busulfan[8]	Phenolphthalein[8]
Captopril[31]	Phenylbutazone[8]
Cephalosporins[8]	Phenytoin[8]
Chloramphenicol[8]	Polymyxin[8]
Chlorpromazine[8]	Protamine[8]
Chlorothiazide[8]	Quinidine[8]
Codeine[8]	Stilbamidine[8]
Dapsone[8]	Streptomycin[8]
Dextran[8]	Sulfonamides[8]
Etretinate[32]	Sulfonylureas[8]
Gold[8]	Tetracycline[8]
Iodides[8]	Thiouracil, propylthiouracil[8]
Isoniazid[8]	Trimethadione[8]
Mercurials[8]	Tubocurarine[8]

IgE fixes to tissue mast cells which, when antigen stimulated, liberate mediators that are chemoattractant for eosinophils. An increased number of mast cells with the presence of MBP has been identified in atopic skin and may be involved in the pathogenesis of this disorder.[4]

INFLAMMATORY DERMATOSES OF INFANCY

Erythema toxicum neonatorum is a condition present at birth or appearing within the first days of life. It is characterized by an erythematous papular-vesicular eruption, which becomes micropustular and is confined to the trunk and proximal extremities. The neonate is often healthy and asymptomatic. Eosinophils are prominent in the vesicles and micropustules, and the condition is associated with blood eosinophilia. The eruption disappears within 1 week to 10 days.

Eosinophilic papulovesicular dermatitis of infancy is characterized by nonpruritic erythematous papules, vesicles, and pustules appearing in children over 2 months of age. The lesions commonly occur on the head and trunk. Skin biopsy of lesions demonstrates numerous eosinophils, and blood eosinophilia is often present. The eruption has a tendency to reoccur over several months.

OTHER INFLAMMATORY DERMATOSES

Eosinophilic pustular folliculitis is associated with tiny pruritic erythematous follicular papulopustules on the face and trunk. Eosinophilia of greater than 5 percent is commonly noted in the peripheral blood. The folliculitis primarily affects the sebaceous areas, with one-fifth of the patients demonstrating palmoplantar lesions. Extracts of stratum corneum reveal a low-molecular-weight ECF.[37]

Well's disease, also known as *eosinophilic cellulitis,* is associated with superficial urticarial papules with subcutaneous edema. The eruption lasts from 3 to 4 weeks and then regresses slowly, leaving a slight gray discoloration and atrophy. It is thought to represent a hypersensitivity phenomenon to an arthropod bite. Eosinophilia is commonly seen. Immunoreactive leukotrienes have been isolated from the skin lesions of patients with eosinophilic cellulitis, which may explain the associated eosinophilia.[38]

Eosinophilia can also be seen in granuloma faciale and sarcoidosis. The cutaneous lesions of *granuloma faciale* consist of reddish brown nodules and are commonly found on the face of middle-aged males. Immunofluorescent studies demonstrate IgG, IgA, and IgM at the dermal-epidermal junction and about dermal blood vessels, suggesting an immune complex vasculitis, which may be involved in the pathogenesis of eosinophilia.

Sarcoidosis is a multisystem noncaseating granulomatous disease affecting young individuals, with a clinical presentation that includes bilateral hilar lymphadenopathy on chest x-ray and cutaneous and ocular lesions. The cutaneous manifestations of sarcoidosis include hyperpigmentation, scarring, keloids, lupus pernio, erythema nodosum, and a maculopapular eruption.

Other dermatoses such as lichen planus, psoriasis, ichthyoses, and exfoliative dermatitis involve sites at which mast cells are most concentrated—around sebaceous glands and eccrine glands, adjacent to blood vessels in the papillary dermis, and in subcutaneous fat and around hair follicles. Release of mast cell granules through

IgE-antigen stimulation may result in eosinophilia through release of chemotactic factors. Elevated levels of ECF-A have been identified in involved skin of psoriasis patients.

Eosinophilia noted in acute urticaria and angioedema can be explained through IgE-mediated mast cell immediate hypersensitivity reactions. Eosinophilia associated with erythema multiforme, erythema nodosum, and urticarial eruptions of serum sickness reactions are secondary to immune complex–complement-mediated mechanisms.

Bullous Diseases

Bullous diseases such as bullous pemphigoid, pemphigus, herpes gestationis, and dermatitis herpetiformis result from autoimmune phenomena involving immune complex–complement activation mechanisms that can produce eosinophilia to some degree.

BULLOUS PEMPHIGOID

Bullous pemphigoid is a subepidermal blistering disease commonly affecting the elderly, which is characterized by tense bullae on erythematous or normal skin. Mucous membrane involvement is present in less than 20 percent of patients. Pemphigoid antigen is produced by epidermal basal cells. Both IgG and C3 are bound to the lamina lucida of the basement membrane zone (BMZ) and the half-desmosomes of epidermal basal cells.[39] Bullous pemphigoid is also associated with elevated serum IgE, ECF-A, and eosinophilia. Extensive mast cell degranulation is noted in the area of bullae as a result of IgE antibodies combining with antigen. This degranulation liberates ECF-A, consequently producing eosinophilia. The eosinophils phagocytize antigen-antibody complexes or, through their cytotoxic potential, induce lysis of BMZ components coated with IgE or C3 in a manner similar to parasite destruction, which results in dissolution of the BMZ and bulla formation.[40] Blood eosinophil levels

revert to normal with clearing of skin lesions after treatment.[40]

HERPES GESTATIONIS

Herpes gestationis usually occurs in the second or third trimester of pregnancy, disappears within 2 months postpartum, and reoccurs with subsequent pregnancies or use of birth control pills. It presents clinically with intensely pruritic bullae, which are usually localized on the trunk and proximal extremities. Direct immunofluorescence studies of perilesional skin reveal linear deposits of C3 in 100 percent of patients and IgG in 30 percent. Properdin and properdin factor have been found as well as IgA and IgM deposits. The herpes gestationis factor is an IgG anti-basement membrane antibody found in the serum, which may cross the placental barrier and cause herpes gestationis in the newborn. Fetal mortality as high as 30 percent has been reported. The occasional eosinophilia observed in herpes gestationis may be the result of mechanisms involving complement activation.

PEMPHIGUS

Pemphigus vegetans consists of the *Neumann type,* in which lesions present as flaccid, weeping bullae similar to those of pemphigus vulgaris, and the *Hallopeau variety,* characterized by hypertrophic, verrucoid granulations arising in denuded areas left by ruptured bullae. Lesions are common in intertriginous areas as well as on mucosal surfaces. Nikolsky's sign is present. Patients' sera demonstrates IgG antibodies to intercellular substance, which subsequently form immune complexes and activate complement through the classical pathway. This results in formation of chemotactic factors, which ultimately can result in eosinophilia. On direct immunofluorescence, lesional skin of patients with pemphigus demonstrates deposits of C3, C3 proactivator, properdin, and C1q in intercellular cement which implicates complement activation through the classical and alternative pathways.[39] Circulating immune complexes have also been detected in the sera of pemphigus patients.

DERMATITIS HERPETIFORMIS

Dermatitis herpetiformis is a chronic, severely pruritic, vesiculobullous disease, which commonly occurs on the elbows, knees, buttocks, face, and scalp. Most patients have an associated gluten-sensitive enteropathy, although gastrointestinal symptoms may be absent. Direct immunofluorescence studies reveal granular IgA deposits in dermal papillae of uninvolved skin. Circulating immune complexes have been demonstrated in the sera of patients with this disease and may be involved in the pathogenesis of eosinophilia in this condition.

Collagen Vascular Diseases

Eosinophilia occurs in 10 percent of patients with *rheumatoid arthritis*.[36] A higher percentage of eosinophils is seen in the presence of rheumatoid nodules, possibly resulting from the increased number of mast cells and ECF found in rheumatoid synovium.[41]

Sjögren's syndrome, or *keratoconjunctivitis sicca,* is an autoimmune syndrome, which presents clinically with keratoconjunctivitis. Xerosis, patchy alopecia, Raynaud's phenomenon, thrombotic thrombocytopenic purpura, cryoglobulinemia, interstitial fibrosis of the lung, and renal tubular acidosis can be associated. Serological abnormalities include: positive antinuclear antibodies (ANAs) in low titer, antisalivary antibodies, Ro and La anticytoplasmic antibodies in one-third of the patients, and eosinophilia in the two-thirds of the patients who present with vasculitis.

Churg-Strauss syndrome, also known as *allergic granulomatosis,* is a chronic illness of unknown etiology characterized by a necrotizing granulomatous vasculitis involving the cardiovascular, pulmonary, hepatobiliary, gastrointestinal, genitourinary, and peripheral nervous systems. Patients present with asthma, hypereosinophilia, and elevated serum IgE levels. Cutaneous lesions are present in two-thirds of the patients and consist of large ecchymotic plaques, tender subcutaneous nodules, and cutaneous infarcts. Death may result from myocardial infarction, congestive heart failure, or, less commonly, renal disease.

Periarteritis nodosa is a disorder caused by a necrotizing vasculitis of small and medium-sized arteries. The cause of the disease is unknown; however, 20 to 40 percent of patients have hepatitis B antigenemia or infection with group A β-hemolytic streptococci. *Staphylococcus aureus* or *Mycobacterium leprae* infections have been associated as well. Systemic symptoms consist of fever, weakness, weight loss, myalgias, and arthralgias. In 25 to 50 percent of patients cutaneous manifestations, limited to the lower extremities, are present. Lesions that are seen include papules, nodules, vesicles, bullae, ulcers, and urticaria. Livedo reticularis can occur in periarteritis nodosa. Effects involving other organs include glomerulonephritis with hematuria and proteinuria, arthritis, gastrointestinal bleeding, peripheral neuropathy, pericarditis, and pneumonitis. Laboratory abnormalities include anemia, leukocytosis with eosinophilia, elevated sedimentation rate, and other abnormalities pertaining to specific organ pathology. Prognosis is poor, with death occurring within weeks in some cases. Causes of fatalities include infection, gastrointestinal bleeding, myocardial infarction, and renal insufficiency.

Eosinophilic fasciitis, also known as *Shulman's syndrome,* is associated with acute swelling and induration of the skin, often following vigorous exercise. Extremities are often affected. Biopsy reveals that skin, subcutis, muscle and overlying fascia are involved by a fibrosing eosinophilic infiltrate. Laboratory examination reveals eosinophilia greater than 2,000/mm^3 and elevated erythrocyte sedimentation rate.[42]

Skin Infections

BACTERIAL AND VIRAL

A number of bacterial infections are characterized by rash associated with eosinophilia. In scarlet fever eosinophilia appears concomitantly with the onset of rash. The mechanism is unknown. In the exanthematous stage of *secondary syphilis* eosinophilia appears as a result of formation of antibody to *Treponema* surface antigen and hypersensitivity to bacterial products.[8] In *lepromatous leprosy* the presence of eosinophilia has been associated with T-lymphocyte dysfunction.[43]

Viral infections are infrequently associated with eosinophilia with the exception of *erythema infectiosum,* also known as *Fifth's disease.* The eosinophilia appears concurrently with onset of the "slapped cheek" skin eruption.

Rash and eosinophilia can occur in a number of fungal infections. Eosinophilia frequently occurs in *chronic mucocutaneous candidiasis* and *coccidioidomycosis* and may be related to the presence of T-lymphocyte immunodeficiency. In *coccidioidomycosis* disrupted sporules and endospores are chemotactic for eosinophils. Cutaneous lesions demonstrate a sporotrichoid pattern, with nodules, ulcers, and lymphadenopathy. Urticaria, erythema multiforme, and erythema nodosum are also seen.

PARASITIC

Protozoal infections are not commonly associated with eosinophilia unless significant tissue destruction occurs. Tissue-invasive helminthic parasitic infections are associated with significant eosinophilia, whereas worms that remain intraluminal in the gastrointestinal tract do not commonly result in increased circulating eosinophils. The eosinophil destroys invading helminths through antibody-dependent cellular cytotoxicity mechanisms involving IgG and complement. Eosinophilia may be generated via immune complex formation, with subsequent complement activation of the classical pathway, or via activation of the alternate pathway by *Schistosoma mansoni;* both generation modes result in the release of ECFs.[44] Helminthic parasite infections with cutaneous involvement and blood eosinophilia are listed in Table 9-1 and are discussed below.

Trematoda (Flukes)

Schistosoma larvae, known as cercariae, are the etiologic agents of *swimmer's itch,* a pruritic papular urticarial dermatitis seen in bathers but which spares the bathing suit area. Death of schistosomes occurs immediately after skin penetration and is associated with eosinophil degranulation.

Platyhelminthes

Cysticercosis results from ingestion of inadequately cooked pork containing *Taenia solium* cysticerci. Ingested eggs develop into larvae, mostly in the subcutaneous tissue and other organs.

Echinococcus granulosus larvae are responsible for hydatid cyst disease. Infection occurs from ingestion of contaminated food and water, resulting in subcutaneous deposits of large cysts. Ruptured cysts can elicit an eosinophilic granulomatous response.[45] Extensive cyst leakage results in pruritus, urticaria, asthma, and anaphylaxis. Larvae migrate to the liver, lungs, and brain, where they encyst.

Nematoda

Cutaneous larva migrans, or creeping eruption, is a mobile serpiginous eruption caused by larvae of *Ancylostoma braziliense* and *Ancylostoma caninum,* the dog and cat hookworms. The larvae penetrate human skin and are unable to complete their life cycles in the abnormal human host. Human hookworms, *Necator americanus* and *Ancylostoma duodenale,* are the etiologic agents of transient creeping eruption. Larva migrans is associated with eosinophilia ranging from 10 to 35 percent.[46]

Visceral larva migrans is caused by infection with *Toxocara canis,* the dog and cat ascarid. Larvae unable to complete their life cycles in the human host elicit blood eosinophilia and a localized granulomatous eosinophilic response, resulting in clinical signs of urticarial papules and hepatosplenomegaly.

Larva currens is caused by infection with *Strongyloides stercoralis,* which has a rapid worm migration rate of 5 to 10 cm/hr. An urticarial eruption may accompany the site of worm infiltration, which is commonly around the genitalia or buttocks and is associated with intestinal strongyloidiasis.

Trichinosis develops as a result of infection with *Trichinella spiralis,* acquired through ingestion of improperly cooked pork. In the stomach the larvae are liberated upon digestion and penetrate the intestinal mucosa. Female and male worms copulate in the small intestine. Fertilized adult female worms deposit larvae in the small intestinal mucosa, which subsequently penetrate through and migrate to skeletal muscle, where they encyst. This phase is accompanied by systemic signs of fever, myalgias, edema, and blood eosinophilia ranging from 10 to 90 percent.[45] Cutaneous manifestations include a maculopapular, urticarial, and petechial eruption. Biopsy of splinter hemorrhages found in fingernail beds demonstrates the organisms.

Filariasis is caused by the nematodes *Wuchereria bancrofti* and *Brugia malayi,* which live in the lymphatics of the extremities and genitalia of humans. Microfilaria are transferred from human to human by the bite of anthropophilic mosquitoes. The microfilariae develop into the adult stage within the mosquito's intestines. The incubation period of filariasis can be up to 1 year before symptoms of lymphadenitis, lymphangitis, and elephantiasis occur. Diagnosis is made by biopsy of enlarged lymph nodes and a positive filarial skin test. *Tropical eosinophilia* consists of asthma-like symptoms with peripheral blood eosinophilia. This results from

the host's development of hypersensitivity to the organism, resulting in the destruction of microfilariae.[47]

Loiasis is a disease caused by the nematode *Loa loa,* transmitted from human to human by the bite of the blood-sucking fly *Chrysops.* Microfilaria appear in the blood 5 months later and adult worms appear after 1 year. The adult wanders around viscera and subcutaneous tissue, causing painful swellings known as *calabar swellings,* which last a few days. The eyes may be involved, with unilateral palpebral swelling. Diagnosis can be made by demonstration of microfilaria on blood smear, complement fixation titers, and a positive skin test. Eosinophilia may be marked.

Onchocerciasis is caused by the worm *Onchocerca volvulus,* transmitted from human to human by the bite of the blackfly *Simulium,* after feeding on infected blood containing *Onchocerca* microfilaria. The microfilaria are commonly found in skin lymphatics and connective tissue and the anterior chamber of the eye in man. They mature into the adult form in the subcutaneous tissue and deep dermis of the face and scalp, forming calcifying nodules known as *onchocercomas.* Other cutaneous manifestations include lichenification, depigmentation, and scarring. Diagnosis is made by the presence of complement fixation titers, a positive filarial skin test and, most significantly, by demonstration of the adult worm on skin biopsy.

Scabies

Eosinophilia is sometimes observed in scabies infections and may result from mechanisms involving immediate hypersensitivity.

Immunodeficiency Diseases

Eosinophilia with skin rash has been described in immunodeficiency diseases involving thymic alymphoplasia, T-lymphocyte dysfunction, combined B- and T-cell deficiencies (as in severe combined immunodeficiency disease), immunoglobulin deficiencies, and diseases with elevated serum IgE levels. Eosinophilia may be related to or enhanced by eczematous skin involvement in Job's syndrome, Wiskott-Aldrich syndrome, and selective IgA deficiency disease.

Selective IgA deficiency disease consists of recurrent sinopulmonary infections, atopic dermatitis, and autoimmune disorders. The latter include systemic lupus erythematosus, dermatomyositis, pernicious anemia, thyroiditis, Coombs' positive hemolytic anemia, Sjögren's syndrome, and chronic active hepatitis. Laboratory findings reveal serum IgA levels below 5 mg/dl, with normal or increased levels of IgG, IgM, or IgE. Levels of B lymphocytes are within normal range, and the cell-mediated immune system is intact. An increased number of T-suppressor cells has been reported in some patients.[48] The mechanism of eosinophilia may be related to or enhanced by the presence of atopic dermatitis.

Severe combined immunodeficiency disease is inherited in two forms: *X-linked* and *autosomal recessive,* also known as *Swiss type.* Clinical signs demonstrate recurrent bacterial, viral, fungal, and protozoal infections with failure of the infant to thrive. Cutaneous manifestations include a morbilliform eruption or a seborrhea-like dermatitis. Onset of symptoms occurs by 6 months of age, and death ensues within 1 year in most instances. Laboratory examination reveals an absence of both T- and B-lymphocytic immunity, resulting from a defect in cell differentiation. Serum demonstrates decreased or absent IgG, IgA, and IgM levels, with leukopenia, eosinophilia, and an absent thymic shadow on x-ray.

Nezelof syndrome, or *thymic alymphoplasia,* is associated with recurrent infections, lymphadenopathy, and hepatosplenomegaly. Laboratory studies reveal abnormal cell mediated immunity with anergy to skin test antigens, decreased T-lymphocyte and normal B-lymphocyte levels, and abnormal immunoglobulin synthesis of all classes.

Wiskott-Aldrich syndrome is an X-linked disorder with recurrent bacterial infections of encapsulated organisms, including pneumococcus, meningococcus, and *Hemophilus influenzae,* resulting in pneumonia, meningitis, and otitis media. An eczematous dermatitis is frequently present. Abnormal laboratory findings include anemia, eosinophilia, thrombocytopenia, absent cell-mediated immunity, decreased serum levels of IgM, and elevated levels of IgA and IgE.

Job's syndrome, also known as the *hyper-IgE syndrome,* is characterized by recurrent "cold" staphylococcal abscesses and occurs in young red-haired girls with atopic dermatitis. Marked elevation of serum IgE levels, defective neutrophil chemotaxis, and eosinophilia have been observed. The defect in chemotaxis is due to the presence of a serum inhibitor.

Graft-versus-host (GVH) reactions occur when differences in histocompatibility between graft (donor) and host (recipient) exist and require the presence of immunocompetent graft cells with immunodeficient host cells.[48] Two forms exist, *acute* and *chronic* GVH reactions. The acute form is often associated with a localized maculopapular eruption of the face, trunk, and hands, which sometimes progresses to a generalized erythroderma. An eruption resembling toxic epidermal necrolysis may also be observed in this phase and is associated with high mortality. Diarrhea, jaundice, hepatosplenomegaly, pulmonary infiltrates, and central nervous system involvement may be observed in this phase. Systemic involvement may occur in the absence of cutaneous signs. Chronic GVH reactions present with an early lichen planus-like eruption or a late sclerodermatous phase. Poikilodermatous skin changes, with discoid lupus-like lesions, have also been observed in this phase, together with lymphadenopathy and hepatosplenomegaly. Circumstances in which GVH reactions occur include maternal-fetal transfusion, immunotherapy with histocompatible bone marrow transplantation, and tranfusion of whole blood, plasma, and platelets in immunosuppressed patients and in those with severe combined immunodeficiency. Blood eosinophilia has been observed in both acute and chronic GVH reactions.

Skin Neoplasia

Tumors can induce antibody responses against tumor antigens,[49] resulting in IgE production with blood eosinophilia.[50] Malignant T-cell lymphomas with cutaneous involvement and mycosis fungoides have been associated with blood eosinophilia. Malignant lymphocytes produce lymphokines, which attract eosinophils and stimulate bone marrow eosinopoiesis. An increased number of mast cells has been observed in enlarged lymph nodes of patients with Hodgkin's disease, mycosis fungoides, Sézary syndrome, and lymphomatoid papulosis. The presence of eosinophilia may be secondary to release of mast cell mediators and/or specific lymphokines elaborated by the tumor cells. Approximately 20 percent of patients with Hodgkin's disease have blood eosinophilia, with eosinophils as high as 95 percent on differential counts in some cases.[36]

Eosinophilia has been described with all cutaneous manifestations of *mycosis fungoides,* including the psoriasiform patch, plaque, tumor, noduloulcerative, and erythrodermic phases. *Sézary syndrome* presents with fever, hepatosplenomegaly, lymphadenopathy, and erythroderma. Laboratory studies reveal leukocytosis with counts greater than 20,000/mm^3, eosinophilia, and elevated serum IgE. Sézary cells can be seen on peripheral smear, and T-cell helper activity is increased.

Clinical signs and symptoms of *angioimmunoblastic lymphadenopathy* include fever, malaise, weight loss, generalized maculopapular rash, lymphadenopathy, and hepatosplenomegaly. The etiology is unknown although viral and drug factors, including penicillin, have been implicated. Laboratory studies reveal anemia, eosinophilia, and polyclonal hypergammaglobulinemia.

Lymphomatoid papulosis has been classified by some as a T-cell lymphoma. The disease is usually benign, but in some reports between 10 and 20 percent of patients subsequently developed a malignant lymphoma. Cutaneous lesions are commonly papuloulcerative. Eosinophilia is occasionally reported.

Plasma cell dyscrasias with skin involvement and eosinophilia include *heavy chain disease*[53] and *Waldenström's primary macroglobulinemia.*[54] The mechanism of eosinophilia may be related to the mast cell infiltration of involved lymph nodes and their subsequent release of mediators. In heavy chain disease cutaneous lesions are not characteristic and result from recurrent bacterial infections. In Waldenström's primary macroglobulinemia cutaneous manifestations include a number of nonspecific findings, as well as infiltrated plaques, nodules, and papules. Other physical findings include signs related to the presence of the hyperviscosity syndrome with congestive heart failure, hepatosplenomegaly, lymphadenopathy, and neurological defects. Laboratory studies reveal homogeneous monoclonal IgM on immunoelectrophoresis, increased serum viscosity, and, occasionally, the presence of cold agglutinins and Bence-Jones proteinuria.

In *Kimura's disease,* also known as *angiolymphoid hyperplasia with eosinophilia,* patients present with purple-red ulcerating nodules of the face, ears, scalp, and subcutaneous tissue. Eosinophilia is present together with elevated levels of serum IgE, and increased numbers of mast cells are noted on biopsy of cutaneous lesions. Immediate hypersensitivity to *Candida* has been demonstrated in some patients and may be involved in the generation of eosinophilia.[8]

In *systemic mastocytosis* blood eosinophilia increases with the increased number of mast cells and release of mast cell granule ECF-A. Organs involved in systemic mastocytosis include skin, bones, blood, liver, and spleen. Cutaneous manifestations reveal multiple reddish-brown macules, papules, and nodules, with telangiectases, pruritus, and dermatographism. Gastrointestinal signs and symptoms include nausea, vomiting, diarrhea, cramping, peptic ulceration, and malabsorption. Hepatosplenomegaly and lymphadenopathy are common. Bone pain, when present, results from lytic lesions secondary to osteoporosis and osteosclerosis. Hematologic abnormalities include anemia, leukopenia, thrombocytopenia, and mast cell leukemia. Tachycardia can be present and results from massive release of histamine. Diagnosis is made by demonstration of increased urine histamine, lytic bone lesions, and skin biopsy. The prognosis is benign for solitary mastocytoma and urticaria pigmentosa and grave for mast cell leukemia.

The *hypereosinophilic syndrome* (HES) is a condition characterized by peripheral blood eosinophilia with eosinophilic infiltration of various organs. Diagnostic criteria for HES include: a blood eosinophil count of 1,500/mm^3 or greater for at least 6 months; multiple organ infiltration of eosinophils; and unexplained etiology for eosinophilia. The pathology of HES results from eosinophil cytotoxicity.

Commonly HES affects men from 20 to 40 years of age; however, the disease has been described in children and in patients well into the ninth decade of life. Organs commonly affected include skin, heart, lungs, and central nervous system; symptoms correspond to the organs involved.

Of patients with HES, 60 percent have cutaneous manifestations, which include macules, papules, nodules, ulcers, and angioedema. Pruritus is common. Skin biopsy demonstrates an eosinophilic infiltrate of the dermis, particularly around dermal blood vessels. In *eosinophilic cutaneous collagenosis,* a variant of HES, biopsy reveals necrosis of dermal collagen, with surrounding palisading granuloma formation as well as an eosinophilic infiltrate.

Hematologic abnormalities include anemia, with the presence of myelocytes and metamyelocytes on peripheral smear, and eosinophil counts often greater than 10,000/mm^3. In its most severe form HES can progress to eosinophilic leukemia. Differentiation of HES from myelocytic leukemia is based on the absence of the Philadelphia chromosome and the presence of normal leukocyte alkaline phosphatase in HES. When eosinophilic leukemia is present, total eosinophil counts can be as high as 50,000 /mm^3.

In HES chest x-ray may reveal cardiomegaly, with pulmonary infiltrates and effusions. Serum abnormalities include elevation of IgE and IgM,

circulating immune complexes, elevation of complement components C3 and C4, alteration of B- and T-lymphocyte levels, and an increased percentage of eosinophils with surface Fc receptors.[8,24] Prednisone has been shown to benefit patients with HES who have elevated serum IgE.[55] Diphenhydramine was shown to provide symptomatic relief.[56] Hydroxyurea is beneficial to some patients unresponsive to corticosteroids.

APPROACH TO THE PATIENT WITH RASH AND EOSINOPHILIA

In evaluating a patient with rash and eosinophilia (Table 9-3), one should pay particular attention to the onset and duration of the patient's symptoms, if any, recent medications, and prior allergic history. Note the distribution and characteristics of the cutaneous eruption: Is it macular, papular, nodular, ulcerative, urticarial, angioedematous, or vasculitic? Observe for accompanying systemic symptoms and signs on physical examination. An eosinophilia of less than 10 percent on differential blood count should be retested. If it persists, a drug or other allergic etiology is most likely. Eosinophilia greater than 10 percent requires a total eosinophil count for confirmation. Once confirmed, a skin biopsy including immunofluorescent studies should be done, especially if bullae are present or autoimmune disease is suspected. Parasitic infestation should always be considered; therefore stool examination for ova and parasites is indicated. A positive stool examination helps confirm the diagnosis while a negative examination does not necessarily exclude infection. Although a *Trichinella* skin test is available, muscle biopsy and stool examination are more definitive for diagnosis. Total serum IgE is often elevated in parasitic infestation, allergic reactions, and some immunodeficiency diseases. When anemia is present with eosinophilia, a bone marrow examination is indicated with an anemia work-up. In patients with skin rash, fever, arthralgias, and myalgias, ANA, lupus erythematosus cell preparation, erythro-

Table 9-3. Approach to the Patient: Evaluation of Patients with Rash and Eosinophilia

History
    Medication
    Allergies
    Symptoms
        Onset
        Duration
        Location

Physical Examination
    Skin eruption
        Type: macular, papular, nodular, ulcerative, petechial, bullous, urticarial
        Location
    Other systemic signs

Laboratory Investigation
    Eosinophilia less than 10%: discontinue all medication, repeat complete blood count and differential, observe patient
    Eosinophilia greater than 10%: discontinue all medication, obtain total eosinophil count, skin biopsy, chest x-ray, antinuclear antibodies, erythrocyte sedimentation rate, LE cell preparation, CH50, C3, C4, rheumatoid factor, SSA-Ro and SSB-La antibodies, cryoglobulins, VDRL, total serum IgE, platelet count, serum protein electrophoresis, serum immunoelectrophoresis, stool for ova and parasites
    When indicated: immunofluorescent studies, trichinella skin test, lymph node biopsy with lymphadenopathy, electrocardiographic/radiographic studies T and B lymphocyte quantitation, skin tests for anergy, blast transformation studies, bone marrow biopsy if anemic, muscle biopsy, T-helper/suppressor assay
    Total eosinophilia count greater than 30,000/mm^3: bone marrow biopsy, leukocyte alkaline phosphatase, serum B$_{12}$, folate level, Philadelphia chromosome

cyte sedimentation rate, rheumatoid factor, Ro and La antibody, and cryoglobulin studies are indicated to determine the presence of collagen vascular disease or vasculitis. Infants with failure to thrive, recurrent skin infections, eczematous dermatitis, and eosinophilia require T- and B-lymphocyte quantitation, total serum immunoglobulin levels, and blast transformation studies to determine the presence of an immunodeficiency syndrome.

Persistent rash with eosinophilia may indicate malignancy. These malignancies usually involve the lymphomatous group, including Hodgkin's disease, mycosis fungoides, Sézary syndrome, and angioimmunoblastic lymph-

adenopathy. When lymphadenopathy is present, a lymph node biopsy is indicated in the work-up, as well as a bone marrow examination, and skin biopsy of cutaneous lesions with appropriate stains. Eosinophilia in association with other internal malignancies may be a sign of existing metastases.[57] Appropriate radiographic studies and invasive studies with tissue biopsy should be included in the work-up.

Elevated eosinophil counts greater than 10,000/mm^3 may indicate the presence of the hypereosinophilic syndrome, including Löffler's endocarditis, Löffler's syndrome, eosinophilic cutaneous collagenosis, and the more severe eosinophilic leukemia. Total eosinophil counts of greater than 30,000/mm^3 require bone marrow examination, determination of leukocyte alkaline phosphatase levels, and search for the presence of the Philadelphia chromosome to confirm the possibility of eosinophilic leukemia.

If the etiology of the eosinophilia cannot be determined, the patient should be treated conservatively and observed periodically until the eosinophilia disappears or its etiology becomes apparent.[24]

REFERENCES

1. Beall GN: Diseases marked by eosinophilia. p. 313. In Beall GN (ed): Allergy and Clinical Immunology. John Wiley & Sons, New York, 1983
2. Gleich GJ, Loegering DA, Mann KG, et al: Comparative properties of Charcot-Leyden crystal protein and major basic protein from human eosinophils. J Clin Invest 57:633, 1976
3. Butterworth AE, Wassom DL, Gleich GJ, et al: Damage to schistosomula of *Schistosoma mansoni* induced directly to eosinophil major basic protein. J Immunol 122:221, 1979
4. Leiferman KM, Ackerman SJ, Sampson HA, et al: Dermal deposition of eosinophil-granule major basic protein in atopic dermatitis: comparison with onchocerciasis. N Engl J Med 313:282, 1985
5. Zucker D: Morphology, biochemistry, and function of eosinophils. p. 816. In Williams WJ,

Beutler E, Erslev AJ (eds): Hematology. 3rd Ed. McGraw-Hill, New York, 1983

6. Wassom DL, Loegering DA, Solley GO, et al: Elevated serum levels of the eosinophil granule major basic protein in patients with eosinophilia. J Clin Invest 67:651, 1981

7. Berretty MD, Cormane RH: Eosinophil granulocytes and skin disorders. Int J Dermatol 20:531, 1981

8. Cohen GC, Ottesen EA: The eosinophil, eosinophilia, and eosinophil-related disorders. p. 701. In Middletown E, Reed CE, Elder V (eds): Allergy, Principles and Practice. CV Mosby, St. Louis, 1984

9. Dahl MV: Phagocytes. p. 44. In Dahl MV (ed): Clinical Immunodermatology. Year Book Medical Publishers, Chicago, 1981

10. Anwar AR, Kay AB: Membrane receptors for IgG and complement (C4, C3b and C3d) on human eosinophils and neutrophils and their relation to eosinophilia. J Immunol 119:976, 1977

11. Hubscher T: Role of the eosinophil in the allergic reactions. I. EDI—an eosinophil derived inhibitor of histamine release. J Immunol 114:1379, 1975

12. Tchnitchin A: Fine structure of rat uterine eosinophils and the possible role of eosinophils in the mechanism of estrogen action. J Steroid Biochem 4:277, 1973

13. Peterson AP, Altmen LC, Hill JS: Glucocorticoid receptors in normal human eosinophils and neutrophils. (Abstract). Clin Res 84:77, 1980

14. Gallin JI, Weinstein AM, Cramer EB, et al: Histamine modulation of human eosinophil locomotion in vitro and in vivo. p. 85. In Mahmoud AF, Austen KF (eds): The Eosinophil in Health and Disease. Grune & Stratton, Orlando, FL, 1980

15. Cline MJ, Hanifon J, Lehrer RI: Phagocytosis by human eosinophils. Blood 32:922, 1968

16. Zeiger RS, Twarog FJ, Colten HR: Histamine release from human granulocytes. J Exp Med 114:1049, 1976

17. Wasserman ST, Goetzl EJ, Austen KF: Inactivation of slow reacting substance of anaphylaxis by human eosinophil arylsulphatase. J Immunol 114:645, 1975

18. Gleich GJ, Loegerung DA, Kueppers F, et al: Physicochemical and biological properties of the major basic protein from guinea pig eosinophil granules. J Exp Med 140:313, 1974

19. Wasserman ST, Whitmer D, Goetzl EJ, et al: Chemotactic deactivation of human eosinophils by the eosinophil chemotactic factor of anaphylaxis. Proc Soc Exp Biol Med 148:301, 1975

20. Hubscher T: Role of the eosinophil in allergic reactions. II. Release of prostaglandins from human eosinophilic leukocytes. J Immunol 114:1389, 1975

21. Koter LA, Goetz EJ, Austen KF: Isolation of human eosinophil phospholipase D. J Clin Invest 57:1173, 1978

22. Weller PF, Wasserman SI, Austen KF: Selected enzymes preferentially present in the eosinophil. p. 115. In Mahmoud AF, Austen KF (eds): The Eosinophil in Health and Disease. Grune & Stratton, Orlando, FL, 1980

23. Colley DG: Eosinophils and immune mechanisms. 1. Eosinophil stimulation promotor (ESP)—a lymphokine induced by specific antigen or phytohemagglutinin. J Immunol 110:1419, 1973

24. Booth BH: Eosinophilia. p. 806. In Patterson R (ed): Allergic Diseases. 3rd Ed. JB Lippincott, Philadelphia, 1985

25. Cohen S, Ward PA: In vitro and in vivo activity of a lymphocyte and immune complex-dependent chemotactic factor for eosinophils. J Exp Med 133:133, 1971

26. Colley DG: Eosinophils and immune mechanisms. IV. Culture conditions, antigen requirements, production kinetics, and immunologic specificity of the lymphokine eosinophil stimulation promotor. Cell Immunol 24:328, 1976

27. Czarnetzki BM, Konig W, Lichenstein LM: Antigen induced eosinophil chemotactic factor (ECF) release by human leukocytes. Inflammation 1:201, 1976

28. Goetzl EJ, Tashjian AH, Rubin RH, et al: Production of a low molecular weight eosinophil polymorphonuclear leukocyte chemotactic factor by anaplastic squamous cell carcinomas of human lung. J Clin Invest 61:770, 1978

29. Goetzl EJ, Rottenberg J, Weber EL, et al: A novel eosinophil chemotactic factor derived from a histiocytic lymphoma of the central nervous system. Clin Exp Immunol 40:249, 1980

30. Kay AB, McVie JG, Stuart AE, et al: Eosinophil chemotaxis of supernatants from cultured Hodgkin's lymph node cells. J Clin Pathol 28:502, 1975

31. Steinman TI, Silva P: Acute renal failure, skin rash, and eosinophilia associated with captopril therapy. Am J Med 75:524, 1983

32. Weiss VC, West DP, Ackerman R, et al: Hepatic reactions in a patient treated with etretinate. Arch Dermatol 120:104, 1984

33. Halla JT, Fallahi S, Koopman WJ: Penicillamine induced myositis. Observations and unique features in two patients and review of the literature. Am J Med 77:719, 1984

34. Zolov DM, Levine BB: Correlation of blood eosinophilia with antibody classes: studies with the penicillin hypersensitivity system. Int Arch Allergy Appl Immunol 35:179, 1969

35. Paton WDM: The mechanism of histamine release. In Wolstenholme GEW, O'Connor CM (eds): Histamine. Little, Brown, Boston, 1956

36. Bass DA: Eosinophilic syndromes. p. 1011. In Wyngaarden JB, Smith LH (eds): Cecil Textbook of Medicine. Vol. 2. WB Saunders, Philadelphia, 1985

37. Takematsu H, Nakamura K, Igarashi M, et al: Eosinophilic pustular folliculitis. Arch Dermatol 121:917, 1985

38. Wong E, Greaves MW, O'Brien T: Increased concentrations of immunoreactive leukotrienes in cutaneous lesions of eosinophilic cellulitis. Br J Dermatol 110:653. 1984

39. Dahl MV: The bullous diseases: pemphigus, pemphigoid, dermatitis herpetiformis, and others. p. 144. In Dahl MV (ed): Clinical Immunodermatology. Year Book Medical Publishers, Chicago, 1981

40. Bushkell LL, Jordan RE: Bullous pemphigoid: a cause of peripheral blood eosinophilia. J Am Acad Dermatol 8:648, 1983

41. Goetzl EJ: Mediators of immediate hypersensitivity derived from arachidonic acid. N Engl J Med 303:822, 1980

42. Cramer SF, Kent L, Abramosky C, et al: Eosinophilic fasciitis. Immunopathology, ultrastructure, literature review, and consideration of its pathogenesis and relation to scleroderma. Arch Pathol Lab Med 106:85, 1982

43. Bulloch WE Jr: Leprosy, p. 630. In Samter M (ed): Immunological Diseases. 2nd Ed. Vol. 1. Little, Brown, Boston, 1971

44. Waksman BH: Cellular hypersensitivity and immunity: inflammation and cytotoxicity. p. 173. In Parker CW (ed): Clinical Immunology. Vol. 1. WB Saunders, Philadelphia, 1980

45. Warren KS: Worms. p. 668. In Samter M (ed): Immunological Diseases. 2nd Ed. Vol. 1. Little, Brown, Boston, 1971

46. Farah FS: Protozoan and helminth infections. p. 1638. In Fitzpatrick TB, Eizen AZ, Wolff K, et al (eds.): Dermatology in General Medicine. 2nd Ed. McGraw-Hill, New York, 1979

47. Donaraj TJ, Pacherco G, Shonmugaratnam K, et al: The etiology and pathology of eosinophilic lung (tropical eosinophilia). Am J Trop Med 15:183, 1966

48. Ammann AJ: Immunodeficiency diseases. p. 384. In Stites DP, Stobo JB, Fudenberg HH, et al. (eds): Basic and Clinical Immunology. 5th Ed. Appleton & Lange, East Norwalk, CT, 1984

49. Broom BC, Alexander P: Rat tumor allografts evoke anaphylactic antibody responses. Immunology 28:1033, 1975

50. Takenada T, Okuda M, Kubo K, et al: Studies on interrelations between eosinophilia, serum IgE and tissue mast cells. Clin Allergy 5:175, 1975

51. Gall EA, Mallory TB: Malignant lymphoma: a clinicopathologic survey of 618 cases. Am J Pathol 18:381, 1941

52. Cyr DR, Geokas MC, Worsley GM: Mycosis fungoides; hematologic findings and terminal course. Arch Dermatol 94:558, 1966

53. Franklin EC: The heavy chain diseases. p. 1109. In Williams WJ, Beutler E, Erslev AS, et al (eds): Hematology. 3rd Ed. McGraw-Hill, New York, 1983

54. Bergsagel DE: Macroglobulinemia. p. 1104. In Williams WJ, Beutler E, Erslev AS, et al (eds): Hematology. 3rd Ed. McGraw-Hill, New York, 1983

55. Parrillo JE, Fauci AS: Human eosinophils, purification and cytotoxicity capability of eosinophils from patients with the hypereosinophilic syndrome. Blood 51:457, 1978

56. Hardy WR, Anderson RE: The hypereosinophilic syndromes. Ann Intern Med 68:1220, 1968

57. Isaacson NH, Rapoport P: Eosinophilia in malignant tumors. Ann Intern Med 25:893, 1946

10

Pustular Disorders in the Neonate

Dorie Hankin
Lawrence Schachner
Shirley Press

Pustular eruptions in neonates present a diagnostic challenge to the skilled dermatologist and pediatrician. A neonate is defined as a newborn less than 28 days of age. Simple diagnostic techniques differentiate those pustular diseases that are transient, benign conditions from those that are serious and life-threatening and require immediate therapy. The discussion below will provide information on history and physical and laboratory findings that help distinguish between transient benign disorders, mild infectious conditions, and serious infectious conditions that can present in the neonatal period as pustular eruptions (Table 10-1). Information about therapeutic intervention will be included where appropriate.

TRANSIENT DISORDERS

Recognition of transient neonatal disorders is of particular importance as it will spare the healthy newborn from an invasive evaluation for sepsis, potentially harmful antibiotic therapy, and prolonged hospitalization. The disorders discussed below are summarized in Table 10-2.

Table 10-1. Neonatal Pustular Eruptions

Noninfectious transient
    Pustular erythema toxicum neonatorum
    Pustular miliaria
    Transient neonatal pustular melanosis
    Acropustulosis of infancy
    Eosinophilic pustular folliculitis of infancy

Infectious, mild
    Candidiasis
        Congenital
        Neonatal
    Staphylococcal impetigo
    Scabies

Infectious, severe
    Bacterial infections
        Staphylococcus aureus
        Group B streptococcus
        Pseudomonas aeruginosa
        Listeria monocytogenes
        Hemophilus influenzae
    Herpesvirus infections
        Herpes simplex
        Varicella
        Cytomegalovirus
    Disseminated candidiasis
    Other
        Neonatal syphilis
        Acquired immunodeficiency syndrome and associated infections

Table 10-2. Neonatal Pustular Eruptions

Disease	Incidence	Age of Onset	Duration	Lesions	Distribution	Pathology	Stains	Treatment
Acropustulosis of infancy	Incidence < 1%, possibly increased in blacks and males	Hours after birth–10 months	2–3 years	Red papules evolving into pustular and vesicular lesions in one day	Hands, feet, both surfaces	Subcorneal pustules with neutrophils and occasionally eosinophils	Gram: neutrophils, no bacteria KOH: negative Wright and Giemsa: neutrophils	Oral antihistamines and/or dapsone in later childhood, ?topical steroids
Candidiasis, congenital	Incidence < 1%, equal among sexes	Birth–24 hours	2 weeks	Pink to red macules and papules evolving into pustules and vesicles	Diffuse	Subcorneal pustules with pseudohyphae and spores	KOH: pseudohyphae and spores Others: negative	Topical nystatin, clotrimazole or miconazole preparation for 10 days
Candidiasis, neonatal	Incidence approximately 4–5%	After the first week of life	2 weeks	Pink to red macules and papules evolving into pustules and vesicles	Oral mucosa, diaper area	Subcorneal pustules with pseudohyphae and spores	KOH: pseudohyphae and spores Others: negative	Topical nystatin, clotrimazole or miconazole for 10 days, plus nystatin suspension if thrush is present
Eosinophilic pustular folliculitis (Ofuji's disease)	Exceedingly rare	From birth; most reported cases is adults	Years	Follicular pustules and papules on an erythematous base	Scalp, trunk, extremities	Epidermal and dermal infiltrate of eosinophils with follicular and perifollicular clusters	Gram: eosinophils and neutrophils Wright and Giemsa: eosinophils and neutrophils KOH: Negative	Topical steroids, systemic steroids and/or sulfones in severe cases in later childhood
Erythema toxicum neonatorum	Approximately ⅓ of full-term newborns	24–72 hours	1 week	Red macules and papules; white to pink pustules, vesicles	Trunk, extremities, face	Subcorneal pustules with eosinophils associated with pilosebaceous system	Gram: eosinophils, no bacteria KOH: negative Wright and Giemsa: eosinophils	None

Disorder	Incidence	Age of onset	Duration	Clinical appearance	Distribution	Histology	Laboratory	Treatment
Impetigo neonatorum	< 1%	2nd day–2nd week	Approx. 5–10 days	Vesicles, pustules, or bullae on an erythematous base	Diaper area, neck, groin, axilla	Subcorneal pustules with gram-positive cocci in clusters and neutrophils	Gram: gram positive cocci in clusters and neutrophils; Wright and Giemsa: neutrophils; KOH: negative	Dicloxacillin, 12.5–25 mg/kg/day for 10 days; cloxacillin, 50 mg/kg/day for 10 days
Miliaria crystallina	Equal among sexes and races	First weeks of life	Hours to days	Clear superficial vesicles	Unclothed skin, neck, axilla, trunk	Subcorneal vesicles associated with sweat ducts	All stains negative	Cooling baths, calamine lotion with 0.25% menthol; air conditioning, removal of excess clothing
Miliaria rubra	Equal among sexes and races	First weeks of life	Hours to days	Grouped erythematous papules	Clothed skin, flexural surfaces	Intraepidermal spongiosis and vesicles associated with sweat ducts	All stains negative	Cooling baths, calamine lotion with 0.25% menthol; air conditioning, removal of excess clothing
Transient neonatal pustular melanosis	5% of all black neonates; < 1% in whites	Birth, indicative of intrauterine involvement	Pustules: days; Macules: 3 months	Vesicles and pustules desquamate leaving brown macules	Chin, neck, palms, soles	Macules: basilar hyperpigmentation; Pustules: intracorneal and subcorneal neutrophils and rare eosinophils	Gram: neutrophils, no bacteria, rare eosinophils; KOH: negative; Wright and Giemsa: neutrophils, rare eosinophils	None

(Modified from Schachner L, Press S: Vesicular, bullous and pustular disorders. Pediatr Clin North Am 30:609, 1983. Reprinted with permission from WB Saunders Co.)

Pustular Erythema Toxicum Neonatorum

First recognized in 1826, erythema toxicum is a benign, self-limited neonatal eruption seen in approximately one-third of all full-term newborns.[1] Black and white infants are affected equally. The condition usually appears after 24 to 72 hours of life although it has been reported at birth as well.[2,3] The etiology of erythema toxicum is unknown although absorption of intestinal toxins, neonatal allergy, viral infection, and chemical or mechanical irritation have all been hypothesized.

The lesions evolve from poorly defined erythematous macules to red, white, or yellow papules to a vesicular and, more rarely, pustular eruption on an erythematous base. They are asymptomatic and evanescent, with individual macular lesions often disappearing in hours. The sites of predilection are the forehead, face, chest, trunk, and extremities (Fig. 10-1). It is unusual to see lesions on the palms or soles.

A Gram, Giemsa, or Wright stain of lesional contents demonstrates numerous eosinophils. Bacteria are not seen, cultures are negative, and potassium hydroxide preparations are negative. Histopathologic examination reveals intrafollicular, subcorneal pustules with dense accumulations of eosinophils. Eosinophils also infiltrate the outer root sheath of the pilosebaceous unit proximal to the sebaceous duct. More macular lesions may present with sparse perivascular accumulations of eosinophils in the dermis.[4,5] Erythema toxicum will resolve spontaneously without residua within days to weeks, the usual duration being less than 1 week. No treatment is necessary other than reassurance to the parents.

Pustular Miliaria

Miliaria is often seen in the first weeks of life. It is a manifestation of sweat retention in which occlusion of the immature eccrine sweat ducts results in rupture of the ducts with escape of sweat into the surrounding epidermis. There are two common types, miliaria crystallina and miliaria rubra.

Miliaria crystallina results from superficial obstruction of the eccrine ducts. The lesions consist of asymptomatic, clear, thin-walled, easily ruptured vesicles, 1 to 2 mm in size. The vesicles appear in a generalized distribution, with an increase in intertriginous areas. On biopsy they appear within or directly beneath the stratum corneum and demonstrate very little perivascular inflammation.

Miliaria rubra results when swelling and inflammation follow rupture of the sweat duct behind a deeper occlusion. The lesions are itchy, small, red papules or papulovesicles, which accounts for the common name of this disorder, *prickly heat*. Although the lesions may occur anywhere, there is a predilection for clothed areas of the body. Biopsy reveals inflammation surrounding the eccrine ductal system in the malpighian layer of the epidermis.

Miliaria rubra may progress to pustular lesions (pustular miliaria or miliaria profunda), particularly in climates with high temperature and humidity or when there has been treatment with occlusive dressings or ointments. Pustular miliaria upon biopsy shows white cells, as well as disruption of the eccrine system. A putative role of *Staphylococcus aureus* in miliaria rubra and pustular miliaria has been cited.[5]

Absorbent, lightweight clothing and regulation of ambient temperature often prevent miliaria and also are important in its treatment. Cool wet to dry soaks provide rapid symptomatic relief. Appropriate medication should be used to treat any suspected bacterial or candidal infection superimposed on miliaria.

Transient Neonatal Pustular Melanosis

Transient neonatal pustular melanosis (TNPM) was first described by Ramamurthy et al. in 1976.[6] The disorder was originally reported to affect approximately 5 percent of full-term black infants and less than 1 percent of white newborns. Males and females are affected

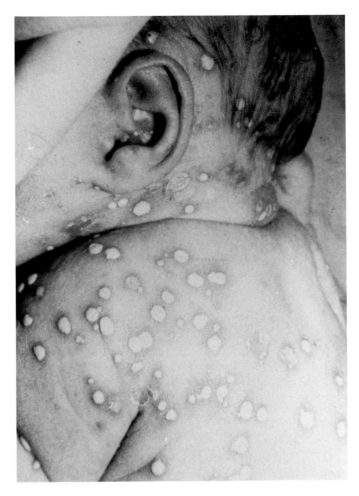

Fig. 10-1. Pustular erythema toxicum. (Schachner L, Press S: Vesicular, bullous and pustular disorders. Pediatr Clin North Am 30:609, 1983. Reprinted with permission from WB Saunders Co.)

equally. The condition is present at birth. The etiology of TNPM is unknown, although an increased incidence of placental squamous metaplasia has been noted in mothers whose infants develop this disorder.[7]

The most common lesion in TNPM is a pigmented macule. Also seen are superficial, easily ruptured vesicles and pustules 3 to 4 mm in size and erosions with a collarette of scale (Fig. 10-2). Lesions occur primarily on the nape of the neck, forehead, lower back, and shins and under the chin. They are occasionally seen on the scalp, palms, and soles. No systemic symptoms are associated with the lesions.

Gram, Giemsa, or Wright stains of lesions in TNPM demonstrate polymorphic neutrophils and occasional eosinophils. Bacteria are absent and cultures are negative, as are potassium hydroxide preparations. On histopathologic examination, intracorneal and subcorneal pustules with collections of polymorphic neutrophils and a few eosinophils are seen under a thickened stratum corneum.[5,6] The dermis is generally uninvolved although in a later stage postinflammatory changes and pigment-laden dermal macrophages may be seen.[8]

The vesiculopustules of TNPM usually rupture within the first few days of life, leaving a brown macule with a fine collarette of scale. The macules may persist for several months but usually fade spontaneously within 3 to 4 weeks. No treatment is necessary.

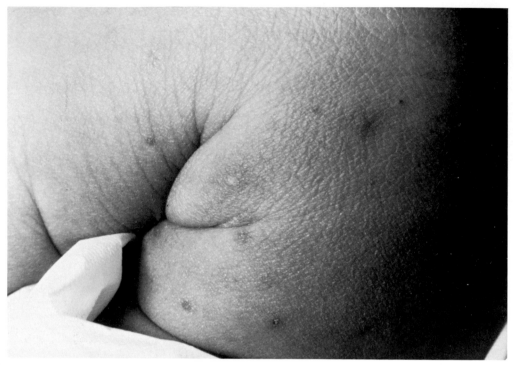

Fig. 10-2. Transient neonatal pustular melanosis. (Schachner L, Press S: Vesicular, bullous and pustular disorders. Pediatr Clin North Am 30:609, 1983. Reprinted with permission from WB Saunders Co.)

Acropustulosis of Infancy

Acropustulosis of infancy is a relatively uncommon disorder first described in 1979 by Kahn and Rywlin[9] and Jarratt and Ramsdell.[10] The condition usually has its onset within the first few months of life but can begin at or shortly after birth.

The lesions begin as small red papules, which evolve within 24 hours into vesicles and pustules several millimeters in diameter (Fig. 10-3). The pustules are intensely pruritic, last for 7 to 10 days, and appear in crops every 2 to 3 weeks. They are found on the hands and feet predominantly and occasionally on the scalp, face, and trunk. Atopy has been reported in two patients.[11]

Gram, Giemsa, or Wright stains of lesions reveal numerous polymorphic neutrophils, occasional eosinophils, and no bacteria.[12,13] Potassium hydroxide preparations are negative for hyphae and spores, and cultures are negative. On histopathologic examination well-circumscribed, subcorneal pustules with polymorphic neutrophils and occasional eosinophils are seen. The underlying dermis is edematous and has a perivascular, chiefly lymphocytic infiltrate.

The etiology of acropustulosis of infancy is unknown. It is a self-limited disease, which exacerbates and remits over 2 to 3 years and then resolves completely. It frequently is worse in the summer months. Topical steroid therapy may be effective. Antihistamines are useful for symptomatic relief of itching in older infants but are contraindicated in neonates because of the undesirable side effect of sedation. Sulfone therapy in the form of dapsone (2 mg/kg/day in two divided doses) may be effective. Dapsone should be reserved, however, for treatment of exceedingly severe cases in older infants because of the possible side effects of methemoglobinemia, hemolysis, crystalluria, and inter-

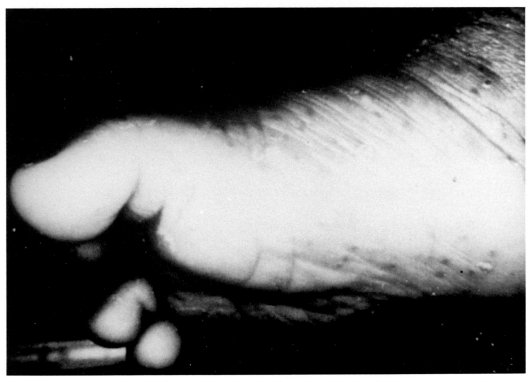

Fig. 10-3. Acropustulosis of infancy. (Schachner L, Press S: Vesicular, bullous and pustular disorders. Pediatr Clin North Am 30:609, 1983. Reprinted with permission from WB Saunders Co.)

ference with liver function.[14] If dapsone is used, monitoring for toxicity is imperative, and the medication should be gradually tapered as soon as a clinical response is seen.

Eosinophilic Pustular Folliculitis of Infancy

Eosinophilic pustular folliculitis was first described in adults in 1970 by Ofuji et al.[15] It has only recently been demonstrated in children, with a description of five cases by Lucky et al. in 1984.[16] This rare disorder has a male predominance and can be present at birth. This disorder is characterized by eosinophilic infiltration of hair follicles, resulting in pruritic grouped follicular papules and pustules. The etiology is unknown although the possibility of an immunologic abnormality[16] or an exagger-

ated allergic response to insects, mites,[17] or parasites[18] has been raised.

In infants, unlike adults with eosinophilic pustular folliculitis, the lesions appear in a perifollicular pattern on the scalp, hands, and feet. They occur as recurrent crops of 1- to 3-mm white to yellow pruritic pustules on erythematous bases (Fig. 10-4). They can also be present on the trunk. Many lesions have secondary crusting. There are no signs of systemic illness.

Cultures for bacteria and fungi are negative. Gram, Giemsa, or Wright stains of the lesions demonstrate eosinophils. Some patients have eosinophilia as well as leukocytosis on blood counts obtained during outbreaks.[16,17,19] Biopsies of the lesions show intraepidermal pustules containing primarily eosinophils, follicular and nonfollicular eosinophilic spongiosis, and a dense dermal perifollicular infiltrate consisting of eosinophils, lymphocytes, and histiocytes.[16,17,20]

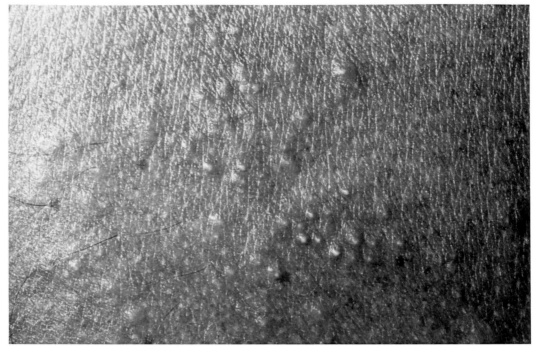

Fig. 10-4. Eosinophilic pustular folliculitis of infancy.

In adult cases the course is variable with exacerbations and remissions. Because the description of eosinophilic pustular folliculitis in children is so recent, the course of the disease is unknown. Topical treatment with high-potency steroids seemed to reduce itching and abort eruptions in the patients described by Lucky et al.[16] Systemic antibiotics, antihistamines, and other topical agents were ineffective. Sulfonamides, sulfones, and systemic steroids have been used in adults.[17,19,21,22]

MILD CUTANEOUS INFECTIOUS CONDITIONS OF INFANCY

All infections in the neonate need prompt attention because of their potential to disseminate and overwhelm the newborn's immune system. Mild infections are defined here as those which under normal circumstances remain confined to the skin, produce few or no systemic symptoms, and are readily resolved with appropriate treatment.

Cutaneous Candidiasis

Cutaneous candidiasis exists in two forms, congenital and neonatal. The congenital form is associated with intrauterine infection, presumably ascending[23] or introduced,[24] and the lesions are present at or shortly after birth. The neonatal form is acquired by passage through an infected birth canal and usually has its onset in the second week of life. In both forms the causative organism is *Candida albicans*, a pathogen found in the vaginal canal of 20 to 25 percent of pregnant women.[23,24]

The congenital form of cutaneous candidiasis begins as diffuse macules, papules, vesicles, and pustules usually affecting the face, chest, back, and extremities (Fig. 10-5). Oral and diaper lesions are generally absent. Signs of systemic disease and hematologic abnormalities are

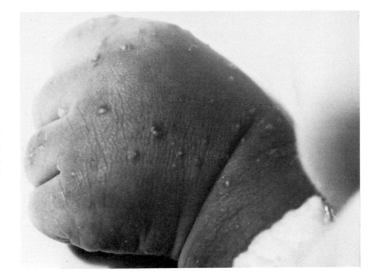

Fig. 10-5. Congenital candidiasis. (Schachner L, Press S: Vesicular, bullous and pustular disorders. Pediatr Clin North Am 30:609, 1983. Reprinted with permission from WB Saunders Co.)

usually absent in most but not all congenital cutaneous candidiasis patients. Stool cultures at birth are sterile.

The neonatal form is usually manifested after the seventh day of life by oral thrush and lesions confined to the diaper area. Pustules and vesicles arising from the perianal area erode and spread peripherally with satellite lesions. The intergluteal fold, perineum, genitalia, suprapubic area, buttocks, and inner thighs[25] are frequently involved. In these areas candidiasis evolves into scaling, confluent plaques of a beefy red color, with distinct pustular and vesicular satellite lesions at the periphery of the plaques. Constitutional signs are absent, and stool cultures are frequently positive for *Candida albicans.*

Diagnosis of cutaneous candidiasis is made by finding pseudohyphae and spores on a potassium hydroxide preparation of a pustule or scale. *Candida albicans* may be cultured from the vesicles and pustules. The histopathology is that of a subcorneal pustule with pseudohyphae or spores.

Candida dermatitis is treated topically for 10 days with nystatin cream. Many physicians also use oral nystatin suspension, particularly if thrush is present. Oral gentian violet is equally effective for thrush but may be unacceptable to parents because of staining. Lesions last approximately 2 weeks, desquamate, and resolve without residua. Disseminated systemic candidiasis can occur rarely and is discussed below.

Staphylococcal Impetigo Neonatorum

Impetigo neonatorum is a term used to describe staphylococcal bullous impetigo appearing as early as the second or third day of life. It consists of vesicles, bullae, or pustules on erythematous bases. When consisting primarily of pustules, the disorder is sometimes termed *staphylococcal pustulosis.* The lesions are superficial and erode easily, leaving a moist, glistening, denuded area, which has a tendency to crust to a mild degree. The diaper region and intertriginous areas of the body, such as the axilla and the neck, are commonly involved (Fig. 10-6).

Polymorphic neutrophils and gram-positive cocci in clusters are seen on Gram stain of lesional contents. Cultures will grow *Staphylococcus aureus.* Histopathology demonstrates subcorneal pustules with gram-positive cocci and polymorphic neutrophils.

The infection is chiefly limited to the epider-

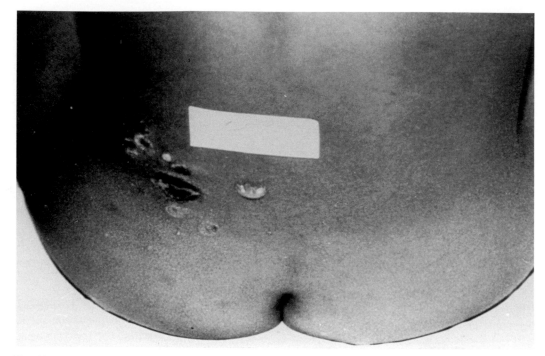

Fig. 10-6. Staphylococcal bullous impetigo. (Schachner L, Press S: Vesicular, bullous and pustular disorders. Pediatr Clin North Am 30:609, 1983. Reprinted with permission from WB Saunders Co.)

mis and does not usually produce systemic manifestations. It responds rapidly to a 10-day course of oral antibiotic therapy with a semisynthetic, penicillinase-resistant penicillin such as dicloxacillin or cloxacillin. Topical antibiotic therapy is not necessary. Hexachlorophene-containing compounds should not be used because of their potential neurotoxicity. If fever, irritability, or other signs of systemic illness are present, the neonate requires admission to the hospital for a complete evaluation for sepsis and intravenous antibiotics. The hospital at which the infant was born should be notified, as the infection may indicate nursery contamination.

Neonatal Scabies

Scabies is a contagious disorder caused by the parasitic mite *Sarcoptes scabiei,* which infests the stratum corneum. Sensitization of the host takes 3 to 6 weeks to create the extremely pruritic dermatitis that accompanies this

infestation.[26,27] If infestation occurs soon after delivery, the disorder may be seen in the neonate.[27] The clinical pattern of scabies in newborns differs from that seen in older infants, children, and adults.

The neonate with scabies presents with red vesicular, pustular, and papular squamous lesions involving the face, neck, scalp, palms, and soles.[27] Pustules from secondary bacterial infection may also be seen in this eruption. Nodular lesions and severe crusting may be seen. The neonates are frequently irritable and feed poorly. A careful history and examination of the baby's caretakers will frequently disclose a history of pruritus and/or typical scabies lesions. Frequent maternal sites of lesions are the periareolar regions of the breasts, as well as the wrists and fingers.

Definitive diagnosis is made by microscopic examination of scrapings from unexcoriated lesions placed in mineral oil. The presence of the adult mite, ova, larva, and/or fecal matter is diagnostic. A biopsy of scabietic lesions may show a mite, eggs, and/or stools beneath the stratum corneum.

Scabies in neonates may best be treated with 5 percent precipitated sulfur in petrolatum.[26] There is less experience, and perhaps less success, with 10 percent crotamiton (Eurax).[27] The neonate should be treated from head to toe, with special attention to those areas most involved with lesions. Repeat treatment 24 hours and 1 week after initial therapy may increase the cure rate.

SEVERE INFECTIOUS CONDITIONS OF INFANCY

Although the incidence of serious neonatal infection varies, newborns may be subject to bacteremia and at risk of serious infection more frequently than is recognized. Of newborns tested on their first day of life in one study, 7 percent had positive blood cultures.[28] Higher percentages have been found in other studies.[29] Rapid diagnosis and aggressive, appropriate treatment of severe infections in the newborn reduce the morbidity and mortality of these diseases. Recognition of the skin manifestations of various severe infectious conditions allows treatment to be instituted while definitive diagnostic studies are still pending. Pustular lesions may be present in a number of bacterial, viral, and yeast neonatal infections. These infections are readily accessible to appropriate diagnostic tests, (e.g., Tzanck smear, Gram stain, and potassium hydroxide preparation).

Bacterial Infections

Bacterial infections can be acquired prenatally, during delivery, or after birth. Group B streptococcus (GBS), *Listeria monocytogenes, Hemophilus influenzae, Pseudomonas aeruginosa,* and *Staphylococcus aureus* are bacterial pathogens that may produce pustules and sepsis in the neonate.

Neonatal disease caused by GBS was uncommon, although present, until the 1960s. For unknown reasons the incidence of the disease has increased, GBS now being the most common agent responsible for bacteremia or meningitis in the first month of life.[30] *L. monocytogenes* is known to be responsible for intrauterine and early neonatal death from fulminating disease. It also has been implicated in neonatal meningitis.

Staphylococcal infections may present with a number of skin findings. Certain strains of *S. aureus* (e.g., phage group II, types 70 and 71) have the ability to elaborate an exfoliative exotoxin. When the infection and toxin remain localized, focal *S. aureus* infections result. When the toxins enter systemic circulation, there is potential involvement of the entire cutaneous surface. This disorder is termed the *staphylococcal scalded skin syndrome.*

The staphylococcal scalded skin syndrome was first described in 1878 by Ritter von Rittershain[31] and is sometimes called *Ritter's disease.* It usually occurs in newborns and infants and is rare past the age of 5 years. The disorder occurs equally among males and females. Most patients present with a prodrome of conjunctivitis and/or purulent rhinitis. They may also present with symptoms of other staphylococcal infections, such as pharyngitis, external otitis, osteomyelitis, omphalitis, or soft tissue abscesses.[32] The prodrome is followed within 2 days by irritability, fever, and diffuse sensitivity and erythema of the skin.[33,34] The perioral or malar area is often the first to be involved. The skin, initially intact, becomes wrinkled, and large flaccid bullae appear in a distribution that may vary from focal to generalized. Pressure applied to the edge of a bulla results in an extension of the lesion (Nikolsky's sign). Exfoliation follows, resulting in moist, raw, denuded areas, which have the appearance of scalded skin (Fig. 10-7). Crusting may be seen around the mouth, nose, and eyes, but mucous membrane involvement beyond the sites of initial prodrome is rare.

Anorexia, low-grade fever, and mild leukocytosis are generally present. Cultures of fluid from intact bullae are sterile since these bullae, in contrast to those of bullous impetigo, result

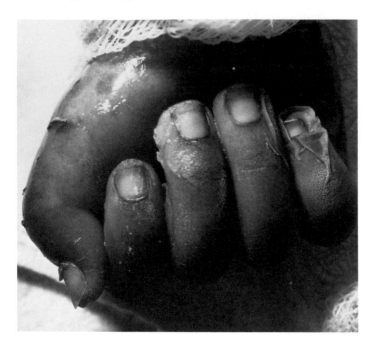

Fig. 10-7. Staphylococcal scalded skin syndrome.

from the circulation of exfoliative toxin. Cultures of prodromal sites of infection will often yield *S. aureus*. Histologically, there is an intact stratum corneum, with cleavage of cells in the stratum granulosum of the epidermis. No dermal inflammation is present.

Treatment of the staphylococcal scalded skin syndrome includes parenteral antistaphylococcal antibiotics, careful fluid management, and supportive care. Corticosteroids should be avoided as they enhance host susceptibility to the toxin.[33–35] Re-epithelialization of the skin without scarring occurs within 2 weeks. The mortality rate is low.

Herpesvirus Infections

The herpesviruses are spherical, enveloped, DNA-containing viruses, which include the human pathogens herpes simplex viruses (types 1 and 2), varicella-zoster virus, Epstein-Barr virus, and cytomegalovirus. The viruses can be transmitted by blood transfusions and organ transplantation as well as by direct contact with infected carriers.

HERPES SIMPLEX VIRUS

Herpes simplex virus (HSV) type 2 may be acquired by the neonate transplacentally by viremia during gestation, intranatally by passage through an infected birth canal, or postnatally by direct contact with infected humans. Prevention of exposure is difficult since history of illness or signs of disease are absent in up to 83 percent of infected mothers at the time of delivery.[36]

The initial symptoms of disseminated HSV are lethargy, hypo- or hyperthermia, irritability, and poor feeding, appearing in the first week of life. Cutaneous findings are the first visible sign in about 70 percent of newborns.[37] Grouped or single vesicles on erythematous bases appear in crops on the skin and mucous membranes. The eyes may also be affected. Vesicles can coalesce to form bullae.[38] Mucosal vesicles may quickly erode or may become pustular and crusted.[5] Neonatal herpes may spread rapidly to involve the central nervous system and/or multiple internal organs. This may progress to rapid deterioration of the neonate's condition.

Wright- or Giemsa-stained smear (Tzanck preparation) of vesicle bases demonstrates multinucleated giant cells. The virus itself can be demonstrated by culture or direct immunofluorescent testing of material obtained from an intact vesicle or a conjunctival swab. Histopathologically, an intraepidermal vesicle produced by ballooning and reticular degeneration of epidermal cells is seen.[5] Marked acantholysis is present. Multinucleated cells and eosinophilic inclusion bodies can be seen. In the dermis there is an inflammatory infiltrate.

Left untreated, disseminated HSV is fatal in 80 percent of cases.[37] Even with treatment survival is not better than 50 to 90 percent, depending on the degree of initial involvement. Survivors often have severe developmental and neurologic deficits. Vidarabine given as a slow intravenous infusion at 15 mg/kg/day for 10 days has been recommended. Acyclovir continues to be studied, with accumulation of favorable experiences, as an alternative therapeutic modality for HSV. Cesarean section is recommended for mothers with active HSV infection at term. Prevention is the best treatment, and newborns should be protected from exposure to HSV whenever possible.

VARICELLA-ZOSTER VIRUS

Varicella-zoster virus (VZ) is the agent responsible for chickenpox and herpes zoster (shingles). Neonates only develop chickenpox (varicella), as the development of herpes zoster would require prior exposure to the virus. Exposure of the neonate to VZ can occur during gestation or postnatally. Exposure in the first trimester of gestation may result in a syndrome of congenital malformations, the major features of which are low birth weight for gestational age, limb hypoplasia, dermal scars, cortical atrophy, ocular lesions, including cataracts and chorioretinitis, and psychomotor retardation.[30,39]

Congenital VZ infection acquired from the second trimester until 5 days prior to delivery usually results in no major sequelae for mother, fetus, or newborn. However, congenital VZ infection acquired from 5 days prior to delivery until 3 days postdelivery may result in a neonatal varicella of increased morbidity and mortality due to insufficient passive transfer of maternal antibody and insufficient active development of neonatal antibody to varicella.[30] Those neonates acquiring chickenpox after the third day of life tend to have a benign course.

The incubation time for chickenpox is approximately 2 weeks (range 10 to 23 days). A mild prodrome of fever, malaise, and upper respiratory symptoms may precede the onset of rash by 1 to 2 days but is generally absent in neonates. The skin lesions erupt in crops over 1 week and evolve within 12 to 24 hours of eruption from small red macules to papules to vesicles and pustules on erythematous bases. The lesions are typically described as umbilicated and appear to sit on top of the skin. Crusting occurs 1 to 3 days following eruption. Viral transmission (contagion) is possible from 1 day before the rash erupts until all lesions are crusted over.

Diagnosis may be aided by the finding of multinucleated giant cells on a Tzanck smear of the base of an intact vesicle. Histopathology is identical to that seen in herpes simplex infections.

Treatment of varicella in uncomplicated cases is supportive and symptomatic. Immunocompromised exposed newborns or neonates who were infected within 5 days prior to or several days after delivery should receive VZ immune globulin (VZIG) immediately. Various antiviral agents (vidarabine, acyclovir, adenine arabinoside) may be used to ameliorate disseminated disease.

CYTOMEGALOVIRUS

Cytomegalovirus (CMV) is a common pathogen transmitted to older infants and adults by blood transfusion and close contact with infected individuals. It causes neonatal disease by in utero transplacental infection, which directly invades fetal organs and results in defects in organogenesis. The congenital CMV syndrome may present with hepatosplenomegaly, jaundice, microcephaly, chorioretinitis, and periventricular intracranial calcifications.[40] Pneumonia and/or meningoencephalitis may also be present. Skin findings include petechiae, purpura, and, more rarely, a papular, vesicular, or pustular rash.

Diagnosis is often made on the finding of intranuclear inclusions in epithelial cells of urine sediment, which accounts for the name *cytomegalic inclusion disease*. Virus may be isolated from placental tissues, amniotic fluid, blood, cerebrospinal fluid (CSF), and urine. Anemia, thrombocytopenia, hyperbilirubinemia, and CSF pleocytosis may be present. Elevated IgM is suggestive, but not diagnostic, of congenital infection.[30]

CMV can persist for months to years postnatally, causing progressive tissue destruction.[30] Sensorineural hearing loss, intellectual compromise, and blindness are late sequelae and may lead to a retrospective diagnosis of congenital CMV infection in infants who were not ill-appearing at birth. There is no effective treatment.

Disseminated Candidiasis

Disseminated candidiasis may occur following ascending infection or infection introduced in utero.[41,42] Aggressive antibiotic treatment and invasive procedures in the sick, high-risk newborn increase the likelihood of disseminated candidiasis.[43–45] This is associated with significant morbidity and mortality.[41,46] Skin findings when present resemble those of congenital cutaneous candidiasis. Candidal abscesses have been seen.[44,45] Persistent candidemia or candiduria, even in the absence of skin findings or systemic symptoms, indicates the presence of disseminated disease in need of systemic therapy.[45–48]

Neonates with suspected or confirmed disseminated candidiasis should be treated with systemic antifungal therapy. The index of suspicion is increased if there is evidence of very low birth weight, respiratory distress, pneumonia, sepsis, antibiotic use, invasive instrumentation (e.g., ventilation, catheterization, hyperalimentation), or immunodeficiency. Amphotericin B and 5-flucytosine are the drugs of choice.[46,47] Some reports of intravenous miconazole and oral ketoconazole therapy of disseminated candidiasis are cited.[45,49] The use of these medications requires careful monitoring as their side effects are considerable.[37]

Other Infections

SYPHILIS

Syphilis is an infectious disease caused by the spirochete *Treponema pallidum*. Congenital syphilis is contracted in utero from an infected mother. Hematogenous spread of the spirochete may lead to infection of all fetal organ systems. Treatment of an infected mother before 16 weeks of gestation will eradicate the spirochete from mother and fetus before damage is done to the growing fetal organs.

Congenital syphilis occurs in an early and late form. The late form appears after 2 years of age and presents with the stigmata of congenital infection, such as Hutchinson's incisors, frontal bossing, interstitial keratitis, and eighth nerve deafness. Early congenital syphilis presents before 2 years of age. In the neonatal period affected infants may be born with a vesicular and/or pustular eruption, which rapidly desquamates during the first days of life. The eruption involves the palms and soles and, when desquamating, may spread to include the mouth, face, and genital region. Lesional fluid is rich in spirochetes. Macular and papular eruptions resembling the rash of secondary syphilis are seen later. The rash, initially pink in color, becomes coppery brown as the lesions age. A mucopurulent nasal discharge (snuffles) is often present. Erythematous or gray-white mucous membrane patches and anogenital condylomata lata are also seen. Hepatosplenomegaly, nephrosis, chorioretinitis, and variably symptomatic long-bone periostitis and osteochondritis may be present.

Table 10-3. Approach to the Patient: Work-Up of Pustular Disorders in the Neonate

History
Maternal: infectious disease
    Candidiasis: history of vaginal and/or uterine infection
    Staphylococcal impetigo: history of maternal lesions
    Scabies: history of maternal (and other close contacts) pruritus and lesions
    Bacterial infections; history of maternal fever, lesions, and/or sepsis
    Herpesvirus infections: history of maternal lesions or symptoms
    Neonatal syphilis: history of maternal lesions, serology
    Acquired immunodeficiency syndrome (AIDS): History of maternal infections, HIV
Neonate
    Age at onset and course
        Pustular melanosis at birth with yellow pustules evolving to brown macules
        Erythema toxicum at one day with evanescent lesions
        Candidiasis at birth to several weeks
        Acropustulosis from birth to 3 months with cyclic eruption of pustules on hands and feet

Physical examination
    Morphology
    Distribution
    Configuration
    Physical techniques of diagnosis (e.g., Nikolsky's sign)

Laboratory investigation
Noninfectious, transient
    Pustular erythema toxicum neonatorum: Giemsa and Wright stains for eosinophils
    Transient neonatal pustular melanosis: Giemsa and Wright stains for neutrophils
    Eosinophilic pustular folliculitis of infancy: Giemsa and Wright stains for eosinophils and neutrophils
    Acropustulosis of infancy: Giemsa and Wright stains for neutrophils and eosinophils
Infectious, mild
    Candidiasis: KOH prep, culture
        Congenital
        Neonatal
    Staphylococcal impetigo: Gram stain, culture and sensitivity
    Scabies: Scabies prep
Infectious, severe
    Bacterial infections: Gram stain, culture and sensitivity
        Staphylococcus aureus
        Group B streptococcus
        Pseudomonas aeruginosa
        Listeria monocytogenes
        Hemophilus influenzae
    Herpesvirus infections
        Herpes simplex: Tzanck preparation viral cultures and titers
        Varicella: Tzanck preparation viral cultures and titers
        Cytomegalovirus: urine sediment stains, cultures and titers
    Disseminated candidiasis: KOH, culture of lesions, blood, urine, spinal fluid
    Other
        Neonatal syphilis: darkfield examination, serology, x-ray
        AIDS: HIV antibody

Diagnosis of syphilis depends on demonstration of the spirochete by darkfield microscopy and/or direct or indirect immunofluorescence. Positive serology (VDRL test) in the neonate is not diagnostic as it may represent passively transmitted maternal antibody. Persistent or rising serologic titers are more diagnostic, as are positive treponemal tests such as the fluorescent treponemal antibody absorption test. The presence of fetal IgM antitreponemal antibody indicates active syphilitic infection in the newborn.

Congenital syphilis is preventable by detection and treatment of infected pregnant women. Once it has been diagnosed in the newborn, prompt treatment will reduce the transmission as well as the morbidity and mortality of this disease. Penicillin remains the drug of choice for treatment of congenital syphilis. The VDRL should be monitored before treatment and serially thereafter to document a decrease in titer.

AIDS

Acquired immunodeficiency syndrome (AIDS) is an infectious disease that was first reported in 1981[50–52] and was first recognized in infants in 1983.[53] It is caused by the human immunodeficiency virus (HIV). In contrast to adults, in whom sexual contact is the major route of virus transmission, 70 percent of infected infants acquire the virus in utero or perinatally from infected mothers.[30,54,55] Transmission of virus by infected blood or blood products also occurs.[56–58] The syndrome in infants is characterized by recurrent viral and opportunistic infections and by specific abnormalities of T-cell function.[30,59] Failure to thrive, hepatosplenomegaly, lymphadenopathy, chronic diarrhea, chronic pulmonary infiltrates and persistent candidiasis are common presenting symptoms.[60,61,62] Encephalitis and/or developmental delay are newly recognized abnormalities. Although the disease in infants usually presents between 3 and 10 months of age, it has been seen in neonates and should be suspected when infants are born to mothers who either are known to have AIDS or belong to a group at high risk of developing AIDS. One should be especially alert for those newborns who present with candidiasis unresponsive to therapy and those neonates with pustular manifestations of other infectious disorders.

APPROACH TO THE PATIENT

An organized approach to the diagnosis of pustular eruptions in the neonate is outlined in Table 10-3. In few other conditions is maternal history so important, since maternal infection should immediately suggest the possibility of transmission to the neonate. Historical features and physical examination of lesions will often yield the correct diagnosis as well. For example, a history of recurring crops of pustules distributed on the hands and feet should immediately suggest a diagnosis of acropustulosis of infancy.

Definitive diagnosis is usually rapidly obtained with smears and stains. *Candida* is readily identified on KOH preparations of pustules, and bacteria can be stained with Gram stain. The Tzanck preparation reveals multinucleated giant cells in herpes simplex and varicella infections. Giemsa and Wright stains are useful in identifying cell types in noninfectious pustular eruptions. When the diagnosis is not immediately apparent, a number of cultures and serologies detailed in Table 10-3 can be helpful.

REFERENCES

1. Jacobs AH, Walton RG: The incidence of birth marks in the neonate. Pediatrics 58:218, 1976
2. Levy HL, Cothran F: Erythema toxicum neonatorum present at birth. Am J Dis Child 103:125, 1962
3. Marino LJ: Toxic erythema present at birth. Arch Dermatol 92:402, 1965
4. Freeman RG, Spiller R, Knox JM: Histopathology of erythema toxicum neonatorum. Arch Dermatol 82:586, 1960
5. Lever WF, Schaumberg-Lever G: Histopathology of the skin. 6th Ed. JB Lippincott, Philadelphia, 1983
6. Ramamurthy RS, Reveri M, Esterly NB, et al: Transient neonatal pustular melanosis. J Pediatr 88:831, 1976
7. Auster B: Transient neonatal pustular melanosis. Cutis 22:237, 1978
8. Caputo RV: Recent advances in pediatric dermatology. Pediatr Clin North Am 30:735, 1983
9. Kahn G, Rywlin AM: Acropustulosis of infancy. Arch Dermatol 115:831, 1979
10. Jarratt M, Ramsdell W: Infantile acropustulosis. Arch Dermatol 115:834, 1979
11. McFadden N, Falk ES: Infantile acropustulosis. Cutis 36:49, 1985
12. Hayden GF, Quackenbush K: Infantile acropustulosis: a ''new'' vesiculopustular eruption of infants and children. J Fam Pract 18:925, 1984

13. Bundino S, Zina AM, Uoertulli S: Infantile acropustulosis. Dermatologica 165:615, 1982

14. Lang PG Jr: Sulfones and sulfonamides in dermatology today. J Am Acad Dermatol 1:479, 1979

15. Ofuji S, Ogino A, Horio T, et al: Eosinophilic pustular folliculitis. Acta Derm Venereal (Stockh) 50:195, 1970

16. Lucky A, Esterly N, Heskel N, et al: Eosinophilic pustular folliculitis in infancy. Pediatr Dermatol 1:202, 1984

17. Cutler TP: Eosinophilic pustular folliculitis. Clin Exp Dermatol 6:327, 1981

18. Czarnetzki BM, Springorum M: Larva migrans with eosinophilic papular folliculitis. Dermatologica 164:36, 1982

19. Colton AS, Schachner L, Kowalczyk AP: Eosinophilic pustular folliculitis. J Am Acad Dermatol 14:469, 1986

20. Dinehart S, Nuppakun N, Solomon AR, et al: Eosinophilic pustular folliculitis. J Am Acad Dermatol 14:475, 1986

21. Steffen C: Eosinophilic pustular folliculitis (Ofuji's disease) with response to dapsone therapy. Arch Dermatol 121:921, 1985

22. Jaliman HD, Phelps RG, Fleischmajer R: Eosinophilic pustular folliculitis. J Am Acad Dermatol 14:479, 1986

23. Chapel TA, Gagliardi C, Nicholas W: Congenital cutaneous candidiasis. J Am Acad Dermatol 6:926, 1982

24. Haberman S, Mandel EB, Hall DK, et al: The incidence of *Staphylococcus aureus* and *Candida albicans* in pregnant women. Obstet Gynecol 20:639, 1962

25. Schachner L, Press S: Vesicular, bullous and pustular disorders in infancy and childhood. Pediatr Clin North Am 30:609, 1983

26. Hurwitz S: Scabies in childhood. Pediatr Rev 1:91, 1979

27. Burns BR, Lampe RM, Hansen GH: Neonatal scabies. Am J Dis Child 133:1031, 1979

28. Ingomar CJ: Bacteremia during the first day of life. Acta Paediatr Scand [Suppl] 206:106, 1970

29. Albers WH, Tyler CW, Boxerbaum B: Asymptomatic bacteremia in the newborn infant. J Pediatr 69:193, 1966

30. Klein JO: Current concepts of infectious diseases in the newborn infant. Adv Pediatr 31:405, 1984

31. Ritter von Rittershain G: Die exfoliative dermatitis jüngerer Säuglinge. Centralz Kinderheilkunde 2:3, 1878

32. Clinical conferences at The Johns Hopkins Hospital: Toxic-shock syndrome. Johns Hopkins Med J 148:14, 1981

33. Ginsburg CM: Staphylococcal toxin syndromes. Pediatr Infect Dis 3: Suppl 3, 523, 1983

34. Melish ME, Glasgow LA: Staphylococcal scalded skin syndrome: the expanded clinical syndrome. J Pediatr 78:958, 1971

35. Rudolf RI, Schwartz W, Leyden JJ: Treatment of staphylococcal toxic epidermal necrolysis. Arch Dermatol 110:559, 1974

36. Jenista JA: Perinatal herpes virus infections. Semin Perinatol 7:9, 1983

37. Levine N: Management of life threatening dermatoses. Emerg Med Clin North Am 3:747, 1985

38. Tunnessen WW Jr: Cutaneous infections. Pediatr Clin North Am 30:515, 1983

39. Stagno S, Whitley RJ: Herpesvirus infections of pregnancy. II. Herpes simplex virus and varicella zoster virus infections. N Engl J Med 313:1327, 1985

40. Naeye RL: Cytomegalic inclusion disease: the fetal disorder. Am J Clin Pathol 47:738, 1967

41. Honore LH: Placental candidiasis: a report of two cases, one associated with an IUCD in situ. Contraception 30:555, 1984

42. Delaplane D, Wiringa KS, Shulman ST, et al: Congenital mucocutaneous candidiasis following diagnostic amniocentesis. Am J Obstet Gynecol 147:342, 1983

43. Dube SD, Bhat GJ: *Candida* septicaemia in a newborn complicating bacterial bronchopneumonia. Cent Afr J Med 29:240, 1983

44. Hensey OJ, Hart CA, Cooke RW: *Candida albicans* skin abscesses. Arch Dis Child 59:479, 1984

45. Tudehope DI, Rigby B: Neonatal systemic candidiasis treated with miconazole and ketoconazole. Med J Aust 1:480, 1983

46. Johnson DE, Thompson TR, Green TP, et al: Systemic candidiasis in very low-birth-weight infants (less than 1500 grams). Pediatrics 73:138, 1984

47. Smith H, Congdon P: Neonatal systemic candidiasis. Arch Dis Child 60:365, 1985

48. Rudolph N, Tariq AA, Reale MR, et al: Congenital cutaneous candidiasis. Arch Dermatol 113:1101, 1977

49. Burke AM, Fitzsimons RB, Kearney PJ: Congenital cutaneous candidiasis and septicaemia treated with miconazole. Ir Med J 78:219, 1985

50. Gottlieb MS, Schroff R, Schanker HM, et al: *Pneumocystis carinii* pneumonia and mucosal candidiasis in previously healthy homosexual men. N Engl J Med 305:1425, 1981

51. Masur H, Michelis MH, Greene JB, et al: An outbreak of community acquired *Pneumocystis carinii* pneumonia. Initial manifestation of cellular immune deficiency. N Engl J Med 305:1431, 1981

52. Siegal FP, Lopez C, Hammer GS, et al: Severe acquired immunodeficiency in male homosexuals, manifested by chronic perianal ulcerative herpes simplex lesions. N Engl J Med 305:1439, 1981

53. Rubinstein A, Sicklick M, Gupta A, et al: Acquired immunodeficiency with reversed T4/T8 ratios in infants born to promiscuous and drug-addicted mothers. JAMA 249:2350, 1983

54. Education and foster care of children infected with human T-lymphotropic virus type III/lymphadenopathy-associated virus. MMWR 34:517, 1985

55. Vilmer E, Fischer A, Navarro J, et al: AIDS in the infant. Rev Fr Transfus Immunohematol 27:423, 1984

56. Wykoff RF, Pearl ER, Saulsbury FT: Immunologic dysfunction in infants infected through transfusion with HTLV-III. N Engl J Med 312:294, 1985

57. Duffy JF, Isles AF: Transfusion-induced AIDS in four premature babies. (Letter). Lancet 2:1346, 1984

58. Ammann AJ, Cowan MJ, Wara DW, et al: Acquired immunodeficiency in an infant: possible transmission by means of blood products. Lancet 1:956, 1983

59. Siegel RL: Clinical disorders associated with T-cell subset abnormalities. Adv Pediatr 31:447, 1984

60. Scott GB, Buck BE, Leterman JG, et al: Acquired immunodeficiency syndrome in infants. N Engl J Med 310:76, 1984

61. Speck WT: Acquired immune deficiency syndrome. J Pediatr 103:161, 1983

62. Joncas JH, Delage G, Chad Z, et al: Acquired (or congenital) immunodeficiency syndrome in infants born of Haitian mothers. (Letter). N Engl J Med 308:842, 1983

11

Neonatal Bullous Diseases

Mark Lebwohl

The differential diagnosis of bullous lesions in the neonate includes a number of conditions that are potentially fatal and may therefore require rapid diagnosis and treatment. Several inherited conditions can also present as bullous disorders that are not easily differentiated by clinical features alone. Although the necessity for a diagnosis may be less immediate, the fears of anxious parents and pediatricians need to be allayed as quickly as possible. Moreover, the diagnosis of inherited bullous conditions must be accurate because of the prognostic implications for the affected infant. Genetic counseling for the parents will also depend entirely on the diagnosis made by the consulting dermatologist.

Definitive diagnosis of these conditions may require a number of tests that are not part of the dermatologist's usual armamentarium. The clinician should know when to send a specimen for electron microscopy and when to order a serum zinc level. The purpose of this chapter is to review those conditions characterized by bullous lesions in newborn infants. Guidelines for the diagnosis and management of these difficult cases are presented, and clinical characteristics of each of the conditions are reviewed.

EPIDERMOLYSIS BULLOSA

The term *epidermolysis bullosa* (EB) encompasses several diseases that can be inherited in autosomal dominant or autosomal recessive fashion. The diseases are linked by a number of common features, including the tendency toward bulla formation and the development of symptoms early in life. The various types of EB are usually subdivided on the basis of whether or not they heal with scarring. The nonscarring, or simplex, forms are characterized by blister formation above the basement membrane zone, while scarring dystrophic forms have a level of separation below the basement membrane.

At least 16 types of EB have been described, including an acquired type that does not have a genetic basis and begins in adulthood. Discussion in this chapter will be limited to those forms of EB that give rise to bullous lesions in infancy[1] (Table 11-1).

Recessive Dystrophic Epidermolysis Bullosa

One of the most severe forms of EB is the recessive dystrophic type. In one study this disease was estimated to occur in approximately 1 in 45,000 births,[2] although lower estimates have also been reported. The etiology of recessive dystrophic EB is controversial. While one group of investigators attributes the disease to a primary defect in the synthesis of anchoring fibrils, a second group has demonstrated excessive collagenase in patients with EB. These investigators believe that destruction of collage-

Table 11-1. Diagnostic Features of Epidermolysis Bullosa in Neonates

Disease	Site of Blister Formation	Diagnostic Features
Recessive dystrophic EB	Subepidermal: beneath PAS-staining basement membrane	Electron microscopy: cleavage beneath basal lamina in upper dermis, loss of anchoring fibrils
Dominant dystrophic EB	Subepidermal: beneath PAS-staining basement membrane	Electron microscopy: cleavage between basal lamina and anchoring fibrils, absent or rudimentary anchoring fibrils
Junctional EB	Subepidermal: above PAS-staining basement membrane	Electron microscopy: cleavage between basal cell plasma membrane and basal lamina, reduced and abnormal hemidesmosomes
EB simplex	Intraepidermal	Light microscopy: vacuolization and degeneration of basal cells

nous structures that attach epidermis to dermis results in blister formation.[3]

CLINICAL FEATURES

Blisters are usually first noted at the time of birth or shortly thereafter. Skin lesions appear at sites of pressure, friction, or trauma, although any area of skin can be affected. Hands, feet, knees, and elbows are characteristically involved. Frank blistering and bulla formation is often noted, although rupture of blisters may leave painful erosions and occasionally large areas of skin may become entirely denuded. Bullae may be hemorrhagic, and mild pressure on the skin may result in enlargement or development of bullae.[4]

Bullae heal with erosions that develop thick crusts. Eventually, lesions resolve with atrophic scars that can be either hyper- or hypopigmented. Milia often develop in areas of resolving bullae.

Recurrent blister formation and scarring can cause crippling deformities. Typically, the hands and feet are most severely affected, resulting in a pseudofusion of the digits, which creates mittenlike hands and flexion contractures of the hands and fingers (Fig. 11-1).

Nail bed involvement is common in recessive dystrophic EB, and fingernails may be severely dystrophic or absent. Involvement of the scalp may leave affected individuals with a scarring alopecia. Repeated involvement of the ears may leave them scarred and matted down to the scalp. Malformation of the teeth occurs, and a tendency to develop dental caries is common. At an early age affected children learn that brushing the teeth leads to the development of intraoral bullae. Repeated intraoral scarring often leads to "puckered" lips and difficulty with mastication[4] (Fig. 11-2).

Unfortunately, other mucous membranes can also be affected. One of the most disabling complications of recessive dystrophic EB occurs when the eyes are involved. Numerous ocular abnormalities can result, including corneal opacities, keratitis, conjunctivitis, symblepharon, and blepharitis.[5]

Laryngeal involvement following blistering of the larynx can lead to soreness or, in rare instances, laryngeal stenosis and airway obstruction.[6] These complications must be stressed to anesthesiologists if the patients are to undergo any surgical procedures with general anesthesia.

Sites in the gastrointestinal tract can also be affected by recessive dystrophic EB. Pyloric and duodenal stenosis can present at birth as a result of intrauterine blistering, and perianal strictures can occur.[7] Pharyngeal and esophageal blisters and erosions can result in dysphagia and, in severe cases, esophageal web formation and stenosis.[8] Patients often become accustomed to avoiding hot foods or irritating rough foods that can cause esophageal blistering due to friction. In severe cases solid foods must be pureed or liquid diets must be instituted.

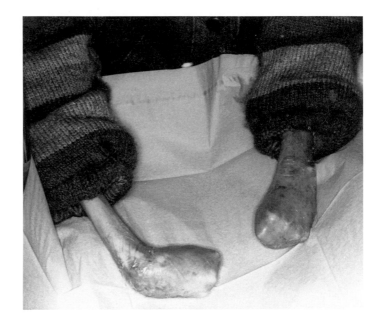

Fig. 11-1. Recessive dystrophic EB. Pseudosyndactyly and mittenlike hands.

Retardation of growth and development are unfortunately typical of recessive dystrophic EB. Nonetheless, many patients with this disease can live to their forties, and with the recent advent of new treatments such as the phenytoins, patients will hopefully live longer and suffer fewer complications.[7]

In severely affected individuals, extensive areas of denuded skin can lead to sepsis or fluid loss, resulting in death in infancy. Malnutrition, anemia of chronic disease, and amyloidosis due to chronic infections often occur in patients who survive until childhood.

The leading cause of death of patients who survive to early adulthood is squamous cell carcinoma of the esophagus.[7] Metastases are unfor-

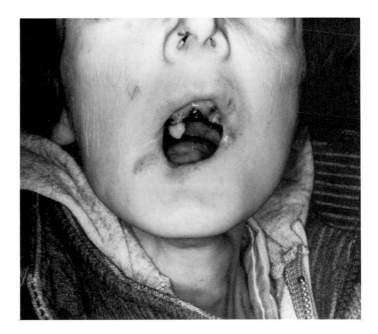

Fig. 11-2. Recessive dystrophic EB. Severe oral and dental involvement.

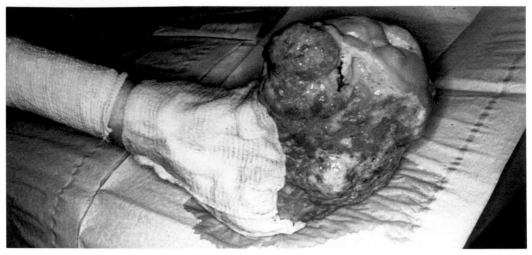

Fig. 11-3. Recessive dystrophic EB. Development of a squamous cell carcinoma on the foot.

tunately common and survival rates are poor. Squamous cells carcinomas also develop in cutaneous scars (Fig. 11-3), and these also tend to metastasize, in contrast to the usually nonmetastasizing squamous cell carcinomas found in sun-damaged skin. An increased incidence of basal cell carcinomas has also been noted.[4]

DIAGNOSIS

Although the mittenlike features and physical findings in adulthood may be pathognomonic of recessive dystrophic EB, the presentation at birth may be clinically indistinguishable from other forms of EB. Mild cases of recessive dystrophic EB may be particularly difficult to diagnose, and both clinical and histologic data may be insufficient to differentiate recessive dystrophic EB, EB letalis, and dominant dystrophic EB.

Histologically, there is separation at the level of the dermal-epidermal junction. It is this deep blistering that accounts for the scarring seen in recessive dystrophic EB. Although the separation occurs below the basal lamina, periodic acid–Schiff (PAS) stains are not always helpful, since the PAS-positive basement membrane can appear hazy. Although the basement membrane can be seen at the top of bullae, it may appear split, with portions appearing at both top and bottom.[3]

Electron microscopy is one of the clinician's most useful tools in the diagnosis of recessive dystrophic EB and should be performed in all cases in which this diagnosis is seriously considered. The basal lamina is seen at the top of the blister, and a reduction in anchoring fibrils is typically noted.

Although electron microscopy is available at many medical centers, it is not a routine procedure, and it may therefore take several weeks before a diagnosis can be made. Immunofluorescence with antibodies directed against basement membrane components can rapidly differentiate dystrophic forms of EB from EB letalis. Antibodies against type IV collagen and laminin are available, and they stain the basement membrane at the roof of the bulla in dystrophic EB and on the floor of the bulla in EB letalis.[3]

MANAGEMENT

Phenytoin is rapidly becoming the mainstay of therapy in recessive dystrophic EB. The drug presumably works by inhibiting the synthesis and/or secretion of collagenase by dermal fibroblasts. It is started at 2 to 3 mg/kg/day in two divided doses and gradually increased until the blood level exceeds 8 mg/ml. Many patients treated this way have a dramatic decrease in blistering. Side effects have been limited, but care must be taken to keep blood levels under 20 mg/ml since lethargy, dizziness, and nystagmus are common at higher levels.[9]

Meticulous skin care from the time of birth is another critical feature in the management of patients with recessive dystrophic EB. Removal of possible causes of friction and trauma is essential. Elastic in diapers and adhesive bandages should be avoided when possible. Soft, smooth material such as lamb's wool can be used to line cribs and carriages. Padding over blister-prone areas such as hands and feet may offer some relief. Nipples with large holes and easy flow may reduce friction on oral mucous membranes by decreasing sucking efforts. Drainage of bullae and application of sterile compresses several times daily can be followed by application of topical antibiotics under nonadherent dressings held in place by rolled gauze. Newer surgical dressings that are supposed to enhance wound healing may ultimately be useful in the management of patients with EB, although more work needs to be done in this area. Addition of chlorhexidine (Hibiclens) to bath water has been suggested for other forms of EB to reduce staphylococcal colonization of the patients.[7,10]

Because of the many complications of recessive dystrophic EB, the expertise of several specialists is often necessary to manage specific aspects of the patient's disease. Nutritional supplements may be needed, and soft, pureed foods should be considered for patients with excessive pharyngeal or esophageal disease. At least one author has advocated involvement of a nutritionist from the time of diagnosis.[7] Surgical repair of the syndactyly that occurs in this condition can restore function to hands, and devices can be made to prevent fusion of digits. Because of the high incidence of squamous cell carcinoma of the esophagus, annual esophageal examinations beginning in early adolescence have been recommended. Colonic-esophageal transpositions may be useful for some patients with esophageal stenosis or carcinoma.[7]

Genetic counseling for the family of a patient with recessive dystrophic EB is an important element that must not be overlooked. Future pregnancies have a 25 percent chance of resulting in a second child with this disease. Fortunately, prenatal diagnosis is possible with fetoscopy and fetal skin biopsy.[11,12]

Dominant Dystrophic Epidermolysis Bullosa

Dominant dystrophic EB is a much milder form of EB than the recessive dystrophic type, although it is more severe than the simplex types. The disease is reported less frequently than recessive EB, but it is possible that milder cases are misdiagnosed.

There are several forms of dominant dystrophic EB, including one which heals with hypertrophic scars (Cockayne-Touraine variant) and one in which white papules develop (Pasini "albopapuloid" variant).

CLINICAL FEATURES

The characteristic skin lesions of dominant dystrophic EB are bullae that may be present at birth, although in milder cases the lesions develop later in life. It is not unusual for bullae to be noted on the elbows and knees when the affected infant begins to crawl. Blisters may also first appear on the feet and ankles when the baby's first shoes are worn. The skin lesions tend to develop in areas of trauma, and bony prominences are particularly prone. Bullae may be tense and are sometimes hemorrhagic. Occasionally, erosions occur without frank bulla formation. Lesions heal with ulcerations that only seldom result in severe scarring. More often, soft, superficial scars with wrinkled surfaces occur. Scars may be hyper- or hypopigmented. Recent lesions are typically studded with milia.

In the hypertrophic form of dominant dystrophic EB, thick keloidal and hyperkeratotic scars can occur. In the albopapuloid variant white papules develop independently of bulla formation[2,4,7] (Fig. 11-4).

DIAGNOSIS

When a family history of dominant dystrophic EB exists, clinical findings alone will suggest the diagnosis. However, a small number of cases can be due to spontaneous mutation, making the diagnosis more difficult to establish. Light microscopy only shows subepidermal bulla formation with the PAS-positive basement membrane on the roof of the blister cavity. Electron microscopy demonstrates a decrease in anchoring fibrils and abnormalities of existing fibrils of lesional and, in some cases, nonlesional skin. It is thought that the defect in these fibrils is a primary pathologic process in dominant dystrophic EB. In contrast to the situation in recessive dystrophic EB, collagenase levels in unaffected skin appear to be normal.[3]

MANAGEMENT

Avoidance of trauma and friction is a fundamental principle of management in dominant dystrophic EB. As in recessive dystrophic EB, adhesive bandages and elastic in diapers should not be used. Affected children should have friction-reducing crib liners and padding to reduce trauma to elbows, feet, and knees in crawling infants. Many of the principles of recessive dystrophic EB management can be applied to dominant dystrophic EB, including the use of chlorhexidine in baths, management of bullae, and use of large-holed nipples when the oral mucosa is involved. Genetic counseling can be offered to families, but it should be stressed that the severity of the disease does not usually approach that seen in recessive dystrophic EB.[7,10]

Junctional Epidermolysis Bullosa

Junctional EB is one of the most severe neonatal bullous diseases. Also called *Herlitz's disease* after Gillis Herlitz, who described it in 1935, this disorder is inherited in an autosomal recessive pattern, affecting males and females with equal frequency. Because of its commonly fatal outcome, this disease has been called *epidermolysis bullosa letalis*.

CLINICAL FEATURES

Skin lesions are almost always present at birth, often occurring on the lower extremities. Bullae can frequently be induced by mild mechanical trauma, and large areas of sloughing

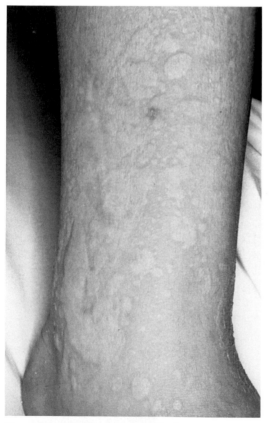

Fig. 11-4. Dominant dystrophic EB, albopapuloid variant. White papules on the leg occurring independently of bulla formation.

or denuded skin can result. Healing occurs without milia formation, and scarring generally does not take place unless severe secondary infection of skin lesions intervenes. Scalp involvement is common, and any area of skin can be affected. Perioral lesions with sparing of the lips have been said to be pathognomonic of junctional EB. Although hands and feet are said to be spared in classic cases, at least several patients have been seen with prominent involvement of the palms and soles. Thus, the finding of acral lesions should not preclude consideration of junctional EB in the differential diagnosis. In fact, hand and foot involvement is demonstrated by the common finding of nails that are thinned, dystrophic, or in some cases entirely lost.[4,7,13]

Mucous membranes can also be affected, and severe intraoral involvement has been noted. Abnormal teeth with a cobblestone appearance can be seen, and enamel deteriorates easily. Gastrointestinal lesions are characterized by epithelial-subepithelial separation similar to that seen in skin lesions. Autopsies have revealed similar findings in the respiratory and urinary tracts. Fortunately, the scarring and stricture formation frequently seen in the esophagus in recessive dystrophic EB does not usually occur in junctional EB, although cases of pyloric and duodenal stenosis and atresia have occurred at birth.[7,14]

Approximately 50 percent of neonates with junctional EB die before the age of 2. Large areas of denudation lead to fluid loss, electrolyte abnormalities, and sepsis, and this is often the mode of death. Beyond the age of 2, junctional EB can improve spontaneously, resulting in a milder chronic blistering, nonscarring eruption.[4,7,13]

DIAGNOSIS

A diagnosis of junctional EB is easily made on the basis of clinical findings when there is a positive family history for the condition. However, the family history is often negative, and clinical features alone do not permit distinction from other neonatal bullous diseases. In fact, even routine histologic data may not suffice to make a definitive diagnosis of junctional EB. As the name of the disease implies, separation of the epidermis from the dermis occurs at the dermal-epidermal junction, with the PAS-positive basement membrane zone remaining on the dermis at the base of the blister. When the basement membrane zone is not clear with PAS staining, immunofluorescent staining with antibodies to type IV collagen, laminin, or bullous pemphigoid antigen will accurately label the basement membrane, thus facilitating a rapid diagnosis.[3,13] It should be noted, however, that staining of the basement membrane only helps identify the site of cleavage. A more definitive but slower diagnosis can be made with the electron microscope, which demonstrates separation between the plasma membrane of the basal cells and the basal lamina. This is thought to be due to a defect of the hemidesmosomes. Even in normal skin of patients with junctional EB, the hemidesmosomes are reduced in number and abnormally developed. Biopsy of normal-appearing skin in these patients can thus be used for diagnosis.

MANAGEMENT

Correction of fluid loss and treatment of sepsis are the most immediate problems that the clinician must face. The necessity of managing these complications must be weighed against the additional skin trauma created by intravenous lines and various monitors and tubes. The use of adhesive tape must be avoided whenever possible. Instead, lines can often be secured with gauze, which can be tied around limbs. As in other forms of EB, meticulous skin care is critical. The steps outlined above for skin care of patients with recessive dystrophic EB can be applied when appropriate. Other important aspects of care include nutritional supplementation, which may be needed to prevent wasting and to support the infant's immune defenses against infection.[7]

Therapeutic trials with phenytoins have been

recommended by some authors because of the beneficial effect that these have had on patients with recessive dystrophic EB.[15] However, definitive proof that phenytoins benefit junctional EB patients is lacking at this time.

Genetic counseling for family members is essential because of the important implications for future pregnancies. As in recessive dystrophic EB, junctional EB is inherited in an autosomal recessive fashion so that one in four future pregnancies can be expected to result in infants with junctional EB. Fortunately, this catastrophic outcome can be diagnosed prenatally by performing fetoscopy with fetal skin biopsy.[16]

Epidermolysis Bullosa Simplex

Epidermolysis bullosa simplex is a much milder form of EB. The level of separation in this disease is higher in the epidermis, and skin lesions heal without scarring. It has been suggested that some families with EB simplex have an inherited deficiency of galactosylhydroxylysyl glucosyltransferase, an enzyme involved in the synthesis of collagen.[17] Inheritance is in an autosomal dominant pattern.

CLINICAL FEATURES

Bullae and erosions of EB simplex are usually noted at birth as a result of trauma incurred during delivery. Areas of rubbing and trauma are principally affected, with prominent involvement of the extremities. Crawling results in blistering of the hands, elbows, and knees. Friction due to clothing can cause bullae on the trunk. Heat can also exacerbate the condition, precipitating formation of bullae. Blistering leads to erosions, which eventually heal without scarring and without development of milia.

Mucous membranes are seldom affected in EB simplex, and when mucosal erosions do occur, they heal without complications. Nails are involved in only 20 percent of patients and are less severely affected than in other forms of EB. Even when nails are lost, they usually grow back normally.

After the age of 3 lesions of EB simplex frequently are limited to the hands and feet. Further improvement usually occurs during adolescence.[4]

DIAGNOSIS

Clinical features combined with routine light microscopy may suffice to make a diagnosis of EB simplex. Vacuolization and degeneration of the basal cell layer results in separation of the epidermis and dermis. The PAS-staining basement membrane remains attached to the dermis on the bottom of the blister. Early blisters can be subepidermal, owing to complete dissolution of the basal layer, but older lesions may appear to be intraepidermal as a result of regenerating epidermis on the floor of the blister.[3]

MANAGEMENT

Although this disease is milder than other forms of EB, the steps outlined above for recessive dystrophic EB should be followed when appropriate in order to minimize blister formation. Genetic counseling can be offered to affected family members, but the benign nature of this disease should be stressed.

Other Forms of Epidermolysis Bullosa

Several other forms of EB exist, including some that do not cause bullous lesions in the neonatal period. However, there have been numerous isolated reports of infants born with bullous diseases that do not fit any of the commonly classified forms of EB.

In 1966 Bart et al. described a new dominantly inherited syndrome in 25 members of a single family. The disease was characterized by congenital aplasia of skin of the lower extremities, blistering of skin and mucous membranes without scarring, and absence or deformity of the nails.[18,19] Since blistering in Bart's syndrome frequently begins in infancy, it should be considered in the differential diagnosis of neonatal vesiculobullous diseases.

Kindler's syndrome, another rare neonatal blistering disease, is characterized by acral blister formation from birth. Other features include progressive poikilodermatous changes, progressive wrinkling, photosensitivity, nail dystrophy, webbing between the fingers and toes, and hyperkeratosis of the palms and soles.[20]

INCONTINENTIA PIGMENTI

Incontinentia pigmenti (IP) is a rare inherited disease, which has numerous systemic manifestations. It appears to be transmitted in an X-linked dominant pattern that is lethal in male fetuses. Consequently, 97 percent of patients are female, and it has been suggested that all males with IP are the result of spontaneous mutations.[21] Although the condition ultimately evolves into verrucous and pigmented lesions, vesicles and bullae are usually present in the first weeks of life.

Skin lesions are present in 90 percent of patients in the first 2 weeks of life. In this early phase of IP, skin lesions are characterized by vesicles and bullae that are filled with eosinophils. The blisters are often found in a linear distribution on the trunk and extremities.

After several weeks or months vesicular lesions resolve and approximately 70 percent of patients develop a verrucous stage characterized by linear, warty lesions. The dorsa of the hands and feet are the most common sites of involvement, and occasionally verrucous and vesicular lesions can be present at the same time.

The verrucous lesions last up to several months and are followed by a stage that is characterized by pigmentary changes. Typical swirls of pigment develop on the trunk and extremities (Fig. 11-5). The pigmentary changes can persist for years, although they frequently fade before adulthood. In some individuals hypopigmented streaks can also develop on the trunk and extremities.

A significant proportion of patients with IP develop extracutaneous manifestations, which can have profound implications for the affected individual. Ocular involvement occurs in 35

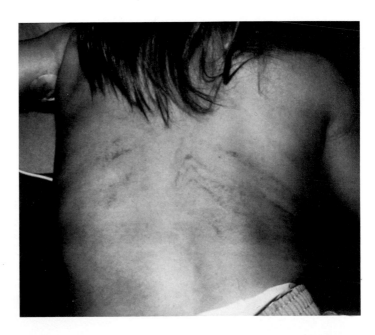

Fig. 11-5. Incontinentia pigmenti. Swirls of pigment on a patient's back.

percent of patients and includes strabismus, cataracts, retrolental fibroplasia, uveitis, retinal detachment, and optic atrophy. Approximately one out of three patients has other neurologic manifestations, including seizures, mental retardation, and spastic or paralytic disorders. Two-thirds of patients have dental abnormalities, and alopecia is found in almost 40 percent. Skeletal abnormalities, dystrophic nails, and cardiac anomalies have been reported. The large majority of patients have eosinophilia, with eosinophil counts reaching as high as 65 percent.[21]

DIAGNOSIS

Because of the severity of systemic manifestations and the implications for future infants born to the same parents, the importance of arriving at an accurate diagnosis must be emphasized. The presence of verrucous lesions in a patient with antecedent or concomitant vesicular lesions should immediately suggest the diagnosis of IP. Eosinophilia in a neonate with vesicular lesions should also prompt the clinician to consider this diagnosis. Fortunately, skin biopsy at this stage is diagnostic. Intraepidermal vesicles containing eosinophils are seen. An infiltrate with numerous eosinophils and mononuclear cells is present in the dermis and epidermis. The epidermis also contains dyskeratotic cells with eosinophilic cytoplasm.

Biopsy during the verrucous stage shows hyperkeratosis, acanthosis, and papillomatosis, with whorling of cells and numerous dyskeratotic cells. In the pigmented stage numerous melanophages are present in the dermis, which contrasts with the frequently hypopigmented basal layer of the epidermis.[3,21]

ACRODERMATITIS ENTEROPATHICA

Acrodermatitis enteropathica (AE) is a rare entity that has a number of findings in common with EB. The bullous nature of the skin lesions in this entity and their acral distribution led early investigators to classify AE as EB of the dystrophic or letalis type.

This disease is probably transmitted in an autosomal recessive fashion since cases of affected siblings have been reported, but there have not been reports of cases occurring in sequential generations. A familial occurrence has been noted in approximately two-thirds of cases. Males and females are affected in equal numbers, and there have only been a few hundred cases reported in the world's literature. Because the clinical presentation can be nonspecific and because the condition is so rarely reported, it is entirely possible that many cases go undiagnosed.[22,23]

CLINICAL FEATURES

The basic lesion in AE is a bulla, and lesions can typically occur on the hands and feet (Fig. 11-6), a characteristic that can easily lead to an incorrect diagnosis of EB. The average age of onset is approximately 9 months, but symptoms can begin from 1 or 2 weeks to up to 20 months after birth. A small number of cases have been diagnosed later in life, but even in these patients mild symptoms had been present since early infancy. Rarely, symptoms have developed as late as 7½ years.[22]

Since the defect in this disease involves an autosomal recessively inherited abnormality of gastrointestinal zinc absorption, it is not surprising that lesions are not usually present at birth and take at least a few weeks to develop. It is also easy to understand why lesions first develop after weaning from breast milk, since human milk contains a factor that enhances zinc absorption.

In early infancy the cutaneous lesions of AE are particularly important in arriving at the correct diagnosis because several characteristic features of the disease may not be apparent. Nail dystrophy may not be present at the onset, and alopecia may go unnoticed in the first year of life.

Lesions can begin as blisters or bullae overly-

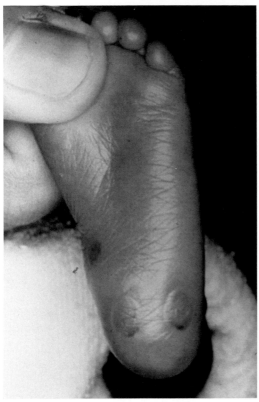

Fig. 11-6. Acrodermatitis enteropathica. Bullous lesions on the heel of an infant.

ing an erythematous base. The vesicles quickly crust, leaving oozing, eroded plaques, which become secondarily infected with *Candida albicans* in 20 percent of cases. The distribution of lesions is primarily acral and periorificial. Paronychial swelling and bulla formation occur, and dystrophic nails can develop as a result. Crusted, often impetiginized plaques develop around the mouth, nose, eyes, ears, and genitals and in the perianal area. Pustules may be present, and in the diaper area the clinical features may simulate moniliasis. Scalp involvement is common and can result in alopecia. Loss of eyebrows and eyelashes can also occur. Glossitis and stomatitis are characteristic of AE, and the tongue and oral mucosa may be covered by white patches resembling oral candidiasis.[22,23]

Infants with AE are typically lethargic and irritable, especially during periods of exacerbation. Diarrhea is a cardinal feature of the disease, and the stool has been likened to the frothy, malodorous stool of patients with sprue. The similarities in stools may not be coincidental since the histologic changes in the duodenal mucosa of both conditions are characterized by flattening of villi and loss of villous architecture.

Failure to thrive, growth retardation, and general debilitation continue if the condition is untreated, and eventually most affected children die of infection. A small number of patients have survived to adulthood without treatment. Skin lesions similar to those observed in AE have been seen in breast-fed infants with transient zinc deficiency caused by low zinc levels in their mothers' milk.[24]

DIAGNOSIS

Diagnosis of AE is based on the demonstration of serum zinc levels below 50 μg per 100 ml. Zinc-contaminated glass syringes and tubes may cause false elevations, which can easily mislead the clinician. The use of plastic syringes and tubes washed in acid has therefore been advocated when a diagnosis of AE is being considered. Decreased zinc levels in red blood cells, hair, and urine have also been found.[4,25]

Histologic examination of skin lesions is not specific and may vary depending on the stage at which the lesion is biopsied. Intraepidermal clefts with acantholytic cells can be seen, creating a histologic picture that can be difficult to distinguish from pemphigus.

MANAGEMENT

Oral zinc gluconate or sulfate in doses of 5 mg/kg/day in two or three divided doses daily brings about complete remission. This treatment is inexpensive and does not have any severe adverse effects. Symptoms usually respond 1 or 2 weeks before the serum zinc reaches normal levels.

Diiodohydroxyquin was used in the treatment of AE until recently. Although this form of treatment was reasonably successful, adverse effects, including optic neuritis, preclude its use now that a safer form of treatment is available.[22,26]

MASTOCYTOSIS

The term *mastocytosis* refers to a group of diseases characterized by mast cell infiltration of the skin and occasionally other organs. It can occur any time from birth to adulthood, but the large majority of cases begin before the age of 2.[27]

The etiology of this group of diseases is unknown. Despite reports of familial cases of mastocytosis, hereditary factors do not appear to play a role in most patients. Males and females appear to be equally affected. Although the condition has been diagnosed in blacks and Orientals, it appears to occur more frequently in whites.[28]

There are many adult forms of mastocytosis but only three types typically involve infants: *urticaria pigmentosa, solitary mastocytoma,* and *diffuse cutaneous mastocytosis.* Bullous variants of these three conditions are common in affected infants under the age of 2. Consequently, these must be considered in the differential diagnosis of neonatal bullous diseases.[7,28]

Urticaria Pigmentosa

Urticaria pigmentosa (UP) is the commonest form of mastocytosis. It can be present at birth, and the majority of cases occur in the first year of life.

CLINICAL FEATURES

Skin lesions are characterized by reddish-brown or orange hyperpigmented macules, papules, or nodules, which are round or oval and range in size from 1 mm to several centimeters. Vesicular and bullous lesions are common

in children, and the condition is then called *bullous urticaria pigmentosa.* Lesions tend to be truncal in distribution, although the extremities can be involved. Scalp, face, palms, and soles are usually clear.[29]

A characteristic feature of the skin lesions is Darier's sign—the production of urticaria within minutes after firmly rubbing or stroking skin lesions. This occurs in 90 percent of patients with cutaneous mastocytosis and has been said to be pathognomonic of this group of diseases. Dermatographism of clinically uninvolved skin occurs in one-third to one-half of patients with UP.[4,27]

Almost half of all patients with UP are asymptomatic. The remaining patients complain of intermittent urticaria, pruritus, and flushing. Symptoms can be induced by rubbing lesions. Other factors that can induce or exacerbate symptoms include exercises, hot baths, spicy foods, and a number of histamine-releasing foods and medications such as alcohol, some cheeses, salicylates, procaine, codeine, morphine, thiamine, quinine, radiographic dyes, scopolamine, atropine, and polymyxin B.[28] Particularly severe reactions have occurred in infants after hot baths followed by vigorous rubbing with a towel. When unusually large amounts of histamine are released, headaches, tachycardia, syncope, and cramps can occur.[7]

Fortunately, the prognosis of UP is good when the condition begins in infancy. Systemic involvement is rare, and lesions clear spontaneously by puberty in over 50 percent of children whose condition began before the age of 2. When UP begins later in life, skin lesions may not disappear and systemic involvement is more common.[7]

Solitary Mastocytoma

Approximately 10 to 15 percent of patients with mastocytosis have one or, in a few patients, several isolated lesions, and this condition is termed solitary mastocytoma. Skin lesions are usually present at birth or develop in early infancy.

CLINICAL FEATURES

Lesions can be present anywhere on the body, and their size can range from 1 to 5 cm in diameter. The characteristic skin finding is a light brown, yellow, or pink plaque or nodule, but bullous lesions commonly occur (*bullous mastocytoma*). As in other forms of mastocytosis, Darier's sign is positive.

After their onset mastocytomas may increase in size for several months, but they usually spontaneously regress within several years. If symptoms occur at all, they are mild and they resolve even before disappearance of the skin lesions.[4,30]

Erythrodermic or Diffuse Cutaneous Mastocytosis

Erythrodermic, or diffuse cutaneous, mastocytosis is a very rare and severe form of mastocytosis.

CLINICAL FEATURES

Of the cutaneous forms of mastocytosis occurring in the neonatal period, diffuse cutaneous mastocytosis has the worst prognosis. Mast cells infiltrate large areas of skin, which become reddened, thickened, and lichenified. The consistency of involved skin is described as being "doughy." The skin surface may be smooth or it may be studded with multiple minute papules. In rare instances generalized bullous lesions may develop (*bullous mastocytosis*), and if this occurs in the neonatal period, systemic mast cell infiltration can be associated.[4,28,29]

Severe pruritus, flushing, and fever can occur. Gastrointestinal symptoms include nausea, vomiting, diarrhea, and abdominal pain. Bronchospasm can lead to compromise of respiratory function. Mast cell infiltration of the reticuloendothelial system is frequently associated with this form of mastocytosis, and other organs may be involved as well. In contrast to other cutaneous forms of mastocytosis, the diffuse form is often fatal.[4,31]

DIAGNOSIS

Clinical features should alert the physician to a diagnosis of mastocytosis, and in fact physical findings may be more accurate in this group of diseases than skin biopsy. In particular, Darier's sign or the ability to produce urticaria in lesional skin by gentle rubbing should immediately suggest the diagnosis of mastocytosis even if the skin biopsy is negative.

Dermatopathologists have called cutaneous mastocytosis an "invisible dermatosis" because the skin biopsy can appear to be entirely normal. Manipulation of lesions during biopsy may cause mast cell degranulation, as may injection of local anesthetic into the area being biopsied. Darier's sign should not be elicited in the lesion to be biopsied. A ring of anesthesia around the lesion, removal of the skin biopsy specimen with a minimum of manipulation, and gentle handling of the specimen may provide a histologic diagnosis.

In all types of cutaneous mastocytosis, biopsy should demonstrate an infiltrate of mast cells in the dermis of lesional skin. Mast cells are recognized by their metachromatic granules, and since these granules are not visible with routine stains, the clinician should request special stains, either Giemsa, azure A, methylene blue, or toluidine blue. This is particularly important in the maculopapular lesions of UP, where mast cells may only be sparsely present in the upper dermis. Several biopsies may be necessary to make a histologic diagnosis in this type of mastocytosis.

In solitary mastocytoma the abnormality is more obvious, with mast cells densely packed in an infiltrate that may fill the dermis. Biopsy of the diffuse, erythrodermic type of mastocytosis typically shows a dense bandlike infiltrate of mast cells in the upper dermis.

Lesions that have been stroked may show a significant number of eosinophils in the dermal infiltrate as well as extracellular mast cell granules. Bullae in all types of mastocytosis are subepidermal and can contain numerous mast cells and eosinophils. As in other bullous diseases, an old lesion may have newly regenerated epidermis at its base, which makes the bulla falsely appear intraepidermal.[3]

MANAGEMENT

Therapy of cutaneous mastocytosis depends on the extent of disease and severity of symptoms. Almost 50 percent of patients are asymptomatic, and these do not require any treatment. In those patients with purely cutaneous symptoms, antihistamines are the mainstay of therapy. Because cyproheptadine (Periactin) has both antihistamine and antiserotonin properties, it has been considered to be the drug of choice by some authors.[4] However, use of most antihistamines will relieve pruritus and flushing in patients with cutaneous mastocytosis. For patients with systemic disease other treatments have been used, including PUVA and oral disodium cromoglycate, a medication that prevents mast cell degranulation.[7,32]

Avoidance of precipitating factors is an important aspect of the treatment of cutaneous mastocytosis syndromes. Patients should be warned to avoid foods and medications that may result in mast cell release. Hot baths and vigorous rubbing must also be avoided.

In infants with the diffuse cutaneous form of mastocytosis other organ involvement must be anticipated and appropriate tests ordered when indicated by history and physical examination.

EPIDERMOLYTIC HYPERKERATOSIS

A chapter on neonatal bullous diseases would not be complete without mentioning *epidermolytic hyperkeratosis*. Since this disease eventuates in a chronic ichthyosiform dermatosis, it will be reviewed in detail in Chapter 13. Discussion in this chapter will be limited to the presentation at birth so that the bullous lesions of epidermolytic hyperkeratosis can be distin-

guished from other neonatal bullous diseases.

Epidermolytic hyperkeratosis is a rare disease, with an incidence of only 1 in 300,000 persons. It is inherited in an autosomal dominant fashion so that a family history should be taken whenever this disorder is considered in the differential diagnosis. A history of an affected parent should immediately suggest a diagnosis of epidermolytic hyperkeratosis to the examining physician.

CLINICAL FEATURES

Epidermolytic hyperkeratosis has been called *congenital bullous ichthyosiform erythroderma* because of the bullous nature of skin lesions in this condition. Bullae are often present at birth or shortly thereafter and can be generalized or localized to limited areas. They are tender and rupture easily, leaving large denuded areas, which can become secondarily infected. Occasionally, an affected infant is encased in a membranous sheath at birth (collodion baby).

DIAGNOSIS

A typical histologic picture is found on skin biopsy. There is granular degeneration, or epidermolytic hyperkeratosis, of the epidermis. Characteristic features include perinuclear clear spaces in the granular layer and upper spinous layer, with indistinct cellular boundaries. There is extensive hyperkeratosis, and the granular layer is thickened. When bullae are biopsied, the level of cleavage is intraepidermal.[33]

MISCELLANEOUS VESICULOBULLOUS ERUPTIONS

A number of conditions and diseases that cause blister formation in adults can do so in neonatal skin as well. In fact, infantile skin is said to be more susceptible to vesicle formation because of less secure attachment of the epidermis to the dermis. Consequently, vesiculation can occur in infants as a result of conditions

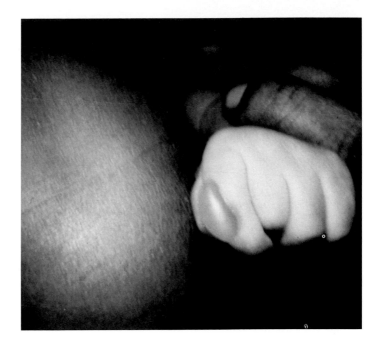

Fig. 11-7. Sucking blister in a neonate. (Photograph courtesy of Neil Prose, M.D. SUNY Health Sciences Center, New York, NY.)

that ordinarily do not result in bulla formation in adult skin. Urticarial wheals, for example, may develop areas of vesiculation in infants, and minor trauma, such as sucking in utero, can result in sucking blisters (Fig. 11-7).

Of the common vesiculobullous diseases, impetigo is found more frequently in infants and children than in adults. Bullous lesions often result when staphylococcal infection is responsible (bullous impetigo). This condition is usually easily distinguished from other bullous diseases because fluid within the bulla is cloudy and the fluid contains numerous staphylococci on culture. On Gram stain the fluid is loaded with clusters of gram-positive cocci.

Allergic contact dermatitis is much less common in infants because the mechanism of contact sensitization is not matured at birth. Primary irritant contact dermatitis, however, does not require an immunologic mechanism. Any irritants, such as powerful acids and alkalis, can produce vesiculation and bulla formation, just as they can in adult skin. A history of exposure to irritants and a vesicular eruption in the distribution of exposure are helpful in diagnosing this condition.

Neonatal herpes is fairly uncommon despite the tremendous attention it has been given by the popular press. However, cases of neonatal herpes that were clinically indistinguishable from EB have been published.[34] It is therefore essential that this condition be considered in the differential diagnosis of vesiculobullous diseases of the neonate. Tzanck preparations should be performed by scraping the base of blisters and staining with methylene blue for a few seconds. Multinucleated giant cells will be seen in a significant proportion of patients, especially when the scraping is taken from fresh vesicles. Viral cultures will be positive for herpes simplex but may take several days for results. Alternatively, immunofluorescence of lesion scrapings using anti-herpes antibodies can provide a rapid and accurate diagnosis.

Burns can also result in vesicle formation, and this diagnosis is simple when a history of contact with a hot object is offered. In a setting of multiple ecchymotic lesions, fractures, or lacerations, child abuse should be suspected, since burns are commonly found in battered children.

Vesiculation and bulla formation are also features of severe sunburn and frostbite. Again, a history of exposure is the most important clue for making the correct diagnosis.

Most of the chronic bullous diseases of adulthood are not apparent in the neonatal period. Dermatitis herpetiformis is rare in infancy and early childhood, and the childhood variant of dermatitis herpetiformis usually occurs after the age of 8. Bullous pemphigoid only rarely affects infants, and the youngest patient reported was 3½ months old.[35] Benign chronic bullous disease of childhood, a condition characterized by linear deposition of IgA along the dermal-epidermal junction, can appear at any time during the first decade of life but generally affects children in the preschool years. Herpes gestationis, a bullous dermatosis of pregnancy, has been reported in infants of affected mothers.[36]

Pemphigus vulgaris is generally a disease of middle age, only rarely affecting children. There have been reports of transient bullous lesions in neonates and in stillbirths of mothers with pemphigus. Circulating antibodies to intracellular substance have been detected in these newborns in some cases. Fortunately, the bullous lesions resolve spontaneously.[37,38] Pemphigus foliaceus also affects middle-aged individuals, although it has been reported in an 18-month-old infant.[39] Other variants of pemphigus, including pemphigus erythematosus and pemphigus vegetans, are also distinctly uncommon in childhood. Familial benign pemphigus does not usually occur before puberty. Fogo selvagem, a variant of pemphigus foliaceus that is endemic in Brazil, can affect children, but the cases reported have generally not occurred in the neonatal period.

Vesiculobullous lesions are also associated with several of the porphyrias, but as a rule these lesions are absent in the neonatal period. The photosensitivity found in patients with Gunther's disease (congenital erythropoietic porphyria) is usually not apparent in the neonatal period.[4] Cutaneous manifestations of erythropoietic protoporphyria usually begin between the ages of 2 and 5, and variegate porphyria generally starts after puberty. Porphyria cutanea tarda most commonly affects adults although it has been reported in a 2-year-old.[40]

A number of conditions characterized by sloughing of large areas of skin are occasionally considered in the differential diagnosis of bullous diseases. Staphylococcal scalded skin syndrome (SSSS) is characterized by a prodrome of fever and malaise, followed by generalized tender erythema, formation of large, flaccid bullae, and sloughing of portions of skin. Skin can be peeled off by gentle rubbing (Nikolsky's sign). Periorifical involvement typically occurs, but mucous membranes are spared. This disease is caused by a circulating staphylococcal exotoxin and, consequently, culture and staining of bullous lesions fail to reveal any organisms. Obvious or occult staphylococcal infection can sometimes be detected. Bullous impetigo, upper respiratory infection, otitis media, and purulent conjunctivitis are potential sources of infection, and group II *Staphylococcus aureus* can occasionally be cultured from the blood or stool as well. Rapid diagnosis of SSSS can be made by examination of a Tzanck preparation, which should reveal the presence of acantholytic cells. Definitive diagnosis may require skin biopsy, which reveals cleavage within the upper epidermis and acantholytic cells within the bulla cavity. For rapid diagnosis frozen sections may be required. Examination of a skin peel may demonstrate necrosis of superficial portions of epidermis.

Toxic epidermal necrolysis (TEN) is most commonly confused with SSSS because it, too, is characterized by sloughing of large areas of skin. It is usually caused by allergic reactions to drugs, but other underlying conditions, including viral, bacterial, and fungal infections, have been implicated. In contrast to SSSS, the incidence of TEN is reduced in neonates and infants. Differentiation between the two diseases is easily made by a number of features. A history of drug intake often precedes TEN, and there is no evidence of staphylococcal infection. In contrast to SSSS, mucous membranes are severely affected, and Tzanck preparations demonstrate only leukocytes and necrotic epidermal cells. Skin biopsy shows necrotic keratinocytes and vacuolization of the basal layer of the epidermis, followed by formation of a subepidermal bulla.[4,41]

APPROACH TO THE PATIENT

Diagnostic features of many of the neonatal bullous diseases are listed in Tables 11-1 and 11-2. Evaluation of the neonate with a bullous eruption should be directed by the history and physical examination. Occasionally, the diagnosis may be obvious from the history alone. A history of exposure to a hot object, for example, would leave little doubt that the infant has a burn. Similarly, a family history of inherited bullous diseases should direct the clinician to the appropriate laboratory tests. Thus, if a history of AE in siblings exists, tissue zinc levels should be examined, whereas skin biopsy for electron microscopy would be indicated if a family history of EB exists.

Maternal history is occasionally important as well. If a diagnosis of neonatal herpes is entertained, a Tzanck preparation and viral cultures should be performed. If the mother has pemphigus or herpes gestationis, immunofluorescent studies should be considered.

Findings on physical examination that may be helpful in establishing a diagnosis are outlined in Table 11-3. Some physical findings are so specific that the diagnosis is easily made (e.g., verrucous or pigmented lesions in IP and Darier's sign in mastocytosis). However, many of these findings may not be present at the time of examination but may evolve over time. Their absence should therefore not be used to preclude the correct diagnosis. For example, the pigmented lesions of IP may develop after the neonatal period. Similarly, the nail changes of acrodermatitis enteropathica are not present at birth but develop months later.

Once history and physical examination have enabled the clinician to formulate a differential diagnosis, the correct diagnosis can be established by the appropriate laboratory findings, as outlined in Table 11-3.

Table 11-2. Diagnostic Features of Neonatal Vesiculobullous Diseases

Disease	Site of Blister Formation	Diagnostic Features
Epidermolytic hyperkeratosis	Upper epidermis	Skin biopsy: "epidermolytic hyperkeratosis"
Incontinentia pigmenti	Intraepidermal	Clinical findings; skin biopsy: eosinophils in vesicle
Mastocytosis	Subepidermal	Darier's sign; skin biopsy: mast cell infiltrate
Acrodermatitis enteropathica	Suprabasal or intraepidermal or subcorneal	Reduced serum zinc
Epidermolysis bullosa	See Table 11-1	Electron microscopy; see Table 11-1
Staphylococcal scalded skin syndrome	Subcorneal	Clinical findings; skin biopsy: acantholytic cells; Tzanck preparation: acantholytic cells
Toxic epidermal necrolysis	Subepidermal	Clinical findings; skin biopsy: epidermal necrosis and vacuolization of basal layer; Tzanck preparation: necrotic epidermal cells and leukocytes
Neonatal herpes	Intraepidermal	Tzanck preparation: multinucleated giant cells; viral cultures; immunofluorescence
Bullous impetigo	Subcorneal	Gram stain: clusters of gram-positive cocci; culture

Table 11-3. Approach to the Patient

History
 Exposure to
  Irritants: contact dermatitis
  Extremes of temperature: sunburn, frostbite
  Hot object: burn
 Diarrhea
  Acrodermatitis enteropathica
 Medications
 Family history
  Epidermolytic hyperkeratosis, epidermolysis bullosa,
   acrodermatitis enteropathica, incontinentia pig-
   menti
 Maternal history
  Herpes, pemphigus vulgaris, herpes gestationis

Physical Examination
 Verrucous or pigmented lesions: incontinentia pig-
  menti
 Milia: dystrophic epidermolysis bullosa
 Bullae heal with scarring: dystrophic epidermolysis
  bullosa
 Dermatographism: mastocytosis
 Darier's sign: mastocytosis
 Nikolsky's sign: staphylococcal scalded skin syn-
  drome, dystrophic epidermolysis bullosa
 Nail abnormalities: epidermolysis bullosa, acroder-
  matitis enteropathica, incontinentia pigmenti
 Mucous membrane involvement: epidermolysis bul-
  losa, acrodermatitis enteropathica
 Ocular abnormalities: incontinentia pigmenti, reces-
  sive dystrophic epidermolysis bullosa
 Neurologic findings: incontinentia pigmenti

Laboratory Investigation
 Skin biopsy: hematoxylin and eosin, PAS stains;
  mast cell stains (mastocytosis); indirect immunofluorescence with antibodies to basement membrane components (epidermolysis bullosa); electron microscopy (epidermolysis bullosa)
 Tzanck preparation: neonatal herpes, staphylococcal
  scalded skin syndrome
 Gram stain: bullous impetigo
 Bacterial cultures: bulla (bullous impetigo); wound,
  respiratory secretions, blood, stool, and urine
  (staphylococcal scalded skin syndrome)
 Viral cultures: neonatal herpes
 Eosinophilia: incontinentia pigmenti
 Reduced serum zinc: acrodermatitis enteropathica

REFERENCES

1. Gedde-Dahl T Jr: Sixteen types of epidermolysis bullosa. Acta Derm Venereol [Suppl] Stockh 95:74, 1981

2. Gedde-Dahl T Jr: Epidermolysis Bullosa: a Clinical, Genetic and Epidemiological Study. Johns Hopkins University Press, Baltimore, 1971

3. Lever WF, Schaumburg-Lever G: Histopathology of the Skin. 6th Ed. JB Lippincott, Philadelphia, 1983

4. Hurwitz S: Clinical Pediatric Dermatology. WB Saunders, Philadelphia, 1981

5. Gorlin RJ, Pindborg JJ, Cohen MM, Jr: Syndromes of the Head and Neck. 2nd Ed. McGraw-Hill, New York, 1976

6. Thompson JW, Ahmed AR, Dudley JP: Epidermolysis bullosa dystrophica of the larynx and trachea. Acute airway obstruction. Ann Otol Rhinol Laryngol 89:428, 1980

7. Schachner L, Press S: Vesicular, bullous and pustular disorders in infancy and childhood. Pediatr Clin North Am 30:609, 1983

8. Hillemeier C, Touloukian R, McCallum R, et al: Esophageal web: a previously unrecognized complication of epidermolysis bullosa. Pediatrics 67:678, 1981

9. Cooper TW, Bauer EA: Therapeutic efficacy of phenytoin in recessive dystrophic epidermolysis. Arch Dermatol 120:490, 1984

10. U.S. Department of Health and Human Services: Living with Epidermolysis Bullosa, National Institutes of Health Publication No. 84–663, 1984

11. Anton-Lamprecht I, Jovanovic V, Arnold ML, et al: Prenatal diagnosis of epidermolysis bullosa dystrophica, Hallopeau-Siemens with electron microscopy of fetal skin. Lancet, 2:1077, 1981

12. Heagerty AHM, Kennedy AR, Gunner DB, et al: Rapid prenatal diagnosis and exclusion of epidermolysis bullosa using novel antibody probes. J Invest Dermatol 86:603, 1986

13. Schachner L, Lazarus GS, Dembitzer H: Epidermolysis bullosa hereditaria letalis. Br J Dermatol 96:51, 1977

14. Peltier FA, Tschen EH, Raimer SS, et al: Epidermolysis bullosa letalis associated with congenital pyloric atresia. Arch Dermatol 117:728, 1981

15. Guill MF, Wray BB, Rogers RB, et al: Junctional epidermolysis bullosa. Am J Dis Child 137:992, 1983

16. Rodeck CH, Eady RAJ, Gosden CM: Prenatal diagnosis of epidermolysis bullosa letalis. Lancet 1:949, 1980

17. Savolainen ER, Kero M, Pihlajaniemi T, et al: Deficiency of galactosylhydroxylysyl glucosyltransferase, an enzyme of collagen synthesis, in a family with dominant epidermolysis bullosa simplex. N Engl J Med 304:197, 1981

18. Bart BJ, Gorlin RJ, Anderson VE, et al: Con-

genital localized absence of skin and associated abnormalities resembling epidermolysis bullosa. Arch Dermatol 93:296, 1966

19. Butler DF, Berger TG, James WD, et al: Bart's syndrome: microscopic, ultrastructural, and immunofluorescent mapping features. Pediatr Dermatol 3:113, 1986
20. Bordas X, Palou J, Capdevila JM, et al: Kindler's syndrome. J Am Acad Dermatol 6:263, 1982
21. Carney RG Jr: Incontinentia pigmenti. Arch Dermatol 112:535, 1976
22. Braverman I: Skin Signs of Systemic Disease. 2nd Ed. WB Saunders, Philadelphia, 1981
23. Wells BT, Winkelmann RK: Acrodermatitis enteropathica—report of 6 cases. Arch Dermatol 84:90, 1961
24. Bye AME, Goodfellow A, Atherton DJ: Transient zinc deficiency in a full-term breast-fed infant of normal birth weight. Pediatr Dermatol 2:308, 1985
25. Hambidge KM, Walravens PA: Acrodermatitis enteropathica. Int J Dermatol 17:380, 1978
26. Neldner KH, Hambidge KM: Zinc therapy of acrodermatitis enteropathica. N Engl J Med 292:879, 1975
27. Sagher R, Even-Paz Z: Mastocytosis and the Mast Cell. Year Book Medical Publishers, Chicago, 1967
28. DiBacco RS, DeLeo VA: Mastocytosis and the mast cell. J Am Acad Dermatol 7:709, 1982
29. Orkin M, Good RA, Clawson CC, et al: Bullous mastocytosis. Arch Dermatol 101:547, 1970
30. Johnson WC, Helwig EB: Solitary mastocytosis (urticaria pigmentosa). Arch Dermatol 84:806, 1961
31. Burgoon CF, Graham JH, McCafree DL: Mast cell disease: a cutaneous variant with multisystem involvement. Arch Dermatol 98:590, 1968
32. Soter NA, Austen KF, Wasserman SI: Oral disodium cromoglycate in the treatment of systemic mastocytosis. N Engl J Med 301:465, 1979
33. Rand RE, Baden HP: The ichthyoses—a review. J Am Acad Dermatol 8:285, 1983
34. Honig PJ, Brown D: Congenital herpes simplex virus infection initially resembling epidermolysis bullosa. J Pediatr 101:958, 1982
35. Gould WM, Zlotnick DA: Bullous pemphigoid in infancy: a case report. Pediatrics 59:942, 1977
36. Chorzelski TP, Jablonska S, Beutner EH, et al: Herpes gestationis with identical lesions in the newborn. Arch Dermatol 112:1129, 1976
37. Terpstra H, de Jong MCJM, Klokke AH: In vivo bound pemphigus antibodies in a stillborn infant. Arch Dermatol 115:316, 1979
38. Ruocco V, Rossi A, Astarita C, et al: A congenital acantholytic bullous eruption in the new-born infant of a pemphigus mother. Ital Gen Rev Dermatol 12:169, 1975
39. Kahn G, Lewis HM: True childhood pemphigus. Pemphigus foliaceus in an 18-month-old child: immunofluorescence as a diagnostic aid. Am J Dis Child 121:253, 1971
40. Kasky A: Porphyria cutanea tarda in a two-year-old girl. Br J Dermatol 90:213, 1974
41. Hansen RC: Staphylococcal scalded skin syndrome, toxic shock syndrome, and Kawasaki disease. Pediatr Clin North Am 30:533, 1983

12

Neonatal and Infantile Erythrodermas

Amy S. Paller

The newborn or young infant with generalized cutaneous erythema risks developing temperature instability, excessive water, protein, and electrolyte loss, secondary cutaneous infection, and sepsis. In addition to managing these concerns, the physician must determine the underlying cause of the erythroderma and treat it appropriately. Erythroderma in the neonatal or young infant may be a manifestation of a variety of conditions, including ichthyosis and ichthyosiform disorders (see also Ch. 13), papulosquamous diseases, graft-versus-host disease, metabolic disorders, infections, and reactions to toxins (Table 12-1).

NORMAL VARIANTS WITH DESQUAMATION

Neonates with normal cutaneous desquamation must be distinguished from neonates with erythrodermas associated with scaling. Newborn infants with a gestational age of 40 or more weeks may occasionally have a marked amount of desquamation, which peaks about 1 week after birth. The dysmature infant has dry, peeling skin but shows additional distinguishing characteristics, including a low birth weight for gestational age and length, little subcutaneous fat, and absence of the vernix caseosa. The hair and nails are long, and dysmature babies are often stained with meconium.

ICHTHYOSIS AND ICHTHYOSIFORM DISORDERS

Neonates with ichthyosis and erythroderma may have cutaneous changes that range from mild thickening of the stratum corneum to marked thickening, as in the harlequin fetus and collodion baby. These infants sweat poorly and have a significantly increased risk of developing temperature instability. Ichthyotic neonates are best managed in a humidified environment with emollient lotions. Thick emollient preparations should not be used because of the already compromised ability to sweat. In patients with thick ichthyotic encasements (harlequin fetus, collodion baby), feeding and respiration may require facilitation.

Harlequin Fetus

The harlequin fetus is the most severely affected of the ichthyotic infants. Although rare, harlequin fetuses have occurred in sibships and

Table 12-1. Differential Diagnosis of Neonatal and Infantile Erythrodermas

Normal variants
    Physiologic desquamation
    Desquamation of dysmaturity
Ichthyosis and ichthyosiform erythrodermas
    Harlequin fetus
    Collodion baby
        Nonbullous congenital ichthyosiform erythro-
            derma
        X-linked recessive ichthyosis
        Ichthyosis vulgaris
        Bullous congenital ichthyosiform erythroderma
        Netherton's syndrome
        Lamellar exfoliation of the newborn
        Trichothiodystrophy with ichthyosiform erythro-
            derma
    Tay's syndrome
    Sjögren-Larsson syndrome
    Rud's syndrome
    KID syndrome
    Chondrodysplasia punctata
    CHILD syndrome
    Ichthyosis hystrix
    Peeling skin syndrome
Papulosquamous disorders
    Seborrheic dermatitis
    Leiner's disease
    Exfoliative psoriasis
    Generalized pustular psoriasis
    Pityriasis rubra pilaris
Graft-versus-host disease
    Generalized maculopapular with desquamation
    Toxic epidermal necrolysis
    Chronic, ichthyosiform
    Transfusion reactions
Metabolic disorders
    Citrullinemia
    Maple syrup urine disease
    Biotin deficiency; multiple carboxylase deficiency
    Essential fatty acid deficiency
Infections
    Staphylococcal scalded skin syndrome
    Congenital candidiasis
Toxins
    Boric acid poisoning

from consanguineous parents, suggesting an autosomal recessive mode of inheritance. The skin is markedly thickened and armorlike, with deep moist fissures that are most prominent overlying joints. The rigid skin around the eyes and chemosis of the palpebral conjunctivae result in marked ectropion, with obscuration of the globes. The lips are everted, and the nose and ears are flattened and distorted. The nails and hair are absent or dysplastic. The hands and feet have poorly developed digits and the joints

have flexion deformities. Histopathologic examination shows marked hyperkeratosis with variable diminution of the epidermal granular cell layer. Four harlequin fetuses have been analyzed for epidermal keratin and lipid abnormalities and have been found to have different underlying defects, which suggests heterogeneity. These alterations include replacement of the normal α-helical pattern of keratin by a cross β pattern,[1] abnormal amino acid pattern of the stratum corneum,[2] poorly oriented α-helical keratin pattern,[2] and abnormal epidermal lipids.[3] The prognosis of the harlequin fetus is extremely poor, and, until recently, no affected neonate had survived beyond 9 months of age.[3] Etretinate therapy improved the condition of one harlequin fetus, however.[4] Nevertheless, most harlequin fetuses die within days after birth as a result of sepsis or of inadequate ventilation and pneumonia.

Collodion Baby

The collodion baby (Fig. 12-1) is encased in a shiny cellophane-like membrane at birth, which distorts facial features and fixes the extremities in flexion. The eyelids (ectropion) and lips (eclabium) are usually everted, and the nostrils and ears are flattened. The hair and nails are usually normal. Soon after birth the scales begin to desquamate and the underlying erythema is revealed. Complete shedding of the membrane takes 15 days to 3 months, and the future course of the dermatosis depends upon the underlying keratinizing disorder. Premature birth occurs with 25 percent of collodion babies.[5] Temporarily, the infants may have difficulty with sucking, requiring nasogastric feeding, and, rarely, with breathing, requiring assisted ventilation. Interference with normal sweating because of the thick scales and temperature instability are other associated problems in the newborn infant. Death may occur in up to one-third of infants, especially within the first 2 weeks of life, and is usually due to respiratory distress or sepsis. During infancy the majority of surviving infants[6] develop the

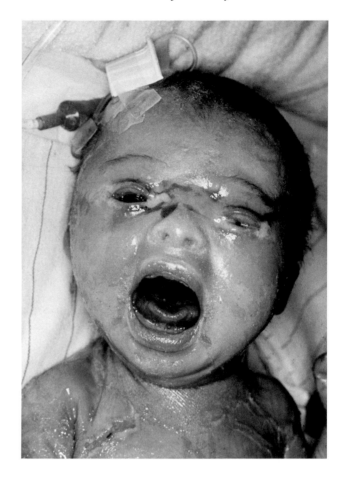

Fig. 12-1. Collodion baby encased in a shiny membrane with mild eclabium and ectropion. The neonate later developed classic lamellar ichthyosis. (Courtesy of Roger W. Pearson, M.D., Rush-Presbyterian-St. Luke's Medical Center, Chicago.)

phenotype of nonbullous congenital ichthyosiform erythroderma (CIE), including lamellar ichthyosis (LI), but bullous CIE (epidermolytic hyperkeratosis), X-linked recessive ichthyosis, ichthyosis vulgaris, ichthyosis linearis circumflexa (Netherton's syndrome), a variant of trichothiodystrophy, and even normal skin[7] (lamellar exfoliation of the newborn), may follow desquamation. Other desquamative ichthyosiform conditions seen at birth that differ in appearance from the collodion baby syndrome include Tay's syndrome, Sjögren-Larsson syndrome, Rud's syndrome, the KID (keratitis, ichthyosis, and deafness) syndrome, chondrodysplasia punctata, the CHILD (congenital hemidysplasia, ichthyosiform erythroderma, and ipsilateral limb defects) syndrome, ichthyosis hystrix, and the peeling skin syndrome.

Any of the four major types of ichthyosis

may manifest as the collodion baby syndrome at birth. Nonbullous CIE is by far the most common outcome of the collodion baby syndrome. This autosomal recessive form of ichthyosis has now been divided into two subgroups, *nonbullous congenital ichthyosiform erythroderma* per se and *classical lamellar ichthyosis* on the basis of the clinical appearance and the elevation of *n*-alkanes in the epidermis of patients with CIE.[8] The erythroderma of nonbullous CIE is generalized, with facial, flexural, and palmoplantar involvement. Ectropion is common, especially in the classical LI form. The nails may be thickened and stippled, and the hair is often absent owing to heavy scaling of the scalp. Histopathologic examination of the skin of collodion babies who develop nonbullous CIE shows marked thickening of the stratum corneum by 15 days after birth, in contrast to those collodion babies who subsequently develop normal skin.[9]

Evolution into the *recessive X-linked form of ichthyosis* (RXLI) is second in frequency to evolution into nonbullous CIE. Affected male infants have thick, dark brown scales with a "dirty" appearance on the face and neck. The trunk and flexural areas are usually affected, but the palms and soles are normal. Corneal opacities of the posterior capsule develop later in childhood or young adulthood in affected male patients and female carriers but do not affect visual acuity. The RXLI syndrome is due to a deficiency of the enzymes steroid sulfatase and arylsulfatase C with accumulation of cholesterol sulfate. The diagnosis may be confirmed by the altered mobility on serum lipoprotein electrophoresis of cholesterol sulfate-enriched serum β-lipoproteins.

Other Forms of Ichthyosis

Infants with *bullous congenital ichthyosiform erythroderma (epidermolytic hyperkeratosis)* and *ichthyosis vulgaris* will rarely present as collodion babies. More commonly, newborn infants with bullous CIE have an exfoliative erythroderma with bullae. The bullae are the most troublesome feature of bullous CIE in infancy, and secondary bacterial infection is common. With advancing age the bullae occur less frequently, and thick, yellow-brown verrucous scales develop, especially over joints and in flexural areas. The palms, soles, and face are usually affected. The hair and nails are not affected, and ectropion is not a feature. The histologic findings of bullous CIE are diagnostic and include extensive vacuolization of the stratum spinosum and stratum granulosum cells, with intraepidermal bullae, dyskeratotic epidermal cells, and large, clumped keratohyaline granules. The disorder is inherited as an autosomal dominant trait. Only 2 percent of collodion babies have ichthyosis vulgaris, despite the frequency of this autosomal dominant disorder; most infants develop its characteristic features after the first 3 months of life. Fine white scales are most prominent on the lower extremities but may occur on the face, trunk, and upper extremities as well. The flexural areas tend to be spared, but the palms and soles are thickened. Histologic examination of ichthyotic skin shows hyperkeratosis, with a decreased to absent granular layer. Filaggrin, a component of the granular layer, is absent or markedly decreased in these patients.[10] Atopic dermatitis and keratosis pilaris may be associated features.

Netherton's Syndrome

Collodion babies and neonates with CIE develop more characteristic features of the various ichthyosiform disorders after exfoliation. Patients with *Netherton's syndrome* usually have scaling erythroderma[11-13] at birth but may manifest as collodion babies. The scaling erythroderma is frequently thought to represent severe seborrheic dermatitis, Leiner's disease, or congenital erythrodermic psoriasis. Histopathologic examination of skin sections shows nondiagnostic changes consistent with those of exfoliative dermatitis or psoriasiform dermatitis. Netherton's syndrome is an autosomal recessive disorder with characteristic scaling, annular, serpiginous, and migratory plaques that are bordered by a distinct double-edged scale (ichthyosis linearis circumflexa) or ichthyosiform erythroderma. The face, trunk, and extremities are most commonly affected. All body hair tends to be short, scant, dry, and lusterless. By microscopic examination the hairs show trichorrhexis invaginata (bamboo hair deformity), as well as other hair shaft defects, especially pili torti. An atopic diathesis, recurrent skin infections, and aminoaciduria are associated features. A similar disorder has been described in siblings who were collodion babies and whose condition evolved into LI with hair shaft abnormalities, aminoaciduria, and no atopic tendency.[14] Jorizzo et al. described a patient who was born as a collodion baby and later developed LI in combination with features of trichothiodystrophy.[15] Abnormalities include dwarfism, mental retardation, nail and dental anomalies, poor sexual maturation, and punctate cataracts. The hair shaft alterations consist of pili torti, transverse fractures of the hairs, alternating light and dark bands under polarizing microscopy, and low sulfur content.

Rud's Syndrome

Patients with Rud's syndrome have ichthyosis in association with seizures, mental retardation, short stature, and hypogonadism. The ichthyosis is almost always present at birth and has been described in the neonatal period as displaying large, coarse scales on the trunk and extremities, with collodion membranes covering the soles.[18] After the neonatal period the ichthyotic scales are large and dark, as in RXLI. The palms and soles tend to be spared. Rud's syndrome is a heterogeneous group of disorders, but most patients have deficient steroid sulfatase activity.[8]

Tay's Syndrome

Infants with Tay's syndrome have a generalized erythematous eruption covered by fine scales at birth. The skin exfoliates during the first months of life, leaving nonbullous ichthyosiform lesions on the face, trunk, and extensor surfaces of the extremities.[16] Other manifestations of this autosomal recessive disorder include growth retardation, mental retardation, short, sparse, brittle hair with pili torti and trichorrhexis nodosa-like hair shaft abnormalities, and a progeric appearance.

Sjögren-Larsson Syndrome

Infants with the autosomal recessive Sjögren-Larsson syndrome almost always have generalized ichthyosiform erythroderma at birth but not collodion membranes.[17] During the first year of life the hyperkeratosis becomes more prominent, but the cutaneous erythema usually decreases. Lamellar scales are most prominent on the neck and lower abdomen and in flexural areas. Histopathologic examination of skin biopsies shows hyperkeratosis, often with thickening of the granular layer and stratum spinosum. During infancy spastic diplegia or tetraplegia and evidence of mental retardation develop.

KID Syndrome

Patients with KID syndrome (keratitis, ichthyosis, and deafness) are born with leathery, erythematous skin that has been likened to elephant skin.[19–21] The thickening and erythema are most prominent on the extensor surfaces of the extremities, the palms, the soles, and the face. The skin rapidly loses its erythema but becomes increasingly verrucous, with development of hyperkeratotic plaques and stippling of the skin in infancy. Marked thickening of the nails and universal alopecia are usually present at birth. Progressive neovascularization of the corneas with resultant blindness and sensorineural deafness develop during infancy. Some patients have recurrent bacterial and candidal infections with immunologic abnormalities.[22] Recently, two children have been described who developed pruritic, migratory ichthyosiform dermatoses within the first month of life, in association with retinal colobomas, conductive hearing loss, seizures, and mental retardation.[23]

Chondrodysplasia Punctata

Chondrodysplasia punctata (Conradi-Hunermann syndrome) (Fig. 12-2) is characterized by stippled epiphyses, cataracts, shortening of the femora and humeri and other skeletal abnormalities, and cutaneous alterations.[9,24] The skin abnormalities are found in 25 percent of patients and are usually noted at birth. Thick, yellow, adherent scales in whorled patterns overlying generalized erythroderma are most common on the trunk and proximal extremities. The palms and soles may be hyperkeratotic, and patchy alopecia is common. The scaling and erythroderma resolve within the first few months of

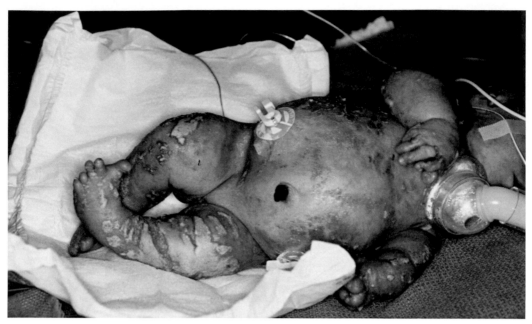

Fig. 12-2. Chondrodysplasia punctata (Conradi-Hunermann syndrome), with whorled patterns of markedly thickened yellow scale overlying erythroderma.

life, with residual follicular atrophoderma in areas of previous scaling.

CHILD Syndrome

The CHILD syndrome is almost always seen in girls and is characterized by congenital hemidysplasia, ichthyosiform erythroderma, and ipsilateral limb defects. The ichthyosiform erythroderma is present at birth or develops within the first few years of life and is unilateral and sharply delineated. Epiphyseal stippling may be present. Patients with ichthyosis hystrix may have unilateral or bilateral patterned erythroderma with overlying hyperkeratotic, verrucous, linear, and whorled plaques[25,26]; these patients should be differentiated from patients with chondrodysplasia punctata by the lack of associated features. With increasing age, the erythema decreases or disappears but the verrucous lesions persist.

Congenital ichthyosiform erythroderma has also been reported in association with late-onset ataxia[27]; with mental retardation, nephropathy, and dwarfism[28]; with progressive neurologic deterioration, renal disease, hypertension, ectodermal dysplasia, short stature, and hypogonadism[29]; and with coarse hair, mental retardation, dwarfism, skin atrophy especially on the dorsum of the hands and feet, and aminoaciduria.[30]

Peeling Skin Syndrome

The peeling skin syndrome is a rare autosomal recessive disorder, which frequently begins at birth. It is characterized by scaling and peeling of the skin overlying erythema.[31,32] The condition is pruritic and is worse during winter months. Examination discloses generalized serpiginous patches of peeling and underlying erythema with hyperkeratosis and erythema of the palms and soles. Occasionally, the face, scalp, palms, and soles are spared. The nails are often thickened and onycholytic. The anagen hairs may be easily removed but are otherwise normal. Short stature, sexual infantilism, and anosmia may be associated. Histopathologic examination of skin biopsy sections shows a psoriasiform dermatitis with a cleavage plane immediately above the stratum granulosum. Patients may have low plasma tryptophan levels and aminoaciduria. Differentiation from the staphylococcal scalded skin syndrome (SSSS) (see below) must be made by the generalized distribution of lesions at the onset and negative nasopharyngeal cultures for *Staphylococcus aureus*.

PAPULOSQUAMOUS DISORDERS

Seborrheic Dermatitis

Seborrheic dermatitis usually begins after the first few weeks of life but occasionally is present at birth. Although the scalp, face, and intertriginous areas are favored sites for the lesions of seborrheic dermatitis, the disorder may be generalized. The lesions are erythematous, with fine white or yellow greasy scaling but with indistinct borders. Secondary bacterial or candidal infections are common. Pruritus is minimal and the child is otherwise well. Most infantile cases either clear spontaneously after weeks to months or respond very quickly to topical medication.

Leiner's Disease

Leiner's disease (Fig. 12-3) is a rare disorder, characterized by severe exfoliative erythroderma, diarrhea, failure to thrive, and recurrent gram-negative bacterial and candidal infections.[33] Most affected infants are breast-fed. Within the first weeks of life, scales and erythema resembling seborrheic dermatitis develop on the scalp, face, and intertriginous areas, followed by a rapid generalized extension of the rash. Concurrently, infants have mucoid diarrheal stools with occasional projectile vomiting. Progressive wasting and death are usually due to gram-negative sepsis. The disorder appears to be due to a dysfunction of the C5 component of complement in opsonization, but

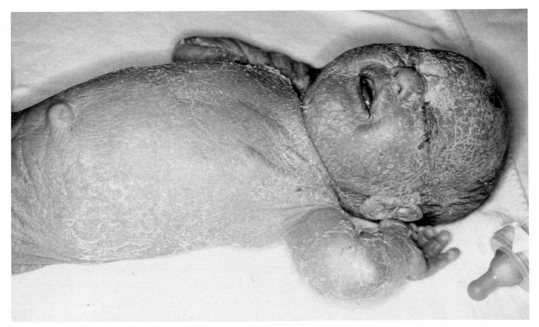

Fig. 12-3. Severe exfoliative erythroderma with diarrhea and failure to thrive in a neonate with Leiner's disease. (Courtesy of Roger W. Pearson, M.D., Rush-Presbyterian-St. Luke's Medical Center, Chicago.)

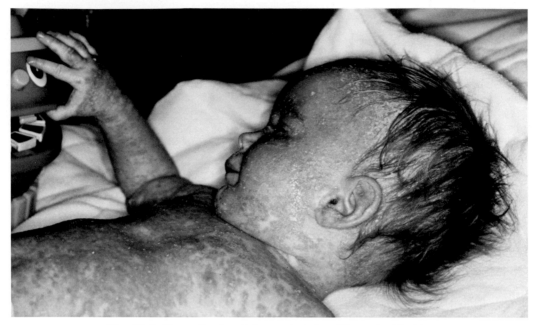

Fig. 12-4. Generalized pustular psoriasis in a 13-month-old girl.

there is no deficiency of C5 nor abnormality in erythrocyte hemolysis (CH50). Infusions of fresh plasma or purified C5 must be given to correct the defect and decrease the mortality from infections. Topical corticosteroids help to clear the dermatitis. Substitution of cow's milk formulas for breast milk is often helpful. The disorder tends to clear spontaneously during infancy if the infant survives.

Psoriasis

The exfoliative and generalized pustular forms of psoriasis (Fig. 12-4) rarely develop in young infants but must be included in the differential diagnosis of neonatal and infantile erythrodermas. *Pustular psoriasis* begins during the first year of life in 27 to 40 percent of patients who develop this condition in childhood.[34] The pustular psoriasis is severe and generalized (von Zumbusch type), with recurrent relapses and associated malaise, irritability, temperature instability, and leukocytosis. The pustular psoriasis is almost always superimposed on seborrheic dermatitis or generalized congenital psoriatic erythroderma. The generalized congenital psoriatic erythroderma must be differentiated from ichthyosiform erythroderma.[35]

Exfoliative erythrodermic psoriasis without pustulosis has also been described in infants.[34,36] Not uncommonly, scattered annular lesions and nail dystrophy are associated and suggest the diagnosis. Familial cases of congenital psoriatic erythroderma have been described.

Erythrodermic or pustular psoriasis in early infancy is often followed by psoriasis vulgaris in later infancy and childhood. The diagnosis may be confirmed by histopathologic examination of lesional skin, which shows hyperkeratosis and parakeratosis, epidermal thickening with elongation and blunting of the rete ridges, a diminished stratum granulosum, increased mitoses in the basal cell layer and lower stratum spinosum, and focal aggregations of polymorphonuclear leukocytes in the stratum corneum or substratum corneum (Munro microabscesses), especially in pustular psoriasis. Most infants with erythrodermic and pustular psoriasis respond to conservative therapy with compresses and mild- to moderate-strength topical corticosteroids. Occasionally, infants require aggressive therapy, such as methotrexate or retinoids. Although bacterial cultures of psoriatic pustules yield no growth of organisms, infants with generalized erythrodermic or pustular psoriasis may develop cutaneous superinfections and sepsis, especially infections due to staphylococcal and streptococcal organisms. These require treatment with systemic antibiotics.

Pityriasis Rubra Pilaris

Fewer than 15 percent of cases of pityriasis rubra pilaris (PRP) occur in infancy as the classical or atypical juvenile forms described by Griffiths.[37] Classical juvenile PRP affects most of these patients and resembles adult PRP except that it starts in infancy. The disorder often begins as erythematous follicular papules, which coalesce to form patches and frequently generalized erythroderma, typically with small islands of sparing. The hyperkeratotic follicular papules are most prominent on the dorsal aspect of the hands and feet, the extensor aspect of the wrists, and the thighs, knees, and elbows. The scalp is often covered with scales and erythema. Salmon-colored hyperkeratosis of the palms and soles is typical and usually associated with painful fissures. The nails often have subungual hyperkeratosis and longitudinal ridges but not onycholysis. Lacy white plaques may cover the oral mucosa. Histopathologic examination of the skin in areas of confluent erythroderma shows hyperkeratosis, spotty parakeratosis, thickening of the epidermis, foci of spongiosis, and liquefaction degeneration of basal cells. Sections from follicular papules show large follicular keratotic plugs surrounded by perifollicular parakeratosis. The microabscesses of psoriasis are not seen.

Classical juvenile PRP must be differentiated from psoriasis and severe seborrheic dermatitis. The typical islands of sparing within the erythroderma, the follicular hyperkeratosis, the lack of nail onycholysis, and the histopathologic appearance of skin sections help to differentiate these conditions. Differentiation from psoriasis may be extremely difficult, and patients have been reported with PRP who later develop typical psoriasis. Drug eruptions, follicular ichthyosis, atypical keratosis pilaris, and symmetric progressive erythrokeratoderma must also be considered in the differential diagnosis.

Infants with atypical PRP have follicular hyperkeratosis and severe palmoplantar keratoderma but do not tend to have the erythroderma of the classical juvenile type. Atypical PRP is often familial and has a chronic course.

The treatment of classical juvenile PRP includes emollients and keratolytic agents, such as salicylic acid or urea. Oral vitamin A and retinoids have also been used in PRP with success but are often associated with considerable toxicity.[38] Classical juvenile PRP spontaneously remits in more than 50 percent of patients within 6 months.[38]

GRAFT-VERSUS-HOST DISEASE

Graft-versus-host disease (GVHD) occurs when an immunoincompetent host receives foreign immunocompetent cells. Most patients with GVHD develop cutaneous abnormalities, and the risk or mortality is high because of associated immunosuppression and resultant infections. The disease may develop in immunologically deficient infants and neonates following blood transfusions, maternal-fetal transfusions, exchange transfusions, and plasma transfusions. In addition, presumably normal infants with Rh isoimmunization who have received intrauterine transfusions and later exchange transfusions and young infants who receive bone marrow transplants (usually for a severe combined immunodeficiency disorder) may develop the cutaneous manifestations of GVHD. Evidence of acute GVHD usually appears a few weeks after contact with the immunocompetent foreign cells, and chronic GVHD begins a few months later. The cutaneous features of GVHD in infants vary considerably and include generalized maculopapular eruptions, often associated with desquamation, a severe seborrheic dermatitis-like eruption, toxic epidermal necrolysis (TEN), and ichthyosiform erythroderma.[39,40] Occasionally, cutaneous features of chronic GVHD that occur in older individuals are seen, including the papulosquamous lesions of lichen planus and sclerodermatous features with a hyperkeratotic, atrophic epidermis, dermal sclerosis, dyspigmentation, and alopecia. Anorexia, failure to thrive, severe diarrhea, hepatosplenomegaly, jaundice, fever, and eosinophilia are the typical noncutaneous abnormalities of acute GVHD. Histopathologic examination of lesional skin biopsies of acute GVHD shows liquefaction degeneration of basal cells and acantholysis, dyskeratosis, and necrosis of individual epidermal cells. *Satellite cell necrosis,* with lymphocytes surrounding the dyskeratotic epidermal cells, is pathognomonic of acute GVHD. Lymphocyte exocytosis, dermal infiltrates of lymphocytes, and epidermal atrophy may also be seen. In severe acute GVHD and especially in patients with the skin manifestations of TEN, clefting occurs between the degenerated basal cells and the dermis. The histopathologic features of chronic GVHD are epidermal hyperkeratosis or atrophy and dermal sclerosis beginning in the papillary dermis, with encasement of adnexal structures.

Generalized maculopapular eruptions are the most common cutaneous manifestation of acute GVHD in infants and characteristically include palmoplantar erythema. Generalized desquamation typically follows the onset of the rash. The maculopapular eruptions must be differentiated from drug reactions and viral or bacterial infections. The posttransfusion syndrome, characterized by a transient generalized maculopapular rash, eosinophilia, thrombocytopenia, and mild lymphopenia, may occur after exchange transfusions (even with irradiated red blood cells) in the first week of life, and may be confused with GVHD.[41] Other features of GVHD are not seen in the posttransfusion syndrome, and the rash of the posttransfusion syndrome develops within days rather than weeks after administration of the transfusion. When the cutaneous eruption of acute GVHD resembles severe seborrheic dermatitis, it must be distinguished from seborrheic dermatitis, Leiner's disease,

histiocytosis X, and exfoliative psoriasis by skin biopsies and testing of opsonization function of C5. The most severe cutaneous alteration associated with GVHD is TEN, which often results in extensive loss of epidermis. The infant is susceptible to fluid and electrolyte imbalances, as well as to sepsis from both the immunologic dysfunction of GVHD itself and the loss of epidermal barrier function. The TEN of GVHD may be confused with TEN due to drug reactions, which is rare in infants,[42] and with the staphylococcal scalded skin syndrome (SSSS) (see below). Skin biopsy and the other clinical and laboratory features of GVHD establish the correct diagnosis. Ichthyosiform erythroderma is an unusual manifestation of chronic GVHD, which usually occurs in infants and neonates who have had intrauterine acute GVHD. The disorder must be distinguished from LI and other ichthyosiform disorders by the associated features and biopsy.

Usually, GVHD responds to immunosuppressive therapy with systemic corticosteroids and azathioprine. Techniques to prevent GVHD from occurring as a sequela to bone marrow transplantation, including elimination of mature T lymphocytes with pan-T-cell antibodies and lectins and the post-transplantation administration of cyclosporin A and methotrexate, are currently under investigation. Blood products with viable lymphocytes should be irradiated prior to administration to immunodeficient or premature infants.

METABOLIC DISORDERS

Citrullinemia and Maple Syrup Urine Disease

Neonatal citrullinemia (Fig. 12-5), a rare autosomal recessive disorder of the urea cycle, has been associated with a generalized exfoliative erythroderma characterized by scaly, moist eroded patches and plaques.[43] The lesions are most prominent in the perioral area, in the perineum, and on the buttocks and lower abdomen. A similar rash occurring with neonatal citrullinemia has been noted to be localized to the

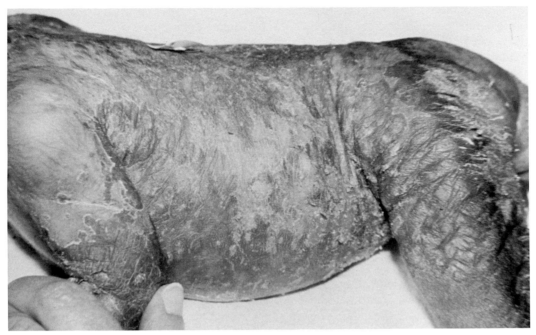

Fig. 12-5. Neonatal citrullinemia with moist eroded patches and generalized exfoliative erythroderma. (Courtesy of Orin M. Goldblum, M.D., Pittsburgh, PA.)

malar area, perineum, and buttocks.[44] Histologic features of the generalized eruption include parakeratosis with crust formation, absence of the stratum granulosum, pallor of the upper stratum spinosum, and mild perivascular mononuclear cell infiltration. The diagnosis is supported by high levels of ammonia and plasma citrulline due to diminished or absent argininosuccinic acid synthetase activity. Plasma arginine levels are low and the rash responds to arginine supplementation. Maple syrup urine disease, an autosomal recessive disorder of branched-chain amino acids, has been associated with an eruption similar to that of neonatal citrullinemia (Mary K. Spraker, M.D., personal communication). Patients have low plasma levels of isoleucine, an amino acid that is also decreased in neonatal citrullinemia.

Biotin Deficiency

The scaly, erythematous eruption and associated alopecia of biotin deficiency may occur in young infants as the result of *juvenile multiple carboxylase deficiency* (MCD) or of inadequate nutritional intake of biotin.[45–47] Although usually periorificial in location, the rash of biotin deficiency may be a generalized exfoliative eruption with accentuation at these sites.[48] Mucocutaneous candidiasis, chronic bacterial and viral infections, keratoconjunctivitis, ataxia, and hypotonia are associated features of juvenile MCD. Juvenile MCD is due to impaired absorption of biotin with dysfunction of the biotin-dependent enzymes of branched-chain amino acid metabolism, namely, β-methylcrotonyl CoA carboxylase, propionyl CoA carboxylase, and pyruvate carboxylase. The diagnosis of juvenile MCD is made by clinical features as well as by laboratory abnormalities, especially organic aciduria, ketonuria, lactic acidosis, hyperammonemia, and hypoglycemia. The rash clears rapidly when adequate biotin is administered.

The more localized eruption of biotin deficiency is commonly confused with acrodermatitis enteropathica and other conditions associated with zinc deficiency. Acrodermatitis enteropathica is an autosomal recessive disorder due to impaired absorption of zinc, with periorificial dermatitis, alopecia, diarrhea, listlessness, and candidal infections. The differentiation from MCD and biotin deficiency may be made by the low plasma levels of zinc and the rapid response to zinc supplementation. Ichthyosis, seborrheic dermatitis, and essential fatty acid deficiency must be considered in the differential diagnosis of infants with generalized exfoliative erythroderma due to biotin deficiency. *Essential fatty acid deficiency* is due to the inadequate intake or absorption (e.g., in cystic fibrosis) of dietary linoleic or linolenic acid and is characterized by generalized dryness, desquamation, and often erythema of the skin.[49,50] Alopecia, growth retardation, diarrhea, increased susceptibility to infections, and thrombocytopenia may be associated. The administration of essential fatty acids by oral, intravenous, or even percutaneous routes corrects the clinical abnormalities.

INFECTIONS

Both *staphylococcal scalded skin syndrome* (SSSS) (Fig. 12-6) and congenital candidiasis may manifest in infants and neonates as generalized erythroderma with scaling. The exfoliative condition characterizing SSSS is most common in young infants because of the diminished ability to excrete the responsible toxin produced by *Staphylococcus aureus* of certain phage groups.[51–53] Three phases occur: erythematous, exfoliative, and desquamative. Cutaneous erythema and tenderness initially develop periorificially and rapidly spread to involve the trunk and limbs. Exfoliation develops 1 to 2 days later, with yellow crusting around the mouth, eyes, umbilicus, perineum, and perianal area. After 2 to 3 days the skin begins to shed spontaneously or with light stroking (positive Nikolsky sign). The palms and soles are involved last. Affected infants are irritable but are often afebrile.

The diagnosis of SSSS is made by the typical clinical course and appearance of affected infants and the superficial blistering seen microscopically in the epidermal granular cell layer, which contrasts with the dermal-epidermal separation of TEN. *S. aureus* is usually recovered from the nasopharynx and occasionally from the conjunctivae and crusted areas of skin, but rarely from the blood or erythematous areas

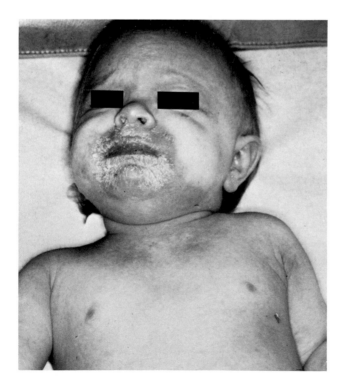

Fig. 12-6. Staphylococcal scalded skin syndrome with accentuation in the perioral area. (Courtesy of Roger W. Pearson, M.D., Rush-Presbyterian-St. Luke's Medical Center, Chicago.)

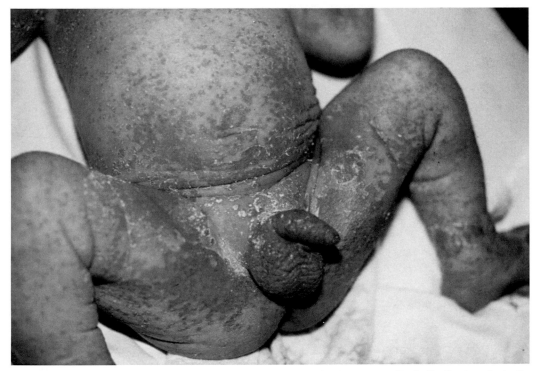

Fig. 12-7. Congenital candidiasis with scaly red papulopustules in a generalized distribution, including palms and soles.

of skin. Systemic antistaphylococcal antibiotics should be administered. Although the mortality is low, infants may have considerable loss of fluid and electrolytes. Systemic corticosteroids are contraindicated.

Cutaneous candidiasis in the young infant usually manifests as diaper dermatitis, with fiery erythema, scaling, and satellite papulovesicles in the diaper area. Occasionally, *congenital candidiasis* (Fig. 12-7) occurs, in which the lesions appear within a few days of birth, presumably from intrauterine exposure to candidal organisms.[54–58] The lesions of congenital candidiasis are found diffusely over the trunk, extremities, scalp, palms, and soles. The oral mucosa is usually not involved. The lesions begin as erythematous macules, which become papulopustules overlying bright erythema. Constitutional symptoms or signs of visceral involvement are extremely rare, and the papulopustules tend to clear spontaneously with residual desquamation in about a week.

Erythema toxicum, staphylococcal pustulosis, transient neonatal pustulosis, neonatal herpes simplex, congenital syphilis, and Letterer-Siwe disease are included in the differential diagnosis of congenital candidiasis and may be distinguished by smears and cultures of pustules and scales, as well as by associated clinical features. Although the eruption clears spontaneously, oral nystatin and topical anticandidal agents (nystatin, miconazole, clotrimazole) should be employed to decrease the number of candidal organisms.

TOXINS

Boric acid poisoning in neonates and young infants is characterized by generalized erythroderma, edema, and desquamation ("boiled lobster appearance"), with accentuation in periorificial and intertriginous sites. The diaper area may show vesiculopustular lesions and gangrene of the genitalia.[59] Other features include alopecia, fever, irritability, vomiting, diarrhea, and dehydration. Poisoning has occurred from sprinkling boric acid powder over the groin area

Table 12-2. Approach to the Patient: Evaluation of the Erythrodermic Infant

History
    Prenatal history
    Onset, course
    Associated abnormalities
    Drug, blood product administration
    Nutritional intake
    Family history

Physical Examination
    Extent of erythroderma
    Areas of accentuation
    Associated cutaneous changes (e.g., scalding, pustules, and crust)
    Hair abnormalities (e.g., trichorrhexis invaginata)
    Other congenital abnormalities

Laboratory Evaluation
Initial Examination
    Stains and cultures
        KOH, candidal
        Bacterial (*Staphylococcus*)
In-Depth Examination
    Skin biopsy
    For metabolic and toxic disorders
        Plasma, urinary amino acids and organic acids
        Levels of lactic acid, ammonia, glucose
        Blood and urine levels of boron
        Response to biotin, arginine, zinc supplementation
        Serum opsonization of yeast (Leiner's disease)

for diaper rash[60] and by the inadvertent addition of boric acid to infant formulas.[61,62] Boric acid poisoning is most easily confused with SSSS, and *S. aureus* may be cultured from skin because of the high frequency of secondary staphylococcal infection. In boric acid poisoning blood, urine, and tissue levels of boron are elevated. The most effective therapy is peritoneal dialysis.

APPROACH TO THE PATIENT

Given the extensive differential diagnosis of neonatal and infantile erythrodermas presented in this chapter, it is imperative that the clinician have an organized approach to the diagnosis of these conditions when the diagnosis is not immediately apparent. A simple approach to the patient is presented in Table 12-2.

REFERENCES

1. Craig JM, Goldsmith LA, Baden HP: An abnormality of keratin in the harlequin fetus. Pediatrics 46:437, 1970
2. Baden HP, Kubilius J, Rosenbaum K, Fletcher A: Keratinization in the harlequin fetus. Arch Dermatol 118:14, 1982
3. Buxman MM, Goodkin PE, Fahrenbach WH, Dimond RL: Harlequin ichthyosis with epidermal lipid abnormality. Arch Dermatol 115:189, 1979
4. Lawlor F, Peiris S: Harlequin fetus successfully treated with etretinate. Br J Dermatol 112:585, 1985
5. Lentz CL, Altman J: Lamellar ichthyosis: the natural course of collodion baby. Arch Dermatol 97:3, 1968
6. Larregue M, Bressieux JM, Fournet JP: Collodion baby. Mod Probl Paediatr 20:40, 1978
7. Reed W, Herwick RP, Harville D, et al: Lamellar ichthyosis of the newborn. Arch Dermatol 105:394, 1972
8. Williams ML, Elias PM: Genetically transmitted generalized disorders of cornification: The ichthyoses. p. 155. In Alper JC (ed): Genodermatoses. Dermatologic Clinics, Vol. 5. WB Saunders, Philadelphia, 1987
9. Rand RE, Baden HP: The ichthyoses—a review. J Am Acad Dermatol 8:285, 1983
10. Sybert VP, Dale BA, Holbrook KA: Ichthyosis vulgaris: identification of a defect in the synthesis of filaggrin correlated with an absence of keratohyaline granules. J Invest Dermatol 84:191, 1985
11. Greene SL, Muller SA: Netherton's syndrome: report of a case and review of the literature. J Am Acad Dermatol 13:329, 1985
12. Caputo R, Vanotti P, Bertani E: Netherton's syndrome in two adult brothers. Arch Dermatol 120:220, 1984
13. Porter PS, Starke JC: Netherton's syndrome. Arch Dis Child 43:319, 1968
14. Yeshudian P, Srinivas K: Ichthyosis with unusual hair shaft abnormalities. Br J Dermatol 96:199, 1977
15. Jorizzo JL, Crounse RG, Wheeler CE: Lamellar ichthyosis, dwarfism, mental retardation, and hair shaft abnormalities. J Am Acad Dermatol 2:309, 1980
16. Tay CH: Ichthyosiform erythroderma, hair shaft abnormalities, and mental and growth retardation. Arch Dermatol 104:4, 1971

17. Liden S, Jagell S: The Sjögren-Larsson syndrome. Int J Dermatol 23:247, 1984
18. Munke M, Kruse K, Goos M, et al: Genetic heterogeneity of the ichthyosis, hypogonadism, mental retardation and epilepsy syndrome. Eur J Pediatr 141:8, 1983
19. Senter TP, Jones KL, Sakati N, Nyhan WL: Atypical ichthyosiform erythroderma and congenital neurosensory deafness—a distinct syndrome. J Pediatr 92:68, 1978
20. Skinner BA, Griest MC, Norins AL: The keratitis, ichthyosis, and deafness (KID) syndrome. Arch Dermatol 117:285, 1981
21. Cram DL, Resneck JS, Jackson WB: A congenital ichthyosiform syndrome with deafness and keratitis. Arch Dermatol 115:467, 1979
22. Harms M, Gilardi S, Levy PM, Saurat JH: KID syndrome (keratitis, ichthyosis, and deafness) and chronic mucocutaneous candidiasis: case report and review of the literature. Pediatr Dermatol 2:1, 1984
23. Zunich J, Esterly NB, Holbrook KA, Kaye CI: Congenital migratory ichthyosiform dermatosis with neurologic and ophthalmologic abnormalities. Arch Dermatol 121:1149, 1985
24. Edidin DV, Esterly NB, Bamzai AK, Fretzin DF: Chondrodysplasia punctata. Arch Dermatol 113:1431, 1977
25. Zeligman I, Pomeranz J: Variations of congenital ichthyosiform erythroderma. Arch Dermatol 91:120, 1965
26. Curth HO, Macklin MT: Genetic basis of various types of ichthyosis in a family group. Am J Hum Genet 6:371, 1954
27. Giroux JM, Barbeau A: Erythrokeratodermia with ataxia. Arch Dermatol 106:183, 1972
28. Passwell JH, Goodman KM, Ziprkowski M, Cohen BE: Congenital ichthyosis, mental retardation, dwarfism and renal impairment: a new syndrome. Clin Genet 8:59, 1975
29. Rayner A, Lampert RP, Rennert OM: Familial ichthyosis, dwarfism, mental retardation, and renal disease. J Pediatr 92:766, 1978
30. Passwell JH, Zipperkowski L, Katznelson D, et al: A syndrome characterized by congenital ichthyosis with atrophy, mental retardation, dwarfism, and generalized aminoaciduria. J Pediatr 82:466, 1973
31. Levy SB, Goldsmith LA: The peeling skin syndrome. J Am Acad Dermatol 7:606, 1982
32. Hacham-Zadeh S, Holubar K: Skin peeling syndrome in a Kurdish family. Arch Dermatol 121:545, 1985
33. Miller ME, Koblenzer PJ: Leiner's disease and C_5 dysfunction. J Pediatr 80:879, 1972
34. Beylot C, Bioulac P, Grupper C, et al: Generalized pustular psoriasis in infants and children: report of 27 cases. p. 171. In Farber EM, Cox AJ (eds): Proceedings of the 2nd International Psoriasis Symposium. Yorke Medical Books, New York, 1976
35. Frost P, Van Scott EJ: Ichthyosiform dermatoses. Arch Dermatol 94:113, 1966
36. Scott RB, Surana R: Erythrodermic psoriasis in childhood. Am J Dis Child 116:218, 1968
37. Griffiths WAD: Pityriasis rubra pilaris. Clin Exp Dermatol 5:105, 1980
38. Gelmetti C, Schiuma AA, Cerri D, et al: Pityriasis rubra pilaris in childhood: a long-term study of 29 cases. Pediatr Dermatol 3:446, 1986
39. Parkman R, Mosier D, Umansky I, et al: Graft-versus-host disease after intrauterine and exchange transfusions for hemolytic disease of the newborn. N Engl J Med 290:359, 1974
40. McCarty JR, Raimer SS, Jarratt M: Toxic epidermal necrolysis from graft-versus-host disease. Am J Dis Child 132:282, 1978
41. Chudwin DS, Ammann AJ, Wara DW, et al: Posttransfusion syndrome. Am J Dis Child 136:612, 1982
42. Hawk RJ, Storer JS, Daum RS: Toxic epidermal necrolysis in a 6-week-old infant. Pediatr Dermatol 2:197, 1985
43. Goldblum OM, Brusilow SW, Maldonado YA, Farmer ER: Neonatal citrullinemia associated with cutaneous manifestations and arginine deficiency. J Am Acad Dermatol 14:321, 1986
44. Thoene J, Batshaw M, Spector E, et al: Neonatal citrullinemia: treatment with keto-analogues of essential amino acids. J Pediatr 90:218, 1977
45. Williams ML, Packman S, Cowan MJ: Alopecia and periorificial dermatitis in biotin-responsive multiple carboxylase deficiency. J Am Acad Dermatol 9:97, 1983
46. Kien CL, Kohler E, Goodman SI, et al: Biotin-responsive in vivo carboxylase deficiency in two siblings with secretory diarrhea receiving total parenteral nutrition. J Pediatr 99:546, 1981
47. Mock DM, Baswell DL, Baker H, et al: Biotin deficiency complicating parenteral alimentation: diagnosis, metabolic repercussions, and treatment. J Pediatr 106:762, 1985
48. Sweetman L, Surh L, Baker H, et al: Clinical and metabolic abnormalities in a boy with dietary deficiency of biotin. Pediatrics 68:553, 1981
49. Caldwell MD, Jonsson HT, Othersen HB: Es-

sential fatty acid deficiency in an infant receiving prolonged parenteral alimentation. J Pediatr 81:894, 1972

50. Friedman Z: Essential fatty acids revisited. Am J Dis Child 134:397, 1980
51. Elias PM, Fritsch P, Epstein EH: Staphylococcal scalded skin syndrome. Arch Dermatol 113:207, 1977
52. Faden HS, Burke JP, Glasgow LA, Everett JR: Nursery outbreak of scalded-skin syndrome. Am J Dis Child 130:265, 1976
53. Margileth AW: Scalded skin syndrome: diagnosis, differential diagnosis, and management in 42 children. South Med J 68:447, 1975
54. Chapel TA, Gagliardi C, Nichols W: Congenital cutaneous candidiasis. J Am Acad Dermatol 6:926, 1982
55. Rhatigan RM: Congenital cutaneous candidiasis. Am J Dis Child 116:545, 1968
56. Delaplane D, Wiringa KS, Shulman ST, Yogev R: Congenital mucocutaneous candidiasis fol-

lowing diagnostic amniocentesis. Am J Obstet Gynecol 147:342, 1983
57. Rudolph S, Tariq AA, Reale MR: Congenital cutaneous candidiasis. Arch Dermatol 113:1101, 1977
58. Kam LA, Giacoia GP: Congenital cutaneous candidiasis. Am J Dis Child 129:1216, 1975
59. Valdes-Dapena MA, Arey JB: Boric acid poisoning. J Pediatr 61:521, 1962
60. Baliah T, MacLeish H, Drummond KN: Acute boric acid poisoning: report of an infant successfully treated by peritoneal dialysis. Can Med Assoc J 101:166, 1969
61. Wong LC, Heimbach MD, Truskott DR, Duncan BD: Boric acid poisoning. Can Med Assoc J 90:1018, 1964
62. Rubenstein AD, Musher DM: Epidemic boric acid poisoning simulating staphylococcal toxic epidermal necrolysis of the newborn infant: Ritter's disease. J Pediatr 77:884, 1970

13

Ichthyosiform Dermatoses

Rhonda E. Rand

The ichthyoses include a varied group of conditions, which are usually inherited and are characterized by the presence of large amounts of scale. These disorders have been classified according to clinical appearance of the skin, mode of inheritance, histopathologic findings, laboratory data, and associated clinical features. Classically, there are four major ichthyoses: ichthyosis vulgaris, X-linked ichthyosis, lamellar ichthyosis, and epidermolytic hyperkeratosis (Table 13-1). However, in a recent report by Williams and Elias[1] lamellar ichthyosis has been divided into two separate entities, classic lamellar ichthyosis and congenital ichthyosiform erythroderma. In addition to these major ichthyoses there are a number of very rare ichthyoses, which will also be discussed (Table 13-2). Several ichthyosiform dermatoses are in the differential diagnosis of infantile erythrodermas, and neonatal aspects of these are discussed in detail in Chapter 12.

HISTORY

The term *ichthyosis* is from the Greek word *ichthys,* which means ''fish,'' and this name appropriately describes the fishlike scale characterizing many of these disorders. The ichthyoses have a distinctive appearance, and they have been recognized and recorded in history almost longer than any other skin disease. Over the past 2,000 years the literature has been sprinkled with many descriptive terms for this large group of related diseases. They were written about in the Charaku Sumhita, an ancient Indian comprehensive medical text dating from about 200 to 300 B.C.,[2] and in ancient Chinese literature people with these disorders were described as having skin like fish scales or snakeskin. Since the turn of the century many publications delineating a wide array of syndromes have emerged. It is the goal of this chapter to categorize and discuss the majority of these diseases.

MAJOR ICHTHYOSES

Ichthyosis Vulgaris

Ichthyosis vulgaris is the most common of the ichthyoses. The disease is dominantly inherited, affects males and females equally, and is estimated to occur in approximately 1 in 250 to 1 in 1,000 persons.[3,4] Frequently, there is a family history of dry skin or fishlike scales on the lower extremities. The majority of cases manifest between the ages of 3 months and 5 years.[3,5] It is important to note that this disease has a wide seasonal variation of appearance and that it may remit entirely in the humid summer months and yet become quite severe in the dry winter season. The scales of ichthyosis are characterized by small, fine, polygonal, whitish to

**Table 13-1. Approach to the Patient: Clinical and Histologic Features
of the Major Ichthyosiform Dermatoses**

Ichthyosis	Mode of Inheritance	Age of Onset	Clinical Appearance	Associated Features	Histology
Ichthyosis vulgaris	Autosomal dominant	Childhood	Fine, light scales; flexures spared; increased palmar and plantar markings; keratosis pilaris	Atopy	Decreased to absent granular layer
X-linked ichthyosis	X-linked recessive	Birth or infancy	Large, dark scales; lateral face and neck commonly involved; flexures variably involved; palms and soles normal	Corneal opacification; steroid sulfatase deficiency	Normal granular layer
Lamellar ichthyosis	Autosomal recessive	Birth	Large, thick scales; uniform, generalized involvement; flexures affected; hyperkeratotic palms and soles	Ectropion; prematurity common	Thickened granular layer
Epidermolytic hyperkeratosis	Autosomal dominant	Birth	Coarse, verrucous scales, particularly in flexures; bullae especially in infancy or childhood	Offensive odor; frequent cutaneous infections; prenatal diagnosis possible	Vacuolization of granular and malpighian layers

(Rand RE, Baden H: The ichthyoses—a review. J Am Acad Dermatol 8:285, 1983.)

translucent scales with turned-up margins resulting in the rough feel of the skin (Fig. 13-1). The extensor surfaces of the arms and legs are usually the skin areas on which the disease is most apparent, the axillae and antecubital and popliteal fossae frequently being spared. The palmar and plantar surfaces can have accentuated linear markings.[6] Keratosis pilaris is also often associated, as well as hay fever, eczema, asthma, or urticaria, and there have been published reports of eczema herpeticum[7] and eczema vaccinatum[8] occurring in ichthyosis vulgaris patients. The kinetics of this form of ichthyosis are normal.[9–11] Therefore it seems that perhaps an increased cohesiveness of the stratum corneum cells would in part explain the thickening of the horny layer.

Skin biopsy reveals mild to moderate hyperkeratosis with occasional parakeratosis (Fig. 13-2). A characteristic histologic finding is that the granular layer is very thin or missing.[12] There may be a slight perivascular and/or periappendageal lymphocytic infiltrate in the dermis.

The prognosis of this disease is really quite good, and some cases may show spontaneous improvement in later childhood or adult life. Treatment consists of emollients alone or containing urea (10 to 20 percent), salicylic acid (up to 6 percent), or lactic acid (up to 6 percent). Propylene glycol, 40 percent in water, is also helpful.[13]

X-Linked Ichthyosis

The distinction of X-linked ichthyosis from ichthyosis vulgaris was not made until 1966.[3,4] The former, as its name implies, is inherited in an X-linked pattern and usually manifests in the first few months of life. The scaling is most severe on extensor surfaces, but the flexural regions are usually involved as well. The sides of the neck and scalp are frequently affected, but in contrast to ichthyosis vulgaris the palms and soles are spared. These scales are also different in that they tend to be large and brown, the brown color being due to the oxidation of keratin (Fig. 13-3). The condition has been found to occur in 1 in 6,000 males[3] and can be identified by slit-lamp detection of corneal opacities on the posterior capsule of

Table 13-2. Approach to the Patient: Clinical Features of the Rare Ichthyoses

Ichthyosis	Mode of Inheritance	Age of Onset	Clinical Appearance	Associated Features
Erythrokeratodermia variabilis	Autosomal dominant	Several months to 3 years	Patches of erythema, plaques of erythema, hyperkeratosis	
Harlequin fetus	Autosomal recessive	Birth	Armor-like skin split by deep fissures into polygonal plates	Ectropion, rudimentary ears
Refsum's disease	Autosomal recessive	Childhood	Mild, variable ichthyosis	Polyneuritis, nerve deafness, retinitis pigmentosa; improves with dietary restriction of phytanic acid
Sjögren-Larsson syndrome	Autosomal recessive	Birth	Mild lamellar ichthyosis	Spastic paralysis, mental retardation, macular retinal degeneration
Rud's syndrome	Probable autosomal recessive	Infancy	Lamellar ichthyosis	Dwarfism, mental deficiency, hypogonadism, epilepsy
Ichthyosis linearis circumflex (Netherton's syndrome)	Unknown	Birth, infancy	Polycyclic eruption with hyperkeratotic margin, trichorrhexis invaginata	?atopy
Tay's syndrome	Autosomal recessive	Birth	Red, scaly skin, sparse hair, keratoderma of palms and soles, brittle hair	Close-set eyes, beaked nose, sunken cheeks
Conradi's disease	Autosomal recessive	Birth, infancy	Scaling of skin in whorl-like pattern, healing with atrophic lesions	Shortening of the humerus and femur, lens opacities, high-arched palate
CHILD syndrome	X-linked dominant	Birth to a few weeks	Unilateral ichthyosiform erythroderma	Congenital hemidysplasia; limb defects
KID syndrome	?	Infancy	Fine, dry scales, follicular hyperkeratotic spines, reticular hyperkeratosis of palms and soles	Vascularizing keratitis, neurosensory deafness
Acquired ichthyosis (associated with malignancy, sarcoid, lupus erythematosus, leprosy, malnutrition, AIDS)			Like ichthyosis vulgaris	
Drug-induced (triparanol, nicotinic acid, butyrophenones, dixyrazine)			Like ichthyosis vulgaris	

(Modified from Rand RE, Baden H: The ichthyoses—a review. J Am Acad Dermatol 8:285, 1983.)

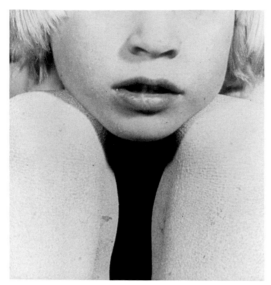

Fig. 13–1. Ichthyosis vulgaris. (Rand RE, Baden H: The ichthyoses—a review. J Am Acad Dermatol 8:285, 1983.)

Descemet's membrane of affected male patients and female carriers. However, these opacities are not usually present until the second or third decade of life,[14] and, most importantly, they

do not affect visual acuity. The kinetics of this disease are normal, as are those of ichthyosis vulgaris.

Light microscopic examination reveals a thickened stratum corneum and a normal to slightly thickened granular cell layer. There is acanthosis with prominent rete ridges, and there can be a slight perivascular lymphocytic infiltrate.[12,15]

The pathogenesis of this disease has recently been clearly defined. The enzymes aryl sulfatase C and steroid sulfatase are deficient in X-linked ichthyosis.[16–18] The microsomal enzyme steroid sulfatase removes sulfate from steroid sulfates. Placental steroid sulfatase deficiency and low serum and urine estriol were observed in women who were unable to normally initiate labor.[19] Shapiro et al noted that all the children that resulted from such pregnancies were males with ichthyosis, suggesting an X-linked recessive mode of inheritance.[20] Baden et al. have also found a steroid sulfatase deficiency in specimens of callous scale from these patients,[21] and steroid sulfatase has also been reported to be deficient in the leukocytes of patients with X-linked ichthyosis.[22] Epstein

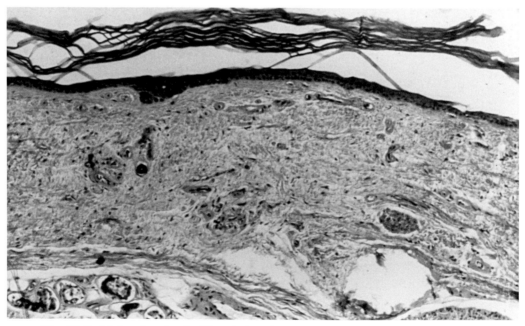

Fig. 13–2. Ichthyosis vulgaris. There is hyperkeratosis with a diminished granular layer.

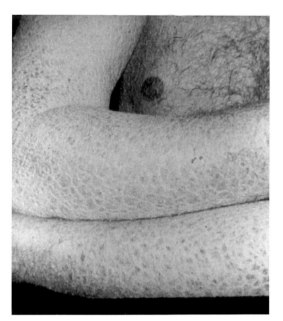

Fig. 13–3. X-linked ichthyosis. Large brown scales are characteristic. (Modified from Rand RE, Baden H: The ichthyoses—a review. J Am Acad Dermatol 8:285, 1983.)

Lamellar Ichthyosis

Lamellar ichthyosis has an estimated incidence of 1 per 300,000 births.[25] It has an autosomal recessive mode of inheritance and is usually apparent at birth. The newborn is frequently encased in a thick stratum corneum membrane called a *collodion membrane,* which is shed in approximately 2 weeks. The skin is erythematous, with large scales usually covering the entire body surface (Fig. 13-4). There may be severe hyperkeratosis of the palms and soles, and fissuring may be a major problem (Fig. 13-5). Around the large joints the skin may be verrucous, and there can be considerable shedding of scale due to the accelerated kinetics of this disease. Sweat glands are often obstructed, and frequently these patients may be heat intolerant with warm weather or exercise. The hair can be matted down with large scales, and a scarring alopecia can result from recurrent infection of the scalp. Ectropion is present in

and co-workers later showed an elevation of cholesterol sulfate in the sera of patients with X-linked ichthyosis[23] and also observed that their low-density lipoproteins (LDL) show greater mobility than the LDL of normals on lipoprotein electrophoresis. This can be explained by an increased negative charge on the LDL due to the large amount of cholesterol sulfate. Therefore lipoprotein electrophoresis is used as a diagnostic test in patients who cannot be diagnosed on clinical grounds.

The locus for X-linked ichthyosis is linked to the gene for steroid sulfatase and the X_g blood group on the short arm of the X chromosome.[24] This region of the chromosome is probably partially inactivated in female patients,[21] but it is unlikely that female carriers of X-linked ichthyosis can be reliably detected by assays of steroid sulfatase.

This disease is quite successfully treated by methods similar to those mentioned for ichthyosis vulgaris.

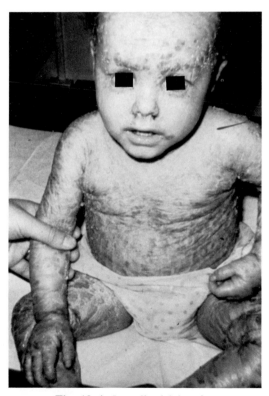

Fig. 13–4. Lamellar ichthyosis.

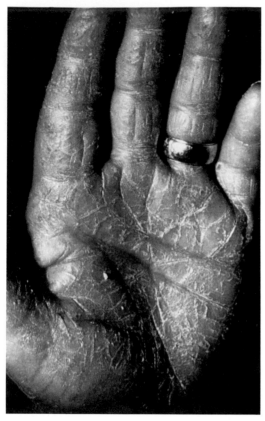

Fig. 13–5. Lamellar ichthyosis. There is hyperkeratosis of the palms and soles, with fissuring.

most patients and can be a diagnostic sign (Fig. 13-6). The nails may be normal or thick with ridges.

Light microscopic examination reveals hyperkeratosis with focal parakeratosis. The granular cell layer is normal to thickened, and there is acanthosis and some follicular plugging. There is often a patchy lymphocytic infiltrate in the upper dermis.[26]

Recently, lamellar ichthyosis has been divided into classic lamellar ichthyosis and nonbullous congenital ichthyosiform erythroderma (CIE).[1] Williams and Elias studied 18 patients who had been followed for treatment of autosomal recessive ichthyosis. These patients, the onset of whose disease reportedly occurred either at birth or shortly thereafter, demonstrated some degree of erythroderma, generalized cutaneous involvement including the flexures, and an absence of other histologic features found in other forms of ichthyosis. All these patients had been instructed not to use any topical treatment for 4 weeks prior to skin biopsy for lipid analysis. Autosomal recessive ichthyosis was then further classified into nonbullous CIE and classical lamellar ichthyosis on the basis of clinical, histopathologic, and biochemical characteristics. Twelve patients reported to have CIE were described as having fine white scales but were heterogeneous with respect to degree of

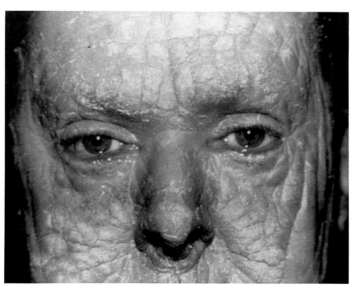

Fig. 13–6. Lamellar ichthyosis. There is extensive facial involvement and ectropion.

erythroderma, ectropion, and prognosis. In contrast, six patients with classical lamellar ichthyosis had large, dark, platelike scales, had severe ectropion, showed no improvement with age, and had minimal erythroderma. Histologically, the stratum corneum of patients with lamellar ichthyosis was two or three times thicker than that of CIE patients. The latter group demonstrated more acanthosis, parakeratosis, and hypergranulosis and less dilated capillaries. However, the most significant finding in Williams and Elias's study was the lipid biochemical evaluation. The percentage of scale lipid weight among the patients was the same as that in normal subjects; however, there was a clear abnormality of lipid distribution between the two patient groups. The patients with CIE demonstrated normal levels of sphingolipids and free sterols, but they expressed elevated amounts of hydrocarbons, namely, *n*-alkanes, in their stratum corneum lipids. Because the increase in amount of *n*-alkanes was accompanied by a corresponding decrease in the level of triglycerides and free fatty acids, it was hypothesized that the alkanes were derived from fatty acid metabolism. The authors further hypothesized that *n*-alkanes may possibly provoke the prominent erythroderma in CIE and also thought that either an overproduction of or a failure to metabolize the *n*-alkanes leads to their accumulation in the epidermis, which stimulates an increase in epidermal cell turnover. In a subsequent report by Hazell and Marks[27] these two diseases, classic lamellar ichthyosis and congenital ichthyosiform erythroderma, were again differentiated, but this time on the basis of labeling indexes using tritiated thymidine. It was found that the two entities could be distinguished on the basis of clinical, histologic, and cell-kinetic data.

Topical treatments for lamellar ichthyosis include treatments similar to those used for other ichthyoses, namely, urea, lactic and salicylic acids and propylene glycol. More importantly, however, this disease may be very successfully treated with oral retinoids, but the bony changes associated with long-term therapy must be considered.

Epidermolytic Hyperkeratosis

Epidermolytic hyperkeratosis, or bullous ichthyosiform erythroderma,[25] is an autosomal dominant disorder occurring with an incidence of 1 in 300,000. Superficial layers of the epidermis are partially sheared off by passage through the birth canal, resulting in skin that is moist, red, and tender at birth (Fig. 13-7). As the stratum corneum reforms, the skin becomes dry and scaly. Bullae, often localized to the legs, are present in childhood but occur only in about 20 percent of adults. The characteristic scales of epidermolytic hyperkeratosis are thick, brown, and often verrucous in areas of flexion over the knees and elbows (Fig. 13-8). Pyogenic infections are frequent, causing a distinc-

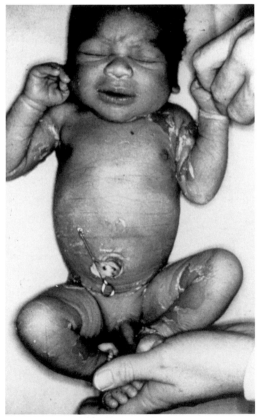

Fig. 13–7. Epidermolytic hyperkeratosis in a neonate. Superficial portions of the epidermis are sheared off during birth.

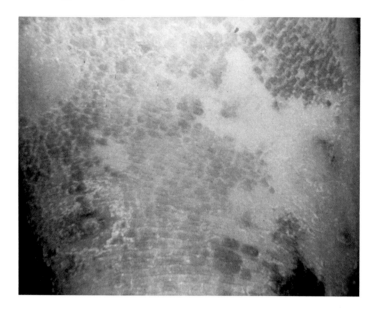

Fig. 13–8. Epidermolytic hyperkeratosis in an adult. There are characteristic thick brown verrucous scales.

tive odor in these patients. The entire skin is rarely involved in this ichthyosis, unlike lamellar ichthyosis.[9–11] The ''porcupine man'' appearance is a variant of epidermolytic hyperkeratosis in which the lesions have a heaped-up, ridgelike appearance resembling a porcupine.[28] The kinetics of this ichthyosis are also acceler-

ated, as they are with lamellar ichthyosis.[9–11]

Light microscopic findings are very characteristic in that there is a vacuolization of the granular and upper prickle cell layer with an increased number of large, very irregularly shaped keratohyalin granules and a thickened granular cell layer (Fig. 13-9). There is variable

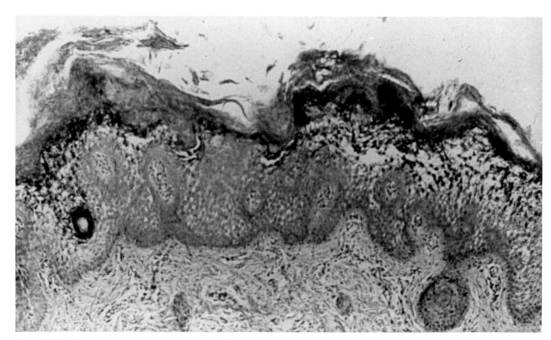

Fig. 13–9. Epidermolytic hyperkeratosis. There is marked vacuolization of cells in the middle and upper portions of the stratum malpighii, with large, irregularly shaped keratohyalin granules.

hyperkeratosis, papillomatosis, and acanthosis.[29]

Epidermolytic hyperkeratosis has been diagnosed prenatally by fetoscopy and fetal skin biopsy. The histologic pattern of the disorder has been demonstrated on fetal skin biopsy performed in the twentieth week of gestation.[30]

Topical treatment for this disease consists of lubricants and keratolytics. This ichthyosis has been successfully treated with oral retinoids. Topical and oral antibiotics are also of value, and sodium bicarbonate baths have been effective in controlling the odor of these patients.

RARE ICHTHYOSES

Erythrokeratodermia Variabilis

Erythrokeratodermia variabilis, first described by Mendes de Costa in 1925,[31] is a rare, autosomal dominant disorder and, as its name implies, has a variety of clinical manifestations. The onset of the lesions usually occurs within the first 3 years of life. There are two types of skin lesions: an erythematous plaque, which may be induced by stress or temperature change and tends to fade in hours or days, and a polycyclic or circinate erythematous hyperkeratotic plaque, which frequently occurs on the face, extremities, and/or buttocks (Fig. 13-10).[32–34] As with other ichthyoses, these lesions tend to improve in summer. It has been noted that women who are pregnant or are on oral contraceptives have an exacerbation of their disease.[33] There is no specific histologic appearance, but hyperkeratosis and irregular acanthosis are often present to a marked degree. There is variable dermal edema and cellular infiltrate. Tritiated thymidine studies show that this disease has a normal transit time.

Treatment of this disorder depends on the clinical manifestations. Topical steroids have been of some benefit. In addition, treatment with vitamin A or its derivatives offers improvement.

Harlequin Fetus

The harlequin fetus syndrome is the most severe form of ichthyosis and is inherited in an autosomal recessive fashion. The infant, often born very prematurely and with low birth weight (Fig. 13-11), is covered with very thick, armorlike skin, which is split into deep fissures shaped like polygonal plates, whence the name *harlequin*. The hands and feet are frequently covered with a very tight keratin encasement. Ectropion and eclabium are present, and the external ears may be very abnormal or even absent. Respiration is often mechanically restricted and infection is a frequent complication. Death usually occurs within the first few weeks after birth, although with the retinoid derivatives this may change. Fetal skin biopsy has also been helpful in prenatal diagnosis of this disease.[35] Light microscopy shows massive hyperkeratosis.

There is apparent heterogeneity in this disorder in view of the fact that the x-ray diffraction pattern and keratin polypeptide composition may vary in different cases.[36]

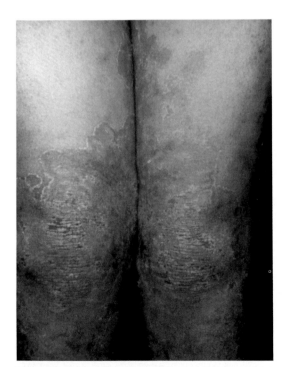

Fig. 13–10. Erythrokeratodermia variabilis. Polycyclic erythematous hyperkeratotic plaques occur on the extremities.

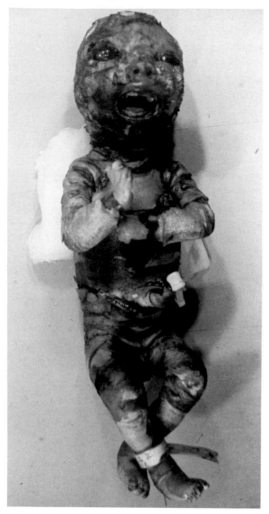

Fig. 13–11. Harlequin fetus.

Collodion Baby

The collodion baby syndrome is not a single genetic disease but the initial presentation of several syndromes. Clinically, the infant at birth is encased in a shiny brown-yellow membrane, which usually is shed by 2 weeks, but complete shedding may take up to several months (Fig. 13-12). Most affected infants will develop lamellar ichthyosis, lamellar exfoliation of the newborn, or one of the rare ichthyoses. In the entity *lamellar exfoliation of the newborn* the collodion membrane is shed and the patient has

a normal skin remaining and will not be affected by ichthyosis at a later time in life.[37] Therefore, in this entity there is spontaneous healing and a normal thickness of stratum corneum, but a basket weave is present and persists. Collodion infants should be treated by placing them in a high-humidity, temperature-controlled incubator. All greases should be avoided since they can increase skin infection. The membrane should not be removed, as to do so might cause scarring or increase the risk of infection.

Refsum's Disease

Refsum first described phytanic acid storage disease in 1946.[38] Subsequently, the biochemical defect was worked out by Klenk and

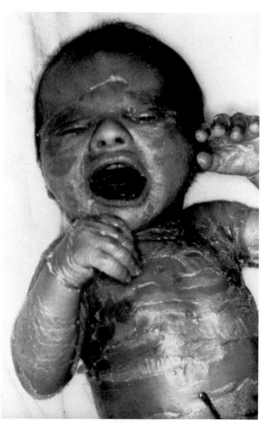

Fig. 13–12. Collodion baby. The neonate is encased in a collodion-like membrane. (Rand RE, Baden H: The ichthyoses—a review. J Am Acad Dermatol 8:285, 1983.)

Kahlke.[39] The actual defect is an accumulation of phytanic acid, a branched-chain fatty acid, resulting from a deficiency of α-phytanic acid α-hydroxylase.[40] The diagnosis can be made by finding excess phytanic acid in the triglyceride portion of the serum lipids.

This syndrome can be quite variable in its clinical presentation. Night blindness caused by atypical retinitis pigmentosa usually begins in childhood. Later, a peripheral neuropathy and cerebellar ataxia develop. Cataracts may also develop, further impeding vision. The skin resembles that seen in ichthyosis vulgaris. Histologically, as with ichthyosis vulgaris, there is hyperkeratosis, with a diminished granular cell layer.[41]

Most patients have a progressive course, with gradual deterioration; respiratory failure, in addition to fatal cardiac arrhythmias, is a frequent cause of death. The disease is inherited as an autosomal recessive trait. Prenatal diagnosis can be done by amniocentesis, with phytanic acid oxidation measured from cultured cells. Patients must reduce the amount of phytanic acid in their diet and must avoid rapid weight loss, as this will tend to raise blood levels of phytanic acid.

Ichthyoses Due to Drugs Affecting Lipid Metabolism

Nicotinic acid and triparanol have been reported to produce ichthyosiform skin changes. Dixyrazine, a phenothiazine tranquilizer, has also been found recently to cause an ichthyosis associated with hair loss, depigmentation of hair, and a blepharoconjunctivitis.[42] This drug lowers cholesterol by approximately 25 percent, and therefore it is postulated that the drug interferes with cholesterol synthesis.

Sjögren-Larsson Syndrome

In 1957 Sjögren and Larsson first described 28 patients with an autosomal recessively inherited syndrome characterized by an ichthyosiform erythroderma present at birth or appearing within the first few months of life.[43] The skin findings are similar to those of lamellar ichthyosis. Ectropion occasionally occurs. The scalp, palms, and soles are variably involved, and it seems that severe acral involvement is associated with a higher degree of mental retardation. The neurologic manifestations consist of mental retardation and spastic diplegia or quadriplegia.[44] Seizures, abnormalities of speech, and skeletal and dental anomalies have been noted as well as retinal changes. There is a specific form of macular degeneration that affects the retina.[43,45] Light microscopy reveals hyperkeratosis and a normal granular cell layer.

Rud's Syndrome

Rud's syndrome, first described in 1927,[46] has features of an ichthyosiform erythroderma, as well as acanthosis nigricans and hyperkeratosis and hyperhydrosis of the palms and soles. In addition, axillary and pubic hair are absent. The distinguishing features of Rud's syndrome are the dermatologic findings described above, hypogonadism, and mental retardation.[47] However, less frequent findings include seizures, short stature, and polyneuritis. Light microscopy shows hyperkeratosis, hypergranulosis, irregular acanthosis, and papillomatosis. The disease is probably inherited in an autosomal recessive fashion, but X-linked inheritance is also a possibility.

Ichthyosis Linearis Circumflex

In 1949 ichthyosis linearis circumflex (ILC) was described by Comel.[48] At birth or shortly thereafter patients were described as having generalized erythema and scaling, which subsequently fade. Later, there are polymorphic and serpiginous erythematous lesions bordered by a double-edged scale. These lesions occur on the trunk and proximal extremities (Fig. 13-13). The antecubital and popliteal fossae as well as the dorsa of the wrists are lichenified. The face

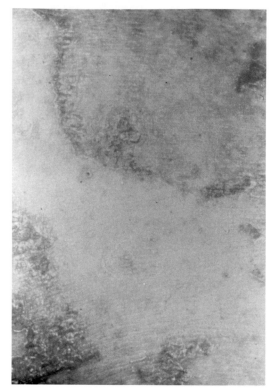

Fig. 13–13. Ichthyosis linearis circumflex. There are erythematous lesions with a serpiginous border and double-edged scale.

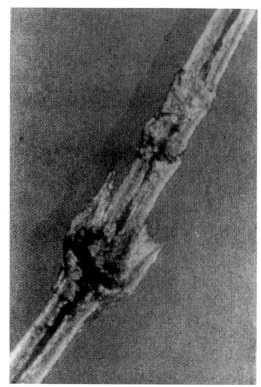

Fig. 13–14. Trichorrhexis invaginata (bamboo hair).

and eyelids are frequently involved. Some patients with ILC have a specific hair shaft abnormality, called *trichorrhexis invaginata* or *bamboo hair* (Fig. 13-14).[49–53] These abnormal hairs show swelling in which there is a ball-and-socket invagination into the shaft itself. The hairs tend to break at these nodal swellings. In addition, some patients may have trichorrhexis nodosa or pili torti. The association of ichthyosiform dermatosis and trichorrhexis invaginata is called Netherton's syndrome.[54] Inheritance of ILC is autosomal recessive, and the course is characterized by partial remission.

Tay's Syndrome

Tay's syndrome is characterized by diffuse red, scaling skin and short, sparse, brittle scalp hair. The palms and soles are hyperkeratotic

and fissured. Children with this condition have a progeria-like appearance due to the absence of subcutaneous fat. Other characteristic facial changes include close-set eyes, sparse eyebrows and eyelashes, beaked nose, sunken cheeks, receding chin, and batlike ears. Mental and growth retardation are associated features. Light microscopic examination shows hyperkeratosis and scattered parakeratosis with follicular plugging and a thin granular cell layer. There is moderate acanthosis, moderate papillomatosis, and a mild perivascular infiltrate. Hairs have pili torti- and trichorrhexis nodosa-like defects. This syndrome is probably inherited as an autosomal recessive trait.[55]

Chondrodysplasia Punctata

Conradi[56] first described chondrodysplasia punctata in 1914. The skin abnormalities in this disease are a thick white-yellow whorl of scales over the trunk and limbs on a background of erythematous skin (Fig. 13-15). There is hyperkeratosis of the palms and soles, but the hair and nails are normal. The associated systemic findings include punctate calcifications of the bone as well as on the tracheal and laryngeal cartilage. There can be shortening of the humerus and femur bones. Other abnormalities that may be present include flexion contractures of the large joints, congenital dysplasia of the hips, scoliosis, clubfoot, frontal bossing, syndactyly, short neck, saddle nose, craniosynostosis, high-arched palate, and micrognathia.[57] Cataracts may also be present, as well as optic atrophy.[58,59] In 1971 this disease was further categorized by Spranger into type 1, which is the Conradi-Hunermann syndrome, and type 2, the rhizomelic dwarf.

The Conradi-Hunermann variant is divided into three types: (1) patients who die early in infancy with small stature, low birth weight, and varying degrees of skeletal abnormality; (2) girls who have a very good prognosis, with moderate asymmetric skeletal involvement, occasional cataracts, and skin manifestations; and (3) children with mild symmetric epiphyseal changes without skin abnormalities or cataracts.[59] The histology of the skin shows marked hyperkeratosis and focal parakeratosis with invagination into the opening of the pilosebaceous units. In addition there is elongation of the rete ridges, with dilation of the dermal papillae. The dermis usually appears normal.

The Conradi-Hunermann syndrome has been associated with advanced paternal age. The inheritance pattern is probably autosomal dominant with the exception of group 2—girls with cataracts, skin manifestations, and a good prognosis—which is inherited as a sex-linked dominant disorder, most likely lethal in male individuals. The rhizomelic type is inherited in an autosomal recessive fashion.

The CHILD Syndrome

The name *CHILD syndrome* is an acronym coined by Happle and co-workers[60] for congenital *h*emidysplasia with *i*chthyosiform erythroderma and *l*imb *d*efects. This syndrome is characterized by a unilateral ichthyosiform dermatosis present at birth or within the first few weeks of life. The ipsilateral defects can vary from hypoplasia of a few fingers to complete absence of the limb. Occasionally there is ipsilateral hypoplasia of other parts of the skeleton, central nervous system, lung, kidney, and heart.

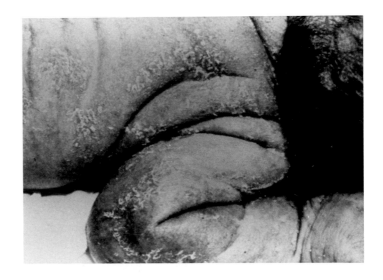

Fig. 13–15. Conradi's disease. There is a thick white-yellow whorl of scales overlying erythematous skin.

The KID Syndrome

An ichthyotic dermatitis has been described in association with keratitis and deafness.[61] The skin reveals mild scaling, with discrete erythematous plaques of the face, extremities, and trunk. There may be a variable verrucous appearance and exaggerated skin markings; other findings may include a scarring alopecia and dystrophic nails. The cornea scars as a result of a vascular keratitis. Histology shows a basket-weave hyperkeratosis, variable slight focal parakeratosis, and an inconsistent presence of a granular cell layer. There is variable acanthosis and papillomatosis.

Acquired Ichthyosis

Acquired ichthyosis is clinically and histologically similar to ichthyosis vulgaris but commences in adult life in association with several diseases. Most commonly, it occurs in association with lymphomas, especially Hodgkin's disease.[62–68] An acquired ichthyosis has also been described with multiple myeloma,[69] Kaposi's sarcoma,[71] leiomyosarcoma,[72] and carcinomas of the lung, breast, and cervix. The acquired ichthyosiform dermatoses usually improve with treatment of the underlying malignancy.[62,63] Most recently, acquired ichthyosis has been seen in association with the acquired immunodeficiency syndrome.[73]

COURSE AND PROGNOSIS

Serious medical problems due to these scaling disorders are not common, but psychiatric problems are not rare. These diseases are lifelong, and psychological counseling beginning in childhood may be beneficial. In addition, genetic counseling may be indicated for certain patients.

REFERENCES

1. Williams ML, Elias PM: Heterogeneity in autosomal recessive ichthyosis: clinical and biochemical differentiation of lamellar ichthyosis and nonbullous congenital ichthyosiform erythroderma. Arch Dermatol 121:477, 1985
2. Menon IA, Hoberman HF: Dermatological writings of ancient India. Med Hist 13:387, 1968
3. Wells RS, Kerr CB: Clinical features of autosomal dominant and sex-linked ichthyosis in an English population. Br Med J 1:947, 1966
4. Wells RS, Jenning MC: X-Linked ichthyosis and ichthyosis vulgaris. Clinical and genetic distinctions in a second series of families. JAMA 202:485, 1967
5. Ziprokowski L, Feinstein A: A survey of ichthyosis vulgaris in Israel. Br J Dermatol 86:1, 1972
6. Uehara M, Hayaski S: Hyperlinear palms association with ichthyosis and atopic dermatitis. Arch Dermatol 117:490, 1981
7. Verbov J, Munro DD, Miller A: Recurrent eczema herpeticum associated with ichthyosis vulgaris. Br J Dermatol 86:638, 1972
8. Verbov J, McCarthy K: Accidental vaccinia in an atopic and her ichthyotic sister. Lancet 8069:870, 1978
9. Frost P, Van Scott EJ: Ichthyosiform dermatoses. Classification based on anatomic and biometric observations. Arch Dermatol 94:113, 1966
10. Frost P, Weinstein GD, Van Scott EJ: The ichthyosiform dermatoses. II. Autoradiographic studies of epidermal proliferation. J Invest Dermatol 47:561, 1966
11. Frost P: Ichthyosiform dermatoses. J Invest Dermatol 60:541, 1973
12. Feinstein A, Ackerman AB, Ziprokowski L: Histology of autosomal dominant ichthyosis vulgaris and X-linked ichthyosis. Arch Dermatol 101:524, 1970
13. Rand RE, Baden H: The ichthyoses—a review. J Am Acad Dermatol 8:285, 1983
14. Jay B, Black RK, Wells RS: Ocular manifestations of ichthyosis. Br J Ophthalmol 52:217, 266, 1968
15. Lever WF, Schaumburg-Lever G: Congenital diseases (genodermatoses). In Histopathology of the Skin. JB Lippincott, Philadelphia, 1975 p. 59.
16. Shapiro LJ, Weiss E, Webster D, France JT: X-Linked ichthyosis due to steroid-sulfatase deficiency. Lancet 1:70, 1978
17. Shapiro LJ, Weiss R, Buxman MM, et al: Enzymatic basis of typical X-linked ichthyosis. Lancet 2:756, 1978
18. Kubilus J, Tarascio AJ, Baden HP: Steroid-sul-

fatase deficiency in sex-linked ichthyosis. Am J Hum Genet 31:50, 1979

19. France JT, Liggans GX: Placental sulfatase deficiency. J Clin Endocrinol Metab 29:138, 1969

20. Shapiro LJ, Cousins L, Fluharty AL, et al: Steroid sulfatase deficiency. Pediatr Res 11:894, 1977

21. Baden HP, Hooker PA, Kubilus J, Tarascio A: Sulfatase activity of keratinizing tissues in X-linked ichthyosis. Pediatr Res 14:1347, 1980

22. Epstein EH, Leventhal ME: Steroid sulfatase of human leukocytes and epidermis and the diagnosis of recessive X-linked ichthyosis. J Clin Invest 67:1257, 1981

23. Epstein E, Krauss RM, Shackleton CHL: X-Linked ichthyosis: increased blood cholesterol sulfate and electrophoretic mobility of low-density lipoprotein. Science 213:659, 1981

24. Race RR, Sanger R: Blood groups in man. Blackwell Scientific Publications, London, 1975

25. Baden HP: Ichthyosiform dermatoses. p. 252. in Fitzpatrick TB, Eisen AZ, Wolff K, et al (eds): Dermatology in General Medicine. Vol. 2. McGraw-Hill New York, 1979

26. Schnyder UW: Inherited ichthyoses. Arch Dermatol 102:240, 1970

27. Hazell M, Marks R: Clinical, histologic, and cell kinetic discriminants between lamellar ichthyosis and nonbullous congenital ichthyosiform erythroderma. Arch Dermatol 121:489, 1985

28. Goldsmith LA: The ichthyoses. Prog Med Genet 1:185, 1976

29. Ackerman AB: Histopathologic concept of epidermolytic hyperkeratosis. Arch Dermatol 102:253, 1970

30. Golbus MS, Sagebiel RW, Filly RA, et al: Prenatal diagnosis of congenital bullous ichthyosiform erythroderma (epidermolytic hyperkeratosis) by fetal skin biopsy. N Engl J Med 302:93, 1980

31. Mendes da Costa S: Erythrodermia and keratodermia variabilis in a mother and a daughter. Acta Derm Venereol (Stockh) 6:255, 1925

32. Cram DL: Erythrokeratoderma variabilis and variable circinate erythrokeratodermas. Arch Dermatol 101:68, 1970

33. Gewritzman GB, Winkler NW, Dobson RL: Erythrokeratodermia variabilis. A family study. Arch Dermatol 114:259, 1978

34. Hacham-Zadeh S, Even-Paz Z: Erythrokcratodermia variabilis in a Jewish Kurdish family. Clin Genet 13:404, 1978

35. Elias S, Mazur M, Sabbagha R, et al: Prenatal diagnosis of harlequin ichthyosis. Clin Genet 17:275, 1980

36. Baden HP, Kubilus J, Rosenbaum K, Fletcher A: Keratinization in the harlequin fetus. Arch Dermatol 118:14, 1982

37. Gosh TK: Collodion baby. Arch Dermatol 100:39, 1969

38. Refsum S: Heredopathia atactica polyneurotiformis. Acta Psychiatr Scand [Suppl] 38:1-303, 1946

39. Klenk E, Kahlke W: Über das Vorkommen der 3.7.11.15-Tetramethylhexadecansäure (Phytansaure) in den Cholesterinestern und anderen lipoid fraktionen der Organe bei einum Krankeitsfall unbekannter Genese (Verdacht auf heredopathia atactica polyneurotiformis—Refsum's syndrome) Hoppe Seylers Z Physiol Chem 333:133, 1963

40. Herndon JH Jr, Shenberg D, Uhlendorf BW, Fales HM: Refsum's disease: characterization of the enzyme defect in cell culture. J Clin Invest 48:1017, 1969

41. Blanchet-Bardon CL, Anton-Lamprecht I, Puissant A, Schnyder UW: Ultrastructural features of ichthyotic skin in Refsum's syndrome. p. 65. In Marks R, Dykes PJ (eds): The Ichthyoses. Spectrum Publications, New York, 1978

42. Poulsen J: Hair loss, depigmentation of hair, ichthyosis and blepharoconjunctivitis produced by dixyrazine. Acta Derm Venereol (Stockh) 61:85, 1981

43. Sjögren T, Larsson T: A clinical and genetic study of oligophrenia in combination with congenital ichthyosis and spastic disorders. Acta Psychiatr Scand [Suppl] 113:1–112, 1957

44. Wallis K, Kalushiner A: Oligophrenia in combination with congenital ichthyosis, spastic disorders and macular degeneration (Sjögren-Larsson syndrome). Ann Pediatr 194:114, 1960

45. Gilbert WR, Smith JL, Nyhan WL: The Sjögren-Larsson syndrome. Arch Ophthalmol 80:308, 1968

46. Rud E: Et tilfailde af infalisme med tetani, epilepsi, polyneuritis ichthyosis og anaemi af pernicious type. Hospitalstidende 70:525, 1927

47. Maldonado RR, Ramaijo L, Carnevale A: Neuro ichthyosis with hypogonadism (Rud's syndrome). Int J Dermatol 14:347, 1975

48. Comel M: Ichthyosis linearis circumflexa. Dermatologica 98:133, 1949

49. Altman J, Stroud J: Netherton's syndrome and ichthyosis linearis circumflexa. Arch Dermatol 100:550, 1969

50. Wilkinson RD, Curtis GH, Hawk WA: Netherton's disease. Arch Dermatol 89:106, 1964

51. Porter PS, Starke JC: Netherton's syndrome. Arch Dis Child 43:319, 1968

52. Julius CE, Keeran M: Netherton's syndrome in a male. Arch Dermatol 104:422, 1971

53. Hurwitz S, Kursch N, McGuire J: Reevaluation of ichthyosis and hair shaft abnormalities. Arch Dermatol 103:266, 1971

54. Netherton EW: A unique case of trichorrhexis nodosa—"bamboo hairs." Arch Dermatol 78:483, 1958

55. Tay CH: Ichthyosiform erythroderma, hair shaft abnormalities, and mental and growth retardation. Arch Dermatol 104:4, 1971

56. Conradi E: Vorzeitiges Aufreten von Knochen und eigenartigen Verkalkungskernen bei Chondrodystrophia fatalis hypoplastica: Histologische und Roentgenuntersuchungen. Johb Kinderheilk 80:86, 1914

57. Josephson BM, Oriatti MD: Chondrodystrophia calcificans congenita. Pediatrics 28:525, 1961

58. Edidnin DV, Esterly NB, Bamzai AK, Fretzin DI: Chondrodysplasia punctata Conradi-Hunermann syndrome. Arch Dermatol 113:1431, 1977

59. Spranger JW, Opitz JM, Biddler U: Heterogeneity of chondrodysplasia punctata. Hum Genet 11:190, 1971

60. Happle R, Koch H, Lanz W: The CHILD syndrome. Congenital hemidysplasia with ichthyosiform erythroderma and limb defects. Eur J Pediatr 134:27, 1980

61. Skinner BA, Greist MC, Norins AL: The keratitis, ichthyosis and deafness (KID) syndrome. Arch Dermatol 117:285, 1981

62. Ronchese F, Gates DC: Ichthyosiform atrophy of the skin in Hodgkin's disease. N Engl J Med 255:287, 1956

63. Glazebrook AJ, Tomaszewski W: Ichthyosiform atrophy of the skin in Hodgkin's disease: report of a case with reference to vitamin A metabolism. Arch Dermatol Syph 50:85, 1944

64. Welsh JL, Epstein E: Acquired ichthyosis in Hodgkin's disease: report of a case. JAMA 148:1221, 1952

65. Sneddon IB: Acquired ichthyosis in Hodgkin's disease. Br Med J 1:763, 1955

66. Stevanovic DV: Hodgkin's disease of the skin. Arch Dermatol 82:96, 1960

67. McCann SR, Barry DP, Temperley J, Weir PG: Ichthyosis and marrow involvement in malignant histiocytosis of the intestine. Br J Haematol 48:281, 1981

68. Cooper MF, Wilson PD, Hartop PJ, Shuster S: Acquired ichthyosis and impaired dermal lipogenesis in Hodgkin's disease. Br J Dermatol 102:689, 1980

69. Bluefarb SM: Cutaneous manifestations of multiple myeloma. Arch Dermatol 75:506, 1955

70. Flint GL, Flam M, Soter N: Acquired ichthyosis; a sign of nonlymphoproliferative malignant disorders. Arch Dermatol 111:1446, 1975

71. Kohn SR: A variant of ichthyosis. Arch Dermatol 112:1616, 1976

72. Majekodunmi AE, Femi-Pearse D: Ichthyosis: early manifestations of intestinal leiomyosarcoma. Br Med J 3:724, 1974

73. Kaplan MH, Sadick N, McNutt NS, et al: Dermatologic findings and manifestations of acquired immunodeficiency syndrome (AIDS). J Am Acad Dermatol 16:485, 1987

14

Alopecia in Children

David S. Orentreich
Norman Orentreich

For the most part children are subject to the same hair and scalp disorders as are adults (see Ch. 15 for the discussion of alopecia in adults). There are, however, such notable exceptions as cradle cap in the infant and male pattern baldness (androgenetic alopecia) of adulthood.

This chapter focuses on the pathogenesis of alopecia and develops the subject using the etiologic classification shown in Table 14-1.[1] Conditions that are prominently associated with alopecia in childhood are reviewed.

THE PHYSIOLOGY OF HAIR AND HAIR GROWTH

Hair is primarily composed of keratin, a specialized fibrous protein remarkable for its strength, elasticity, and relative resistance to chemical damage.[2]

The hair shaft itself is not a living structure but the protein end product of a very dynamic living structure, the hair follicle. The follicle is a down-pocketing from the epidermis, which differentiates from the epidermis between the third and fourth fetal months.[3] Living cells at the base of the follicle grow and divide rapidly, pushing a compact column out toward the surface of the skin. Directly above the area of active cell division is the zone of keratiniza-tion.[4] In this region, by a process of dehydration and chemical change, the living cells die and are converted into dense masses composed almost entirely of keratin. This complex process of cell growth, division, death, and chemical specialization requires the rich supply of oxygen and nutrients provided by the relatively dense capillary network that supplies the active base of the follicle.[5]

The dermal papilla, located directly beneath the mitotically active matrix area, plays a vital regulatory function in the control of the cycle of hair growth. With the rare exception of angora variants, there is a regular sequence of activity and rest in every hair follicle.[6,7] During the growth period, called the *anagen phase,* follicular cells are actively growing, dividing, and keratinizing, thus producing a growing hair. The follicle then undergoes a 10- to 14-day period of partial degeneration, termed the *catagen phase.* During the resting period, or *telogen phase,* the follicle is quiescent and hair growth temporarily ceases. The anagen phase for each scalp hair in human beings varies ordinarily from 2 to 5 years, or approximately 1,000 days, probably lasting somewhat longer for females and shorter for males. This phase is followed by the telogen phase of some 3 to 6 months' duration, during which the hair does not increase in length and the attachment of the hair

Table 14-1. Classification of Alopecia in Children

Congenital and inherited alopecia
    Aplasia cutis congenita
    Incontinentia pigmenti
    Leiner's disease
    Menke's kinky hair syndrome
    Oral-facial-digital syndrome I
    Hallerman-Streiff syndrome
    Marie Unna hypotrichosis
    Tay's syndrome
    Monilethrix
    Pili torti
    Pili annulati
    Trichorrhexis nodosa
    Trichorrhexis invaginata
Neoplastic alopecias
    Hemangioma
    Nevi
    Nevus sebaceus of Jadassohn
Acquired alopecias
    Traumatic alopecia
        Physical trauma
        Thermal, chemical, and radiation damage
    Hormonal factors
    Infectious alopecia
    Neurologic and psychiatric factors
        Trichotillomania
        Neurodermatitis
    Toxic alopecia
    Nutritional factors
Dermatologic alopecias
    Alopecia areata
    Keratosis pilaris atrophicans
    Alopecia mucinosa
    Other

to the base of the follicle becomes progressively weaker. Finally, as a result of ordinary wear and tear, its own weight, or a push from a new growing hair coming up under it, the old hair is shed.

Hair follicles are capable of producing three types of hair, namely, lanugo, vellus, and terminal. Lanugo hairs are normally seen only in fetal and neonatal life. They are fine, soft, unmedullated, and poorly pigmented and appear as a dense growth over the entire cutaneous surface of the fetal infant. The first hair coat of long lanugo is shed in the uterus approximately 1 month before birth at full term[8] but may cover the entire cutaneous surface of the newborn premature infant. The second coat of shorter lanugo, in all areas except the scalp, where the hair may be both longer and of larger caliber, is shed during the first 3 or 4 months of life, almost imperceptibly or as a wave termi-

nating in almost complete alopecia.[9] The more or less unsynchronized mosaic pattern of hair growth then becomes established. Lanugo hair is seen during postnatal life in the rare hereditary syndrome *hypertrichosis lanuginosa.*

Vellus hairs are fine, soft, short, hypopigmented, unmedullated, and almost invisible. They are seen on the arms and faces of children, the faces of most women, and the forehead and bald scalp of adult men. Terminal hair is relatively thick, coarse, long, often medullated, and usually pigmented. It is seen on normal scalp, eyebrows, eyelashes, and areas of secondary sexual hair distribution. Between classic vellus and terminal hairs lies a spectrum of subtypes. The duration of anagen relative to telogen determines whether a follicle produces a vellus or terminal hair and the length the hair shaft will attain. Some vellus hairs become terminal hairs, as in the development of a beard in adolescent males; terminal hairs may become vellus, as in male pattern balding.

The average human scalp has approximately 100,000 hairs, with slightly more in blonds and fewer in redheads. Roughly 90 percent of these hairs are in the anagen phase. Since hair grows approximately 1 inch in 3 months,[10,11] the daily production of scalp hair placed end to end would produce a single strand almost 100 ft long. With 100,000 hairs, of which approximately 90 percent are growing for 1,000 days, the average daily hair loss for normal individuals is about 100 hairs.

In many mammalian species a distinctly seasonal profuse shedding of hair is normal. In man shedding retains a seasonal pattern but occurs more gradually and is continuous rather than abrupt, with telogen and anagen hairs present in any given area.[12,13] In the north temperate zone, a natural increase in hair loss (telogen) occurs during the months of October, November, and December and a compensating decrease in hair loss during the months of April, May, and June.[13] The reverse holds true in the southern hemisphere.

The ratio between resting and growing hairs[6,7,14] can be an important diagnostic tool and is easily determined. Approximately 50 hairs are plucked from each posterolateral side of the patient's scalp. The 100 hairs are examined microscopically for the typical anagen and telogen root characteristics. Normal scalps show about 10 percent of the hairs to be in the telogen phase. A telogen count of much higher magnitude, for example 20 percent or more, indicates abnormal and excessive hair loss. Allowance must be made for a slight seasonal variation.

Where there is hair loss, either the living hair follicle or the keratinized hair shaft may be involved. When the dead hair shaft alone is affected, hair loss is temporary since the unaffected follicle continues to produce normal hair. If the living follicle is damaged or diseased but not destroyed, this may be followed by: (1) the immediate initiation of regrowth of hair (e.g., anagen effluvium), (2) the temporary failure to regrow a hair (e.g., telogen effluvium), or (3) the persistent inability to regrow hair (e.g., alopecia areata). However, if the follicle is destroyed (cicatricial alopecia), the resultant alopecia is always permanent since no regeneration of hair follicles takes place in postfetal life.[15,16]

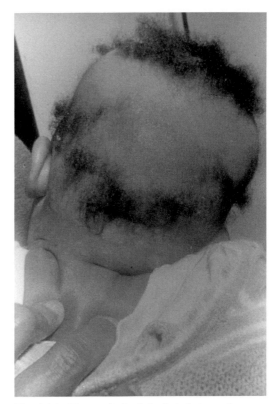

Fig. 14-1. Neonatal physiologic hair loss of unusually marked extent.

CONGENITAL AND INHERITED ALOPECIA AND HAIR SHAFT DEFECTS

A complete or partial absence of hair can be present from birth owing to aberrant differentiation of hair follicles.[17] This is completely different from the common hair loss in the newborn child (Fig. 14-1), which is no cause for alarm. This physiologic alopecia is spontaneous and temporary and is caused by the synchronous shedding of the telogen hairs that at birth constitute the majority of scalp hair.[18] Postnatal shedding is normally diffuse, but friction of the occiput (for example, from a pillow) can accelerate the shedding and produce a temporarily bald area. If the crib is situated so that the infant's head is constantly turned in one direction (attracted by the source of light, sound, or move-

ment), then the accentuation of the alopecia may be unilateral.

True Alopecia

True congenital alopecia (Fig. 14-2), in contrast to normal postnatal hair loss, is usually permanent although, rarely, some initiation of hair growth may occur at puberty. Congenital alopecia[17] can take the form of complete absence of hair, patches of alopecia (congenital triangular alopecia)[9] (Fig. 14-3), or simple sparse hair or hypotrichosis of a diffuse or patterned nature. Congenital alopecia may be associated with other congenital ectodermal anomalies, such as defective teeth, nails, or sweat glands, and even localized absence of skin covering.

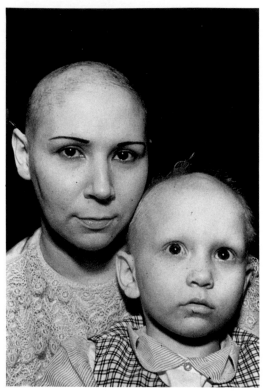

Fig. 14-2. Congenital alopecia in a mother and child, illustrating the hereditary nature of the defect. (Orentreich N: Disorders of the hair and scalp in childhood. Pediatr Clin North Am 18:953, 1971. Reprinted with permission of WB Saunders Co.)

APLASIA CUTIS CONGENITA

Aplasia cutis congenita is a rare, localized, congenital skin defect, which may involve only absence of skin appendages but usually involves absence of the epidermis, dermis, and subcutaneous tissues. Most cases are sporadic, whereas others show autosomal dominant inheritance.[19] There is a wide variation in extent and depth of lesions, ranging from trivial cosmetic disability to gross deformity incompatible with life. Aplasia cutis presents at birth as a variably shaped but sharply circumscribed ulcer, usually 1 to 3 cm in diameter, with a granulating base. Healing takes place gradually to leave an atrophic, smooth, alopecic scar. Over 60 percent of cases involve the scalp,[20] usually near the vertex; the remaining cases are located on the skin of the face, trunk, and extremities. Rare complications include erosion of the sagittal sinus with fatal hemorrhage,[21] meningitis, and other developmental defects.[9,22,23] Aplasia cutis congenita must be differentiated from forceps injury at birth, morphea, discoid lupus erythematosus, epidermal nevus, and nevus sebaceus. Control of infection until healing takes place is the primary concern early in life. If the defect is cosmetically unacceptable, correction by multiple punch graft transplants with or without scalp reduction is possible.

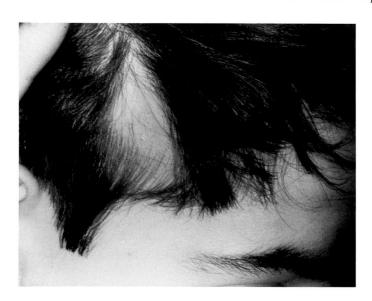

Fig. 14-3. Congenital alopecia limited to characteristic wedge-shaped frontal patch.

INCONTINENTIA PIGMENTI

Incontinentia pigmenti is a rare, probably X-linked dominant, trait, usually lethal in males. In about 90 percent of cases the skin changes are present at birth or develop within the first 2 weeks of life.[23] In patients showing the entire sequence of dermatologic changes, the disease may be classified into four stages: inflammatory, hypertrophic, pigmented, and involutionary. Incontinentia pigmenti is usually accompanied by neurologic, mental, bony, ocular, and other dermatologic changes. Cicatricial alopecia has been present in at least 25 percent of reported cases; it appears in early infancy and ceases to extend after a variable period of up to 2 years, but the loss of hair is, of course, permanent. Other hair defects present in some cases have been hypoplasia of the eyebrows and eyelashes and woolly hair nevus of the scalp.[24]

LEINER'S DISEASE

Leiner's disease has its onset during infancy and is characterized by severe diarrhea, failure to thrive, recurrent infections, and a severe, generalized dermatitis that resembles seborrheic dermatitis. The scalp is covered with thick, greasy, yellow crusts, and a patchy or total alopecia may present. Patients with Leiner's disease have dysfunctional complement component C5 and respond to dietary supplements of vitamin B complex, including biotin.[25]

MENKES' KINKY HAIR SYNDROME

Menkes' kinky hair syndrome (trichopoliodystrophy) is a rare, X-linked recessive, neurodegenerative disorder, which affects infant males and is usually fatal prior to 5 years of age.[26,27] Although originally thought to be a disorder of copper deficiency, it now appears to be a copper storage disease, with the observed defects resulting from inappropriate systemic copper distribution. Disorders in the metabolism of metallothionein, a metalloprotein involved in cellular copper transport, may be the primary defect in this syndrome.[28]

Hair present at birth is normal.[29] As this is shed, it is replaced by short, brittle, light-colored, dull, kinky hair, which stands on end and feels like steel wool. On microscopy the hair has the features of pili torti. Study of the hairs shows several different patterns of hair twisting.[30] Other less frequently reported hair abnormalities include monilethrix and trichorrhexis nodosa.

ORAL-FACIAL-DIGITAL SYNDROMES

Oral-facial-digital syndrome I is a rare, X-linked dominant disorder limited to females and lethal to males.[31] The syndrome is characterized by multiple oral and skeletal defects. There are numerous milia on the skin at birth, and the hair is coarse, lusterless, and brittle, varies in diameter, and shows many broken shafts. The hair is normal in oral-facial-digital syndrome II.

HALLERMAN-STREIFF SYNDROME

The Hallerman-Streiff syndrome (mandibulo-oculo-facial dyscephaly) is characterized by dwarfism, malformation of the skull, low-set ears, beaked nose, and mandibular hypoplasia, which combine to give the patient a birdlike profile. Also associated are microphthalmia, congenital cataracts, physical and mental retardation, frontal and parietal bossing, thin, small lips, and dental defects. Hypotrichosis occurs in practically all cases. The scalp hair may be normal at birth but soon becomes thin, diffusely sparse, brittle, and sometimes whitish, with frontal baldness and baldness of the lateral and posterior scalp margins. A more distinctive feature is the occurrence of baldness following the lines of the cranial sutures. Alopecia areata may occur. Eyebrows and eyelashes are scanty or absent, and pubic and axillary hair may be sparse. The skin of the face is atrophic, particularly in the central area, where telangiectasia may be marked; the subcutaneous veins may be conspicuously prominent.[9,23,32]

TRICHODYSPLASIA

Hereditary trichodysplasia (Marie-Unna hypotrichosis) is a rare, autosomal dominant disorder manifested by almost complete congenital absence of scalp hair, eyebrows, and eyelashes, decreased body hair, and widespread facial milia; otherwise, affected individuals are normal. In early childhood fine, sparse hair growth may occur, but the hair soon becomes coarse, flattened, or twisted. With the approach of puberty hair is progressively lost, particularly on the vertex and scalp margins. The ultimate extent of the scarring alopecia shows some variation, is often patchy, and tends to be more severe in males. Histologic examination reveals an abnormal proliferation of the internal root sheath in the region of the keratogenous zone. When examined under the dissecting microscope, abnormal hairs are seen as flat, twisted, and ribbonlike. Electron microscopic examination of hair may reveal peeling of the cuticle, increased interfibrillar cortical matrix, and intracellular fractures of the cuticular cells, cortical cell fibrils, and medullary cells. There is no effective treatment. The disorder has also been reported in association with Noonan's syndrome.[33]

TAY'S SYNDROME

In Tay's syndrome the hair of the scalp, eyebrows, and eyelashes is short, sparse, and brittle. Examination of the hairs reveals pili torti and trichorrhexis nodosa-like changes. These individuals are affected with diffuse, red, scaling skin; keratoderma of the palms and soles; and a progeria-like appearance with close-set eyes, beaked nose, and sunken cheeks.

Other Inherited Hair Shaft Defects

Monilethrix, pili torti, and pili annulati[34,35] are inherited defects involving abnormal hair shafts but not true alopecia.

MONILETHRIX

With monilethrix (Fig. 14-4) the child usually appears normal at birth but several months later develops brittle hair, which is rapidly broken to a short length. Under magnification the hair appears beaded. Monilethrix of the occiput and nape and occasionally other scalp areas is associated with follicular keratosis (horny follicular papules). Scalp involvement may be widespread or circumscribed, and the eyelashes, eyebrows, or pubic or axillary hair may occasionally be involved. Intermittent argininosuccinic aciduria has been reported in a few patients and suggests a possible related underlying metabolic disorder.

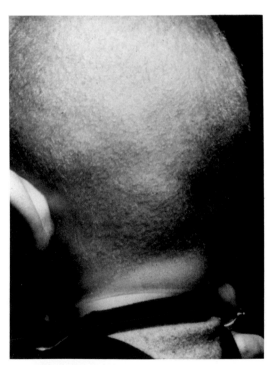

Fig. 14-4. Monilethrix showing hairs broken very short and marked follicular keratosis.

PILI TORTI AND ANNULATI

Pili torti is usually clinically evident by the second or third year of life and is characterized by sparse, brittle hairs broken short. It is more common in females and blonds and has been known to occur in conjunction with monilethrix. In pili torti the hair shimmers in reflected light since the inherited defect causes the hair to be flattened and twisted on its own long axis. Eyelash, eyebrow, pubic, and axillary hairs sometimes are also affected. Examination may reveal only stumps of broken hair. Pili torti is found in Björnstad's syndrome, Menkes's kinky hair syndrome, and in familial hypotrichosis of the Marie-Unna type.

Pili annulati is easily confused clinically with pili torti because in both the hair shimmers in reflected light and because pili annulati is sometimes associated with increased fragility and breakage of the hair shaft. Magnification distinguishes the two entities, showing pili annulati to have alternating dark and light bands. The condition, present in some or all of the scalp hair, may be evident at birth or manifest itself later in early childhood.

TRICHORRHEXIS DEFECTS

Trichorrhexis nodosa is the most common defect of the hair shaft. Trichorrhexis is best regarded as a distinctive response of the hair shaft to injury. If the degree or frequency of the injury is sufficient, it can be induced in normal hair. However, it is well established that congenital and hereditary defects of the hair shaft can predispose to trichorrhexis nodosa. It may occur in certain families as an apparently isolated defect or in association with abnormalities of the teeth and nails. Trichorrhexis nodosa is a feature of the rare metabolic defect argininosuccinic aciduria, in which it is associated with mental retardation. Gross examination of the hair reveals the presence of grayish white nodules (nodes), which microscopically show segmental longitudinal splitting of fibers without fracture, resembling two inter-locking brushes or brooms. If fracture occurs transversely through a node (trichoclasis), the end resembles a small paint brush. In the congenital or hereditary forms the hair is dry and lusterless. It breaks easily so that variable portions of the scalp show only short broken stumps.

In the much commoner acquired forms of trichorrhexis nodosa, trauma plays a proportionately larger role and the predisposing inadequacy of the shaft a proportionately smaller one.[36] Proximal trichorrhexis nodosa occurs in blacks, and distal trichorrhexis nodosa occurs mostly in whites and Orientals. The avoidance of all unnecessary trauma may be followed by marked improvement.

Trichorrhexis invaginata (bamboo hair) is a rare nodular defect caused by abnormal intussusception or telescope-like invagination along the hair shaft, which microscopically resembles the ball-and-cup joints of bamboo. It may involve all body hairs and clinically is characterized by dry, lusterless, brittle, sparse, and short hair. Trichorrhexis invaginata is associated with the rare, apparently autosomal recessive Netherton's syndrome (a combination of trichorrhexis invaginata, various forms of ichthyosis, and atopy).

The hair defect appears in infancy, and all hair is affected to some degree. Protecting the hair from excessive physical and chemical trauma may result in considerable cosmetic improvement. Although spontaneous remission of the hair defect can occur (generally between 6 and 15 years of age), many cases will persist into adulthood.[37]

NEOPLASTIC ALOPECIAS

Benign and malignant neoplasms[38] can produce hair loss by pressure, displacement, replacement, or systemic influences. Pressure on the overlying hair follicles from a pilar cyst (trichilemmal cyst or wen) of the scalp may produce temporary or permanent alopecia depending on the duration and degree of pressure (see Fig. 15-3, p. 309).

Hemangioma

The hemangioma, especially in its cavernous form, is a common form of benign neoplasm producing alopecia in children. Since most cavernous hemangiomas spontaneously involute in childhood, the most difficult problem is to convince the parents to allow observation without treatment. Hemangiomas may continue to enlarge with the growth of the child and are proportionately alarming. Photographing the site at intervals with careful measurement procedures and regular 3- to 6-month checkups is the usual way to restrain the parents from precipitating unnecessary and possibly detrimental treatment. The best cosmetic results are usually accomplished by spontaneous involution rather than by such techniques as cryotherapy, electrodesiccation, surgery, sclerosing solutions, or ionizing radiation. However, treatment may ultimately be required if the rate of growth of the hemangioma greatly and persistently exceeds that of the child; if the bulk of the lesion impinges on a vital anatomic site; or if a Kasabach-Merritt syndrome (thrombocytopenia and disseminated intravascular coagulation) results. After the hemangioma has involuted, the site of residual alopecia may be filled in with transplanted hair-bearing scalp plugs.

The nevus flammeus nuchae (Unna's nevus), in its simplest and most frequent form seen on the nape of the neck and the occiput, is not associated with any hair loss. Hemangiomas of this type may disappear spontaneously; only a small percentage persist throughout life.

Epithelial Nevi

Epithelial nevi are not infrequently seen in children. Verrucous, sebaceous, and apocrine nevi are the more common types. They usually appear at birth or in infancy or early childhood and are characterized by partial or complete hair loss at the site. Melanocytic nevi, on the contrary, tend to have abnormally coarse and dense hair at the site.

Nevus Sebaceus of Jadassohn

The nevus sebaceus of Jadassohn is an organoid nevus (hamartoma) of epidermis, dermis, and epidermal appendages, particularly sebaceous glands. It occurs most commonly near the vertex of the scalp and may occasionally involve the face and periorbital skin. The lesion is a sharply circumscribed, yellow-orange-brown, alopecic, verrucous, round, oval, or linear plaque, which may vary in size from a few millimeters to several centimeters. The hamartoma is generally solitary, but multiple and extensive lesions have been reported.[39] Nevus sebaceus is present at birth or appears shortly thereafter and becomes more verrucous, raised, thickened, or nodular with puberty. It affects both sexes and all races equally.

The histopathology of this disorder depends on its stage of development, i.e., infantile or adolescent, and whether or not there is an associated neoplasm. Beginning with puberty and during adulthood, various types of cutaneous tumors develop secondarily within lesions of nevus sebaceus. In order of frequency these include: basal cell carcinoma (approximately 10 percent), syringocystadenoma papilliferum, squamous cell carcinoma, keratoacanthoma, nodular hidradenoma, apocrine cystadenoma, syringoma, sebaceous epithelioma, and apocrine carcinoma. Associated ocular malformations and external oculomotor nerve dysfunction have been reported.[40,41]

In young individuals the clinical differential diagnosis includes juvenile xanthogranuloma, solitary mastocytoma, xanthoma, juvenile melanoma (Spitz nevus), pilomatricoma, and nevus unius lateralis. The likelihood of recurrence and the residual bald scar after electrodesiccation and curettage make full-thickness surgical excision more acceptable and the treatment of choice. Excision is recommended prior to puberty before the sebaceous elements enlarge and malignancy develops.

A number of other benign or malignant tumors can uncommonly give rise to localized areas of alopecia. In children multiple bluish red nodules, which may be devoid of hair, may be indicative of leukemia.

ACQUIRED ALOPECIAS

Acquired alopecias may be of several types: traumatic, hormonal, infectious, neurologic, psychiatric, nutritional, metabolic, related to poisons or drugs, or strictly dermatologic.

Traumatic Alopecia

Traumatic alopecias can be caused by physical, chemical, or radiation damage. The attachment of an electrode to the scalp for monitoring the fetal heartbeat during labor may occasionally cause some superficial damage to the scalp, and, particularly if secondary infection supervenes, this may be followed by a small alopecic scar. Aplasia cutis has sometimes been mistaken for such a lesion.[42] Aplasia cutis may also be falsely attributed to a forceps injury at childbirth.[9] An unusual case of cicatricial alopecia in a boy aged 13 was due to injury to the scalp by an intravenous infusion given in infancy for gastroenteritis.[43] Exceptionally, self-inflicted injuries may involve the scalp and may leave scars.

PHYSICAL TRAUMA

Physical trauma from acute traction by plucking, combing, or brushing can cause breakage of the hair shaft or evulsion from the follicle. Breaking of the shaft does not interfere with continuity of growth. Evulsion usually produces a temporary cessation of hair growth. A plucked anagen hair enters into the telogen phase. Nevertheless, for every 100 hairs plucked, one dermal papilla is epilated, producing permanent alopecia for that follicle. Combing and brushing only for grooming purposes is acceptable. The comb should be wide-toothed and the brush loosely bristled so that neither forcibly pulls

out or breaks the hair. There is no therapeutic value in brushing the hair beyond the necessity of grooming. The "100 brush strokes a day" practice, alleged to increase the blood supply to the scalp and promote hair growth, is actually detrimental, putting undue and unnatural strain on the hair shaft and its attachment. Excessive or improper brushing or combing can induce trichorrhexis nodosa and fracture of the shaft. This condition can also be caused by heat, bleaches, and other chemicals or by the friction of rubbing an area of lichen simplex chronicus.

It is not uncommon to see a child who in play or "combat" has had a hank of hair pulled from the scalp. This produces particular alarm when hairs fail to regrow over a period of weeks. Regrowth is delayed because it takes approximately 3 months for the follicles of forcibly epilated or evulsed anagen hairs to return to the growing phase.

Chronic traction by tight ponytails, cornrows, braids, curlers, barrettes, hair pins, headbands, or rubber bands can cause hair loss at the site(s) of tension. Alopecia is temporary if the traction is not prolonged; however, permanent follicular destruction by avascular necrosis can result from prolonged traction.

Avulsion, or the forcible tearing off of scalp tissue, can cause not only loss of the hair-bearing follicles and thus permanent alopecia but also injury to the skull. If the site is small, immediate replacement of the avulsed skin may be successful. When doing such autografting,[44-46] if the aponeurosis and subcutaneous fat are trimmed with care so as not to damage the hair follicles, this will increase the probability of the autograft's viability and ability to regrow hair. Regrowth of hair from the graft may be partial or complete.

Prompt microvascular anastomosis of an entire avulsed scalp can prevent avascular scalp necrosis and permanent alopecia. Laceration may cause permanent alopecia at the site of injury if there is scarring. Punch autografts are a suitable therapy for acquired traumatic alopecia and scars of the scalp.

Friction can cause breakage of the hair shaft

close to the scalp in addition to producing trichorrhexis nodosa. Physiologic neonatal alopecia is often enhanced by friction of the head against the pillow or crib. Occupational or recreational sports headgear can cause hair shaft breakage close to the scalp. The condition invariably improves after removal of the eliciting agent. Lichen simplex chronicus (neurodermatitis) can produce a self-inflicted frictional alopecia. Physical pressure factors may be internal or external; either type produces possible hair loss.

THERMAL, CHEMICAL, AND RADIATION DAMAGE

Electric burns that are severe enough to destroy hair follicles produce permanent scarring hair loss in the affected area. Thermal trauma—burns from fire or scalding liquids—are not infrequent in children. With deep damage, hair loss will be permanent.[46] Extreme cold can also cause destruction of hair follicles. Caustic chemicals may accidentally come into contact with the scalp of the child. Only if their action destroys the follicle-bearing tissue will there be permanent hair loss.

Hair cosmetics[47] are now more frequently used by preadolescents than in previous generations. They may contain the following chemicals: thioglycolates in cold-wave permanent wave preparations, used with oxidizing agents to control their action; strong alkalies, such as sodium and barium hydroxide, ammonia, triethanolamine, or monethanolamine in hair straighteners, with formalin or permanganate as fixatives; hydrogen peroxide in bleaches; vegetable dyes, such as henna, rhubarb root, nut galls, chamomile, and indigo; metallic hair dyes of silver, copper, iron, and lead (these have been reported to cause systemic poisoning); synthetic organic dyes, such as those based on paraphenylenediamine, used with an oxidizing agent such as hydrogen peroxide or sodium perborate to form the dye; soap and detergent shampoos; and gum resins and lacquers in hair sprays and dressings.

All chemicals usually affect the hair shaft—some beneficially, others detrimentally—causing fragilitas crinium (abnormal brittleness of the hair shaft) and breakage. A chemical allergen may cause eczematous contact dermatitis without affecting hair growth since the scalp is relatively resistant to chemical trauma. The glabrous skin adjacent to or even distant from the scalp is frequently more severely involved than the scalp itself. However, a severe acute chemical dermatitis may cause temporary hair loss. Only the severest primary irritation or secondary bacterial infection with cicatrization of the damaged areas can explain the permanent alopecia that is seen on such rare occasions.

In practice true allergic reactions interfering with hair growth are quite rare. More commonly the misuse of a product by improper compounding or application is responsible for the reaction and hair damage. Many innocuous procedures, such as shampooing, are often falsely accused of having harmful effects. Shampooing is a safe, effective means of cleaning the hair and controlling dandruff. Frequent, even daily, shampooing is generally not harmful to hair or hair growth. It should be noted, however, that there is a natural increase in shedding of hair immediately following a shampoo because the physical massage eases out the already loose telogen hairs that would have been shed the following day. On the day of shampooing total hair loss may be 150 instead of 100, while on the day after, the loss may be about 50 hairs.

Exposure to x-rays, radium, radioisotopes, atomic explosions, or radiation accidents can produce either temporary or permanent baldness. In temporary alopecia from radiation, the follicles are thrown into a period of inactivity. After 3 to 5 weeks the hair loss is almost complete; however, after about 10 weeks a new anagen phase begins. When radiation destroys the more resistant dermal papilla (more than 1,500 rads of a single dose of superficial x-rays with a half-value layer of 0.9 mm Al or more), alopecia is permanent. The same degree of radiation that produces permanent alopecia will also invariably produce some degree of radiodermatitis and an increased predisposition

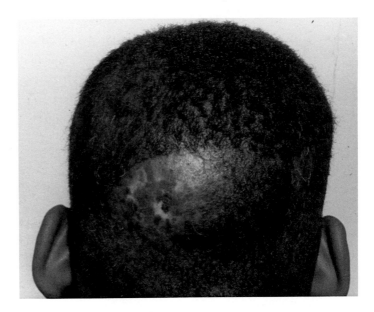

Fig. 14-5. Permanent alopecia 2 years after x-ray epilation, showing radiodermatitis.

to skin cancers; there is no safe permanent epilating dose (Fig. 14-5).

Hormonal Factors

Hormonal factors may be involved in acquired alopecias. The most common form of hair loss in adult life is androgenetic alopecia (AGA), in which each hair follicle is genetically predisposed to respond or not to respond to androgenic and other hormonal influences that either inhibit or stimulate the follicle's production of hair.[14] Male pattern baldness is the most prevalent example of a hereditary predisposition to hair loss precipitated by androgens. In the female scalp AGA usually manifests itself in a diffuse manner but sometimes with patterned features. A form of AGA can occur in late childhood: with adrenarche (sometimes even before but certainly with pubarche) the body can produce enough androgens to cause temporary AGA.

The following endocrinopathies can produce alopecia or hirsutism: thyroid dysfunction, pituitary dysfunction, hypoparathyroidism, hypocorticoidism, diffuse adrenocortical hyperplasia, benign or malignant androgenic adrenocortical tumors, adrenogenital syndrome, and benign and malignant androgenic ovarian tumors. Occasionally these conditions can be helped by surgery or appropriate hormonal adjustment, but hair regrowth may not occur for many months after surgery or institution of appropriate drug therapy. In some cases, such as the adrenogenital syndrome, correction of the hormonal imbalance will only prevent further hair loss without restoring already lost hair.

Infectious Alopecia

Localized infection[38] of a superficial nature rarely causes permanent hair loss although it can damage the scalp. With impetigo, for example, hairs become encrusted, fall out with the crusts, but regrow. Deeper infection, such as ecthyma, can cause temporary hair loss due to breakage of the hair shaft or direct involvement of the follicles. If the follicle is destroyed, scarring is produced and the alopecia is permanent. Organisms that affect the follicle and can cause alopecia include viruses (such as herpes simplex, zoster, varicella, and variola) and bacteria (such as tuberculosis, leprosy, and pyogenic organisms). The follicles can also be destroyed in folliculitis decalvans and in acne varioliformis (acne necrotica), although these disorders

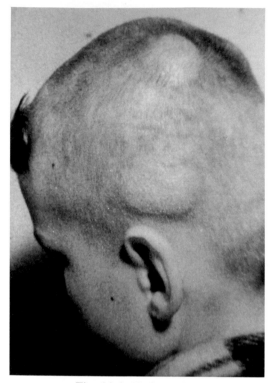

Fig. 14-6. Kerion celsi.

are rarely seen in childhood. Fungi that produce tinea capitis usually cause temporary hair loss due to breakage of the involved hair shaft, but particular fungal infections such as favus may destroy the follicles. Kerion (Fig. 14-6) may produce permanent hair loss. The treatment of choice for tinea capitis is adequate doses of griseofulvin administered orally until the culture and Wood's light fluorescence are negative. Oral corticosteroids may be indicated to reduce destructive inflammation.

Hair loss of the telogen effluvium variety has been noted, beginning about 10 weeks after systemic infections producing high fever. The following systemic infections can be associated with postfebrile temporary hair loss: viral, such as measles and influenza; bacterial, such as typhoid, scarlet fever, erysipelas, and pneumonia; treponemal; yeast; and protozoal. Extended periods of high fever can produce *Beau's lines* on the nails, which can be diagnostically help-

ful. A corresponding narrowing of the hair shaft is called the *Pohl-Pinkus mark*.

Neurologic and Psychiatric Factors

Contrary to popular opinion, there is little evidence that neurogenic and psychogenic factors directly influence the hair follicle. However, psychiatric factors in hair loss are very frequently overlooked.

TRICHOTILLOMANIA

Trichotillomania is the most commonly misdiagnosed cause of alopecia, both in children and adults. Trichotillomania (hair pulling tic)[48,49] is the preconscious pulling out of hair by the patient and may be patterned or diffuse (Fig. 14-7). Scalp hair and occasionally eyelashes and eyebrows are the areas attacked.[50]

Self-inflicted hair loss can be brought about by hair pulling, rubbing, twisting, cutting, shaving, sucking, biting, mutilating with a comb, brush, or other instrument, or applying noxious substances. Indeed, these activities are not always self-inflicted but may be performed by a "partner in neurosis."[51]

Trichotillomania can be associated with trichocryptomania (hiding of the hairs so removed) or trichophagy (swallowing of the hairs) with the possibility of trichobezoar formation. A bizarre configuration of hair loss in trichotillomania will often engender suspicion if not outright diagnosis on the part of the clinician. Trichotillomania appears clinically as irregularly shaped, partially alopecic areas containing hairs broken off at different lengths. The involved areas may show erythema, edema, and postinflammatory hyperpigmentation. Persistent, localized hair loss of prolonged duration (approximately 1 year) accompanied by onychophagia in a young female favor a diagnosis of the self-inflicted neurotic manifestation called trichotillomania.[52] A critical diagnostic aid is the painting of a small affected area with collodion or other occlusive (sometimes su-

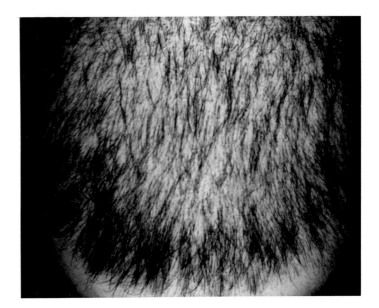

Fig. **14-7** Trichotillomania, showing a diffuse pattern.

tured) dressing.[53] When the protected area is examined 2 weeks later and hair growth is present, the diagnosis of trichotillomania is confirmed (Fig. 14-8).

If trichotillomania is stopped soon enough, no permanent hair loss occurs. However, prolonged trichotillomania may result in permanent hair loss. In children 4 to 10 years of age the phenomenon is usually simply a nervous tic of pulling or twisting the hair about the fingers. Hair loss is usually limited to one or two small areas, frequently near the temples. Such children tend to be nervous and under emotional stress. They are not aware of their tic, which frequently occurs when the child is preoccupied with something else, such as reading or watching television. Generally, bringing the habit to the attention of the child and reassuring him is enough to stop the tic, especially if some of the aggravating stress is removed.

In older children, especially females, trichotillomania is usually associated with neurosis and requires psychiatric help. There is considerable, sometimes persistent, denial of the self-inflicted hair loss, which is more extensive in scope for this older group, the entire scalp being epilated occasionally (Fig. 14-8). Psychiatrists have found that the family constellation of older children with trichotillomania is usually malev-

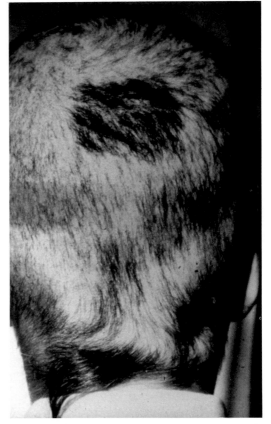

Fig. 14-8. Positive test results from trichotillomania occlusion test on a totally epilated scalp.

olent, including power struggles and psychological torture. Mothers tend to be aggressive, fathers relatively passive. Strong feelings on the part of one or both parents regarding hairstyle of the child is common.[48]

NEURODERMATITIS

Neurodermatitis[53] (lichen simplex chronicus) is not uncommonly seen, especially in retarded children. Scratching or rubbing of an area and the resultant hair breakage can produce temporary localized alopecia. On the other hand, repeated rubbing or biting of an area can occasionally produce localized hypertrichosis, also not infrequently seen in retarded children.[54]

Toxic Alopecia

Many organic and inorganic chemicals entering the system by inhalation, injection, ingestion, or transepidermally may affect hair growth and produce toxic alopecia. Such alopecia may be divided into two groups: toxic nonspecific chemical alopecia and toxic follicle-specific chemical alopecia. The nonspecific type may be caused by heavy metals such as lead, arsenic and related compounds, potassium thiocyanate, quinacrine (Atabrine), quinine, ethyl carbamate, and the general anesthetic agents. Follicle-specific toxic alopecia can be caused by antineoplastic compounds, such as cyclophosphamide; folic acid antagonists, such as aminopterin and methotrexate; radiomimetic chemicals, such as nitrogen mustard; thallium; unsaturated lipid-soluble compounds, such as chlorothene (chlorobutadiene); substituted amino acids, such as leucenol; vitamin A in high doses; 13-cis-retinoic acid; and androgenic compounds in genetically predisposed individuals. Baldness produced by the above compounds is not likely to be permanent.

Nutritional Factors

Nutritional deprivation must be relatively severe to produce hair loss, as in kwashiorkor, sprue, or celiac disease. The common alopecias are not associated with nutritional deficiencies, but anemia, hypervitaminosis A, or hypovitaminosis A may be factors in producing alopecia.

Protein-calorie malnutrition is characterized by a spectrum of conditions from the relatively mild state of growth retardation to the extremes of marasmus and kwashiorkor.[55] *Kwashiorkor,* a Ghanian word meaning "the sickness of the weanling,"[56] occurs as the result of a low-protein, high-carbohydrate diet in the weaning and postweaning periods. The condition is characterized by anemia, edema, depigmentation of the skin, and alterations in hair color and texture. The hair is typically short and dry and shows increased cuticular weathering.[57] The hair is usually reddish brown to rusty in color and may exhibit the flag sign (i.e., alternating bands of dark and pale hair along a single strand, recording alternating periods of good and poor nutrition).[56] There is an increase in hair loss due partly to a raised telogen count but mainly to atrophy of anagen hair bulbs[55]; the bulb diameters are reduced so that the products are short hairs of reduced diameter.[58]

Marasmus is the result of an extremely low caloric diet in children; they utilize amino acids from skeletal muscles and other less essential tissues to maintain essential body functions. Clinically, the marasmic child is emaciated and shows extreme muscle wasting and atrophy of most organs, although histologic changes are minimal. Hair changes are less severe than those seen in kwashiorkor. The most consistent finding is an overall shift to the telogen phase (up to 50 percent of anagen follicles); the remaining bulbs often show various degrees of atrophy of bulb diameter. The hair is dry and lusterless, with a reduction in shaft diameter. Changes in hair color do not always occur.[55]

Abnormalities of vitamin metabolism also can affect the hair follicle. Hyperkeratosis due to vitamin A deficiency may result in plugging of the follicle, thereby preventing the hair shaft's emergence from the follicular canal.[55] High doses of vitamin A (hypervitaminosis A) may cause dryness and itching of the skin together with sparseness of most body hair due to telogen effluvium.[59] Two siblings with vitamin D-resistant rickets had complete and persistent alopecia in addition to orthopedic and radiographic findings of bowed thighs and legs, widened metaphyseal plates, and other signs of active rickets.[60] Treatment with exogenous calcitriol (1,25-dihydroxyvitamin D_3) did not produce hypercalccmia, further suggesting organ unresponsiveness. Defective cytoplasmic and nuclear receptors for the active vitamin D metabolite calcitriol has been reported in four children with total alopecia and severe, treatment-resistant rickets.[61] A biopsy specimen of scalp skin taken from one of the children at age 6 years revealed a normal number and normal light microscopic appearance of the hair follicles and normal gross and microscopic appearance of the hair shafts. Other vitamin deficiencies (e.g., vitamins K and E) are not known to cause any hair abnormalities in man.[55]

A biotin-responsive form of immunodeficiency (biotin-dependent multiple carboxylase enzyme deficiency) with associated total alopecia has been described in two recent reports.[62,63] Clinically, the children with this disorder manifested alopecia, blepharitis, conjunctivitis, corneal ulceration, "skin rashes," neurological deficits, and organic aciduria. Oral biotin therapy rapidly caused a fall in the organic acids and improvement in the dermatitis, hair growth, neurologic symptoms, and immunologic abnormalities. This type of alopecia has also responded to unsaturated fatty acid administration in a case of multiple carboxylase deficiency.[64]

Biotin is found in egg yolks and binds with very high affinity to avidin in egg whites. Biotin is required in branched-chain amino acid catabolism. Isoleucine and valine are metabolized via propionylcoenzyme A (CoA) carboxylase, and if that enzyme is deficient, propionic aciduria occurs. Leucine is catabolized via β-methylcrotonyl-CoA carboxylase, and when that enzyme is absent, β-methylcrotonylglycinuria occurs. Relative deficiencies of both these enzymes were present in white blood cells of children with biotin-dependent multiple carboxylase enzyme deficiency, which suggests that biotin metabolism and transport may be the primary abnormal factor in the disease and that the enzyme deficiencies are secondary. The response of the enzymes to biotin therapy is con-

sistent with this suggestion.[65] Biotin deficiency in man does not occur naturally.

Copper is thought to be necessary for the oxidation of thiol groups to the dithio cross-links so essential in producing the resilient properties of keratin fibers in hair and wool.[55] Sheep fed on copper-deficient pastures produce wool that is weak, shows abnormal dyeing and processing qualities, and lacks crimp.[66,67] Copper supplementation rapidly restores wool quality to normal. Similarly, in Menkes' syndrome[27] the hair is typically short, brittle, and light in color and exhibits pili torti-type twisting.

Zinc deficiency may occur as a result of an inborn defect of zinc absorption (acrodermatitis enteropathica), from dietary deficiency, or as the result of long continued incomplete parenteral alimentation. Acrodermatitis enteropathica is an autosomal recessive disorder of zinc metabolism.[68] The triad of dermatitis, diarrhea, and alopecia often coincides with weaning from breast to cow's milk. There are erythema and scaling plaques, partially covered with bullae and vesicles. These skin changes characteristically occur periorificially around the mouth and anus and acrally on the extremities. The hair may be sparse, dry and brittle, or completely shed. Alopecia may involve the scalp, eyebrows, or eyelashes, and the hair color often becomes red. The child is listless and apathetic and growth is retarded. The liver and spleen are enlarged and there is hypogonadism. The symptoms may respond rapidly to oral zinc sulfate; hair growth returns to normal even if severe alopecia has been present for many years prior to treatment.[55]

Hair zinc concentration was determined by atomic absorption spectrophotometry in 308 normal newborn infants and 199 normal infants aged 1 to 12 months. Hair zinc concentration declined from 204 μg/g at birth to 112 μg/g at age 8 months and then rose to 144 μg/g at age 12 months. Diaper rash was significantly associated with reduced hair zinc, and infants with the least hair had lower zinc levels than infants with the most hair. The data indicate that hair loss and diaper rash found in normal infants is significantly associated with a reduction in hair zinc concentration.[69]

universalis, and alopecia areata produced a clinical response, as judged by total or partial hair growth, in 9 of the 14 patients treated. Seven of the nine responders had autoantibodies prior to treatment. These autoantibodies disappeared or decreased with Isoprinosine therapy. In contrast, only one of five nonresponders had serum autoantibodies. After treatment, both groups showed an increase in blood-active T rosettes. These results suggest that alopecia areata is a heterogeneous disease subdivided by the presence or absence of autoantibodies since clinical response was mainly obtained in patients presenting autoantibodies.[96] Early reports of successful (cosmetically satisfying) topical minoxidil therapy of alopecia areata[97] have not been supported by our clinical experience or subsequent reports,[98] but this modality is still under investigation.

Keratosis Pilaris Atrophicans

Keratosis pilaris atrophicans is an encompassing term for a group of three related disorders, all having in common the same pathogenic mechanism of follicular hyperkeratosis, inflammation, and atrophy.[99]

Keratosis pilaris atrophicans faciei (KPAF) (also called ulerythema ophryogenes or keratosis pilaris rubra atrophicans faciei) refers to an inflammatory process beginning in the eyebrows. Onset occurs a few months after birth in the lateral third of the eyebrows with follicular papules surrounded by an erythematous halo. Eventually, there is loss of hair in the involved follicles. The process subsequently involves the cheeks and forehead. This entity is accompanied by keratosis pilaris of the extensor surface of the arms and occasionally of the thighs and buttocks. It is rare and has been observed in several family members, but the mode of inheritance has not been defined.

Atrophoderma vermiculatum (acne vermoulanti, honeycomb atrophy, or folliculitis ulerythema reticulata) is a related syndrome. It is morphologically distinct, leaving pitlike depressions of the cheeks (reticulate atrophy). The preceding lesion is an erythematous follicular papule, and therefore some authors view this entity as the end stage of KPAF. The disease is rare and manifests itself when the patients are between the ages of 5 and 12 years.

Keratosis follicularis spinulosa decalvans refers to diffuse keratosis pilaris associated with scarring alopecia of the scalp. During infancy keratosis pilaris begins on the face, and by childhood it progresses to involve the trunk and extremities. Sometime during childhood or up to the early teenage years a cicatricial alopecia of the scalp and eyebrows develops, which is the hallmark of this disorder. Hyperkeratosis of the palms and soles is a frequently associated finding, usually manifested during adolescence. Other features occurring with this syndrome include atopy, photophobia, and corneal abnormalities. Sex-linked inheritance has been proposed by several authors.

Alopecia Mucinosa

Alopecia mucinosa, also referred to as follicular mucinosis, is characterized clinically by occasionally pruritic, grouped, follicular papules; erythematous, raised, infiltrated plaques; and loss of hair from the involved areas. The lesions are distributed mostly on the face, neck, and scalp but may appear elsewhere as well.[100,101] The plaques tend to be 2 to 5 cm in diameter.

Histologically there are mucinous changes in the outer root sheaths and sebaceous glands. In the primary, or idiopathic, benign form the lesions tend to be localized and to resolve spontaneously in 2 months to 2 years. In some cases the lesions are more extensive and persistent or continue to develop at intervals for years without any evidence of associated disease. These benign forms occur at any age from early childhood onward but are not frequent between 10 and 40.[9] When alopecia mucinosa occurs secondary to lymphoma, the individual is usually elderly, the lesions more widespread, and the histologic appearance that of mycosis fungoides or lymphoma.

Other Dermatologic Alopecias

Cicatricial alopecias, other than those already mentioned, that occasionally occur in childhood include those due to pseudopelade, lupus erythematosus, lichen planopilaris, and scleroderma. Once the active inflammatory phase has subsided, hair transplantation by the punch auto-

graft technique can be used to fill in the cosmetically disturbing area.[44-46]

CONCLUSION

In the preceding pages many scalp disorders have been discussed in relationship to alopecia. However, the discussion would be incomplete without touching upon some common scalp disorders of childhood that are unassociated with alopecia.

As mentioned before, hair follicles and seba-

Table 14-2. Approach to the Patient:
Alopecia in Children

History
Age of onset
   At birth: common (physiologic) alopecia of the newborn; congenital absence of hair follicles; aplasia cutis congenita
   Postnatal: frictional
Fetal heart monitoring
Scalp intravenous infusion
Plucking, combing, brushing
Acute traction—''combat''
Chronic traction—tight ponytails, cornrows, braids, curlers, etc.
Headgear use (recreational)
Electric or thermal burn
Hair cosmetics
Radiation exposure
Recent (1–3 months) high fever
Systemic exposure to toxic chemicals
Medicines: quinacrine, quinine, general anesthetics, antineoplastic compounds, high doses of vitamin A, 13-cis-retinoic acid, androgenic medications

Hair Shaft Examination
Lanugo: hereditary hypertrichosis lanuginosa
Vellus
Terminal: examine roots
   Telogen (bulb)
   Anagen (pigmented)
   Bayonet or tapered (Pohl-Pinkus line; alopecia areata)
Monilethrix
Pili torti
Pili annulati
Trichorrhexis nodosa
Trichorrhexis invaginata

Physical Examination
Pattern of scalp hair loss: patchy, diffuse, unilateral, bizarre (trichotillomania), alopecia along lines of cranial sutures (Hallerman-Streiff syndrome)

Presence or absence of scarring
Presence of hairs broken off at different lengths (trichotillomania)
Hair color: red (acrodermatitis enteropathica), light color (Menkes' kinky hair syndrome)
Nutritional status (protein calorie malnutrition, marasmus)
Skin lesions: absence of cutis, milia, dermatitis, tumor/neoplasia, infection (kerion)
Associated hair loss of eyebrows, eyelashes, or body hair
Associated hirsutism (adrenogenital syndromes)
Nail change: onychophagia (trichotillomania), pitting and ridging (alopecia areata), Beau's lines (recent illness)
Dermatoglyphics: abortive loops and arches (alopecia areata)
Associated abnormalities: neurologic, mental, bony, ocular, endocrinologic (signs of masculinization)

Laboratory Investigation
Wood's lamp examination of hair and skin: dermatophyte infections
Complete blood count: decreased hematocrit/hemoglobin (iron deficiency anemia, pernicious anemia associated with alopecia areata)
Chemistry screen: increased glucose (diabetes mellitus with alopecia areata); zinc (decreased in acrodermatitis enteropathica)
C5: dysfunctional in Leiner's disease
Thyroid function testing: alopecia areata, hypothyroidism, hyperthyroidism, androgenetic alopecia
Cortisol
Dehydroepiandrosterone sulfate
Total testosterone
Sex hormone binding globulin
Free testosterone
Urine: organic aciduria (biotin dependent multiple carboxylase deficiency); argininosuccinic aciduria

ceous glands appear between the third and fourth months of fetal life. Since keratin, sebum, and hair debris are actively forming in the scalp area during the remaining 5 months of intrauterine life, debris keeps accumulating and is seen at birth as the vernix caseosa. In the neonatal period hygienic measures will usually correct the ''cradle cap'' variety of seborrheic dermatitis. Throughout life shampooing is the most effective way of reducing seborrheic dermatitis of the scalp.[102,103] Studies have shown an inverse relationship between frequency of shampooing and this disorder. When simple shampoos alone fail to control seborrhea capitis, tar, sulfur, selenium sulfide, zinc pyrithione, and salicylic acid are quite effective shampoo additives. In addition, topical scalp lotions containing corticosteroids, tar, or sulfur are quite useful.

Psoriasis, atopic dermatitis, ichthyosis, and, rarely, lichen planopilaris can affect the scalp and produce the appearance of dandruff. Examination of the total child will help in the differential diagnosis (Table 14-2). The clinical features of these dermatologic disorders help differentiate their appearance on the child's scalp. Medicated shampoos[102,103] and topical preparations[81] are useful in controlling such conditions. It is not unusual to see simultaneous combinations of the most prevalent dermatoses, for example, seborrheic dermatitis and psoriasis. Pruritus, particularly on the back and the sides of the scalp, can be symptomatic of pediculosis capitis, often confused with impetigo of the scalp. Although seen much less frequently now than in previous decades, the possibility of a pedicular infection should not be omitted. A magnifying lens and Wood's light will quickly give the answer.

REFERENCES

1. Orentreich N: Pathogenesis of alopecia. J Soc Cosmetic Chemists 11:479, 1960
2. Flesch P: Hair growth. In Rothman S (ed): Physiology and Biochemistry of the Skin. University of Chicago Press, Chicago, 1954
3. Pinkus H: Embryology of hair. p.1. In Montagna W, Ellis R (eds): The Biology of Hair Growth. Academic Press, Orlando, FL, 1958
4. Matoltsy AG: The chemistry of keratinization. p.135. In Montagna W, Ellis R (eds): The Biology of Hair Growth. Academic Press, Orlando, FL, 1958
5. Montagna W, Ellis R: The vascularity and innervation of human hair follicles. p.219. In Montagna W, Ellis R (eds): The Biology of Hair Growth. Academic Press, Orlando, FL, 1958
6. Van Scott EJ: Responses of hair roots to chemical and physical influence. p.441. In Montagna W, Ellis R (eds): The Biology of Hair Growth. Academic Press, Orlando, FL, 1958
7. Van Scott EJ, Reinerston RP: Detection of radiation effects on hair roots of the human scalp. J Invest Dermatol 29:205, 1957
8. Kligman AM: Pathologic dynamics of hair loss. Arch Dermatol 83:175, 1961
9. Rook A, Dawber R: Diseases of the hair and scalp. Blackwell Scientific Publications, Oxford, 1982
10. Myers RJ, Hamilton JB: Regeneration and rate of growth of hairs in man. Ann NY Acad Sci 53:562, 1951
11. Saitoh M, Uzuka M, Sakamoto M: Rate of hair growth, p.183. In Montagna W, Dobson RL (eds): Hair Growth. Pergamon Press, Oxford, 1969
12. Kligman A: The human hair cycle. J Invest Dermatol 33:307, 1959
13. Orentreich N: Scalp hair replacement in man. p.99. In Montagna W, Dobson RL (eds): Hair Growth. Pergamon Press, Oxford, 1969
14. Orentreich N: Hair problems. Am Med Women's Assoc 21:481, 1966
15. Billingham RE: A reconsideration of the phenomenon of hair neogenesis with particular reference to the healing of cutaneous wounds in adult mammals. p. 451. In Montagna W, Ellis R (eds): The Biology of Hair Growth. Academic Press, Orlando, FL, 1958
16. Miller SA: Hair neogenesis. J Invest Dermatol 56:1. 1971
17. Cockayne EA: Inherited Abnormalities of the Skin and Its Appendages. Oxford University Press, London, 1933
18. Pecoraro V, Astore I, Barman JM: Cycle of scalp hair of the newborn child. J Invest Dermatol 43:145, 1964

19. Bart BJ, Gorlin RJ, Anderson VE, et al: Congenital localized absence of skin and associated abnormalities resembling epidermolysis bullosa. Arch Dermatol 93:296, 1966
20. Boureau M: Les aplasies cutanées congenitales du nouveau-né. Presse Med 69:2175, 1961
21. Peer LA, Duyn JV: Congenital defect of the scalp. Plast Reconstr Surg 3:722, 1948
22. Hurwitz S: Clinical Pediatric Dermatology. WB Saunders, Philadelphia, 1981
23. Butterworth T, Ladda RL: Clinical Genodermatology. Vol. 1. Praeger Publishers, New York, 1981
24. Wiklund DA, Weston WL: Incontinentia pigmenti. Arch Dermatol 115:701, 1960
25. Domonkos AN, Arnold HL, Odom RB: Andrews' Diseases of the Skin. 7th Ed. WB Saunders, Philadelphia, 1982
26. Danks DM, Stevens BJ, Campbell PE, et al: Menkes' kinky-hair syndrome. Lancet 1:1100, 1972
27. Menkes JH, Alter M, Steigleder GK, et al: A sex linked recessive disorder with retardation of growth, peculiar hair and focal cerebral and cerebellar degeneration. Pediatrics 29:764, 1962
28. Hart DB: Menkes' syndrome: an updated review. J Am Acad Dermatol 9:145, 1983
29. Danks DM, Campbell PE, Stevens BJ, et al: Menkes's kinky hair syndrome: an inherited defect in copper absorption with widespread effects. Pediatrics 50:188, 1972
30. Dupre A, Enjobras O: Syndrome de Menkes an pilotorten alternant. Ann Dermatol Venereol (Paris) 102:269, 1980
31. Gorlin RJ, Psaume J: Orodigitofacial dysostosis: a new syndrome: a study of 22 cases. J Pediatr 61:520, 1962
32. Golomb RS, Porter PS: A distinct hair shaft abnormality in the Hallerman-Streiff syndrome. Cutis 16:122, 1975
33. Pierini DO, Pierini AM: Keratosis pilaris atrophicans faciei (ulerythema ophryogenes): a cutaneous marker in Noonan syndrome. Br J Dermatol 100:409, 1979
34. McCarthy L: Diseases of the Hair. CV Mosby, St. Louis, 1960
35. Pillsbury DM, Shelley WB, Kligman AM: Diseases of the hair. In Dermatology. WB Saunders, Philadelphia, 1956
36. Price V: Office diagnosis of structural hair anomalies. Cutis 15:231, 1975
37. Hurwitz S, Kirsch N, McGuire J: Reevaluation of ichthyosis and hair shaft abnormalities. Arch Dermatol 103:266, 1971
38. Leider M: Practical Pediatric Dermatology. CV Mosby, St. Louis, Missouri, 1961
39. Demis DJ, Dobson RL, McGuire J: Clinical Dermatology. 10th Revision. Harper & Row, Philadelphia, 1983
40. Haslam RHA, Wirtschafter JD: Unilateral external oculomotor nerve palsy and nevus sebaceus of Jadassohn. Arch Ophthalmol 8:293, 1972
41. Lantis S, Thew M, Heaton C: Nevus sebaceus of Jadassohn. Part of a new neurocutaneous syndrome? Arch Dermatol 98:117, 1968
42. Brown ZA, Jung AL, Stenehuver MA: Aplasia cutis congenita and the fetal scalp electrode. Am J Obstet Gynecol 129:351, 1977
43. Strong AMM: Extensive cicatricial alopecia following a scalp vein infusion. Clin Exp Dermatol 4:197, 1979
44. Orentreich N: Autografts in alopecias and other selected dermatological conditions. Ann NY Acad Sci 83:463, 1959
45. Orentreich N: Hair transplants—long-term results and new advances. Arch Otolaryngol 92:576, 1970
46. Stough DB, Berger RA, Orentreich N: Surgical improvement of cicatricial alopecias of diverse etiology. Arch Dermatol 97:331, 1968
47. Harry RG: Modern Cosmeticology. Vol. 1. Leonard Hill, Ltd., London, 1955
48. Graham F: Trichotillomania, a symptom of adolescent identity crisis. Psychosom Med 21:239, 1966
49. Greenberg HR, Sarner C: Trichotillomania. Arch Gen Psychiatry 12:482, 1965
50. Orentreich N: Etiology of loss of eyelashes in a child. JAMA 207:961, 1969
51. Selmanowitz VJ, Orentreich N: Cosmetic treatment of factitial defects. Cutis 6:549, 1970
52. Muller FA: Trichotillomania. p. 305. In Brown AC, Crounge RG (eds): Hair, Trace Elements, and Human Illness. Pragen, New York, 1980
53. Orentreich N, Selmanowitz VJ: Cosmetic improvement of factitial defects. Med Trial Tech Q 172, Dec. 1970
54. Ressmann AC, Butterworth T: Localized acquired hypertrichosis. Arch Dermatol 65:458, 1952
55. Gummer CL: Diet and hair loss. Semin Dermatol 4:35, 1985

56. Fitzpatrick TB, Eisen AZ, Wolff K et al (eds): Dermatology in General Medicine. 2nd Ed. McGraw-Hill, New York, 1979

57. Gummer CL, Dawber RPR, Harman RM, et al: Kwashiorkor: an electron histochemical study of the hair shaft. Br J Dermatol 106:407, 1982

58. Bradfield RB, Bailey MA, Margen S: Morphological changes in human scalp hair roots during deprivation of protein. Science 157:438, 1967

59. Soler-Bechara J, Soscia JL: Chronic hypervitaminosis A. Arch Intern Med 112:58, 1963

60. Rosen JF, Fleischman AR, Finberg L, et al: Rickets with alopecia: an inborn error of vitamin D metabolism. J Pediatr 94:729, 1979

61. Hochberg Z, Gilhar A, Haim S, et al: Calcitriol-resistant rickets with alopecia. Arch Dermatol 121:646, 1985

62. Charles BM, Hosking G, Green A, et al: Biotin-responsive alopecia and developmental regression. Lancet 2:118, 1979

63. Cowan MJ, Wara DW, Packman S, et al: Multiple biotin-dependent carboxylase deficiencies associated with defects in T-cell and B-cell immunity. Lancet 2:115, 1979

64. Munnich A, Saudubray JM, Coude FX, et al: Fatty-acid responsive alopecia in multiple carboxylase deficiency. Lancet 1:1080, 1980

65. Goldsmith LA: Vitamins and alopecia. Arch Dermatol 116:1135, 1980

66. Marston HR: Studies on the relationship between nutrition and wool production of Merino sheep. J Agric Sci (Camb) 25:113, 1955

67. Burley RW, Horden FWA: Experiments on wool from copper deficient sheep. Nature 184:1725, 1959

68. Moynahan EJ: Acrodermatitis enteropathica: a lethal inherited human zinc deficiency disorder. Lancet 2:339, 1974

69. Collipp PJ, Kuo B, Castro-Magana M, et al: Hair zinc, scalp hair quantity, and diaper rash in normal infants. Cutis 35:66, 1985

70. Verbov J: Fingertip arches. Lancet 1:1090, 1968

71. Safai B, Orentreich N, Good RA: Immunological abnormalities in patients with alopecia areata (AA). Clin Res 27:244A, 1979

72. Todes-Taylor N, Turner R, Wood GS, et al: T cell subpopulations in alopecia areata. J Am Acad Dermatol 11:216, 1984

73. Friedman PS: Alopecia areata and auto-immunity. Br J Dermatol 105:153, 1981

74. Igarashi R, Morohashi M, Takeuchi S, et al: Immunofluorescence studies on complement components in the hair follicles of normal scalp and of scalp affected by alopecia areata. Acta Derm Venereol (Stockh) 61:131, 1981

75. Orentreich N: Hair loss in young boy: trichotillomania or alopecia areata? JAMA (Questions and Answers) 234:761, 1975

76. Brown AC, Pollard ZF, Jarrett WH II: Ocular and testicular abnormalities in alopecia areata. Arch Dermatol 118:546, 1982

77. Berger RA, Orentreich N: Abrupt changes in hair morphology following corticosteroid therapy in alopecia areata. Arch Dermatol 82:408, 1960

78. Dillaha CJ, Rothman S: Therapeutic experiments in alopecia areata with orally administered cortisone. JAMA 150:546, 1952

79. Dillaha CJ, Rothman S: Treatment of alopecia areata totalis and universalis with cortisone acetate. J Invest Dermatol 18:5, 1952

80. Dougherty TF, Schneebeli GL: Use of steroids as anti-inflammatory agents. Ann NY Acad Sci 61:328, 1955

81. Orentreich N: Clinical efficacy of triamcinolone acetonide and hydrocortisone acetate in dermatological patients. Monogr Ther 3:161, 1958

82. Orentreich N, Sturm H, Weidman AI, et al: Local injections of steroids and hair regrowth in alopecias. Arch Dermatol 82:894, 1960

83. Rony HR, Cohen DM: The effect of cortisone in alopecia areata. J Invest Dermatol 25:285, 1955

84. Orentreich N, Orentreich D: Diseases of the hair. p. 611. In Rakel RE (ed): Conn's Current Therapy. WB Saunders, Philadelphia, 1986

85. Orentreich N: Treatment of alopecia areata. JAMA (Questions and Answers) 238:347, 1977

86. Happle R, Hausen BM, Wiesner-Menzel L: Diphencyprone in the treatment of alopecia areata. Acta Derm Venereol (Stockh) 63:49, 1983

87. de Prost Y, Paquez F, Touraine R: Dinitrochlorobenzene treatment of alopecia areata. Arch Dermatol 118:542, 1982

88. Case PC, Mitchell AJ, Swanson NA, et al: Topical therapy of alopecia areata with squaric acid dibutylester. J Am Acad Dermatol 10:447, 1984

89. Happle R, Kalver KJ, Buchner U, et al: Contact allergy as a therapeutic tool for alopecia areata: application of squaric acid dibutylester. Dermatologica 161:289, 1980

90. Barth JH, Darley CR, Gibson JR: Squaric acid

dibutyl ester in the treatment of alopecia areata. Dermatologica 170:40, 1985

91. Arrazola JM, Sendagorta E, Harto A, et al: Treatment of alopecia areata with topical nitrogen mustard. Int J Dermatol 24:608, 1985

92. Mitchell AJ, Douglass MC: Topical photochemotherapy for alopecia areata. J Am Acad Dermatol 12:644, 1985

93. Amer MA, El Garf A: Photochemotherapy and alopecia areata. Int J Dermatol 22:245, 1983

94. van der Schaar WW, Sillevis Smitt JH: An evaluation of PUVA-therapy for alopecia areata. Dermatologica 168:250, 1984

95. Galbraith GMP, Thiers BH, Fudenberg HH: An open-label trial of immunomodulation therapy with inosiplex (Isoprinosine) in patients with alopecia totalis and cell-mediated immunodeficiency. J Am Acad Dermatol 11:224, 1984

96. Lowy M, Ledoux-Corbusier M, Achten G, et al: Clinical and immunologic response to Iso-prinosine in alopecia areata and alopecia universalis: association with autoantibodies. J Am Acad Dermatol 21:78, 1985

97. Weiss VC, West DP, Fu TS, et al: Alopecia areata treated with topical minoxidil. Arch Dermatol 120:457, 1984

98. Frentz G: Topical minoxidil for extended areata alopecia. Acta Derm Venereol (Stockh) 65:172, 1985

99. Rand R, Baden HP: Keratosis follicularis spinulosa decalvans. Arch Dermatol 119:22, 1983

100. Emmerson RW: Follicular mucinosis. Br J Dermatol 81:35, 1969

101. Kim R, Winkelmann RK: Follicular mucinosis (alopecia mucinosa). Arch Dermatol 85:490, 1962

102. Orentreich N, Berger RA: Selenium disulfide shampoo. Arch Dermatol 90:76, 1964

103. Orentreich N, Taylor EH, Berger RA, et al: Comparative study of two antidandruff preparations. J Pharm Sci 58:1279, 1969

15

Alopecia in Adults

David S. Orentreich
Norman Orentreich

Adults are subject to many of the same hair and scalp disorders that afflict children, including congenital and inherited disorders that persist in adulthood, alopecia areata, and some of the acquired alopecias. These have been discussed in Chapter 14, Alopecia in Children.

Several conditions are seen almost exclusively in adults, for example, male pattern hair loss, a variety of inflammatory conditions, and several acquired disorders, and these are examined in this chapter (Table 15-1).

The number of hair follicles is the same in both sexes.[1] The wide range of hair patterns observed in men and women of different races is thus dependent on the distribution of the type (terminal or vellus) of hair present in each follicle. The total number of hair follicles in an adult human is estimated at about 5 million.[2] Approximately 1 million are on the scalp, of which only about 100,000 are terminal hairs. The number of terminal hairs varies somewhat depending on the color: light-haired persons have approximately 140,000, dark-haired persons 102,000, and redheads 88,000 hairs.[3]

Certain common events can alter physiologic shedding. For example, during pregnancy more follicles are maintained in the growing phase and there is less shedding than usual. After delivery, approximately 30 percent of the follicles simultaneously go into the resting phase, causing a temporary, self-correcting, profuse shedding of hair generally about 3 months postpartum. A prolonged febrile episode induces an increase in telogen hairs, with a period of shedding noticeable about 3 to 12 weeks later. The hair cycle is also subject to chronobiologic influences; in the north temperate zone daily hair shedding may double in the fall months, and there is diminished shedding in the spring.[4] Both the duration of hair growth[5] and the daily growth rate[6] are greater in summer than in winter. Temperature as well as duration of light (photoperiod) may play a role, since visitors to the tropics have noticed an accelerated rate of beard growth there. It can be noted here that although it is possible to increase the rate of hair growth by increasing blood supply and thus skin temperature, common hair loss is not caused by diminished blood supply.

ANDROGENETIC ALOPECIA

Androgenetic alopecia (AGA)[7] is the most common type of hair loss in both sexes; *male pattern baldness* is its common name. This alopecia is caused by the gradual conversion of terminal to vellus hairs; it occurs only in those scalp follicles that have the genetic potential to be inhibited by androgens over a period of

Table 15-1. Types of and Factors Involved in Adult Alopecia

Androgenetic alopecia
Hair changes associated with aging
Acquired alopecias
    Traumatic alopecia
        Friction and pressure
        Thermal and chemical trauma
    Neoplastic factors
    Toxic alopecia
    Nutritional factors
Dermatologic alopecias
    Dissecting cellulitis
    Folliculitis decalvans
    Lichen planopilaris
    Pseudopelade
    Acne keloidalis nuchae

time. It is perhaps more appropriately called *androchronogenetic alopecia.*[8] A converse of this condition is the gradual conversion of vellus to terminal hairs in the beard skin of males or in facial hirsutism of females.

For both men and women the androgenic dermatoses include AGA, oily skin, and acne. Women may also exhibit varying degrees of hirsutism: darker, longer, coarser hair of the chin, upper lip, sideburns, body, arms, and legs; a masculinized pubic hair distribution (male escutcheon), including midline hairs from pubis to umbilicus; and periareolar breast hair. Menstrual irregularity and other symptoms may also be present.

Relative hyperandrogenic states that can trigger androgen-dependent alopecia in genetically predisposed individuals are puberty, menopause, the postpartum period, the polycystic ovarian syndrome, post-estrogenic contraceptive therapy, and relatively androgenic oral contraceptive therapy.

Genetic Factors

Androgenetic alopecia is controlled by a single dominant, sex-limited, autosomal gene and may be influenced by polygenic modifying factors affecting expressivity of the trait (Fig. 15-1). The expression of this gene is dependent on the level of circulating free androgens. Although genetic and chronobiologic influences

are operative at the genome level, there is no expression of baldness in the absence of circulating androgens.

In the year 400 B.C. Hippocrates (in the *Hippocratic Corpus*)[9] made an astute observation: "Eunuchs are not subject to gout nor do they become bald." He himself was completely bald except for the classic narrow horseshoe-shaped fringe of hair covering the lower parietal and occipital scalp. To this day this advanced stage of male pattern baldness is called *calvities Hippocratica,* or Hippocratic baldness. Aristotle, too, was aware of the association of baldness and androgenicity; he noted that neither eunuchs nor [normal] women went bald and that both were unable to grow hair on their chests.[10]

In a seminal identical twin study,[11] one twin, who had been castrated before puberty, at age 40 retained his original full complement of scalp hair. The uncastrated twin had gradually gone bald over a period of more than 20 years. At age 40 the castrated twin received injections of testosterone and within 6 months (!) became as bald as his twin brother. That decades of exposure to androgens were not required to reach this degree of baldness indicated that time-dependent gene alteration was operative, though not expressed, in the absence of essential hormonal influence: thus the term *androchronogenetic alopecia.*

The genetic potential is expressed if the appropriate androgen enters the androgen-sensitive target cells of the hair papilla and/or matrix and binds with a specific androgen-receptor protein that interacts with the cell's genetic material.

The influence of inheritance is further shown by the fact that a eunuch whose normal male relatives are not bald does not become bald simply by treatment with androgens. On the other hand, a eunuch whose normal male relatives tend to be bald will develop baldness when treated with the same amount of androgens.[11]

The hair follicles most typically subject to AGA are in the temporofrontal (temple) and crown regions of the scalp.[12] Balding is a gradual process: the anagen period, and thus the maximum achievable hair length, becomes

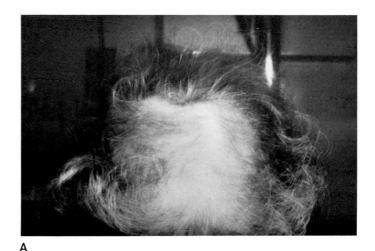

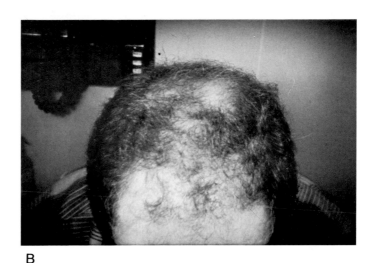

Fig. 15–1. Androgenetic alopecia in **(A)** a mother and **(B)** a son.

A

B

shorter with each successive hair cycle; it has not been established if the telogen phase becomes longer. When baldness is attained, each genetically susceptible terminal scalp hair has been reduced to its almost imperceptible vellus state. This process must affect approximately half the follicles in any given area of the scalp before hair loss becomes clinically evident.

In women AGA tends to be less severe, later in onset, slower to develop, and more diffuse although no less patterned; these differences are probably because women have less circulating free androgen available to inhibit the follicles.

Receptor-Mediated Control

The mode of androgen action in AGA has been elucidated in studies of persons with mutations influencing androgen target cell responsiveness. The clinical and biochemical findings in patients with testicular feminization syndrome and in 5-α-reductase (5αR)-deficient type 2 pseudohermaphrodites strongly suggest that dihydrotestosterone (DHT), not testosterone (T), is the androgen that must be bound to target cells for the expression of beard growth and AGA in genetically predisposed individuals, whereas pubic and axillary hair growth is dependent upon T.

Androgenetic Alopecia in Normal and Hyperandrogenized Women

Some women with AGA have an endocrinopathic basis for their alopecia. They may have ovarian and/or adrenal hyperandrogenism; they may also show signs of virilism in severe hyperandrogenism or only hirsutism and/or acne with mild to moderate hyperandrogenism.

Acne, hirsutism, and AGA can and frequently do occur in patients without frank plasma hyperandrogenism. There are several explanations:

1. The affected hair follicles and sebaceous glands may be hypersensitive to normal adult female blood androgen levels. This explanation has been invoked to account for idiopathic unilateral facial hirsutism.[13] There may be increased androgen receptor affinity and/or capacity for DHT and/or enhanced nuclear retention of the DHT-receptor complex, which may lower the threshold for androgen expression. According to this explanation, these are genetically transmitted traits and explain individual and racial variations in androgen-dependent hair growth and distribution.

2. Because the production rate and metabolic clearance rate of T determine blood T concentration,[14–16] if both rates are elevated, the net is probably a normal blood T concentration; however, increased metabolic utilization of T and its conversion by the skin to DHT could lead to AGA.

3. There may be a low circulating level of the primary plasma androgen transport protein, known as *androgen-binding globulin* (ABG) or sex hormone-binding globulin, which is produced by the liver.[17] A low level of ABG results in more unbound (free) T and DHT, and it is only free T or DHT that is active on (able to enter) target organs. If there is insufficient ABG to bind either normal or excessive amounts of androgens, AGA can occur. Deficient production of ABG by the liver can be caused by a deficiency of estrogen or thyroid hormone, an excess of androgens, obesity, or a hepatic defect.

Acne, hirsutism, and AGA may be exacerbated by androgenic medications, including certain oral contraceptives that contain progestins with androgenic properties (norethindrone, norgestrel, norethindrone acetate).

Cutaneous Androgen Metabolism and Androgenetic Alopecia

Testosterone secreted by the testis is the principal androgen circulating in the plasma in men, whereas in women the adrenal and ovarian steroids 4-androstenedione and dehydroepiandrosterone sulfate are the most abundant circulating proandrogens. A prohormone is a 19-carbon steroid that arrives at the target tissue and is converted to an active hormone. Human skin is an important site for the biotransformation and metabolism of androgens.[18,19] It has the potential to enzymatically convert the primary adrenal androgen, dehydroepiandrosterone sulfate, to dehydroepiandrosterone[20] and to convert dehydroepiandrosterone to androstenedione, then to T, and then to DHT.[21,22] The primary ovarian proandrogen, 4-androstenedione, can also be converted by the skin to T.[23] We agree with published reports that pretestosterone androgens contribute significantly to the total androgenization of women, especially in the second and third decades of life, when dehydroepiandrosterone and its sulfate are at their highest levels in the life span.[24,25]

The skin is also one of the major sites of peripheral conversion of T to DHT by 5αR, and 5αR activity is especially high in areas of high sebaceous gland density.[26] Activity of 5αR has been demonstrated in plucked pubic hair,[27] and DHT formation is elevated in hirsute women.[28]

Plasma androgen studies were performed on adult female patients with hirsutism (17 to 51 years) and AGA (18 to 46 years), and these results were compared with those from normal adult females.[29] Androgens measured included 5α-androstane-3α,17β-diol sulfate, 4-androstenedione, dehydroepiandrosterone sulfate, T, and DHT. The findings of elevated 5α-androstane-3α,17β-diol sulfate together with elevated T and normal DHT levels in patients with hirsutism and AGA suggest that 5α-androstane-3α,17β-diol sulfate may be of physiopathological importance, providing information on androgen metabolism occurring within the liver and/or peripheral target cells.[29]

The skin may be hyperandrogenic as the result of enhanced 5αR activity; such an increase, although slight, was found in balding hair roots compared with nonbalding hair roots from the frontal scalp of persons with AGA.[30] However, it is not necessary to postulate increased enzyme activity in the actual hair follicles. The scalp has an abundance of sebaceous glands, and these may be a major source of DHT to hair follicles because of their close proximity. Because 5αR activity is high in human scalp skin (Rizer and Orentreich, unpublished observations) and because it may be highest in balding sites,[31] this alone could induce AGA in genetically susceptible individuals.

Those genetically susceptible to AGA may be similar to those genetically susceptible to acne and seborrhea, in whose skin androgen receptors were detected by "exchange assay" although not detected in subjects without seborrhea or acne.[32]

Androgenetic Alopecia and Vascular Supply

For the past 30 years the punch hair transplant technique has clearly demonstrated that diminished blood supply, tight hat bands, and muscle pull are not the cause of common male pattern alopecia. Hair transplanted from the persistent hair-bearing areas of the back and sides of the scalp continues to grow after 30 years with the same vigor in totally bald areas as well as in scarred areas of diminished vascularity.[33] Histologic examination of male pattern bald sites

show intact miniaturized hair follicles; there is no diminution in the number of follicles when corrected for age. Diminished vascularity in areas of AGA is thus a secondary phenomenon. Male pattern alopecia, therefore, is not a loss of follicles but a time- and steroid hormone-dependent genetic expression, with diminution in the growing phase of the hair and possibly also a prolongation of the resting phase.

Androgenetic Alopecia and Hygiene

Frequent shampooing (preferably daily) reduces surface sebum containing high levels of DHT and T,[34] which may reenter the skin and adversely affect the hair follicle. Although regular shampooing and conditioning can create a cleaner, healthier looking head of hair, AGA is not related to too frequent or infrequent shampooing. Furthermore, mild to even moderate local skin conditions (e.g., seborrheic dermatitis and contact dermatitis) do not cause AGA. If not performed daily, shampooing is accompanied by increased shedding because it harvests several days' accumulation of telogen hairs.

Androgenetic Alopecia and Diet

Diet plays a minor role in AGA. While it is conceivable that consuming androgen-containing foods might exacerbate AGA in some women, it is unlikely that men (because of their high levels of endogenous androgens) would experience any deleterious effects.

Prevention and Early Medical Treatment of Androgenetic Alopecia

Prescriptions for the treatment of baldness date back over 5,000 years to the Egyptian papyri, the pharmacopeias of their day. Hippocrates, around 400 B.C., prescribed opium mixed with essence of roses or lilies to be made into an ointment with wine and oil of unripe olives or acacia juice. For more severe cases he suggested a poultice of cumin, pigeon droppings, crushed horseradish, and beetroot or nettles. The Bible offers no cure but admonishes scoffing at bald pates. For example (2 Kings 2:23): "there came forth little children and mocked him [Elisha], and said unto him, go up, thou bald head; go up, thou bald head." Elisha, bald and sensitive, promptly cursed the children in the name of the Lord. Whereupon "there came forth two she-bears out of the wood, and tore forty and two children of them."

To this day the medical treatment of AGA still cannot effectively be directed against the genetic or time-dependent factors. However, androgen inhibition of the growing phase of the hair follicle on the scalp is amenable to treatment.

Optimal medical treatment is directed against DHT, reducing its production from T and preventing its binding to androgen receptors and induction of genetic expression. Because of the inherent lag time in hair response, no clinically noticeable effect from therapy can be expected in less than 3 months. Also, allowance should be made for the normal increase in hair shedding from September through December in the north temperate zone.

Pathogenesis and Related Treatment of Androgenetic Alopecia

Plasma hyperandrogenism is not rare in women with multiple androgenic dermatoses; AGA and other cutaneous and systemic symptoms of hyperandrogenism can occur from excess androgen production, low levels of ABG, and/or increased androgen metabolism and utilization by the target sites. Laboratory studies of differential, contributory, and pathogenetic factors include the following: complete blood count with differential, Venereal Disease Research Laboratory testing, bilirubin, alkaline phosphatase, cholesterol, triglycerides, serum glutamic oxaloacetic transaminase, uric acid, and creatinine; adrenal function tests, including cortisol and dehydroepiandrosterone sulfate; androgen function tests, including T, ABG, and

free T; and thyroid function tests, including free thyroid index (T4-RIA and T3 uptake), and possibly T3 and thyroid-stimulating hormone.

Plasma Androgens

Both T and DHT circulate in the blood mostly bound to plasma proteins, especially ABG. Only the unbound (free) hormone can enter a cell; T and DHT bound to serum protein are inactive. Symptoms can occur if there is too little ABG to bind either normal or excessive amounts of androgens. Plasma ABG and T levels were measured in a study of eight women aged 21 to 41 years, who complained of diffuse hair loss, and subsequently in a larger group of 15 patients of a similar age range.[35] There was a significant reduction in ABG levels in both groups of patients when compared with controls, but T values were normal. Deficient liver production of ABG results in higher levels of free T and DHT and may be caused by a deficiency of estrogens or thyroid hormone or by an excess of androgens.

Adrenal androgens can significantly contribute to androgenization of women, especially in the second and third decades of life, when dehydroepiandrosterone and its sulfate (DHEAS) are at their highest levels. Excessive adrenal production of androgens (as measured by serum DHEAS) can be effectively and safely reduced by glucocorticoids in the appropriate oral dosage (e.g., prednisone, 2.5 mg taken orally at bedtime); there is no significant change in cortisol levels or adrenal reserve capacity. When both the adrenals and ovaries are producing excess androgen, glucocorticoid combined with estrogen treatment suppresses both adrenal and ovarian production of androgen. Estrogens in the form of contraceptive pills that contain nonandrogenic progestins may be prescribed after gynecologic consultation.

Estrogens and thyroids also stimulate liver production of ABG. If ABG is low, L-triiodothyronine (Cytomel 37.5 to 75 μg orally in the morning) or other thyroids (Synthroid, Choloxin) have been administered to healthy euthyroid women to stimulate production of ABG; relative contraindications are hypertension, arteriosclerotic heart disease, tachycardia, cardiac arrhythmia, and tremulousness. Estrogen therapy for contraception or postmenopausal replacement also has the beneficial effect of increasing ABG.

Elimination of exogenous androgens that may precipitate or aggravate AGA is beneficial. Exogenous sources are androgenic drugs and androgenic contraceptive pills.

Androgen Receptor Binding

Cyproterone acetate,[36] originally developed as an antiandrogen for treatment of male sex offenders (because it inhibits spermatogenesis and depresses libido and potency), is available in Europe for the treatment of hirsutism, alopecia, and acne in women.[37] Taken with estrogen to prevent conception (a male fetus would be feminized), it is a remarkably effective antiandrogen. The mechanism of action is interference with binding of both T and DHT to their receptors and hence to genetic material. Decreased libido is noticed by some patients.

There is ample evidence available to show that oral antiandrogen and estrogen therapy may benefit acne and hirsutism, but efficacy of this treatment in AGA has not been established unequivocally.

In order to evaluate the efficacy of oral antiandrogen treatment of common baldness in women, 49 patients with AGA were studied,[38] of whom 29 received combined therapy with 50 μg ethinyl estradiol and 100 mg cyproterone acetate daily, and the other 20 were followed but received no specific treatment. Progress was assessed: (1) subjectively by both patient and physician, and (2) objectively by regular shedding counts and standardized hair diameter measurements and telogen counts. Of the treated group, 18 were subjectively improved during treatment, compared with 7 of the untreated group. In 24 treated subjects the objective measurements significantly improved. Two patients

stopped treatment because of fluid retention and menorrhagia.

To determine whether low-dose therapy can maintain improvement obtained from high-dose regimens, 17 of the treated group showing subjective and objective improvement from the above treatment were changed to Diane (50 μg ethinyl estradiol and 2 mg cyproterone acetate daily). In only three cases was the improvement maintained. It is possible that AGA requires higher doses of cyproterone acetate for clinical effectiveness than does acne or hirsutism.[37]

In another study endocrine profiles were established in 19 women, aged 18 to 43 years, with common baldness.[39] Reduced plasma levels were found for ABG (68 percent), luteal phase progesterone (52 percent, indicating subfertility), luteinizing hormone (42 percent), estradiol (37 percent), and follicle-stimulating hormone (21 percent), while total plasma T was raised in only one patient.

Of this group three women with a history of diffuse loss of scalp hair of 2, 13, and 23 years' duration (two of whom had a familial history of premature balding) were treated with cyclic antiandrogen therapy for 52 weeks. Therapy was cyclic cyproterone acetate (50 mg daily for 10 days) and ethinyl estradiol (40 μg daily for 21 days following withdrawal bleeding. Cyclic antiandrogen therapy was introduced to suppress ovarian androgen secretion and to increase plasma ABG concentrations, thereby causing a fall in circulating free T and consequently DHT, with inhibition of the peripheral effects of these hormones. All patients showed an increase in hair density (hairs per square centimeter)[40] and meaningful density (hairs greater than 40 μm diameter per square centimeter) after 24 to 28 weeks. The percentage of hairs in the anagen growth phase increased during therapy. During cyclic antiandrogen therapy each patient showed an increase in plasma ABG and a fall in plasma total T levels. Three control patients, untreated for 26 weeks, showed no significant improvement in hair density, meaningful density, or percentage of hair in anagen.

Previously, cyproterone acetate (100 mg

daily from day 5 to 14) and ethinyl estradiol (50 µg from day 5 to 25 of each menstrual cycle) had been used, but unwanted side effects were common.[41]

Male patients taking the histamine H_2 antagonist cimetidine have been reported to develop such side effects as gynecomastia and impotence. These typically antiandrogenic side effects are now thought to be due to cimetidine competing with DHT for its receptor as assayed in vitro in the human prostate.[42] Cimetidine has been reported to be effective in hirsutism.[43] Although we have not found any publications on its effects in alopecia, there is at least a theoretical basis for its use.

The aldosterone antagonist spironolactone (Aldactone) is used in the treatment of primary aldosteronism and low-renin essential hypertension and produces antiandrogenic side effects, such as decreased libido, impotence, and gynecomastia in males and menstrual irregularity and breast enlargement in females. Its use as a treatment for hirsutism has been reported,[44,45] and improvement of acne in the same subjects was also noted. Female patients treated with oral spironolactone, 200 mg daily, showed objective improvement in their acne and hirsutism and subjective improvement in AGA by the end of 6 months.[46] The drug appears to interact with androgen receptors to block nuclear uptake of DHT,[47–49] decrease T biosynthesis,[50] and increase estrogen synthesis.[51,52]

Supplementary zinc therapy (zinc gluconate 60 mg/day) has been used to potentially inhibit $5\alpha R$ activity. There is a significant inverse relationship between zinc and $5\alpha R$ activity of the human hyperplastic prostate.[53] The concentrations of DHT were shown to be inversely proportional to zinc in benign hypertrophy and carcinoma of the human prostate.[54] However, it was not clear whether the zinc inhibits the $5\alpha R$ activity leading to reduced formation of DHT or influences DHT binding at the cellular level.[54] Inhibition by zinc ions of $5\alpha R$ reduction of both T to DHT and androstenedione to androstanedione could be demonstrated in $5\alpha R$ extracts from hamster prostate tissue or frozen and homogenized hamster ear tissue (sebaceous glands).[55] While there have been reports both for and against the benefit of zinc in acne, its (beneficial) role in AGA remains hypothetical.

Local Therapy

Local therapy is an alternative or supplement to systemic therapy. Although there are several compounds that systemically inhibit the reduction of T to DHT by $5\alpha R$ and/or inhibit the binding of DHT to its target cell receptor protein, there are few (and none clinically available in the United States) that meet the criteria of adequate percutaneous absorbability and action limited to the site of application.

Natural steroids such as progesterone safely reduce the production of DHT from T. Both T and progesterone contain a C4-C5 double bond in the steroid A ring; in vitro and in vivo studies have shown that they compete with each other for the $5\alpha R$ enzyme that converts T to DHT. Tinctures and locally injected aqueous suspensions of progesterone have been used safely for 20 years.[56]

Progesterone was found to be a natural and significant $5\alpha R$ inhibitor when tested in the human skin microsome system,[57] a rich source of $5\alpha R$. Progesterone also inhibits $5\alpha R$ in human scalp hair follicles.[19] When a solution of progesterone in alcohol was applied to the pubic skin of normal males, it produced a decrease of 75.2 percent in $5\alpha R$ activity when assayed after 24 hours of treatment.[58]

Moreover, while less DHT is made in the presence of progesterone, more dihydroprogesterone (DHP, 5α-pregnane-3,20 dione) is made. The DHP competes with the residual DHT for the intracellular androgen binding protein, resulting in a further reduction in the amount of DHT interacting with genetic material.[59,60]

Because of the reversible enzyme kinetics, progesterone would need to be present at the active site of $5\alpha R$ continuously; thus a lapse in treatment results in the resumption of DHT production from T. Further, since progesterone only *partially* inhibits DHT production and since DHP only *partially* inhibits binding of residual DHT, local progesterone at best can only ameliorate the progression of AGA.

Because more than 70 percent of topically supplied progesterone is metabolized in the skin to weak, nonandrogenic by-products,[58,61] it can be used in women at the rate of 1 ml of a 2 percent solution bid (40 mg); higher doses may result in menstrual irregularities. It may be combined with other percutaneously acceptable antiandrogens (e.g., spironolactone or its active metabolite canrenone).[45]

Animal studies have demonstrated that the rate of hair growth can be increased by application of thyroid hormones to hair-bearing skin.[62] The most active thyroid hormone for this purpose is L-triiodothyronine, commonly called L-T3. A tincture with an L-T3 concentration of 50 μg/ml has been used and produces no systemic side effects when applied at the rate of 1 ml bid.

TREATMENT IN MEN

Systemic Therapy

Transsexual medicine has taught us that physical or chemical castration of males arrests but does not reverse the balding process. Even in noncastrates, a reduction of plasma androgen levels sufficient to stop hair loss is also sufficient to produce a decrease in both libido and sexual potency which appear to be dependent on plasma levels of free T.

Endocrinologic reversal of AGA in males is possible, but the psychoneuroendocrinologic price is high and generally acceptable only to male-to-female transsexuals. Therapy entails complete chemical gonadal castration, suppression of adrenal androgen production with corticosteroids, reduction of free plasma androgens by increasing ABG with thyroid and/or estrogen supplements, and local therapies to reduce both 5αR activity and DHT receptor binding. When androgens are reduced to less than normal female levels, hair regrowth has been noted.[8] Both cyproterone acetate and megestrol acetate taken orally will reverse AGA in men, but there

is no true safe therapeutic range. All effective doses produce diminished libido and impotence.

Local Therapy

Scalp skin production of DHT from T may be reached and DHP production increased with application of progesterone in males as well as females. For males the dosage is usually 1 ml of a 4 percent progesterone tincture bid; no systemic antiandrogenic effects have been noted, and plasma androgen levels remain normal (Orentreich, unpublished results). The progesterone may be combined with other antiandrogens (e.g., spironolactone). Topical estrogens are ineffective unless applied in doses high enough to achieve pharmacologic systemic levels; they then operate through a systemic mechanism (increasing ABG and reducing gonadotropins and total T production), not through a direct local action on the hair follicle.

MINOXIDIL

Minoxidil (Loniten) is a piperidinopyrimidine derivative and a potent peripheral arteriolar vasodilator[63] used in the treatment of resistant hypertension.[64] Hypertrichosis is a frequent (30 to 100 percent in different reports) side effect of oral therapy in adults[65–71] and even children.[72] Using the laser Doppler technique, it was demonstrated that increased blood flow occurs following topical application of minoxidil to the bald scalps of men.[73] Although the mechanism of action by which hair growth is stimulated has not been established, whether taken orally or applied topically, minoxidil presumably works in AGA by locally increasing cutaneous perfusion of the scalp and thereby reducing the difference between core and skin temperature. By raising skin temperature the rate of hair growth is increased. Cutaneous hyperemia is well known to be responsible for localized acquired hypertrichosis.[74] The hypertrichosis of minoxidil does not appear to be due to androgenic or antiandrogenic mechanisms.[75,76]

Cutaneous or systemic side effects from topical application of minoxidil in concentrations of 1 to 5 percent have not been reported in most trials.[11] Local tolerance has been good, with only a few reports of contact irritation or possible contact sensitization[77] at the application sites.

Reports of treatment of AGA have shown mixed results. Three of five patients with AGA using 5 percent minoxidil for 12 months noted hair regrowth, ranging from minimally observable hair in two patients to an appreciable restoration of larger, pigmented, terminal hair in one.[77] A double-blind study showed no statistically significant difference at 15.7 weeks between three groups of healthy bald males (seven per group) treated either with 1 percent minoxidil or the vehicle alone.[79] In a double-blind study of 56 males with AGA, "cosmetically acceptable" hair growth was achieved in 18 (32 percent) treated with 2 to 3 percent topical minoxidil.[80] The most notable prognosticators for regrowth of hair were the number of "indeterminate" hairs initially present (more than 100 in a 2.5-cm diameter circle in the center of the bald area), the duration of baldness (less than 10 years), and the size of the balding area (less than 10 cm). Most recently, 0.5 percent minoxidil has been studied in combination with topical tretinoin for AGA.

SURGICAL TREATMENT OF ANDROGENETIC ALOPECIA

Despite the wide array of pharmacologic agents used to grow hair on bald scalps, there is not a single agent that has been shown to be reliably effective in the majority of patients treated. However, sites of advanced AGA can be effectively and permanently corrected with full-thickness, hair-bearing punch autografts obtained from the AGA-resistant occiput. In their new location transplanted follicles continue to produce hair of the same texture and color at the same rate as they did in the occipital scalp.[81] When indicated, bald scalp reduction can reduce the area requiring hair transplants.

HAIR CHANGES ASSOCIATED WITH AGING

The changes in hair associated with aging are related to an interplay of endocrinologic, chronologic, and physiologic factors. Each hair type responds differently, most diminishing but some inexplicably increasing in their growth function with age. Many of the changes can be related to the altered endocrine function, but some seem to be related to chronologic and physiologic aging, such as the inexorable gradual decrease in scalp hair diameter.

With age, a significant loss of hair follicles occurs throughout the scalp. The number of follicles in adults aged 20 to 30 years is about 615 per square centimeter of scalp. This figure drops to 485 in adults aged 30 to 50, and 435 in those aged 80 to 90; bald scalps in adults between 45 and 85 years have an average of 305 follicles per square centimeter.[82]

In the aging adult the quality of hair undergoes a change that results in an increase in the number of vellus hairs on the scalp, a decrease in facial hair in men, and an increasing thickness of hair on the face of women. In men the eyebrows become thicker and longer.[83] Both the duration of the growth phase and the size of hair follicles change with age. For example, from the third decade on there is a progressive transition of vellus hairs into terminal hairs on the tragus and antitragus of male ears. The opposite transition, from terminal to vellus, occurs in both sexes in age-associated common baldness of the scalp.[84] In general, the order of loss of terminal hair with advancing age on the trunk and limbs, pubes, and axillae reverses that of its appearance, but axillary and pubic hair are lost earlier and more completely in females than in males.[85]

In all races the incidence and degree of baldness increases with age. Baldness was studied and correlated positively with age in 77 normal Chinese males in New York[86] and in 312 males and 214 females who were students or staff members at Yale University, the University of Missouri, or the State University of New York, or who were inmates or staff members at Riker's Island Prison, New York; Fairfield State Hospital, Newton, Connecticut; or Jewish Sanatorium, Brooklyn, New York.

Studies of organ functions show that it is the reserve capacity that changes most with age. For the hair follicle, reserve capacity can be evaluated by measuring the regeneration time after plucking anagen hair. Regeneration time after plucking increases with age for chin, axillary, and thigh hair.[87] Many women who repeatedly pluck the hair of the glabellar area and the eyebrows report the occasional regeneration of gray hairs and the eventual cessation of regrowth after multiple pluckings.

Because of the difficulties in avoiding nutritional variations and environmental contamination, the conflicting results obtained in elemental analyses of hair and their correlation with aging have been of little use. Although hair analysis has limited value in screening for heavy metal exposure, its correlation with specific deficiency or disease states remains unproven. Most experts feel that the chemical condition of the hair and the state of health of the body are so unreliably related that hair analysis provides little useful information.[88] Nonetheless, many commercial laboratories claim hair analysis can provide valuable clues to deficiency states and diseases and offer this service, along with detailed recommendations for therapy, to health stores, beauticians, nutrition consultants, and physicians. A recent report suggests that commercial use of hair analysis is unscientific, economically wasteful, and of little clinical utility.[89]

On the other hand, a change as obvious as graying has proved to be a measurable parameter useful in studies of aging and is related to longevity. Hair grayness in 480 adult Mexicans was recorded in 1948. By 1969, 21 years later, 101 of the original sample had died. Those

between 35 and 69 years of age in 1948 who had died from natural causes in the intervening years were significantly grayer than average for their respective sex and 5-year age group.[90] Approximately 50 percent of the population will have about 50 percent gray hairs by age 50.[91]

ACQUIRED ALOPECIAS

Traumatic Alopecia

FRICTION AND PRESSURE

Fastening and removal of hair pieces can cause alopecia due to friction and evulsion of hair at the sites of attachment. Prolonged general anesthesia, especially in the Trendelenburg position, may cause a temporary alopecia in the area of dependent edema. Postoperative localized alopecia has been reported most commonly after certain gynecologic and open heart surgical procedures, the likelihood of hair loss and the chance of permanence correlating with the length of the anesthesia and intubation. Some cases of pressure-induced alopecia have been described after prolonged coma from other causes. Coma blisters have been reported after drug overdoses, but clinically similar blisters have been seen in other cases of coma. Both coma blisters and postoperative alopecia probably arise from the same phenomenon, pressure-induced ischemia.[92]

THERMAL AND CHEMICAL TRAUMA

Cryotherapy of cutaneous scalp malignancies may produce permanent hair loss. Industrial or cosmetic chemical contactants usually produce only partial or complete disintegration of the hair shaft, which results in hair breakage and temporary alopecia (Fig. 15-2). Severe primary irritant reactions that destroy hair follicles will produce permanent alopecia. Allergic eczematous contact dermatitis does not ordinarily produce permanent alopecia.

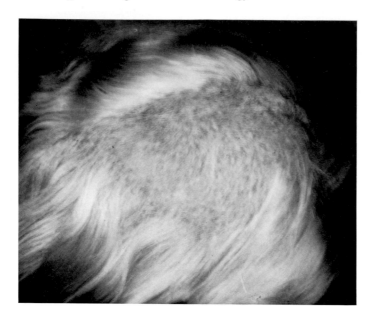

Fig. 15–2. Temporary hair loss due to chemical breakage.

Neoplastic Factors

In adults, as in children, benign and malignant neoplasms can produce hair loss by pressure, displacement, replacement, or systemic influences. Pressure on the overlying hair follicles from a pilar cyst (trichilemmal cyst or wen) of the scalp may produce temporary or permanent alopecia depending on the duration and degree of pressure (Fig. 15-3).

Toxic Alopecia

Many organic and inorganic chemicals entering the system by inhalation, injection, ingestion, or transepidermally may affect hair growth and produce toxic alopecia.

In general, adults use medications more frequently than children and are more likely to experience drug-induced alopecia. Drug-induced hair loss may be classified as anagen effluvium, telogen effluvium, or idiopathic effluvium. Antimetabolites provide a classic example of drug-induced anagen effluvium. These drugs interfere with hair in the active, proliferating anagen phase and induce attenuation of the hair shaft, with breakage, rapid shedding, and prompt regrowth when the inciting agent is removed.

Anticoagulants, anticholesterolemics, and β-blockers are a few examples of medications that induce telogen effluvium. Hair loss occurs after a latent period of about 100 days (2 to 4 months), which is the typical duration of telogen. Telogen effluvium hair loss occurs coincidently with the onset of the next anagen phase, with the new hairs pushing out the old telogen hairs. The topic of drug-induced alopecia has been well reviewed.[93,94] Terfenadine (Seldane), an antihistamine,[95] and Captopril (Capoten), an antihypertensive,[96] have also recently been reported to induce hair loss.

Examples of drugs that may cause hair loss are found in nearly all therapeutic classes: antikeratinizing, antimitotic, anticoagulant, antithyroid, anticonvulsant, hormonal, antibiotic, nonsteroidal anti-inflammatory, and many others. Occupational and medicinal exposure to heavy metals (arsenic, lead, bismuth, gold, lithium, mercury) has also been implicated.

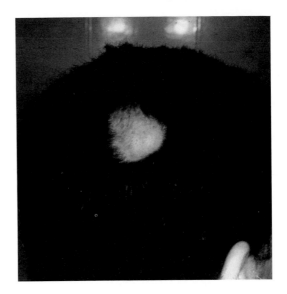

Fig. 15–3. Alopecia overlying a pilar cyst.

Nutritional Factors

Although proteins, carbohydrates, vitamins, and minerals are essential for normal hair growth, their absence produces not AGA but a rather characteristic diffuse hair loss. Concordantly, supplementation can reverse alopecia secondary to a true deficiency of one or more of these dietary constituents, but it cannot reverse AGA that has a hormonal-genetic pathogenesis.

Nevertheless, many alleged hair loss remedies exist that claim to contain the essential nutritive factors necessary for regrowth of AGA. There is, however, little if any evidence to support claims of increased hair growth by increasing diet content for a normal person.[97] Some studies relating to wool growth suggest that certain amino acids (methionine, cystine) and minerals may increase the diameter of the hair shaft,[98] but these do not alter the number of actively growing follicles.[97]

The effect of protein-calorie malnutrition on hair growth in adults has also been studied. Male subjects aged 24 to 29 years were fed equicaloric (2,800 kcal) diets with or without 75 g protein per day.[99,100] In subjects deprived of protein, severe atrophy occurred, up to 50 percent of the anagen hair bulbs being affected.

As to "crash" dieting, nine adults experienced profuse hair loss 2 to 5 months after starting a vigorous weight reduction program which resulted in weight loss of 11.7 to 24.75 kg.[101] Telogen counts of 25 to 50 percent were observed (normal scalp telogen count is about 10 percent). Regrowth of hair occurred within several months. Three of these patients had experienced hair loss closely following a successful weight reduction program on several occasions. Rigorous caloric restriction with consequent inadequate energy supply for the hair matrix is thought to cause the telogen defluvium of the crash dieter. A contributing factor may be release of androgens from the mobilized fat depots. Adequate energy supply appears to determine the rate of epidermal mitotic activity. Since the hair matrix is known to have the highest rate of cell turnover of human tissue,[102] it is not surprising that a drastic reduction in caloric intake might adversely affect the cellular kinetics of the hair matrix and precipitate a telogen phase.

Iron deficiency may be accompanied by diffuse hair loss, although the reduction in iron is often difficult to detect accurately owing to the wide range of normal serum iron levels; iron-binding capacity and serum ferritin measurements may therefore be useful. Patients exhibiting a number of other disease states unrelated to diet may show low serum iron levels without iron deficiency.[97] Iron-deficiency diffuse alopecia is uncommon in western countries although proven cases respond well to iron therapy; for example, routine iron supplementation is required following gastrectomy, in which iron deficiency produces a telogen-type diffuse alopecia and itching. Similarly, menorrhagia may cause anemia and diffuse hair loss; both symptoms may be corrected with dietary iron supplementation. Increasing the iron content of an already adequate diet does not, however, promote hair growth.[97]

An acquired form of acrodermatitis enteropathica and zinc deficiency has been described in patients receiving total parenteral nutrition.[103-105] The clinical presentation is characterized by dermatitis, diarrhea, apathy, and sparseness of scalp and eyebrow hair. This condition is reversed by zinc supplementation.

Scurvy, or vitamin C deficiency, is characterized by capillary hemorrhages surrounding hyperkeratotic follicular papules, swollen and bleeding gums, petechiae, ecchymoses, and weakness and tenderness in the lower extremities. The most significant skin manifestation is keratotic plugging of the hair follicles, chiefly on the anterior forearms, abdomen, and posterior thighs. The hairs are curled in follicles capped by keratotic plugs. These distinctive lesions have been named "cork-screw hairs."[106]

A lack of vitamin B12 may be associated with premature graying although vitamin B12 supplements do not delay the process.[97]

DERMATOLOGIC ALOPECIAS

Dissecting Cellulitis

Dissecting cellulitis of the scalp (or perifolliculitis capitis abscedens et suffodiens) is rare, more common in blacks than in whites, and is of unknown etiology. It occurs predominantly in males between 18 and 40.[107,108] A scarring alopecia results from destruction of hair follicles by an intense folliculitis (Fig. 15-4). A dissecting cellulitis leads to formation of interconnecting burrowing abscesses and fluctuant nodules. Crusted sinuses exude bloodstained pus and keloid formation is frequent. The disease is occasionally seen in patients with hidradenitis sup-

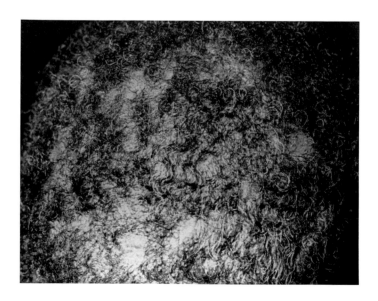

Fig. 15–4. Dissecting cellulitis of the scalp in a 55-year-old black male.

purativa and acne conglobata. It usually runs a chronic intermittently remitting course. Treatment is difficult and consists of oral and topical antibiotics, oral and/or intralesional corticosteroids, and judicious surgical drainage of fluctuant areas.

Folliculitis Decalvans

Folliculitis decalvans is a patchy, scarring alopecia, in which pustular folliculitis of the advancing margin is a conspicuous feature.[93] The cause is uncertain, although *Staphylococcus aureus,* seborrheic dermatitis, and an immune deficit have been suspected. Hairy regions other than the scalp may be involved. Folliculitis decalvans of the scalp occurs in both sexes. It affects women aged 30 to 60 and men from adolescence onwards.[93] When the pustules have healed and the erythema and scaling have resolved, the clinical presentation is identical to that of pseudopelade.

Lichen Planopilaris

Lichen planopilaris (LPP) is thought to be a form of lichen planus with a sharp localization to the hair follicles of the scalp or other hair-bearing areas. If present, classical lesions of lichen planus, with associated nail and mucosal changes, are helpful in making the diagnosis. Scalp involvement occurs in over 40 percent of patients.[93] Most patients are middle-aged or older adults. Active LPP of the scalp is manifested clinically by a patchy eruption of follicular, violaceous, spiny papules, with erythema and scaling, which progresses to follicular plugging and finally scarring with permanent alopecia. As the follicular plugs are shed, the irregularly shaped scarred areas appear white and smooth, and the clinical and histologic picture is indistinguishable from that of the pseudopelade of Brocq. Histopathologically, LPP can usually be identified in the early inflammatory stage.[109] The disorder tends to run a chronic course, with activity often lasting for years. Injections of triamcinolone acetonide (5 mg/ml in 0.1 ml aliquots) may slow its progression. Patients with severe, rapidly progressive disease may benefit from a trial of antimalarial (Plaquenil) or sulfone (dapsone) therapy. Quiescent cases are correctable by hair transplantation.

The Graham-Little syndrome consists of an LPP-like inflammatory condition of the scalp, which progresses to patchy cicatricial alopecia, loss of pubic and axillary hair, and rapid development of keratosis pilaris on glabrous skin.

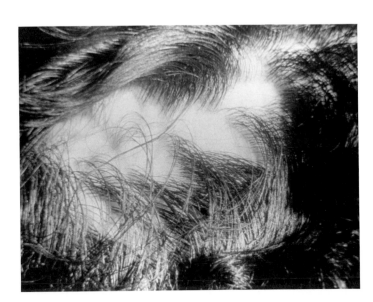

Fig. 15–5. Pseudopelade.

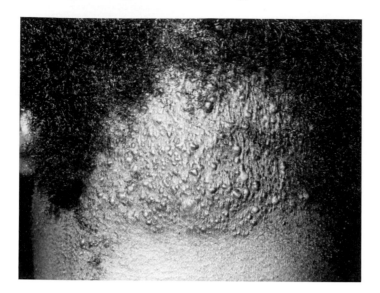

Fig. 15–6. Acne keloidalis nuchae showing scarring alopecia and keloidal papules.

Table 15-2. Approach to the Patient: Alopecia in Adults

	Type of Alopecia			
	Physiologic	Androgenetic	Gerontologic	Acquired
History	Seasonal Postpartum Postfebrile After oral contraceptive Puberty Gerontologic	Family history Menstrual irregularity (polycystic ovarian syndrome, menopause) Onset with adrenarche or pubarche	Old age	Hair pieces General anesthesia Thermal or chemical trauma Medications (anticoagulants, anticholesterolemics, β-blockers, etc.) Marked precipitous weight loss (crash dieting) Menorrhagia (iron deficiency) Total parenteral nutrition (decreased zinc)
Scalp and hair examination	Increased numbers of telogen hairs	Patterned (temporofrontal and crown) and diffuse (gradual change from terminal to vellus hairs)	Decreased hair follicle number Decreased hair shaft diameter Decreased regeneration time after plucking Graying	Neoplasia (benign and malignant) Dissecting cellulitis Cicatricial alopecias
Associated skin findings		Oily skin Acne Hirsutism (female)		
Laboratory investigation		DHEA-S SHBG T Free T Complete blood count Chemistry screen T3 T4		Complete blood count Fe/TIBC Serum ferritin

Pseudopelade

The pseudopelade of Brocq is best regarded as a slowly progressive form of cicatricial alopecia, which may be the end result of any one of a number of different pathological processes, both known and unknown. Clinically, there are smooth alopecic patches on the scalp often said to resemble "footprints in the snow" (Fig. 15-5). Therapy depends on whether pseudopelade can be shown to be secondary to a treatable condition. Intralesional triamcinolone acetonide may be helpful in early stages, and hair-bearing punch autografts from uninvolved to involved areas can be cosmetically beneficial in quiescent cases.

Acne Keloidalis Nuchae

Acne keloidalis nuchae is a chronic, inflammatory, cicatricial folliculitis of the nape of the neck which occurs almost exclusively in postpubertal males, especially blacks, between the ages of 14 and 25. The condition progresses from follicular papules, pustules, and discharging sinuses to firm keloidal papules, nodules, and plaques, with destruction of hair follicles (Fig. 15-6). Topical and intralesional corticosteroids and topical and oral antibiotics may help arrest the process; excision of keloids or injection of triamcinolone acetonide suspension are helpful in advanced situations.

APPROACH TO THE PATIENT

The approach to examining the adult patient with alopecia is outlined in Table 15-2. Particular aspects of the history, physical examination, and laboratory studies pertaining to the various types of alopecia are detailed.

REFERENCES

1. Szabo G: The regional frequency and distribution of hair follicles in human skin. p.33. In Montagna W, Ellis RA (eds): The Biology of Hair Growth. Academic Press, Orlando, FL, 1958
2. Ferriman D: Human Hair Growth in Health and Disease. Charles C Thomas, Springfield, IL, 1971
3. Friedenthal H: Das Dauerhaarkleid des Menschen. G. Fisher, Jena, 1908
4. Orentreich N: Scalp hair replacement in man. p.99. In Montagna W, Dobson RL (eds): Hair Growth. Pergamon Press, Oxford, 1969
5. Pinkus F: The story of a hair root. J Invest Dermatol 9:91, 1947
6. Casey JH, Burger HG, Kent JR, et al: Treatment of hirsutism by adrenal and ovarian suppression. J Clin Endocrinol Metab 26:1370, 1966
7. Orentreich N: Pathogenesis of alopecia. J Soc Cosm Chemists 11:479, 1960
8. Orentreich N, Rizer RL: Medical treatment of alopecia androgenica. p.294. In Brown AC, Crounse RA (eds): Hair, Trace Elements and Human Illness. Pt 4. Hirsutism and Alopecia. Praeger, New York, 1980
9. Chadwick J, Mann WN (trans): The Medical Works of Hippocrates. p.171. Blackwell Scientific Publications, London, 1959
10. Rothman S: Introduction. p.xi. In Montagna W, Ellis RA (eds): The Biology of Hair Growth. Academic Press, Orlando, FL, 1958
11. Hamilton JB: Male hormone stimulation is prerequisite and an incitant in common baldness. Am J Anat 71:451, 1942
12. Hamilton JB: Patterned loss of hair in man: types and incidence. Ann NY Acad Sci 53:708, 1951
13. Thomsen RJ, Webster SB: Idiopathic unilateral facial hirsutism. Arch Dermatol 115:99, 1979
14. Mahoudeau JA, Bardin CW, Lipsett MB: The metabolic clearance rate and origin of plasma dihydrotestosterone in man and its conversion to the 5α-androstanediols. J Clin Invest 50:1338, 1971
15. Bardin CW, Lipsett MB: Testosterone and androstenedione blood production rates in normal women and women with idiopathic hirsutism or polycystic ovaries. J Clin Invest 46:891, 1967
16. Kirchner MA, Bardin CW: Androgen production and metabolism in normal and virilized women. Metabolism 21:667, 1972

17. Anderson DC: Sex-hormone binding globulin. Clin Endocrinol 3:69, 1974

18. Price V: Testosterone metabolism in the skin. Arch Dermatol 11:1496, 1975

19. Rizer RL, Orentreich N, Finch CE: Testosterone metabolism in human scalp and beard hair follicles. p. 346. In Brown AC (ed): The First Human Hair Symposium. Medcom Press, New York, 1974

20. Hay JB, Hodgins MB: Metabolism of androgens in vitro by human facial and axillary skin. J Endocrinol 59:475, 1973

21. Cameron EHD, Baillie AH, Grant JK, et al: Transformation in vitro of 7α-3H-dehydroepiandrosterone to 3H-testosterone by skin from men. J Endocrinol 35:19, 1966

22. Hay JB, Hodgins MB: Metabolism of androgens by human skin in acne. Br J Dermatol 91:123, 1974

23. Gomez EC, Hsia SL: Studies in cutaneous metabolism of testosterone-4-^{14}C and 4-androstene-3-17-dione-4-^{14}C in human skin. Biochemistry 7:24, 1968

24. Migeon CJ, Keller AR, Lawrence B, et al: Dehydroepiandrosterone and androsterone levels in human plasma: effect of age and sex; day-to-day and diurnal variations. J Clin Endocrinol Metab 17:1051, 1957

25. Yamaji T, Ibayashi H: Plasma dehydroepiandrosterone sulfate in normal and pathological conditions. J Clin Endocrinol Metab 29:273, 1969

26. Sansone G, Reisner RM: Differential rates of conversion of testosterone to dihydrotestosterone in acne and in normal human skin: a possible pathogenic factor in acne. J Invest Dermatol 56:366, 1971

27. Northcut RC, Island DP, Liddle GE: An explanation for the target organ unresponsiveness to testosterone in the testicular feminization syndrome. J Clin Endocrinol Metab 29:422, 1969

28. Kuttenn F, Mauvais-Jarvis P: Testosterone 5-α-reductase in the skin of normal subjects and of patients with abnormal sex development. Acta Endocrinol (Copenh) 79:164, 1975

29. Montalto J, Callan A, Smith P, et al: Plasma androgens in females with hirsutism and androgenetic alopecia. (Abstract No. 1623). 7th International Congress of Endocrinology, International Congress Series, No.652, Excerpta Medica, Amsterdam, 1984

30. Schweikert HU, Wilson JD: Regulation of human hair growth by steroid hormones. I. Testosterone metabolism in isolated hairs. J Clin Endocrinol Metab 38:811, 1974

31. Bingham KD, Shaw DA: The metabolism of testosterone by human male scalp skin. J Endocrinol 57:111, 1973

32. Bonne C, Saurat J, Chivot M, et al: Androgen receptor in human male scalp skin. J Invest Dermatol 8:256, 1977

33. Stough DB III, Berger RA, Orentreich N: Surgical improvement of cicatricial alopecia of diverse etiology. Arch Dermatol 97:331, 1968

34. Rizer RL, Wheatley VR, Orentreich N: Androgens in human skin surface lipids: a radioimmunoassay analysis. (abstract). J Invest Dermatol 76:327, 1981

35. Miller JA, Darley CR, Karkavitsas KK, et al: Low sex-hormone binding globulin levels in young women with diffuse hair loss. Br J Dermatol 106:331, 1982

36. Neumann F: Pharmacology and potential use of cyproterone acetate. Horm Metab Res 9:1, 1977

37. Ekoe JM, Burckhardt P, Ruedi B: Treatment of hirsutism, acne and alopecia with cyproterone acetate. Dermatologica 160:398, 1980

38. Dawber RPR, Sonnex T, Ralfs I: Oral antiandrogen treatment of common baldness in woman. Br J Dermatol 107:suppl. 22, 20, 1982

39. Mortimer CH, Rushton H, James KC: Effective medical treatment for common baldness in woman. Clin Exp Dermatol 9:342, 1984

40. Rushton H, James KC, Mortimer CH: The unit area trichogram in the assessment of androgen-dependent alopecia. Br J Dermatol 109:429, 1983

41. Hammerstein J, Meckies J, Leo-Rossberg I, et al: The use of cyproterone acetate (CPA) in the treatment of acne, hirsutism and virilism. J Steroid Biochem 6:827, 1975

42. Winters SJ, Lee J, Troen P: Competition of histamine H2 antagonist cimetidine for androgen binding sites in man. J Androl 1:111, 1980

43. Vigersky RA, Mehlman I, Glass AR et al: Treatment of hirsute women with cimetidine. N Engl J Med 303:1042, 1980

44. Shapiro G, Evron S: A novel use of spironolactone: treatment of hirsutism. J Clin Endocrinol Metab 51:429, 1980

45. Nielsen PG: Treatment of moderate idiopathic hirsutism with a cream containing canrenone (an anti-androgen). Dermatologica 165:636, 1982

46. Burke BM, Cunliffe WJ: Oral spironolactone therapy for female patients with acne, hirsutism, or androgenic alopecia. Br J Dermatol 112:124, 1985

47. Corvol P, Michaud A, Menard J, et al: Antiandrogenic effect of spironolactones: mechanism of action. Andocrinology 97:52, 1975

48. Pita JC, Lippman E, Thompson EB, et al: Interaction of spironolactone and digitalis with the 5α-dihydrotestosterone (DHT) receptor of rat ventral prostate. Endocrinology 97:1521, 1975

49. Steelman SC, Brooks JR, Morgan ER, et al: Antiandrogenic activity of spironolactone. Steroids 14:449, 1969

50. Menard RD, Stripp B, Gillette JR: Spironolactone and testicular cytochrome P-450: decreased testosterone formation in several species and changes in hepatic drug metabolism. Endocrinology 94:1628, 1974

51. Pentikainen PL, Pentikainen LA, Huffman DH, et al: The effect of spironolactone on plasma levels and excretion of testosterone and estrogens in the urine in males. J Int Med Res 2:439, 1974

52. Rose LI, Underwood RH, Newmark ST, et al: Pathophysiology of spironolactone-induced gynecomastia. Ann Intern Med 87:398, 1977

53. Wallace AM, Grant JK: Effect of zinc on androgen metabolism in the human hyperplastic prostate. Biochem Soc Trans 3:540, 1975

54. Habib FK, Hammond GL, Lee IR, Dawson JB: Metal-androgen interrelationships in carcinoma and hyperplasia of the human prostate. J Endocrinol 71:133, 1976

55. Wilms H, Schleusener A: The effect of zinc ions on the 5 alpha-reductase of the sebaceous gland in hamster ears. Acta Endocrinol (Copenh) 94:suppl. 234, 112, 1980

56. Orentreich N: Medical treatment of baldness. Ann Plast Surg 1:116, 1978

57. Voigt W, Fernandez EP, Hsia SL: Transformation of testosterone into 17β-hydroxy-5α-androstan-3-one by microsomal preparations of human skin. J Biol Chem 245:5599, 1970

58. Mauvais-Jarvis P, Kuttenn F, Baudot N, et al: Inhibition of testosterone conversion to dihydrotestosterone in men treated percutaneously by progesterone. J Clin Endocrinol Metab 38:142, 1974

59. Mowszowics I, Riahi M, Wright F, et al: Androgen receptor in human skin cytosol. J Clin Endocrinol Metab 52:338, 1981

60. Wright F, Kirchoffer MO, Mauvais-Jarvis P: Antagonistic action of dihydrotestosterone on the formation of the specific dihydrotestosterone–cytoplasmic receptor complex in the rat ventral prostate. J Steroid Biochem 10:419, 1979

61. Mauvais-Jarvis P, Baudot N, Bercovici JP: In vivo studies on progesterone metabolism by human skin. J Clin Endocrinol Metab 29:1580, 1969

62. Berman A: Peripheral effects of L-thyroxine on hair growth and coloration in cattle. J Endocrinol 20:288, 1960

63. DuCharme DW, Freyburger WA, Graham BE, et al: Pharmacologic properties of minoxidil; a new hypotensive agent. J Pharmacol Exp Ther 184:662, 1973

64. Mehta PK, Mamdani B, Sharsky RM, et al: Severe hypertension: treatment with minoxidil. JAMA 233:249, 1975

65. Burton JL, Marshall A: Hypertrichosis due to minoxidil. Br J Dermatol 101:593, 1979

66. Zappacosta AR: Reversal of baldness in patient receiving minoxidil for hypertension. N Engl J Med 303:1480, 1980

67. Devine BL, Fife R, Trust PM: Minoxidil for severe hypertension after failure of other hypotensive drugs. Br Med J 2:667, 1977

68. Dargie HJ, Dollery CT, Daniel J: Minoxidil in resistant hypertension. Lancet 2:515, 1977

69. Jacomb RG, Brunnberg FJ: The use of minoxidil in the treatment of severe essential hypertension: a report on 100 patients. Clin Sci Mol Med 51:579, 1979

70. Hull AR, Long L, Prati RC, et al: The control of hypertension in patients undergoing regular maintenance hemodialysis. Kidney Int Suppl., 57:184, 1975

71. Seidman M, Westfried M, Maxey R, et al: Reversal of male pattern baldness by minoxidil. Cutis 28:551, 1981

72. Pennisis AJ, Takahashi M, Bernstein BH, et al: Minoxidil therapy in children with severe hypertension. Paediatr Pharm Ther 90:813, 1977

73. Wester RC, Maibach HI, Guy RH, et al: Minoxidil stimulates cutaneous blood flow in human balding scalps: pharmacodynamics measured by laser doppler velocimetry and photopulse plethysmography. J Invest Dermatol 82:515, 1984

74. Ebling FJ, Rook A: Acquired circumscribed hypertrichosis. p.1757. In Rook AJ, Wilkinson DS, Ebling FJ (eds): Textbook of Dermatology.

3rd Ed. Vol. 2. Blackwell Scientific Publications, Oxford, 1979

75. Earhart RN, Ball J, Nuss DD, et al: Minoxidil-induced hypertrichosis: treatment with calcium thioglycolate depilatory. South Med J 70:442, 1977

76. Parker LN, Lifrak ET, Odell WD: Lack of gonadal or adrenal androgenic mechanism for the hypertrichosis produced by diazoxide, phenytoin and minoxidil. Biochem Pharmacol 31: 1948, 1982

77. Vanderveen EE, Ellis CN, Kang MPH, et al: Topical minoxidil for hair regrowth. J Am Acad Dermatol 11:416, 1984

78. Weiss VC, West DP, Mueller CE: Topical minoxidil in alopecia areata. J Am Acad Dermatol 5:224, 1981

79. Headington JT, Novak E: Histological findings in androgenic alopecia treated with topical minoxidil. Br J Dermatol 107: suppl. 22, 20, 1982

80. DeVillez RL: Topical minoxidil therapy in hereditary androgenetic alopecia. Arch Dermatol 121:197, 1985

81. Orentreich N: Autografts in alopecias and other selected dermatological conditions. Ann NY Acad Sci 83:463, 1959

82. Giacometti L: The anatomy of the human scalp. p. 97. In Montagna W (ed): Advances in Biology of the Skin. Vol. 6. Aging. Pergamon Press, Oxford, 1965

83. Soloman LM, Virtue C: The biology of cutaneous aging. Int J Dermatol 14:172, 1975

84. Barman JM, Pecararo V, Astore I: Biological basis of the inception and evolution of baldness. J Gerontol 24:163, 1969

85. Rook A: Endocrine influences on hair growth. Br Med J 1: 609, 1965

86. Hamilton JB: Patterned loss of hair in man: types and incidence. Ann NY Acad Sci 53:708, 1951

87. Myers RJ, Hamilton JB: Regeneration and rate of growth of hairs in man. Ann NY Acad Sci 53:562, 1951

88. Commercial hair analysis—unscientific and misleading. Intern Med Alert 7:74, 1985

89. Barrett S: Commercial hair analysis; science of scam? JAMA 254:1041, 1985

90. Lasker GW, Kaplan B: Graying of the hair and mortality. Soc Biol 21:290, 1974

91. Ebling FJ: The physiology of hair growth. p.181. In Breuer MM (ed): Cosmetic Science. Vol. 2. Academic Press, London, 1980

92. Wiles JC, Hansen RC: Postoperative (pressure) alopecia. J Am Acad Dermatol 12:195, 1985

93. Rook A, Dawber R: Diseases of the hair and scalp. Blackwell Scientific Publications, Oxford, 1982

94. Stroud JD: Drug-induced alopecia. Semin Dermatol 4:29, 1985

95. Jones S, Morley W: Terfenadine causing hair loss (unreviewed report). Br Med J 291:940, 1985

96. Leaker B, Whitworth H: Alopecia associated with captopril treatment. (Letter). Aust NZ J Med 14:886, 1984

97. Gummer CL: Diet and hair loss. Semin Dermatol 4:35, 1985

98. Reis PJ: The growth and composition of wool. Aust J Biol Sci 20:809, 1967

99. Bradfield RB, Bailey MA, Margen S: Morphological changes in human scalp hair roots during deprivation of protein. Science 157:438, 1967

100. Calloway DH, Margen S: Physiological evaluation of nutrient defined diets for space flight metabolic studies. University of California Press, Berkeley, 1966

101. Goette DK, Odom RB: Alopecia in crash dieters. JAMA 235:2622, 1976

102. Weinstein GD, Frost P: Replacement kinetics. p. 84. In Fitzpatrick TB, Arndt KA, Clark WH (eds): Dermatology in General Medicine. McGraw-Hill, New York, 1971

103. Kay RG, Tasman-Jones C: Acute zinc deficiency in man during intravenous alimentation. Aust NZ J Surg 292:879, 1975

104. Weismann K, Hjorth N, Fischer A: Zinc depletion syndrome with acrodermatitis during long-term intravenous feeding. Clin Exp Dermatol 1:237, 1976

105. Wexler D, Pace W: Acquired zinc deficiency disease of the skin. Br J Dermatol 96:669, 1977

106. Domonkos AN, Arnold HL, Odom RB: Andrews' diseases of the Skin. 7th Ed. WB Saunders, Philadelphia, 1982

107. Moschella CL, Klein MH, Miller RJ: Perifolliculitis capitis abscedens et suffodiens. Arch Dermatol 96:195, 1967

108. Moyer DG, Williams RM: Perifolliculitis capitis abscedens et suffodiens. Arch Dermatol 85:378, 1962

109. Lever WF, Schaumburg-Lever G: Histopathology of the skin. 6th Ed. JB Lippincott, Philadelphia, 1983

16

Chronic Urticaria

Bernard R. Adelsberg

The skin lesions of urticaria are usually easily recognized, and although frequently troublesome to the patient, they are often self-limited. In isolated instances of acute urticaria the precipitating cause is easily identified, and the symptoms generally resolve whether or not the cause is known. The term *chronic urticaria* has been coined for recurrent episodes of urticarial lesions that come and go over a period of more than 6 weeks.[1] This definition is useful since it allows a reasonable amount of time for brief viral infections to pass and for ingested allergens such as drugs to be excreted. Identifying the cause of chronic urticaria can involve an extremely difficult, prolonged, and expensive evaluation, which is better avoided in those patients whose symptoms are limited to a few weeks.

This chapter will divide the clinical urticarias into their two basic pathophysiological mechanisms: (1) urticaria caused by mast cell degranulation as the final common pathway; (2) urticaria caused by vasculitis as the final common pathway. The rationale for this arbitrary separation is based particularly on the different therapies required for the two groups. The treatment of the effects of mast cell degranulation may be accomplished by antihistamines (of both the H_1 and H_2 class) or by inhibitors of mast cell degranulation (cromolyn sodium or ketotifen), with corticosteroids reserved for only the most resistant cases. The treatment of vasculitis occasionally requires steroids as the first-line therapy and may require additional cytotoxic modalities. Thus, discriminating between the two mechanisms may be of more than academic interest.

URTICARIA CAUSED BY MAST CELL DEGRANULATION

The causes of mast cell degranulation are usually classified as immunologic or nonimmunologic. Occasionally this distinction is unclear owing to overlap between definitions. It may be easier to divide the causes of mast cell degranulation into four categories:

1. IgE-mediated (allergic)
2. Complement-mediated (immunologic)
3. Direct degranulating effects of drugs, neurohormones, opioid peptides, or other chemicals, which may be physiologic, pathophysiologic, toxic, hypersensitive, or idiosyncratic reactions (toxic)
4. Direct (or indirect) effects of physical stimuli (direct)

Urticaria Mediated by Immunoglobulin E

The surfaces of mast cells contain receptors that are specific for the Fc portion of the IgE molecule. Cross-linking of contiguous IgE molecules by an antigen serves as the trigger for a series of biochemical events leading to mast cell degranulation and urticaria. The offending substance can be a food, drug, pollen, infectious agent, or any other antigenic material capable of eliciting an immunologic response of the IgE type. Exposure to the antigen via inhalation, ingestion, or contact can result in urticaria.

Medications are particularly common causes of urticaria, and a detailed history of drug ingestion or injection should be sought in every patient. The list of drugs capable of causing an urticarial reaction is quite long, and it has been stated that almost any drug can cause urticaria.[2] Penicillin has received the most attention, being the commonest medication to cause urticaria by an IgE-mediated mechanism. Positive intracutaneous tests with penicillin have been found in 33 of 152 patients (21.5 percent) with chronic urticaria, compared with 3 to 8 percent of the general population.[3] This has led to the suggestion that traces of penicillin in food may be responsible for chronic urticaria. Consequently, diets omitting all milk and other dairy products and many meat products have been suggested for chronic urticaria patients with positive intracutaneous tests for penicillin.[3] This diet was allegedly effective in more than 50 percent of 42 patients with positive penicillin skin tests. Moreover, penicillinase has been successfully used in the treatment of patients with chronic urticaria and a history of penicillin allergy.[4,5]

Other substances implicated in causing urticaria include inhalants such as dusts, pollens, animal danders, and molds[6]; foods, especially milk,[7] shellfish, fruit, nuts, eggs, and food additives[8]; and a variety of insect venoms.[6] Mechanisms mediated by IgE have also been suggested for urticaria associated with a number of infections, especially helminthic infections. While IgE levels can be elevated in patients with parasitic infections, a type I IgE-mediated mechanism remains to be proved.[9]

In discussing IgE-mediated urticaria, patients with atopic symptoms deserve special mention. It seems logical that patients with ''allergic'' rhinitis or ''allergic'' asthma should also develop ''allergic'' urticaria, and this has been

discussed by several investigators.[10] However, urticaria seldom accompanies an exacerbation of other atopic symptoms, and in fact atopic patients do not have an increased prevalence of urticaria.[9]

Complement-Mediated Mast Cell Degranulation

Activation of the complement cascade leads to mast cell degranulation and urticaria or angioedema. The classical pathway is activated by antibody-antigen interactions (immune complexes), and its role in the production of urticarial vasculitis will be discussed below. The alternate pathway may also be activated directly, both by specific immunologic mechanisms and by nonspecific polysaccharide repeating structures, as on bacterial and fungal cell walls or on the cellophane membranes of dialyzers and oxygenators. Other substances, such as venoms and radiocontrast dyes, may cause mast cell degranulation by direct activation of the alternate pathway, resulting in urticaria.

Complement-mediated mast cell degranulation has not been shown to play a major role in chronic urticaria. In fact, hypocomplementemia seldom occurs in chronic urticaria with the exception of urticarial vasculitis.[11,12]

Direct Effects of Drugs and Other Agents

A number of substances appear to be able to foster release of granules from mast cells by direct, nonimmunologic action. Those substances that do this by destroying the cell will not be considered here. Enzymes found in bee venom may activate the complement system or cause direct mast cell degranulation.[13] Substances isolated from beans, wheat, and lentils (lectins) have been shown to cause direct histamine release in vitro.[14,15] The prescribed opiates morphine, codeine, and meperidine, as well as endogenous opioid peptides, have been recognized as capable of causing direct mast cell degranulation.[16] A whole host of basic polypeptides, including polymyxin B, bradykinin, substance P, neurotensin, somatostatin, ACTH (residues 1 through 24), protamine sulfate, and PTH (residues 1 through 34) have direct mast cell degranulating activities.[17-24] Several types of muscle relaxants, including succinylcholine and D-tubocurarine, may also cause direct mast cell degranulation.[25] Agents usually associated with aggravation of existing urticaria rather than being identified as the sole cause of urticaria include aspirin, other salicylates and nonsteroidal anti-inflammatory agents, azo dyes, and tyramine-containing foods (chocolate, cheese, wine, and shellfish).[26-29] The food additives benzoic acid, benzoate salts, monosodium glutamate, and sulfiting agents are often cited as capable of causing mast cell degranulation directly.[30] A recent report described urticaria caused by aspartame, although no mechanism for its activity has been established.[31]

Effects of Physical Stimuli

Physical stimuli are perhaps the most easily recognized causes of urticaria. Physically induced urticarias frequently occur in the younger population and may be directly demonstrated under controlled conditions in the office or laboratory. Despite the reproducible nature of these lesions, mechanisms are still not entirely clear for each type of physical stimulus. Physical stimuli may cause urticaria by direct effects on mast cells, or they may require a cofactor, usually a serum protein such as IgE or IgM. Occasionally, they may cause urticaria through vasculitis or through other, unknown mechanisms.

TRAUMA

Trauma may be the cause of several different types of urticaria. Dermatographism is defined as an exaggerated, transient wheal and flare response after firm stroking of the skin.[32] Although the presence of wheals at sites of tight clothing or mild trauma (such as that caused by leaning against a rail) is common, it is relatively rare for patients to describe pruritus as part of this response. Symptomatic dermatographism, then, refers to a group of patients who itch when they develop wheals after mild trauma. The subsequent scratching that is provoked may perpetuate and extend the areas of involved skin. In some cases, IgE has been implicated in symptomatic dermatographism,[33] while in others, substances such as adenosine triphosphate or substance P, released by the axon reflex, may be responsible.[19,34] Delayed dermatographism is a rare condition in which patients first exhibit a normal or dermatographic response to a stimulus. This disappears rapidly, but 1 to 8 hours later a wheal may return at the test site associated with angioedema. This subsequent reaction may last up to 48 hours and can be associated with a burning or painful sensation.[35,36] A satisfactory explanation of this delayed type of urticaria has yet to be advanced.

Pressure-associated urticaria also presents in a more delayed form. Application of pressure may cause a wheal to develop, which ordinarily disappears rapidly, but 4 to 8 hours later painful but not pruritic erythematous lesions develop, often associated with fever, chills, and arthralgias.[37] Biopsies of these lesions are not consistent from patient to patient. A mononuclear cell infiltration of the mid-dermis is the usual picture, but more than 50 percent of the specimens show a concomitant infiltration with eosinophils. There is no evidence of vasculitis but there is some endothelial thickening of capillaries.[36] This syndrome has been variably associated with chronic urticaria,[36,37] and, interestingly, one set of authors suggests that the pressure lesions are responsive to nonsteroidal anti-inflammatory drugs, which possibly implicates arachidonic acid metabolites in the pathogenesis of these lesions.

TEMPERATURE

Changes in temperature are occasionally associated with the development of urticaria. Reactions to cold may require local and/or generalized exposure; they may also be immediate, delayed, or both. Cold exposure may include eating or handling of cold foods and beverages, exposure to drafts of cold air, or immersion in cold water as in showers or swimming. Systemic symptoms are infrequently present in patients with cold-induced urticaria but are serious if present, since they include bronchospasm, hypotension, and flushing.[32] Death from drowning has even been reported in one case.[38] In patients with essential acquired cold urticaria, passive transfer experiments have documented that IgE is the immunoglobulin most commonly associated with symptoms, although IgM has been implicated in at least two patients. There are also at least two forms of familial cold-induced urticaria. Both are inherited in a dominant fashion, but they appear to differ in the length of time from cold exposure to development of symptoms.[42,43] The pathophysiology of the lesions produced in the familial forms of cold-induced urticaria is as yet unknown. Even though IgE and IgM may passively transfer cold sensitivity and increased histamine levels are present in the venous effluent of cold-challenged limbs, mast cell degranulation may not be the sole mechanism by which urticaria occurs. In at least one study, leukocytoclastic vasculitis could be induced by repeated cold challenges in five of eight patients thought to have essential acquired cold urticaria.[44] Vasculitis may also be present as urticaria in other syndromes relating to the cold, such as cryoglobulinemia[45] and paroxysmal cold hemoglobinuria.[46]

Exposure of parts of the body to heat or generalized warming of the patient as by exercise may also result in urticaria. The former is called *localized heat urticaria* and the latter *cholinergic urticaria.* Localized heat urticaria may exist in a sporadic, immediate form or in a familial, delayed manner. In the immediate type there may be associated nausea, diarrhea, abdominal cramps, and headache lasting for about 1 hour.[47] In the delayed form, lesions begin after 1½ to 2 hours and may persist for 12 to 14 hours.[48] It is not clear at present whether direct effects of heat on mast cells are sufficient

to explain these lesions or whether heat affects other immunologic or nonimmunologic pathways leading to mast cell degranulation as a secondary phenomenon. Generalized overheating of the body can lead to a form of urticaria called *cholinergic urticaria.* Other stimuli that may induce this mechanism include exercise, ingestion of hot and/or spicy food, and emotional stress. The skin lesions are distinctive, with punctate wheals surrounded by erythematous flares that often coalesce. Nausea, vomiting, salivation, abdominal cramps, diarrhea, headaches, and syncope occasionally are present during severe attacks.[49] Angioedema may be a prominent symptom as well.[50] Some patients may demonstrate concomitant airway hyperreactivity or may mimic patients with exercise-induced anaphylaxis.[51,52] Mast cell degranulation is thought to be responsible for this syndrome since products of mast cell degranulation may be present after an attack.[51] As with many other forms of urticaria, it is not clear at present whether this is a primary event or secondary, in this case, to a sympathetic cholinergic reflex.[53]

Other, rarer forms of physically induced urticarias include aquagenic,[54,55] vibratory,[56] and solar[57,58] urticarias. The mechanisms responsible for aquagenic and vibratory urticaria are unclear, whereas in solar urticaria recent evidence suggests that a "photoallergen" may be involved and that specific IgE-generated in response to it may be the cause of the mast cell degranulation in some patient populations.[59,60] However, solar urticaria can also occur in patients with erythropoietic protoporphyria, presumably on a nonimmunologic basis.[61]

VASCULITIS AS A CAUSE OF URTICARIA

It is not always possible to separate true urticaria from urticarial vasculitis on clinical grounds alone (Fig. 16-1). The clues to the presence of vasculitis are that (1) the lesions last for more than 24 hours; (2) they burn, sting, or may be asymptomatic; (3) they do not blanch

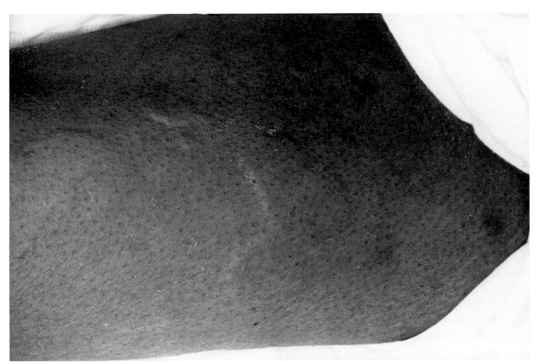

Fig. 16–1. Urticarial vasculitis morphologically indistinguishable from true urticaria on the thigh of a patient with systemic lupus erythematosus.

upon pressure; and (4) upon resolution they leave a red or brownish discoloration from extravasated red cells. However, the lesions of urticarial vasculitis may also itch and disappear within 24 hours.[62]

Histologically, urticaria caused by mast cell degranulation may show only vascular dilatation, dermal edema, and a sparsely cellular perivascular infiltrate. At the other end of the spectrum, some urticarial lesions will demonstrate the picture of necrotizing vasculitis. Histologically this appears as venular endothelial cell swelling, neutrophilic perivascular infiltrates, extravasation of red blood cells, fibrinoid deposits in and necrosis of venules, and leukocytoclasis.[63,64] A more liberal view defines vasculitis as the presence of neutrophils within the walls of affected vessels.[62] As might be imagined, using these different histologic criteria different authors have found very different incidences of vasculitis in their patients with chronic urticaria. If criteria were strict, 20 percent of patients with chronic urticaria might

be identified as having vasculitis, as against 52 percent if criteria were more liberal.[62,65]

Another type of stratification of patients was offered by Jones et al., who recognized a third histologic category, namely, a dense perivascular mixed-cell infiltrate, which was predominantly mononuclear but contained neutrophils and/or eosinophils without deposition of fibrinoid material within vessel walls and without leukocytoclasis.[66] Recent studies have concentrated on this type of nonnecrotizing perivascular mononuclear cell infiltrate and have demonstrated that the infiltrate consists of mast cells and mononuclear cells.[67] Further analysis has demonstrated that the mononuclear cells are mostly T4-positive cells, the so-called helper cells, implicating cell-mediated immune responses in this form of urticaria.[68] Immunohistologic analysis often reveals deposits of immunoglobulin and complement in lesional skin, particularly in and around blood vessels and along the dermal-epidermal junction.[62,65,66] Interestingly, positive immunofluorescent studies are occasionally found in patients without histologic evidence of exuberant cellular infiltration[65,66] or depressed complement levels.[69] Patients may then be further stratified by the presence or absence of hypocomplementemia[64,69] and by the presence or absence of additional extracutaneous symptoms and findings.[62,63,65,66] Alterations in the complement system seem to be centered on the classical complement pathway and include decreased levels of CH50, C1q, C4, and C3, although some patients with depressed levels of terminal components have been noted.[70,71] The alternate pathway appears to be variably involved.[63,72] Circulating immune complexes, as detected by a variety of assays, are often found in hypocomplementemic patients and in normocomplementemic patients with systemic manifestations.[65,69]

Both hypocomplementemic and normocomplementemic patients may also be divided into those with and those without extracutaneous symptoms. Clinically, arthralgias, arthritis, abdominal or chest pain, asthma, chronic obstructive pulmonary disease, uveitis, conjunctivitis, nausea, vomiting, fever, and unexplained lymphadenopathy have all been reported as associated findings.[62,65,66,69] Aside from hypocomplementemia, other laboratory abnormalities often include an elevated sedimentation rate, hematuria, proteinuria, increased creatinine levels, and alterations of pulmonary function tests.[65,69,73] Renal biopsies, when performed in both hypo- and normocomplementemic patients, have demonstrated a variety of histologic findings, including focal necrosis, both focal and diffuse proliferation, mesangiopathy, and tubulointerstitial involvement.[69] The deposition of immunoglobulin and complement in these areas has been noted on occasion.[71] Tests for cryoglobulins, rheumatoid factor, syphilis, antinuclear antibodies, anti-DNA antibodies, hepatitis B surface antigen, and immunoglobulins have also been noted to be occasionally abnormal.[63–65,69] A unique 7S immunoglobulin that precipitates with C1q has been associated with the hypocomplementemia-vasculitis-urticaria syndrome.[74,75]

Some systemic diseases have demonstrated a frequent association with urticarial vasculitis. In patients with systemic lupus erythematosus, biopsies of urticarial lesions demonstrated vasculitis in 70 to 80 percent of specimens examined.[76,77] Sjögren's syndrome may also present with urticarial vasculitis,[78] as may relapsing polychondritis.[79] Viral infections such as those caused by hepatitis B and Epstein-Barr virus have been associated with urticarial vasculitis.[80,81]

APPROACH TO THE PATIENT

There are different philosophies about the evaluation of patients with chronic urticaria. One approach states that since the treatment of urticaria is the same regardless of the cause and since routine evaluations rarely discover a cause, evaluation of the patient is unnecessary and unwarranted. In fact, in several series of patients with chronic urticaria, specific causes have been found in fewer than 20 percent of cases.[2,5,82] A second, very different school of thought recommends a major effort to determine the cause of chronic urticaria, including numerous diagnostic tests. If these fail, elimination routines to remove offending allergens from the diet and therapeutic trials to treat possible occult infections are attempted.[83]

Unfortunately, repeated diagnostic tests and trials are often unhelpful and expensive. How then should the clinician approach a patient with chronic urticaria? Certainly a thorough history and physical examination are indicated in any patient with chronic urticaria that does not have an obvious cause. More in-depth evaluation must be individualized and the extent of workup determined by the frequency and severity of urticaria and by any clues that are found on history and physical examination (Table 16-1).

There are two compelling reasons for pursuing the cause of chronic urticaria. The first is that by performing some tests looking for systemic diseases one may be able to reassure the patient that no systemic or life-threatening problem exists, even if one cannot pinpoint the exact

Table 16-1. Approach to the Patient: Diagnostic Steps in the Patient with Chronic Urticaria

General
    Sedimentation rate
    Complete blood count with differential
    Chemistry screen
    Thyroid function tests

    Infectious
        Stool for ova and parasites
        Indicated cultures
        Serum hepatitis antigens
        Indicated x-rays: sinus, chest, dental, others

IgE mediated
    Total IgE by PRIST
    Antigen specific IgE by RAST
    Skin tests
    Challenges

Vasculitis/immune complex mediated
    Complement levels or CH_{50}
    Antinuclear antibodies
    Immune complex assay (C1q, conglutinin, C3d)
    Complement activation studies
    Biopsy with immunofluorescence
    Cryoglobulins

Non-immunologically mediated
    Challenge with relevant food, additive, drug or physical stimulus (dermatographism, ice cube test for cold urticaria, phototesting for solar urticaria, exercise challenge for cholinergic urticaria)

cause or mechanism of the urticaria. On the other hand, both negative and positive test results may point the physician and patient toward either avoidance of offending agents or toward the most appropriate therapies. The purpose of an evaluation for patients with chronic urticaria should consist of efforts directed at establishing whether the lesions are caused by the effects of mast cell degranulation or by active vasculitis.

History and Clinical Evaluation

In the assessment of the patient with chronic urticaria there is no substitute for a thorough history obtained by a knowledgeable physician, although questionnaires abound and may be quite useful.[5] This history may even have to be repeated regularly after the patient's awareness of the wide range of provocative agents lurking in his environment has been increased.

A moment-by-moment daily diary is occasionally necessary to pinpoint exposures that the patient takes for granted. A discussion with the patient of possible triggers of urticaria in the home, such as molds in heating or cooling systems, may abrogate the need for extensive and expensive work-ups.

An example is worth discussing. A 28-year-old white female had just returned from a vacation in Spain when, upon her arrival at her apartment, she developed urticaria. The history revealed that she was atopic but that she and other members of her family had suffered from a diarrheal illness just prior to their departure from Europe. Stool cultures and assorted serologic tests for parasites were all negative. Further history suggested that her urticaria, although now present constantly for 8 weeks, was exacerbated in her apartment. A discussion of potential sources of exposure led her to a careful look around her apartment. In one closet she found a patch of damp, moldy plaster. While she had been away in Europe and without her knowledge, a bathtub in the floor above had overflowed, causing the water damage and subsequent mold overgrowth. Removal of the damaged plaster ended her urticaria entirely. This example is presented to demonstrate that when looking for causes of chronic urticaria, the physician must: (1) have an open mind about alternative possibilities; (2) be persistent about questioning the patient repeatedly and exploring new avenues suggested by these discussions; and (3) realize that if the physician can enlist the patient's cooperation, together they may often discover the source of the patient's urticaria. It is not unusual to have the patient call the doctor's office at some interval after the initial visit, describing a likely culprit responsible for his or her urticaria.

The physical examination is often diagnostic in patients whose urticaria is caused by one of the several varieties of physical trauma or by cholinergic stimuli. Many patients may also have severe dermatographism. This is particularly important to recognize since skin tests may be uninterpretable in such patients. Their skin reactivity is so exaggerated that even the saline control will cause the rapid development of a large wheal and flare. Other easily discernible physical findings include the tiny hives with large flares that may be diagnostic of cholinergic urticaria and the yellow-brown macules of urticaria pigmentosa which form wheals on light stroking. Examination of the ears and nose may strongly suggest the possibility of allergies or chronic sinusitis. The neck should be evaluated for lymphadenopathy and tender thyromegaly. Enlargement of the liver and spleen should be sought. Careful inspection of the hands and feet should be made for evidence of fungal infections, and the joints should also be examined if vasculitis is being considered. Other physical findings should be sought if suggested by the history.

Laboratory Work-Up

The extent of the laboratory work-up depends upon the results of the history and physical examination and the severity of the patient's symptoms. An algorithm for the evaluation of patients with chronic urticaria is presented in Figure 16-2. As indicated earlier, one approach is to try to separate patients into those whose lesions are caused by vasculitis and those whose lesions are caused by mast cell degranulation. There are many cases in which a careful history reveals the source of the lesions, particularly for the allergic and physical urticarias. Laboratory tests in allergic urticaria might be useful to confirm the presence of atopy (total IgE levels) and to confirm specific allergic sensitivities (RAST or skin tests). In a patient with a physical urticaria, immunoglobulin analyses and passive transfer studies (if available) might be useful tests to perform. As indicated earlier, some patients with cold-induced urticaria may have vasculitis and low complement levels.[44,84] Additional studies of complement levels, complement activation products, or hemolytic activity might be indicated in such a situation.

If the history and easily available laboratory tests are not helpful, a skin biopsy is indicated as the next step to distinguish between mast cell degranulation and vasculitis. The analysis of the biopsy must include immunofluorescent studies for the presence of immunoglobulins and complement, as well as standard stains for light microscopy. If vasculitis is found, a more extensive evaluation for systemic disease is warranted. This should include determinations of sedimentation rate; antinuclear antibodies and other autoantibodies, such as rheumatoid factor or antithyroglobulin antibody; immunoglobulin levels; cryoglobulins and cryofibrinogens; complement component levels and an assay for functional integrity of the complement system (CH50); circulating immune complex levels; hepatitis B and Epstein-Barr virus analysis, etc.

On the other hand, if there is no reason to suspect a systemic process and if the biopsy shows no evidence of vasculitis, the lesions are most likely related to mast cell degranulation. If IgE-mediated reactions can be excluded, these lesions are often related to nonimmunologic toxic or hypersensitivity reactions, such as those seen with food additives or preservatives. Double-blind challenges with opaque capsules might be considered if absolute proof is required, but diets that eliminate exposure to the offending substances rather than challenges can be recommended in troublesome cases. Laboratory tests are often not very helpful in defining any abnormalities in these patients, and the primary goal of using the laboratory should be to reassure the physician and patient that there are no serious systemic causes of, or sequelae from, the mast cell degranulation.

Therapy

Therapy should be based on the proven or presumed cause of the urticaria. Avoidance, where possible, should be the mainstay of therapy for the allergic, toxic, and physical urticarias linked to mast cell degranulation. Medications interfering with mast cell degranulation and products of mast cell degranulation, i.e., H_1 and H_2 antihistamines, are likely to be effective. Steroids should be reserved for the most

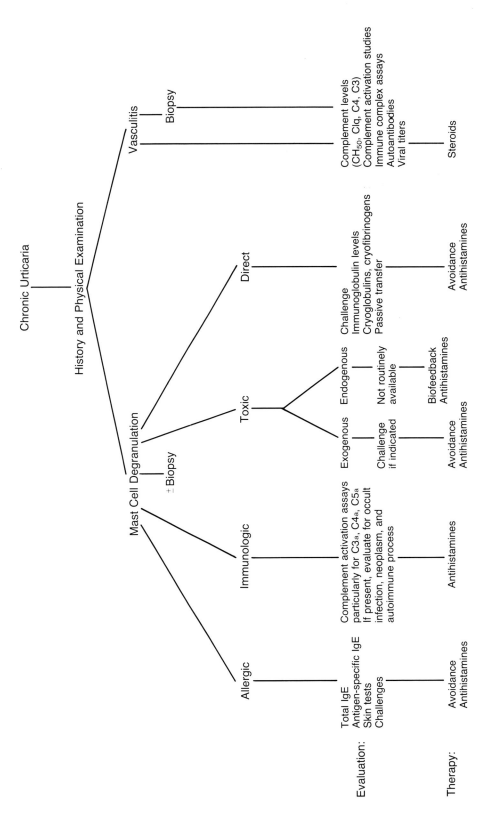

Fig. 16–2. Approach to the patient: algorithm for evaluation of patients with chronic urticaria.

recalcitrant of cases. In patients with urticarial vasculitis and no recognized systemic disease antihistamines may be tried first, but in some cases steroids will be necessary.

Conclusion

An approach to the problem of establishing a diagnosis in patients with chronic urticaria rather than a complete listing of every cause has been suggested by this chapter. In some patients it is easy to determine the cause of the urticaria. For many others both the physician and patient must invest considerable effort before a diagnosis is established. Sometimes the urticaria vanishes as it arrived, without explanation. As our understanding of mast cell pathophysiology and its role in the inflammatory process has grown, so has our understanding of the causes of urticaria. Urticaria, whether related to the products of mast cell degranulation or to the effects of necrotizing vasculitis, must always have a cause. More and more often, the discerning physician, through a careful evaluation, may be able to discover the cause and treat the urticaria.

REFERENCES

1. Champion RH, Pye RJ: Urticaria—clinical aspects. p. 135. In Champion RH, Greaves MW, Kobza Black A, et al (eds): the Urticarias. Churchill Livingstone, Edinburgh, 1985
2. Monroe EW: Investigation of chronic urticaria. p. 89. In Champion RH, Greaves MW, Kobza Black A, et al (eds): The Urticarias. Churchill Livingstone, Edinburgh, 1985
3. Van Ketel WG, Boonk WJ: The role of penicillin in chronic urticaria p. 113. In Champion RH, Greaves MW, Kobza Black A, et al (eds): The Urticarias. Churchill Livingstone, Edinburgh, 1985
4. Zimmerman MC: Chronic penicillin urticaria from dairy products; proved by penicillinase cures. Arch Dermatol Syphil 79:1, 1959
5. Guin JD: The evaluation of patients with urticaria. p. 29. In Jorizzo JL (ed): Dermatologic Clinics. Vol. 3, No. 1. WB Saunders, Philadelphia, 1985
6. Champion RH, Muhlemann MF: A list of the potential causes of urticaria. p. 125. In Champion RH, Greaves MW, Kobza Black A, et al (eds): The Urticarias. Churchill Livingstone, Edinburgh, 1985
7. Coombs RRA: Milk allergy. p. 101. In Champion RH, Greaves MW, Kobza Black A, et al (eds): The Urticarias. Churchill Livingstone, Edinburgh, 1985
8. Juhlin L: Food additives in urticaria. p. 105. In Champion RH, Greaves MW, Kobza Black A, et al (eds): The Urticarias. Churchill Livingstone, Edinburgh, 1985
9. Soter NA, Wasserman SI: IgE-dependent urticaria and angioedema. p. 1282. In Fitzpatric TB, Eisen AZ, Wolff K, et al (eds): Dermatology in General Medicine. 3rd Ed. Vol. 1, McGraw-Hill, New York, 1987
10. Barnetson RS, Benton EC: Immediate, dual and late reactions in atopic eczema. p. 98. In Champion RH, Greaves MW, Kobza Black A, et al (eds): The Urticarias. Churchill Livingstone, Edinburgh, 1985
11. Champion RH, Highet AS: Investigation and management of chronic urticaria and angioedema. Clin Exp Dermatol 7:291, 1982
12. Brown DL: The role of the complement anaphylatoxins in urticaria, angio-oedema and other forms of vascular damage. p. 39. In Champion RH, Greaves MW, Kobza Black A, et al (eds): The Urticarias. Churchill Livingstone, Edinburgh, 1985
13. Habermann E: Bee and wasp venoms. Science 177:314, 1972
14. Ennis M: Histamine release from human pulmonary mast cells. Agents Actions 12:60, 1982
15. Hook WA, Brown H, Oppenheim JJ: Histamine release from human leukocytes by concanavalin A and other mitogens. Proc Soc Exp Biol Med 147:659, 1974
16. Casale TB, Bowman S, Kaliner M: Induction of human cutaneous mast cell degranulation by opiates and endogenous opioid peptides: evidence for opiate and nonopiate receptor participation. J Allergy Clin Immunol 73:775, 1984
17. Norton S, DeBeer EJ: Effect of some antibiotics on rat mast cells in vitro. Arch Int. Pharmacol 102:352, 1955
18. Johnson AR, Erdos EG: Release of histamine from mast cells by vasoactive peptides. Proc Soc Exp Biol Med 142:1252, 1973
19. Jorizzo JL, Coutts AA, Eady RAJ, et al: Vascular responses of human skin to injection of sub-

stance P and mechanism of action. Eur J Pharmacol 87:67, 1983

20. Cochrane DE, Emigh C, Levine G, et al: Neurotensin alters cutaneous vascular permeability and stimulates histamine release from isolated skin. Ann NY Acad Sci 400:396, 1982

21. Theoharides TC, Betchaker T, Douglas WW: Somatostatin-induced histamine secretion in mast cells. Characterization of the effect. Eur J Pharmacol 69:127, 1981

22. Jasani B, Kreil G, Macker BF, et al: Further studies on the structural requirements for polypeptide-mediated histamine release from rat mast cells. Biochem J 181:623, 1979

23. Schnitzler S, Renner H, Pfuller U: Histamine release from rat mast cells induced by protamine sulfate and polyethylene imine. Agents Actions 11:73, 1981

24. Wilhelms O-H, Kreusser W, Ritz E: Parathyroid hormone elicits histamine release from mast cells. Miner Electrolyte Meth 6:29, 1981

25. Moss J, Roscow CE: Histamine release by narcotics and muscle relaxants in humans. Anesthesiology 59:330, 1983

26. Moore-Robinson M, Warin RP: Effect of salicylates in urticaria. Br Med J 4:262, 1967

27. Michaelson G, Juhlin L: Urticaria induced by preservatives and dye additives in food and drugs. Br J Dermatol 88:525, 1973

28. Weltman JK, Szaro RP, Settipane GA: An analysis of the role of immunoglobulin E in intolerance to aspirin and tartrazine. Clin Allergy 33:273, 1978

29. Kaplan AP: Urticaria and angioedema. p. 1341. In Middleton E Jr, Reed CE, Ellis EF (eds): Allergy: Principles and Practices. 2nd Ed. CV Mosby, St Louis, 1983

30. Anderson JA, Sogn DD: Adverse reactions to foods. p. 103. In American Academy of Allergy and Immunology Committee on Adverse Reactions to Foods. National Institute of Allergy and Infectious Diseases, 1984

31. Kulcycki A Jr: Aspartame induced urticaria. Intern Med 104:207, 1986

32. Jorizzo JL, Smith EB: The physical urticarias: an update and review. Arch Dermatol 118:194, 1982

33. Newcomb RW, Nelson H: Dermatographia mediated by immunoglobulin E. Am J Med 54:174, 1973

34. Coutts AA, Jorizzo JL, Eady RAJ, et al: Adenosine triphosphate-evoked vascular changes in human skin: mechanism of action. Eur J Pharmacol 76:391, 1981

35. Baughman RD, Jillson OF: Seven specific types of urticaria: with special reference to delayed persistent dermatographism. Ann Allergy 21:248, 1963

36. Ryan TJ, Shim-Young N, Turk JL: Delayed pressure urticaria. Br J Dermatol 80:485, 1968

37. Sussman GL, Harvey RP, Schocket AL: Delayed pressure urticaria. J Allergy Clin Immunol 70:337, 1982

38. Siegel C, Mitchell JC: Essential cold urticaria (a potential cause of death while swimming). Can Med Assoc J 91:609, 1964

39. Houser DD, Arbesman CE, Koki ITO, et al: Cold urticaria (immunological studies). Am J Med 49:23, 1970

40. Wanderer AA, Maselli R, Ellis EF, et al: Immunologic characterization of serum factors responsible for cold urticaria. J Allergy Clin Immunol 48:13, 1971

41. Inoue S, Teshuma H, Ago Y: Cold urticaria associated with immunoglobulin M serum factor. J Allergy Clin Immunol 66:299, 1980

42. Tindall JP, Becker SK, Rosse WF: Familial cold urticaria. Arch Intern Med 124:129, 1969

43. Soter NA, Joshe NP, Twarog FJ, et al: Delayed cold induced urticaria. J Allergy Clin Immunol 59:294, 1977

44. Eady RAJ, Greaves MW: Induction of cutaneous vasculitis by repeated cold challenge in cold urticaria. Lancet 1:336, 1978

45. Brouet JC, Clauvel JP, Danon F, et al: Biologic and clinical significance of cryoglobulins. Am J Med 57:775, 1974

46. Miescher PJ, Dayer JM: Autoimmune hemolytic anemias. p. 649. In Miescher PJ, Muller-Eberhard HJ: Textbook of Immunopathology. Grune & Stratton, Orlando, FL, 1976

47. Delorme P: Localized heat urticaria. J Allergy 53:284, 1969

48. Michaelson G, Ross A: Familial localized heat urticaria of delayed type. Acta Derm Venereol (Stockh) 51:279, 1971

49. Kounis NG, MacMahon RG: Cholinergic urticaria with systemic manifestations. Ann Allergy 35:243, 1975

50. Lawrence CM, Jorizzo JL, Kobza Black A, et al: Cholinergic urticaria with associated angioedema. Br J Dermatol 105:543, 1981

51. Soter NA, Wasserman SI, Austen KF, et al: Release of mast cell mediators and alterations

in lung function in patients with cholinergic urticaria. N Engl J Med 302:604, 1980

52. Lewis J, Lieberman P, Treadwell G, et al: Exercise-induced urticaria, angioedema and anaphylactoid episodes. J Allergy Clin Immunol 68:432, 1981

53. Herzheimer A: The nervous pathway mediating cholinergic urticaria. Clin Sci Mol Med 15:195, 1956

54. Chalamidas SL, Charles CR: Aquagenic urticaria. Arch Dermatol 104:541, 1971

55. Bonnetblanc JM, Andrieu-Pfahl F, Meraud JP, et al: Familial aquagenic urticaria. Dermatologica 158:468, 1979

56. Patterson R, Mellies CJ, Blankenship ML, et al: Vibratory angioedema: a hereditary type of physical hypersensitivity. J Allergy Clin Immunol 50:174, 1972

57. Harber LC, Holloway RM, Wheatley VR, et al: Immunologic and biophysical studies in solar urticaria. J Invest Dermatol 41:439, 1963

58. Ramsay CA: Solar urticaria. Int J Dermatol 19:233, 1980

59. Sams MW: Solar urticaria studies of the active serum factor. J Allergy Clin Immunol 45:295, 1970

60. Horio T: Photoallergic urticaria induced by visible light: additional cases and further studies. Arch Dermatol 114:1761, 1978

61. Magnus IA, Janett A, Prankerd TAJ, et al: Erythropoietic protoporphyria: a new porphyria syndrome with solar urticaria due to protoporphyrinemia. Lancet 2:448, 1961

62. Phanuphak P, Kohler PG, Standord RE, et al: Vasculitis in chronic urticaria. J Allergy Clin Immunol 65:436, 1980

63. Monroe EW: Urticarial vasculitis: an updated review. J Am Acad Dermatol 5:88, 1981

64. Soter NA: Chronic urticaria as a manifestation of necrotizing venulitis. N Engl J Med 296:1440, 1977

65. Monroe EW, Schulz CL, Maize JC, et al: Vasculitis in chronic urticaria: an immunopathologic study. J Invest Dermatol 76:103, 1981

66. Russell Jones R, Bhogal B, Dash A, et al: Urticaria and vasculitis: a continuum of histological and immunopathological changes. Br J Dermatol 108:695, 1983

67. Nathony SF, Phillips ME, Elias JM, et al: Histologic studies of chronic idiopathic urticaria. J Allergy Clin Immunol 71:177, 1983

68. Mikori YA, Giorno RC, Anderson BS, et al: Lymphocyte subpopulations in the skin of patients with chronic urticaria. J Allergy Clin Immunol 72:681, 1983

69. Sanchez NP, Winkelman RK, Schroeter AZ, et al: The clinical and histopathologic spectrum of urticarial vasculitis: study of forty cases. J Am Acad Dermatol 7:599, 1982

70. McDuffie FC, Sams WM Jr, Maldonado JE, et al: Hypocomplementemia with cutaneous vasculitis and arthritis. Mayo Clin Proc 48:340, 1973

71. Feig PU, Soter NA, Yager HM, et al: Vasculitis with urticaria, hypocomplementemia and multiple system involvement. JAMA 236:2065, 1976

72. Mathison DA, Arroyave CM, Bhat KN: Hypocomplementemia in chronic idiopathic urticaria. Ann Intern Med 86:534, 1977

73. Schwartz HR, McDuffie FC, Black LF, et al: Hypocomplementemic urticarial vasculitis. Association with chronic obstructive pulmonary disease. Mayo Clin Proc 57:227, 1982

74. Marder RJ, Burch FX, Schmid FR, et al: Low molecular weight C1q precipitins in hypocomplementemic vasculitis urticaria syndrome: partial purification and characterization as immunoglobulin. J Immunol 121:613, 1978

75. Zeiss CR, Burch FX, Marder RJ, et al: A hypocomplementemic vasculitis urticarial syndrome. Report of four new cases and definition of the disease. Am J Med 68:867, 1980

76. O'Laughlin S, Schroeter AL, Jordon RE: Chronic urticarial-like lesions in systemic lupus erythematosus: a review of 12 cases. Arch Dermatol 114:879, 1978

77. Provost TT, Zone JJ, Synkowski E, et al: Unusual cutaneous manifestations of systemic lupus erythematosus. I. Urticaria-like lesions: correlation with clinical and serological abnormalities. J Invest Dermatol 75:495, 1980

78. Alexander I, Provost TT: Cutaneous manifestations of primary Sjögren's syndrome. A reflection of vasculitis and association with anti Ro (SSA) antibodies. J Invest Dermatol 80:386, 1983

79. Michet CJ Jr, McKenna CH, Luthra HS, et al: Relapsing polychondritis associated with urticaria. Ann Intern Med 104:74, 1986

80. Gower RG, Sausker WF, Kohler PF, et al: Small vessel vasculitis caused by hepatitis B virus immune complexes. J Allergy Clin Immunol 62:222, 1978

81. Wands JR, Perrotto JL, Isselbacher KJ: Circulating immune complexes and complement sequence activation in infectious mononucleosis. Am J Med 60:269, 1976

82. Champion RH, Roberts SOB, Carpenter RG, et al: Urticaria and angioedema: a review of 554 patients. Br J Dermatol 81:588, 1969

83. Akers WA, Naverson DN: Diagnosis of chronic urticaria. Int J Dermatol 17:616, 1978

84. Wanderer AA, Nuss DD, Tormey AD: Urticarial leukocytoclastic vasculitis with cold urticaria. Report of a case and review of the literature. Arch Dermatol 119:145, 1983

17

Pruritus

James Herndon, Jr.

Itching is the most common and distressing symptom of skin disease and may occur in a variety of illnesses affecting other parts of the body. When confined to a few areas or to a short period of time, itching can sometimes be tolerated, but generalized pruritus quickly becomes unbearable, compelling the patient to seek medical care.

Occasionally the cause of pruritus is easily identified and readily treated. Eczematous or urticarial skin lesions, for example, quickly lead the clinician to the appropriate diagnosis and therapy. Several other conditions, however, can cause very subtle skin lesions, making diagnosis more difficult. Scabies and dermatitis herpetiformis, for example, may present with severe pruritus but sparse cutaneous eruptions; in advanced cases, excoriations may obscure the burrows of scabies and the vesicles of dermatitis herpetiformis. Pruritus without primary skin lesions may be even more difficult to diagnose and treat. It has been stated that half the patients with generalized itching without primary skin lesions will eventually get better without a more definitive diagnosis than *idiopathic generalized pruritus.*[1] Nevertheless, it is important that pruritus be taken seriously not only because of the severity of the symptom but because of a possible association with occult systemic disease.

Localized pruritus can also occur without any clinically apparent skin lesions in a number of common dermatoses, such as pruritus ani and pruritus vulvae. Several unusual conditions have been reported in association with both localized and generalized pruritus. Severe itching of the nose has been recorded in patients with brain tumors,[2] and atypical angina has also presented as nasal pruritus.[3] *Hereditary localized pruritus* has been reported in multiple members of two generations of a family.[4] In all affected patients the pruritus was localized over the lower scapula. This entity appears to represent a familial susceptibility to mild injury to sensory nerve fibers. In sporadic cases it is called *notalgia paresthetica. Aquagenic pruritus,* which can also affect more than one family member, is a condition characterized by intense skin discomfort that occurs shortly after contact with water. Skin lesions are absent and pruritus is usually generalized.[5] *Prodromal itching* can occur in almost one-third of children with asthma. The itching occurs in the same site between 1 and 30 minutes before an episode of wheezing.[6] Premenstrual and pregnancy-associated pruritus due to recurrent cholestasis has also been reported.[7] Recognition of syndromes associated with itching and exclusion of associated systemic diseases are an important part of the clinician's approach to the management of patients with pruritus.

Table 17-1. Pruritus with and without a Rash

Skin Completely Normal	Excoriations Only	Prominent Rash
Atopic complex	Scabies	Urticaria
Fiberglass	Dermatitis herpetiformis	Contact allergy
Elderly or debilitated skin		Insect bites, etc.
Systemic pruritogens		

PATHOPHYSIOLOGY OF ITCH

At the molecular level histamine and proteases released in the course of allergic and inflammatory reactions act directly on nerve endings to create the sensation of itch. Much can happen to the sensation before it registers at the conscious level, however. Inputs such as cold, heat, and vibration regularly suppress or reinforce the perception of itch. Emotional responses such as anxiety or excitement or, occasionally, just attention given to some other activity may influence its expression. The threshold for itching also seems to vary widely; some patients complain of severe itching with little or no provocation, while others display almost superhuman tolerance for discomfort.

Unfilled psychological needs also modify the perception of itch and other sensations.[8,9] The need to somaticize, that is, to translate unacceptable feelings into acceptable physical complaints, produces its share of difficult diagnostic and therapeutic problems. The physician, absorbed in the medical challenge of the patient's condition, may find it difficult to sort through these other factors but must acknowledge their importance.

CRITICAL FACTORS IN THE CLINICAL APPROACH TO PRURITUS

Presence or Absence of Rash

The first question for the clinician is: Does the patient have a rash? As shown in Table 17-1, many severely affected patients show no visible rash while others display only self-inflicted signs of excoriation. When a rash is present, its morphologic features may suffice, enabling the clinician to recognize the disorder

and proceed with therapy without further work-up. Patients with normal or excoriated skin, however, usually require more detailed evaluation. It should be noted that great overlap exists between conditions associated with specific rashes and conditions without skin lesions. Atopic patients, for example, may have typical flexural skin lesions or may have completely normal-appearing skin. Alternatively, the wheals of urticaria may be so evanescent that the patient may have severe pruritus without apparent lesions at the time of examination.

Based on the outcome of the first and most important objective question above, the evaluation of an itching patient can be divided into several stages (Tables 17-2 and 17-4).

Duration of the Itch

The second critical factor to consider is: How long has the itch been present? As in other algorithms of diagnosis, the question of acute versus chronic pruritus affects the clinical approach to the patient. The atopic complex produces repeated and prolonged pruritus. Pruritus produced by systemic medical illness also tends to occur with a longer history, as noted in Table 17-3. This category includes systemic disorders in which hormonal agents (hyperthyroidism), cellular proteases, or other products of cellular

Table 17-2. Approach to the Patient: History and Physical Examination

Presence or absence of rash	Relevant medical history
Diagnostic features	Illness
Distribution	Surgery
Evolution with time	Allergies
History of pruritus	Atopic complex
Circumstances of onset	Physiologic state
Triggering factors	Infancy
Relieving factors	Old age
Prior treatment	Pregnancy

Table 17-3. Medical Illness Producing Pruritus without Rash

Polycythemia vera
Lymphomas, especially Hodgkin's disease
Thyroid disease
Cholestatic liver disease
Chronic renal failure

breakdown (polycythemia, lymphoma), biologic detergents (bile acids or other biliary derivatives in cholestatic liver disease), or the nitrogenous breakdown substances of chronic renal failure play a role.

In various series reviewing patients with generalized pruritus, the incidence of underlying systemic disease has ranged from 10 to 50 percent.[10–12] One study that compared 44 patients with generalized pruritus with 44 age- and sex-matched psoriatic controls found a statistically significant increase in kidney disease, liver disease, and internal malignancies. Hypothyroidism was slightly increased in the pruritus group, but in contrast to earlier studies diabetes was not found to be associated with pruritus.[13] The association between kidney disease and pruritus is well established although the mechanism is unknown. While some correlation between blood urea nitrogen and pruritus exists, patients with acute renal failure do not develop pruritus, and some patients note an exacerbation of pruritus when they begin dialysis. Others notice intense pruritus during dialysis itself. Calcium, phosphate, bilirubin, parathyroid hormone, magnesium, cutaneous mast cells, histamine, and sweat gland abnormalities have all been implicated in the mechanism of uremic pruritus, but proof of the mechanism has eluded investigators.[14–16] Uremic pruritus does respond to phototherapy with ultraviolet B[17] and to renal transplantation, and some centers report a response to oral activated charcoal.[18] Short-term measures to which some patients have responded are diets low in protein and high in carbohydrates, infusion of salt-poor albumin, and dialysis. Several patients with secondary hyperparathyroidism have also responded dramatically to parathyroidectomy.[19]

Obstructive liver disease is also associated with generalized pruritus, but again the mechanism is unknown.[20] Pruritus is often the first symptom of primary biliary cirrhosis. Treatment of this condition with ultraviolet B phototherapy results in a reduction of bile acids in the skin and a concomitant improvement in symptoms, which suggests that cutaneous bile acids play a role in the pruritus of cholestasis. This view is supported by the observations that oral bile salts exacerbate pruritus in patients with liver disease; cholestyramine reduces bile acids and improves pruritus; and topically applied bile acids cause local pruritus.[21–23] However, a 1981 study failed to show any relationship between serum or skin bile acid levels and pruritus.[24] Moreover, methyltestosterone can relieve the pruritus although it exacerbates the cholestasis.[25]

The association between endocrinopathies and pruritus has been less conclusively established. As already mentioned, one study failed to show any association with diabetes mellitus.[13] It has been suggested that diabetics complaining of pruritus should be investigated for monilial infections. Pruritus has been reported in patients with hyper- and hypothyroidism, but the strength of this association does not approach that found between kidney disease and pruritus.

Even more controversial is the association between generalized pruritus and malignancies. Pruritus is certainly a recognized symptom of Hodgkin's disease, occurring in approximately 25 percent of patients and as the presenting symptom in 5 to 10 percent.[10] It occurs less frequently in non-Hodgkin's lymphomas, although pruritus can precede the premycotic phase of mycosis fungoides and is a common feature of the Sézary syndrome. A striking association between itching of the nostrils and brain tumors has already been mentioned, and the sign of Leser-Trélat, a sudden development of numerous seborrheic keratoses in association with a malignancy, has been reported with severe pruritus in a patient with a uterine carcinoma.[26] Numerous case reports have documented an association between solid tumors and generalized pruritus, and often the pruritus is associated with stinging. In many of these cases

Table 17-4. Approach to the Patient: Laboratory Investigation of Patients with Persistent Generalized Pruritus

Complete blood count with differential
Liver function tests
Blood urea nitrogen, creatinine
Urinalysis[a]
Chest x-ray[a]
Thyroid function tests[a]

[a] Because of limited yield of some tests and the questionable association between conditions such as thyroid disease and pruritus, all tests do not have to be ordered routinely in all patients with persistent generalized pruritus.

the temporal relationship between the onset of tumor-related symptoms and pruritus has led physicians to the conclusion that the two are associated. Even more convincing is the response of pruritus to tumor removal and return of pruritus upon tumor recurrence. While there is no doubt of an association between pruritus and internal malignancy in some cases, this association is probably not common, and a simple complaint of pruritus should not warrant an extensive malignancy work-up.

A number of other systemic disorders have been associated with generalized pruritus, including carcinoid, hemochromatosis, and polycythemia vera.[10,27] After a hot shower severe itching occurs in 20 to 50 percent of patients with polycythemia vera. The pruritus has been attributed to elevated serum histamine levels and increased numbers of basophils.[10] At least one group of investigators has attributed the itching of polycythemia vera to iron deficiency in some cases.[28] Iron deficiency itself has been thought to cause pruritus, but this association has recently been disproved.[29]

In view of the real but uncommon association between pruritus and systemic diseases, how should the physician evaluate a patient with generalized pruritus? A thorough history and physical examination as outlined in Table 17-2 should enable the clinician to diagnose and treat a substantial proportion of his patients. Prolonged and expensive work-ups are seldom warranted for pruritus, but if symptoms persist, the diagnostic tests outlined in Table 17-4 have been suggested. Because of the known association of pruritus with Hodgkin's disease, physi-

cal examination should include a thorough search for lymphadenopathy and hepatosplenomegaly.

NONSYSTEMIC SOURCES OF PRURITUS

The Atopic Complex

Even in persons free of systemic disease, however, itching can reach distracting severity. The commonest reason for itching without a rash in young and/or otherwise healthy individuals is the *atopic complex* (Table 17-5). This still poorly understood state usually involves persons with personal or family histories of hay fever or other seasonal allergies. Most sufferers complain of dry skin in winter, coin-sized patches of loss of suntan, irritation from application of underarm deodorant, and itching from wool clothing or lace at the neckline. This form of pruritus often presents in those who begin a program of swimming or other exercise, move to a drier climate, or simply enjoy long hot showers, particularly during cold weather, when indoor humidity falls to low levels. This underlying hyperirritable state helps account not only for a major portion of patients who itch all over but also helps explain most examples of pruritus ani and vulvae, as well as other localized itches.

While the fundamental defect involved in the atopic complex remains obscure, recent study implicates elevated levels of leukocyte phosphodiesterase, detectable even in cord blood of newborns destined to show the trait. Clinically the skin behaves as if a critically important system for quenching itch sensations has been deleted. Thus, weak irritants cause prolonged

Table 17-5. The Atopic Complex: Eczema

Primary Features	Secondary Features
Respiratory allergies	Frequent skin infection
Circles of loss of tan	Ichthyosis vulgaris
Sensitivity to wool, lace	Rare contact dermatitis
Itching after desiccation, bathing	

and magnified pruritus. The skin thickens readily into lichenified areas marked by accentuation of normal skin markings and easy irritability. Therapy for pruritus of the atopic state[30,31] is summarized in Table 17-6.

Itching with Minimal Rash and/or Excoriations: Scabies

Especially in the sexually active teenager and adult, one must also suspect early scabies (Table 17-7 and Fig. 17-1). The history of itching predominantly at night and the presence of itching of the genitals and central trunk should raise particular suspicion since these areas become affected less often in other conditions. Scraping with a scalpel blade of barely visible burrows on thicker areas of skin such as sides of the fingers and feet can yield the diagnostic eight-legged parasite, but the clinical picture is usually dominated by excoriations, often secondarily infected ones. Close contacts and partners are usually involved, although they may not have complained of itching if the 3-week incubation period has not passed. Topical or systemic corticoids, often prescribed when the diagnosis is not yet apparent, usually worsen the infestation while simultaneously making it easier to diagnose by suppressing the pruritus and allowing the mites to proliferate. For adults topical application of 1 percent lindane lotion remains the standard treatment, but careful instruction is needed for proper use. The main

Table 17-6. Therapy for Pruritus of the Atopic Complex

1. Prevention of irritation: shorter, cooler bathing; substitutes for soap (Cetaphil lotion)
2. Nonspecific antipruritics: lotions containing pramoxine (Prax, Pramosone), menthol, phenol
3. Anti-inflammatory agents
   Topical: corticoid creams, lotions, ointments
   Oral: phosphodiesterase inhibitor (papaverine); antihistamines (doxepin, terfenadine)
4. Mechanism not fully understood
   Evening primrose seed oil as a source of omega-3 fatty acids
   Ultraviolet B light
5. Anti-infective: for frequent staphylococcal pyoderma (penicillinase-resistant penicillin)

Table 17-7. Scabies

Itching severe, disturbing sleep
Excoriations dominate rash
Short history in well individual
In men, genitals usually involved
Corticoids, a provocative test
Close contacts often involved

danger is overuse, since itching does not stop for 2 to 4 weeks after successful treatment. Most cases of central nervous system toxicity following percutaneous absorption have occurred in infants and young children, who should receive an entirely different medication, 3 to 5 percent sulfur in eucerin or comparable hydrophilic ointment base. To suppress needless misery after definitive therapy, one should prescribe ade-

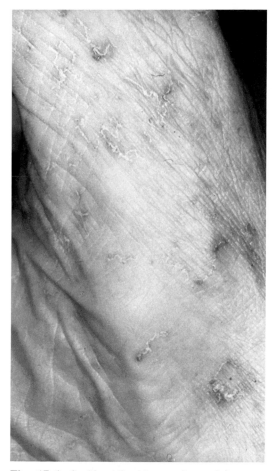

Fig. 17–1. Scabies. Pruritic papules and burrows on the lower leg.

quate topical and sytemic antipruritic therapy. The patient's contacts should always be treated and the family examined.

Itching with Prominent Rash: Urticaria/Drug Rash

Raised red wheals, erythematous maculo-papular lesions and even vesiculobullous lesions with accompanying intense pruritus may develop with overwhelming speed in the course of allergic reactions to foods, drugs, infectious antigens, serum sickness, etc. Histamine mediates many of the changes in patients whose urticarial lesions come and go in 12 hours or less, but cellular and other mediators exert control in longer-lasting reactions. Since the great majority of cases are self-limiting, extensive diagnostic studies are best deferred in favor of energetic suppressive therapy. A history of recent illness or medication should suggest appropriate treatment or change to a chemically unrelated alternative medication. Oral antihistamines, topical antipruritic preparations, and, in severe cases, systemic steroids may be needed.

Itching with Prominent Rash: Bullae Due to Poison Ivy

In many parts of the United States, blisters and itching mean poison ivy until proved otherwise. Even in winter, contact with vegetation, often roots and stems as part of clean-up operations, or with the family pet who has been in the vegetation, often leads to the characteristic splotchy, sometimes linear streaks of redness and vesicles. An important but often overlooked point is that the examiner must know whether the current episode is the patient's first attack of a lifetime or a later attack. A first attack requires 8 to 10 days to develop and frequently recurs if corticoid therapy is stopped too soon (2 to 4 weeks of treatment being usually required), while a subsequent attack develops within a day or two following contact with the plant and resolves more rapidly. Localized ivy

dermatitis can be treated successfully with topical moist compresses, shake lotions, and the most potent of the corticoid creams such as clobetasol propionate and oral antihistamines, but more generalized and severe cases require systemic corticoid. A representative course for a 70-kg adult with normal blood pressure and glucose tolerance might begin at 40 to 80 mg daily and taper rapidly to half and then a quarter of the starting dose. Treatment should include maximal use of cool moist compresses, antipruritic lotions, and doxepin in order to reduce the dose of corticoid needed.[31]

Other blistering disorders that produce itching include dermatitis herpetiformis, bullous pemphigoid, herpes simplex and zoster in some patients, occasional blistering sunburns, insect bites, and impetigo.

Pustules and Pyoderma as a Source of Pruritus

A number of bacterial and viral conditions can cause severe pruritus. Antibiotic treatment of the bacterial disorders in Table 17-8 is neces-

Table 17-8. Pustules and Pyoderma as a Source of Pruritus

Bacterial causes
- Impetigo
  - Usually face or neck
  - Honey-colored crusts or flaccid blisters
  - Intense itching
- Perinasal and perioral folliculitis
  - Tiny, less than 1 mm whitish blisters on bright red base
  - Scaling, flaking predominant
- Hot tub folliculitis
  - Larger, separate nodules with soreness as well as itching
  - Usual location on thighs, buttocks, lower trunk
- Eosinophilic folliculitis of scalp
  - Wright stain shows no organisms
  - Predominantly eosinophils
  - Maddening pruritus common

Viral causes
- Herpes simplex
  - Often mistaken for impetigo
  - Smears or cultures needed
- Herpes zoster
  - Often misdiagnosed in the scalp

of itching also cause increased pore plugging, the process typically spreads and worsens as long as such creams continue in use. Therapy requires oral and topical erythromycin or tetracycline. Unfortunately, neither of these standard antibiotics has a favorable effect on eosinophilic scalp folliculitis. Here, the sulfa derivative dapsone usually clears the process although it may be necessary to give the material for an extended period. Sulfones can, rarely, cause agranulocytosis, so periodic white cell and platelet counts are warranted.

Special Categories of Itching: Influence of Age and Pregnancy

Both extremes of age and the physiologic and immunologic influences of pregnancy affect the evaluation of itching, as shown in Tables 17-9 and 17-10. In infants the infectious and allergic causes of pruritus predominate, with atopic eczema the usual answer to otherwise difficult to explain chronic pruritus. In the aged a marked reduction in skin resistance heads the list; this is expressed as exaggerated pruritus following use of weak primary irritants such as soap, commercial lotions (purchased to relieve itch but paradoxically able to foment it), mistaken self-therapy with alcohol, calamine, or other drying agents, etc.

In pregnancy a series of physiologic and immunologic events involving hormones and pla-

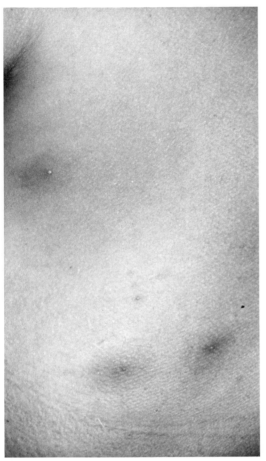

Fig. 17–2. *Pseudomonas* folliculitis. Painful and pruritic pustules with prominent surrounding erythema after use of a hot tub.

sary but not sufficient to relieve pruritus. Hot-tub folliculitis presents a difficult choice. Most cases of this form of gram-negative folliculitis clear slowly (1 to 2 weeks) but spontaneously. This is fortunate since cultures often show organisms resistant to antibiotics used by mouth, but itching may be intense to a degree rivaling poison ivy dermatitis and require systemic corticoid. For this reason culture and determination of sensitivity patterns should be done at first, since antibiotics may be required later. In perioral folliculitis the pathogenesis is complex, depending on keratinous plugs in the facial follicles along with growth of bacteria. Since topically applied corticoid creams given for relief

Table 17-9. Itching in Infancy and Old Age

Infants	Aged
Eczema	Reduced resistance to irritants
Impetigo	Medical illness
Scabies	Drug reactions
Viral exanthem	Immunologic derangements
Urticaria due to food, drugs	Psychologic factors

Table 17-10. Pruritus and Eruptions of Pregnancy

Herpes gestationis
Toxic erythema of pregnancy
Cholestatic pruritus of pregnancy

cental antigens can make for miserable pruritus.[32] Other than traditional antihistamines, physicians have become more reluctant to prescribe oral medication for pregnant patients, placing greater burdens on topical therapy and diagnosis. Lacking a rash, an itching pregnant patient should undergo liver function studies to detect the cholestatic changes. In severe cases treatment with oral bile-sequestering agents (cholestyramine, charcoal) to remove pruritogenic metabolites via the intestine should be considered. Oral corticoid may be needed in a few patients who fail to respond completely but should be used cautiously, with consultation from the obstetrician.

An erythematous or edematous rash with itching points either toward the inflammatory but topically manageable toxic erythema of pregnancy (Fig. 17-3), a milder urticaria-like variant (also called pruritic urticarial papules and plaques of pregnancy), or the more threatening herpes gestationis, in which blistering, intractable itching, and increased fetal mortality dictate aggressive oral therapy with corticoster-

Table 17-11. Recommendations for Emergency Topical Management of Severe Inflammatory Pruritus in Pregnancy

1. Cool moist compresses, rotating exposure region by region.
2. Potent topical corticoid cream applied after each compress.
3. To each area 15–30 minutes following corticoid, apply anti-itch lotion (such as 1% pramoxine lotion with or without 0.5% phenol and 0.25% menthol).

oids. To distinguish these conditions early in the course may require immunofluorescent processing of biopsy material and plasma, but all respond acutely to a regimen of cool compresses, nonspecific topical antipruritic lotions, and potent topical corticoids (Table 17-11).

SUMMARY

The severely itching patient presents one of the most subjectively acute medical crises and deserves rapid and aggressive management. Clinical judgment hinges on distinctions of (1)

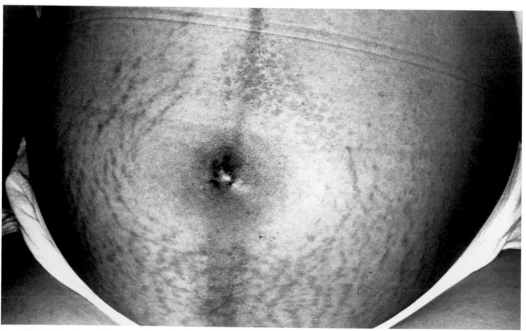

Fig. 17–3. Toxic erythema of pregnancy (pruritic urticarial papules and plaques of pregnancy). Characteristic involvement of abdominal striae in the last days of pregnancy.

rash versus no visible eruption; (2) acuteness of onset; (3) relevant medical history; and (4) age and physiologic state (e.g., pregnancy). Most patients can be managed easily with topical or oral antipruritic therapy and without extensive diagnostic work-up. In unusually severe or persistent cases limited laboratory investigation should suffice to examine those systemic disorders associated with pruritus.

REFERENCES

1. Champion RH: Clinical algorithms: generalised pruritus. Br Med J 289:751, 1984
2. Andreev V, Petkov I: Skin manifestations associated with tumours of the brain. Br J Dermatol 92:675, 1975
3. Reichstein RP, Stein WG: Nasal pruritus as atypical angina? N Engl J Med 309:311, 1983
4. Comings DE, Comings SN: Hereditary localized pruritus. Arch Dermatol 92:236, 1965
5. Steinman HK, Greaves MW: Aquagenic pruritus. J Am Acad Dermatol 13:91, 1985
6. David TJ, Wybrew M, Hennessen U: Prodromal itching in childhood asthma. Lancet 2:154, 1984
7. Dahl M: Premenstrual pruritus due to recurrent cholestasis. Trans St John Hosp Dermatol Soc 56:11, 1970
8. Herndon JH Jr: Itching: the pathophysiology of pruritus. Int J Dermatol 14:465, 1975
9. Gilchrest BA: Pruritus: pathogenesis, therapy, and significance in systemic disease states. Arch Intern Med 142:101, 1982
10. Jorizzo JL: The itchy patient: a practical approach. Primary Care 10:339, 1983
11. Lyell A: The itchy patient: a review of causes of pruritus. Scott Med J 17:334, 1972
12. Rajka G: Investigation of patients suffering from generalized pruritus, with special reference to systemic diseases. Acta Derm Venereol (Stockh) 46:190, 1966
13. Kantor GR, Lookingbill DP: Generalized pruritus and systemic disease. J Am Acad Dermatol 9:375, 1983
14. Gilchrest BA, Stern RS, Steinman TI, et al: Clinical features of pruritus among patients undergoing maintenance hemodialysis. Arch Dermatol 118:154, 1982
15. Cawley EP, Hoch-Ligeti C, Bond GM: The eccrine sweat glands of patients in uremia. Arch Dermatol 84:51, 1961
16. Young, AW Jr, Sweeney EW, David DS, et al: Dermatologic evaluation of pruritus in patients on hemodialysis. NY State J Med 73:2670, 1973
17. Gilchrest BA, Rowe JW, Brown RS, et al: Relief of uremic pruritus with ultraviolet phototherapy. N Engl J Med 297:136, 1977
18. Pederson JA, Matter BJ, Czerwinski AW, et al: Relief of idiopathic generalized pruritus in dialysis patients treated with activated oral charcoal. Ann Intern Med 93:446, 1980
19. Hampers CL, Katz AI, Wilson RE, et al: Disappearance of "uremic" itching after subtotal parathyroidectomy. N Engl J Med 279:695, 1968
20. Garden JM, Ostrow JD, Roenigk HH: Pruritus in hepatic cholestasis, pathogenesis and management. Arch Dermatol 121:1415, 1985
21. Varco RL: Intermittent external biliary drainage for relief of pruritus in certain chronic disorders of the liver. Surgery 21:43, 1947
22. Carey JB, Williams G: Relief of the pruritus of jaundice with a bile acid sequestering resin. J Am Acad Dermatol 176:432, 1961
23. Varadi DP: Pruritus induced by crude bile and purified bile acids. Arch Dermatol 109:678, 1974
24. Freedman MR, Holzbach RT, Ferguson DR: Pruritus in cholestasis: no direct causative role for bile acid retention. Am J Med 70:1011, 1981
25. Lloyd-Thomas HGL, Sherlock S: Testosterone therapy for the pruritus of obstructive jaundice. Br Med J 4:1289, 1952
26. Ronchese F: Keratoses, cancer and the sign of Leser-Trélat. Cancer 18:1003, 1965
27. Hamilton DV, Gould DJ: Generalized pruritus as a presentation of idiopathic haemochromatosis. Br J Dermatol 112:629, 1985
28. Salem HH, Van der Weyden MB, Young IF, Wiley JS: Pruritus and severe iron deficiency in polycythemia vera. Br Med J 285:91, 1982
29. Tucker WFG, Briggs C, Challoner T: Absence of pruritus in iron deficiency following venesection. Clin Exp Dermatol 9:186, 1984
30. Hanafin JM, Butler JM, Chan SC: Immunopharmacology of the atopic diseases. J Invest Dermatol, 85:suppl.1, 1615–1645, 1985
31. Mangla JC: Doxepin in pruritus. Clin Res 33:300A, 1985
32. Holmes RC, Black MM: The specific dermatoses of pregnancy. J Am Acad Dermatol 8:405, 1983

18

Annular Erythemas

Nelson Lee Novick

Annular erythematous lesions are the predominant clinical feature in a number of dermatologic conditions. Moreover, many other cutaneous disorders not generally considered among the annular erythemas may likewise demonstrate annular, erythematous phases somewhere during the course of their natural histories. This chapter is devoted to those conditions in which annular erythema either represents the major cutaneous manifestation of a disease or may appear somewhere in its evolution. Before beginning any discussion of the differential diagnosis of annular erythemas, the terms *annular* and *erythema,* and their pathophysiologic correlations, merit some clarification.

Annular is defined as "circular, round, or like a ring" and *erythema* is used to designate the "sign of redness."[1] The terms *gyrate* and *polycyclic* refer to variations of the annular pattern in which the rings are either incomplete and/or multiple and contiguous. Siemens[2] contended that in inflammatory conditions each individual erythematous area initially corresponds to a region of direct blood supply and hence is oval in shape. The variety of annular shapes observed among the various annular erythemas may subsequently arise as a consequence of both peripheral spreading and central recession within individual lesions or may result from an aggregate circular configuration of many individual lesions.[3]

Lesional erythema is due primarily to capillary, venular or arteriolar dilation. The precise shades of "erythema," such as pink, purple, or fawn-colored, that may be observed in the various annular erythemas reflect the interplay of a number of modifying factors. These factors include: the thickness and type of the associated cornified layer; the amount of epidermal melanin present; the degree of involvement either of the superficial dermal vascular plexus alone or of both the superficial and deep dermal plexuses; the presence of dermal edema, melanophages, or extravasated red blood cells; and the type, nature, and extent of any associated deposits or neoplastic or inflammatory cell infiltrates. By keeping these fundamental concepts in mind throughout the remainder of this chapter one will not only be better able to diagnose the various annular erythemas but also will be better equipped to appreciate the diversity and subleties of their various clinical presentations.

DIFFERENTIAL DIAGNOSIS OF ANNULAR ERYTHEMA

Despite the variety of clinical conditions that may be considered among the annular erythemas, for purposes of facilitating diagnosis it is useful to classify them according to etiologic categories (Table 18-1). Furthermore, to facilitate comparison between the various diseases to be covered the format for the discussion of

341

each entity will uniformly parallel the suggested approach to patient diagnosis outlined in Table 18-2 (see p. 357). This approach will be used in considering both the patient and his condition first in overview and then in specific detail.

Hereditary Diseases

FAMILIAL ANNULAR ERYTHEMA

Familial annular erythema is a rare disorder occurring within specific families. This condition first presents within a few days of birth and is occasionally associated with other developmental abnormalities, such as geographic tongue, nystagmus, and mental retardation.[4] Individual lesions are occasionally pruritic and always transitory, but patients are seldom free from them and the condition typically persists for many years.

Clinically, the lesions may be widespread, particularly involving the trunk. Individual lesions may begin as one or more papules, which enlarge by peripheral spreading into annular, arciform, or polycyclic shapes and are reddish in color. They may exhibit a vesicular border as well as peripheral collarettes of scaling. Lesions are generally flat but, if edematous, may be palpable. Laboratory studies are nonspecific and diagnosis rests upon the family history and the clinical examination. Treatment is symptomatic.

PSORIASIS ANNULARIS (CIRCINATA, GYRATA)

Psoriasis vulgaris is a chronic, papulosquamous disorder typified by a rapid rate of keratinocytic cell turnover and epidermal hyperplasia. Genetic studies indicate a familial inheritance pattern, which is both polygenic and multifactorial and which reflects variable phenotypic penetrance and expression. The major human leukocyte histocompatibility antigens HLA-B13 and HLA-Bw17 have been found to be significantly increased in psoriasis. According to Braun-Falco,[5] environmental factors operating upon the genetically predisposed patient account for the appearance of the initial psoriatic lesions, and to that end the dermis and epidermis in such patients act in an integrated fashion.

Psoriasis exhibits equal incidence between males and females and may initially manifest at any age, frequently in association with minor skin trauma (Koebner, isomorphic response). The course of psoriasis is variable. For most patients the disease remains mild, affecting few sites; some patients experience spontaneous improvement, while others experience marked exacerbation. Psoriasis has a prevalence in the

United States of approximately 2 percent, affecting between 3 and 5 million people.

Psoriasis may involve any or all areas of the integument. Lesions often vary in size, are symmetrical, and are ordinarily fixed rather than transitory. Sites of particular predilection are the scalp, elbows, sacral region, and knees. Psoriatic lesions may assume a variety of morphologies: they are most frequently large and plaque-type, or guttate, and less often they are of annular, gyrate, and circinate forms. The lesions are reddish, owing largely to a pronounced capillary dilation within the affected dermal papillae and to the appearance of these vessels through the overlying thinned suprapapillary epidermis. The lesions are palpable above the surrounding skin as a consequence of epidermal hyperplasia and dermal vascular dilatation and are characteristically covered by loosely adherent thick micaceous scales. In annular psoriasis pustules may also be seen at the borders of the lesions. The appearance of punctate bleeding points after the scale has been scraped off (Auspitz sign) is a useful, although not pathognomonic, diagnostic sign.

Other than testing for hyperuricemia, which may be observed with severe, widespread involvement, and an elevated erythrocyte sedimentation rate in erythrodermic psoriasis, routine laboratory studies are nondiagnostic. Biopsy findings are characteristic, consisting of parakeratosis, subcorneal focal accumulations of neutrophils (Munro microabscesses), acanthosis, elongation of the dermal papillae, thinning of the suprapapillary plate, diminished or absent granular layer, and a mixed lymphohistiocytic infiltrate in the superficial dermis.

Although no cure for psoriasis exists, a variety of therapies have been found effective. Treatment may be tailored in each patient to the type of psoriasis and its severity. Among the successful therapies are topical corticosteroids, tars, and anthralin; ultraviolet light therapy, using either the conventional Goeckerman regimen (UVB) or psoralen and high-intensity ultraviolet A light (PUVA); and chemotherapeutic agents, such as methotrexate, hydroxyurea, and, most recently, the oral retinoid etretinate.

Infectious Diseases

DERMATOPHYTOSIS

During the past 50 years the anthropophilic fungus *Trichophyton rubrum* has become the most widely encountered dermatophyte, accounting for the majority of all superficial "ringworm" infections. Wartime troop movements, migration of labor, and increased intercontinental travel are felt to have played important roles in the present geographic distribution of this fungus.[6] More common in males but with no racial predilection, *T. rubrum* generally affects the feet, interdigital areas, nails, medial aspects of the thighs, and hands. Moisture, frictional irritation, and intimate skin-to-skin contact with infected individuals predispose to ringworm infections. Infected patients may be asymptomatic or may experience pronounced itching or burning, usually depending upon the particular sites of involvement. *T. rubrum's* capacity for autoinoculation through pruritus-induced scratching, its capacity for asymptomatic nail involvement, and its ability to spread well beyond the initial site of infection account, at least in part, for its maintenance and spread within the community at large.

Tinea corporis may affect large areas of the trunk, face, and extremities. Lesions may be annular, gyrate, or polycyclic (hence the name *ringworm*) and are ordinarily asymmetric in distribution. They may be reddish, reddish brown, or brown. They have sharp, scaly, irregular borders and may occasionally demonstrate central clearing. Although ordinarily flat, lesional borders may be slightly raised.

Routinely serologic laboratory studies are nondiagnostic. Microscopic demonstration of septate hyphae by use of a 10 percent potassium hydroxide (KOH) preparation supports a clinical diagnosis of dermatophytosis. Although species identification cannot be made in this way, the KOH preparation is nonetheless useful since it permits the rapid recognition of dermatophytosis and makes possible early institution of antifungal therapy. Growth of colonies of pure *T. rubrum* on appropriate fungal media, which usually requires an incubation period of between 10 and 14 days, constitutes the definitive diagnostic examination for tinea. Biopsy of suspected fungal lesions is generally unnecessary, although the demonstration of abundant hyphae within the stratum corneum would be supportive.

The use of broad-spectrum topical preparations, such as miconazole, clotrimazole, econazole, and ciclopirox, as well as oral griseofulvin and ketoconazole, has been found to be particularly effective in treating most ringworm infections of the glabrous skin.

SECONDARY SYPHILIS

Syphilis, or lues, is a worldwide largely venereally transmittable disease caused by the spirochete *Treponema pallidum.* It affects all strata of society, most commonly sexually active individuals between the ages of 20 and 39 years; its estimated annual incidence in the United States is approximately 3.5 per 100,000.

The natural history of syphilis has been divided into four stages based upon clinical manifestations: primary, secondary, latent, and tertiary syphilis (which includes late benign and cardiovascular syphilis and neurosyphilis). The syphilitic chancre, the hallmark of primary lues, forms at the site of contact on intact mucous membranes or abraded skin about 3 weeks following inoculation, persists for between 1 and 5 weeks, and then spontaneously resolves. Between 2 and 24 weeks later the signs and symptoms of secondary lues begin and last for approximately 4 weeks before spontaneous resolution. Approximately one-third of untreated patients will subsequently enjoy perfect health, another one-third will remain asymptomatic but will retain serologic evidence of lues, and the remaining one-third will manifest signs of tertiary lues.[7]

In secondary syphilis patients may experience nonspecific constitutional symptoms of low-grade fever, malaise, headache, arthralgias, myalgias, anorexia, and weight loss, as well as symptoms related to specific organ involvements.

The cutaneous lesions reflect host reaction to hematogenously and lymphatogenously deposited *T. pallidum.* Such lesions are frequently generalized, most often papular, and rarely pruritic. Palmar and plantar involvement is typical and is an extremely helpful diagnostic sign. Papular lesions may be annular, concentric, arciform, or serpiginous in configuration (Fig. 18-1). The skin lesions of secondary lues are red or reddish brown and covered with a fine scale (hence their usual inclusion in the differential diagnosis of papulosquamous eruptions); mucosal lesions may present as elevated "mucous patches."

Associated findings may be macular, follicular, and nodular lesions; hypopigmentation; palmar/plantar hyperkeratosis; paronychia; patchy ("moth-eaten") alopecia; moist, papular, mucosal, and intertriginal lesions (condylomata lata); and generalized, occasionally painful lymphadenopathy. Multivisceral disease, including hepatitis, gastric ulceration, glomerulonephritis, arthritis, myositis, uveitis, and central nervous system and cranial nerve involvement, may also occur.

The highly sensitive, nontreponemal, Venereal Disease Research Laboratories (VDRL) screening test is invariably elevated in secondary lues (above 1:16). The fluorescent treponemal-antibody test (FTA), which is more specific, is used to eliminate the possibility of a false positive VDRL. A positive FTA confirms the diagnosis of lues in a patient with no prior history of lues or related treponemal diseases. Dark field examination of moist or intentionally abraded lesions of secondary lues will often reveal the presence of live treponemes. Biopsy is nondiagnostic. Anemia, leukocytosis, lymphocytosis, and an elevated erythrocyte sedimentation rate are commonly observed during the secondary stage. In addition, other serum and urine tests may be abnormal, depending upon the particular organ systems affected.

Treatment consists of intramuscular benzathine penicillin or, alternatively, oral tetracycline or erythromycin. In most cases if appropriate therapy is instituted early, that is, within 3 months of primary infection, rapid sero-reversal can be achieved.

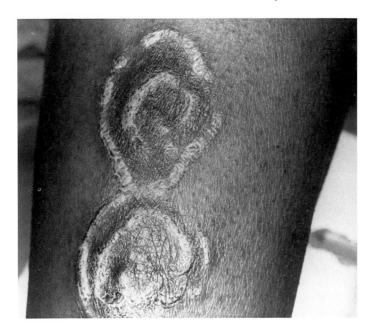

Fig. 18–1. Polycyclic lesions of secondary syphilis on the thigh of an affected patient.

BORDERLINE (DIMORPHOUS) LEPROSY

Hansen's disease, or leprosy, is a chronic granulomatous disease, primarily involving the dermis, upper respiratory mucosa, and peripheral nerves, and is caused by the obligatory bacterial human parasite *Mycobacterium leprae*. The disease is endemic in the tropics and affects an estimated 11 million patients with leprosy worldwide. Increased immigration to the United States from the Far East during the past decade accounts for the significantly increased number of cases of leprosy seen here recently.

Slightly more common in men and showing no racial or age predilections, leprosy is presumed to spread through prolonged intimate contact between patients with open or bacterially laden lesions and susceptible hosts. The incubation period varies from 2 to 5 years and is followed by a period characterized by complaints of paresthesias and the appearance of a transitory, faint macular eruption. The disease may be self-limited or progressive, depending upon host immunologic factors.

Leprosy has been traditionally classified into three basic types on the basis of the host's immunologic response to the organisms: polar tuberculoid, in which cell-mediated immunity is preserved; polar lepromatous, in which the patient is anergic; and borderline (dimorphous), representing an intermediate spectrum.[8]

The clinical manifestations of dimorphous leprosy are intermediate between those of polar lepromatous and polar tuberculoid leprosy. More often, it is the lesions of the near lepromatous type that may most resemble annular erythemas. Such lesions may be widespread or localized. In addition, violaceous or brownish plaques, reddish or light-colored macules, and dimpled nodules may be seen. The earlobes and intertriginous areas are usually also affected. Annular lesions typically have an ''inverted saucer'' appearance, with central hypopigmentation, hypoesthesia or anesthesia, and peripheral erythema and induration.

Routine laboratory studies are nonspecific, although diffuse hyperglobulinemia is usually present. A biopsy is essential. Definitive diagnosis rests upon demonstration of the causative organisms within the biopsy specimen using the Fite-Faraco stain and demonstration of granulomatous nerve involvement. A second method of demonstrating the acid-fast mycobacteria, the slit-smear technique, involves obtaining tissue fluid by making a small incision in a typical lesion and staining it with the Ziehl-Neelsen stain. The Mitsuda-type lepromin test, an intradermal skin test employing impure antigen, is not helpful in diagnosing leprosy but has been found useful for assessing the level of host immune responsiveness.

The drug of choice for treating leprosy remains dapsone. Other drugs that have been successfully employed are rifampin, clofazimine, ethionamide, and streptomycin. For borderline leprosy the rate of relapse is high and lifelong treatment is therefore recommended.

ERYTHEMA CHRONICUM MIGRANS (LYME DERMATITIS)

Erythema chronicum migrans (ECM), one of the so-called gyrate erythemas, usually follows by days to weeks the bite of the tick *Ixodes dammini*.[9] Cases have also been reported following a mosquito bite or thorn prick, as well as cases having no relation to prior bites or scratches. The spirochetal bacterium *Borrelia burgdorferi* has most recently been associated with this condition. The gyrate lesions are generally asymptomatic but may occasionally be pruritic. Primarily seen in northern, central, and eastern Europe, ECM has more recently been reported in North America.

Patients frequently experience a variety of associated constitutional symptoms, including headache, chills, fever, malaise, myalgias, and arthralgias. Ten percent of patients with ECM may also suffer from any or all of the following conditions: lymphocytic meningitis; cranial and peripheral neuropathies; myocarditis, pericarditis, and heart block; and Lyme arthritis, which is an acute, sterile, large-joint, mono- or oligoarticular arthritis, first described in Lyme County, Connecticut but since reported in many forested areas of North America.

Lesions of ECM most often involve the trunk or proximal extremities. They begin as small macules or papules and then expand peripherally, clear centrally, and develop sharp, some-what irregular borders. A central punctum is sometimes also observed. Most lesions are several centimeters in width but some have even exceeded 50 cm. Where multiple bites have occurred, crisscrossed patterns may be seen. Lesions are red or bluish red, are nonscaling, and have palpable borders (Fig. 18-2).

The erythrocyte sedimentation rate, serum immunoglobulins, and cryoglobulins are frequently elevated, particularly in those patients with pronounced constitutional symptoms or arthritis. Elevated specific IgM and IgG antibodies have been found in more than 90 percent of all patients with Lyme disease. Depending

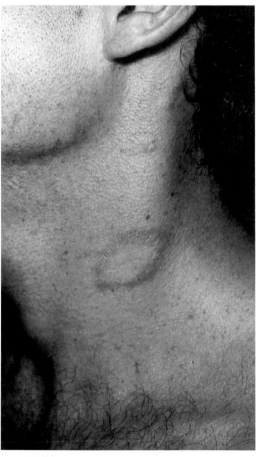

Fig. 18–2. Lesions of erythema chronicum migrans, characteristically large, have somewhat sharp, irregular borders and central clearing. This patient had an associated arthritis of the shoulder.

upon the particular organ systems involved, other nonspecific serologic, cerebrospinal fluid, and electrocardiographic abnormalities may be observed. Demonstration of spirochetes in the cerebrospinal fluid or blood is diagnostic of Lyme disease.

Biopsy of the center of the lesion frequently demonstrates the characteristic tick bite findings, while the active rim of the lesion displays a superficial and deep perivascular lymphohistiocytic infiltrate beneath a normal epidermis. Spirochetes, when occasionally observed either in the center or rim of the lesions, are diagnostic.

The early institution of oral penicillin leads to a rapid resolution of ECM within days and appears to prevent or decrease the severity of ensuing arthritis. Tetracycline has also been effective and has been considered the drug of choice by some investigators. Antibiotics, however, may not prevent the neurologic or cardiac sequelae. If untreated, ECM may persist for years.

TINEA VERSICOLOR

Tinea versicolor is a worldwide fungal infection of the skin due to the obligate parasitic species *Pityrosporum ovale* and *Pityrosporum orbiculare* and accounts for approximately 5 percent of all fungal infections. Lesions primarily involve the trunk, neck, and extremities. Usually annular and macular, they may coalesce to form large patches and may vary in color—hence the name *versicolor*. Typically, lesions are tan, brown, white, or pink and are covered by fine scales. The demonstration of a green to orange fluorescence upon Wood's ultraviolet light examination is supportive; the finding of the so-called meatballs and spaghetti pattern of hyphae in a KOH preparation of lesional scrapings is diagnostic.

LUPUS VULGARIS

Lupus vulgaris, a slowly progressive, destructive, postprimary, cutaneous tuberculosis seen more commonly in northern Europe and England, usually results from direct extension, lymphatogenous, or rarely hematogenous spread to the skin from a visceral source.

The head and neck regions are most often affected. Lesions, usually solitary, most frequently initially arise on the nose or cheek and then spread to contiguous areas. Rarely, when multiple foci are present, large, gyrate lesions may result from the coalescence of several smaller lesions. Individual lesions may be ulcerative, hypertrophic, or, less commonly, annular; brown or brownish red in color; and either smooth, scaly, or even vegetative. Typically, lesional centers are atrophic and the borders are sharply marginated and composed of multiple soft nodules. A biopsy revealing typical noncaseating tubercles is supportive; cultural isolation of *Mycobacterium tuberculosis* is confirmatory.

IMPETIGO CONTAGIOSA

Impetigo contagiosa is an acute, often self-limited, superficial pyoderma caused most frequently by group A β-hemolytic streptococci and *Staphylococcus aureus* and most often affecting children in the late summer and autumn. Pruritus is common. Lesions generally affect exposed areas of the extremities and may be solitary or multiple. They are oval or annular and red to reddish brown and may show central clearing. The lesions, which are initially vesicular and then pustular, typically rupture and form a thick, amber, stuck-on crust, the hallmark of the condition. Gram stain and bacterial culture are confirmatory.

Allergic Disorders

FIXED DRUG ERUPTION

Adverse cutaneous drug reactions, defined as unwanted or unanticipated cutaneous sequelae of medication administration, have been estimated to occur in up to 3 percent of all hospitalized patients. Such reactions may result from allergic, toxic, or pharmacologic mechanisms and may take a number of different forms. The *fixed drug eruption* is an unusual variety of drug-related adverse cutaneous reaction. The adjective *fixed* refers to the remarkable ability of the offending drug to induce the same reaction in the same location each time the medication is administered. The pathogenesis of fixed drug eruptions is unknown. A number of drugs, such as phenolphthalein, once commonly found in laxatives, and tetracyclines, have been frequently associated with this form of drug reaction. Other commonly prescribed agents that have been associated with fixed drug eruptions are barbiturates, phenylbutazone, salicylates, and sulfonamides.[10]

Fixed drug eruptions may occur anywhere on the skin, but most commonly occur on the palmar/plantar regions, penile glans, and lips. Although lesions are most often solitary, multiple lesions may also occur, and subsequent reexposure to the causative drug may result in an increased number of lesions. Lesions are well circumscribed, are oval or annular, and may or may not have a vesicular or bullous component. They may acutely be dusky red to violaceous in color and slightly elevated. Upon spontaneous resolution, usually within 1 week following discontinuation of the causative drug, postinflammatory hyperpigmentation results, which may persist for months or years.

Routine laboratory studies are nondiagnostic. Biopsy of an early suspected lesion reveals a mixed superficial and deep perivascular inflammatory cell infiltrate, marked epidermal and dermal edema, vacuolar alteration at the dermoepidermal junction, and necrotic keratinocytes.

Other than discontinuation and future avoidance of the causative medication, no therapy is usually required.

INSECT BITES

Insects are strictly defined as any of the numerous small invertebrates having an adult body form with three major segments, two pairs of wings, and six legs. This discussion is limited primarily to mosquitos, fleas, and bedbugs, blood-feeding insects whose saliva contains toxins responsible for eliciting the bite reaction. Patients should be questioned about travel to endemic areas and recent contact with animals, old furniture, or strange beds. Initial bite reactions are thought to be nonallergenic; subsequent bite reactions, however, are felt to reflect allergic sensitization.[11] While the occurrence of the bites themselves may go unnoticed, patients often subsequently complain of intense pruritus, burning, or pain at the site.

Mosquito bites may affect any region of the body. Flea bites, in general, are restricted to the exposed and extensor areas, while sparing the trunk and intertriginous regions. Bedbug bites are likewise found on non-clothing-covered regions. Bites from these insects may be linearly arranged or grouped, and may give rise to papules, vesicles, and erythematous wheals. The typical linear grouping of three lesions seen with flea bites has been referred to as "breakfast, lunch, and dinner." The presence of a central punctum on the peak of a papule is strong supportive evidence of insect bite reaction.

Routine serologic studies are unhelpful. Biopsy of a lesion may be helpful when a diagnosis of insect bite reaction is suspected but a history of exposure cannot be elicited. Typical histopathologic findings consist of a dense, wedge-shaped, mixed superficial and deep perivascular inflammatory cell infiltrate; papillary edema; and the presence of interstitial eosinophils and extravasated erythrocytes.

Treatment is symptomatic, consisting of cool compresses, topical corticosteroid creams, and oral antihistamines. For prophylaxis against mosquitos and fleas, repellents containing diethyltoluamide have been found most effective. Control of bedbugs may be achieved through the application of a pesticide, such as hexachlorocyclohexane, to floors, wall crevices and furniture. Insect bite lesions generally resolve within 48 hours. In some patients, however, lesions may become granulomatous and persist for many months.

ERYTHEMA ANNULARE CENTRIFUGUM

Erythema annulare centrifugum (EAC), considered the paradigm of annular erythemas, is a relatively uncommon chronic, recurrent hypersensitivity reaction pattern. Having no age, sex, or racial predilections, EAC in most instances has been associated with a diverse group of underlying conditions, such as malignancy, food and drug ingestion, and bacterial, viral, dermatophytic, and candidal infections.[12]

Most often, EAC involves the trunk and extremities. It begins as papules, which enlarge peripherally and clear centrally, resulting in gyrate, arcuate, serpiginous, or polycyclic configurations (Fig. 18-3). Lesional centers may be yellowish and covered by fine scaling. Lesional borders are pink or reddish in color and may be hivelike or vesicular, finely scaling, and palpable.

Since there are numerous causes of EAC, laboratory evaluation should be directed toward detecting the most probable antecedent etiologies based upon the history. Peripheral eosinophilia is occasionally observed. Biopsy reveals a superficial perivascular, lymphohistiocytic infiltrate, slight papillary edema, focal spongiosis, and occasional parakeratosis.

The course of EAC generally parallels that of the underlying condition. When no specific etiology has been determined, the empiric use of broad-spectrum antibiotics, antifungals, and anticandidal agents may be of use. Although oral steroids may effect dramatic clearing of EAC, recurrence is common following their discontinuation.

ERYTHEMA MULTIFORME

Erythema multiforme (EM) is a relatively common acute, self-limited, often recurrent cutaneous reaction pattern. Lesions of EM may symmetrically involve the extensor aspects of the extremities, palmar/plantar regions, face, and oral mucosa. The iris, or target lesion, which is most often acrally located and consists of a central vesicle or purple-red macule sur-

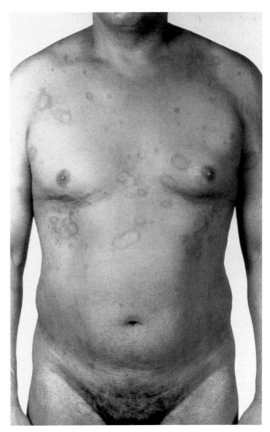

Fig. 18–3. The prototype of the annular erythemas, erythema annulare centrifugum, gradually spreads peripherally with central clearing.

rounded by concentric whitish and red rings, is pathognomonic of EM. In addition, macules, papules, vesicles, bullae, and urticarial lesions may be present—hence the name *multiforme*. The disorder has a characteristic histopathology, consisting of a superficial perivascular, lymphohistiocytic infiltrate, extravasated erythrocytes, epidermal and papillary edema, necrotic keratinocytes, and subepidermal vesicle formation.

URTICARIA

Urticaria is a largely histamine-related cutaneous reaction pattern estimated to affect approximately 20 percent of the population at some point during their lifetimes. Urticarial lesions may appear anywhere, are usually multiple and sharply marginated, and range in size from several millimeters to several centimeters in diameter. They may have annular, polycyclic, or serpiginous borders, with a faint surrounding halo and a pale central area. Lesions may be pink or reddish in color and, owing to the presence of intradermal edema, are firm to palpation. Biopsy findings reveal dermal edema and otherwise normal architecture.

Neoplastic Disorders

PARAPSORIASIS EN PLAQUES, LARGE PLAQUE TYPE AND MYCOSIS FUNGOIDES, PATCH STAGE

Parapsoriasis en plaques has been divided into two varieties: parapsoriasis en plaques, small plaque type, a wholly benign entity, and parapsoriasis en plaques, large plaque type. The large plaque type, which has no sexual predilection and largely affects middle-aged whites, may be either a benign condition or a premalignant condition. Malignant transformation, most frequently to mycosis fungoides, occurs in approximately 12 percent of these patients. Patients with nonmalignant lesions are generally asymptomatic but occasionally complain of mild pruritus. Those in whom malignancy has supervened generally experience severe pruritus.[13]

Lesions of large-plaque parapsoriasis are usually symmetrically distributed or, less commonly, localized to portions of the trunk, proximal extremities, buttocks, hips, and breasts. Lesions are generally oval with indistinct borders and covered by fine scaling (Fig. 18-4); their color may vary from reddish blue to blue-red. Particularly in patients with the premalignant variety of the disorder, the lesions may be associated with the poikilodermatous findings of telangiectasia, mottled hyperpigmentation, and atrophy. Initially, however, lesions may be slightly indurated.

In the premalignant stage routine laboratory

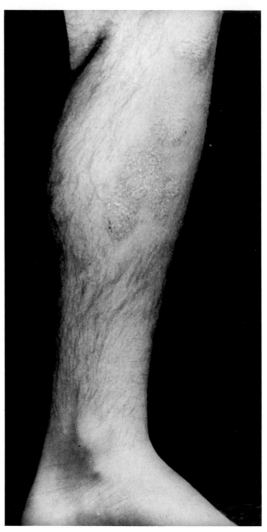

Fig. 18–4. Lesions of large-plaque parapsoriasis are oval or annular, indistinctly bordered, and symmetrically distributed and may be associated with poikilodermatous changes.

studies are nondiagnostic. Biopsy findings are also nonspecific, consisting of a perivascular, lymphohistiocytic dermatitis, and, when present, the histopathologic changes of poikiloderma. Following malignant transformation, atypical mononuclear cells, analogous to mycosis cells, may be seen within the dermal infiltrate or singly within the epidermis.

Mycosis fungoides is an uncommon progressive, cutaneous T-cell lymphoma, accounting for 1 percent of lymphoma deaths annually in the United States. Worldwide in distribution and displaying no racial predilection, mycosis fungoides usually affects middle-aged individuals and affects men twice as frequently as women. Patients most commonly complain of severe pruritus.[14]

Cutaneous lesions have been clinically and histologically classified into three stages: stage 1, patch stage; stage 2, indurated plaque stage; and stage 3, tumor stage. Stage 1 and 2 lesions of mycosis fungoides may be clinically confused with a number of benign annular erythemas.

Stage 1 and 2 lesions chiefly involve the trunk and extremities, are morphologically annular, arcuate, serpiginous, or generalized, and are typically reddish in color. Many of these lesions undergo either central clearing or total spontaneous involution, both of which are felt to be related to changing levels of host resistance. Initially some patches may be atrophic, but within months to years they generally undergo transition to indurated plaques or tumors.

As a rule, both the large plaque-type of parapsoriasis en plaques and mycosis fungoides follow chronic, unremitting courses. In general, patients with large-plaque parapsoriasis whose lesions manifest poikilodermatous changes appear at greatest risk for the development of lymphoma and should be closely followed. Palliative therapy for parapsoriasis, using emollients and topical steroid creams to alleviate dryness and itching, may be of some use. PUVA and topical nitrogen mustard therapies for mycosis fungoides may result in temporary clinical and symptomatic improvement. Infiltrated plaques may benefit from grenz ray or superficial x-ray therapy.

ERYTHEMA GYRATUM REPENS

Erythema gyratum repens (EGR), a superficial gyrate erythema, is a rare disorder almost invariably associated with the presence or later development of underlying internal malignancy. The lesions of EGR may occasionally

be pruritic. Pulmonary, prostatic, gastric, and bladder carcinomas are among the variety of malignancies that have been associated with EGR.[15] The lesions of this paraneoplastic disorder are characteristically rapid-moving, usually enlarging in waves within a matter of hours.

Lesions most often are multiple and involve the trunk and proximal extremities. The so-called wood-grain or zebralike festooning configurations are distinctive (Fig. 18-5). Lesions are reddish, possess a collarette of scale, and are most often flat but may occasionally be slightly indurated.

The distinctive clinical picture is diagnostic. Biopsy reveals a superficial perivascular, lymphohistiocytic infiltrate, papillary edema, and

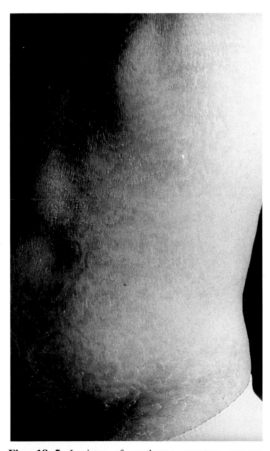

Fig. 18–5. Lesions of erythema gyratum repens characteristically display a "wood grain" or "zebralike" pattern. (Photograph courtesy of Ernest Ast, M.D., Bronx VA Medical Center, Bronx, NY.)

overlying epidermal acanthosis, spongiosis, and hyperkeratosis. The results of routine and special laboratory investigations depend upon the nature of the underlying disorder.

Therapy consists of treating the underlying malignancy, and the overall prognosis parallels that of the underlying disorder. Removal of the malignancy results in complete resolution of the cutaneous lesions.

NECROLYTIC MIGRATORY ERYTHEMA (GLUCAGONOMA SYNDROME)

Patients with glucagon-secreting pancreatic tumors may experience a rare, but striking, superficial, migratory eruption. Lesions of necrolytic migratory erythema are generally confined to the dependent and frictionally irritated intertriginous regions, particularly the lower abdomen, groin, and lower extremities. Lesions are usually annular and reddish, and vesiculation, scaling, and erosion are common. Diagnosis rests upon the findings of an elevated plasma glucagon level in the appropriate clinical setting and demonstration of the pancreatic tumor.

Collagen-Vascular Disorders

ERYTHEMA MARGINATUM RHEUMATICUM

Erythema marginatum rheumaticum (EMR) is a superficial gyrate erythema seen in approximately 18 percent of patients with acute rheumatic fever; it is one of the five major Jones criteria for the diagnosis of acute rheumatic fever, a disease that occurs as a delayed sequel to a prior group A β-hemolytic streptococcal pharyngitis. Other major Jones criteria include carditis, migratory polyarthritis, Sydenham's chorea, and subcutaneous nodules.

Lesions of EMR are recurrent, asymptomatic, or occasionally mildly pruritic; rapidly migratory (between 2 and 10 mm in 12 hours); and transitory, usually lasting no more than several hours. Although EMR is uncorrelated with rheumatic fever severity, it usually follows the onset of arthritis and is frequently associated with rheumatic carditis.[16]

Lesions generally are multiple and involve the trunk, axillae, and proximal extremities, but they may also involve the hands. Beginning as small patches or papules, they may assume polycyclic or festooned configurations (Fig. 18-6). These lesions are pink or faintly reddish and nonscaling; they may be flat or slightly indurated.

Laboratory studies are not diagnostic for EMR, or for rheumatic fever for that matter, and usually reflect the accompanying manifestations of the rheumatic fever. Depending upon the specific circumstances, one may find elevations in both the erythrocyte sedimentation rate

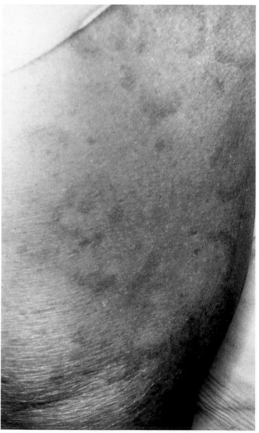

Fig. 18–6. Arising as small pink or faintly reddish scaling patches or papules, lesions of erythema marginatum assume polycyclic or festooned appearances.

and antistreptococcal antibody titers, as well as electrocardiographic abnormalities. Biopsy of a lesion of EMR usually demonstrates a superficial perivascular, lymphohistiocytic infiltrate with little overlying epidermal change.

Although EMR seldom lasts more than several days, it may persist for several weeks. The eruption neither requires nor responds to topical or systemic anti-inflammatory therapies.

DISCOID AND SUBACUTE CUTANEOUS LUPUS ERYTHEMATOSUS

Lupus erythematosus (LE) is a connective tissue disease with a broad spectrum of clinical presentations, ranging from a benign strictly cutaneous disorder, chronic discoid LE (CDLE), to a potentially fatal cutaneous and multivisceral disease, systemic LE. Subacute cutaneous LE (SCLE), conceptually an intermediate disorder, is characterized by a cutaneously distinct entity associated with a milder form of systemic illness and characteristic serologic findings.

Displaying no racial predilection and affecting women twice as frequently as men, CDLE is an uncommon cutaneous connective tissue disease most often affecting adults in their third to fifth decades of life. In approximately 50 percent of patients the onset of CDLE, or flares in predisposed individuals, have been related to ultraviolet light exposure, hot weather, trauma, and menstruation. Lesions are generally asymptomatic or may be slightly pruritic.[17]

Recently a number of patients described with what has been referred to as SCLE have shown skin lesions that possessed the characteristic histologic findings of CDLE but were clinically distinguishable from those of CDLE. In addition, these patients generally complained of such constitutional symptoms as fever, myalgias, and arthralgias. Oral mucosal lesions are also more common in SCLE than in CDLE. Although sharing some of the serologic findings of systemic LE, none of these patients has been reported to have significant renal or central nervous system involvement.[18] To date, the major-

ity of patients with SCLE have been white women.

The lesions of CDLE are most commonly located on the face, ears, and scalp, are often multiple, and demonstrate little tendency to coalesce. Beginning as small, scaly plaques, they slowly enlarge into annular patterns, maintaining disease activity at the active, well-circumscribed lesional borders. Such lesions are generally purple or purple-red. As they evolve, the lesions of CDLE become centrally depigmented, owing to the development of scarring and atrophy. Central telangiectasia and follicular plugging are also prominent features.

By contrast, the lesions of SCLE are widespread and symmetrical in distribution and most often involve the upper trunk and proximal upper extremities. They begin as small papules and may either remain papulosquamous in appearance or enlarge and merge into annular or polycyclic configurations. Either or both patterns may be observed in any patient. Lesional borders are reddish and superficially scaly or vesicular; lesional centers are grayish and may also be telangiectatic. Similar lesions can be seen in neonatal lupus (Fig. 18-7).

Laboratory investigation of patients with CDLE is usually unremarkable but occasionally may reveal mild leukopenia, mild hypergammaglobulinemia, a false-positive VDRL, minimally positive antinuclear antibody titer, positive rheumatoid factor, and minimally depressed complement levels. These laboratory studies are more commonly positive in patients with SCLE. In addition, patients with SCLE have frequently been found to have positive anti-Ro and anti-La antibodies and minimally elevated anti-double-stranded DNA antibodies.

Biopsy of a lesion of CDLE reveals a superficial and deep perivascular, lymphohistiocytic infiltrate, vacuolar alteration at the dermoepidermal junction, a thickened basement membrane, epidermal hyperkeratosis, and follicular plugging. Biopsy of a lesion of SCLE demonstrates the same dermoepidermal pathology as that seen in CDLE; however, the inflammatory infiltrate, hyperkeratosis, and follicular plugging are less prominent. Interestingly, in contrast to the majority of patients with CDLE, in whom deposits of immunoglobulin and complement at the dermoepidermal junction may be found on direct immunofluorescence examination of lesional skin, only about 50 percent of patients with SCLE may be observed to have similar findings.

Both SCLE and, especially, CDLE may respond to the use of topical steroids under occlusion and to oral antimalarials. In unresponsive SCLE systemic corticosteroids and nonsteroidal anti-inflammatory agents may be of value.

Idiopathic Diseases

GRANULOMA ANNULARE

Granuloma annulare (GA) is an asymptomatic benign granulomatous disorder, which affects women twice as often as men. In more than two-thirds of the patients onset of the disease occurs before the age of 30. By contrast, in the disseminated form patients are frequently in the fifth decade of life. The relationship of GA to heredity, diabetes mellitus, or prior trauma remains unconfirmed. Lesions usually enlarge over the course of weeks to months. Several clinically distinguishable but histologically similar types of GA exist: papular, subcutaneous, perforating, disseminated, and, most frequently encountered, plaque form.[19] Only the latter two forms figure prominently in the differential diagnosis of annular erythemas and need concern us here.

Lesions of GA, multiple in about 50 percent of patients, most often affect the dorsa of the hands and feet but may appear elsewhere on the extremities. They vary in size but usually do not exceed 5 cm in diameter and are generally composed of a group of papules or nodules in oval or arciform arrangement. Often flesh-colored, they may be reddish or purplish and firm to palpation. Lesions of disseminated GA tend to be symmetrical and may coalesce into large gyrate lesions.

Routine laboratory studies are unhelpful. Histopathologic analysis reveals granulomas in the upper dermis composed of peripheral palisading

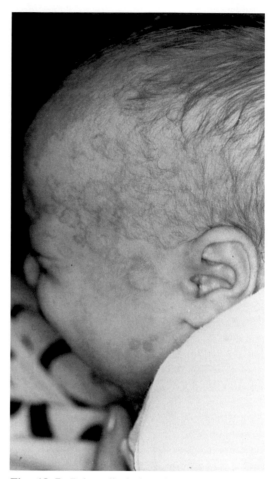

Fig. 18–7. Polycyclic lesions in a newborn infant with neonatal lupus.

histiocytes, central degenerated collagen bundles, and mucinous deposition.

Intralesional or topical corticosteroids under occlusion have been found effective in GA. In general, the disease is self-limited, resolving spontaneously in most patients within 2 years. The disseminated variety tends to follow a more chronic course, lasting for years, and is characterized by remissions and exacerbations.

ERYTHEMA DYSCHROMICUM PERSTANS (ASHY DERMATOSIS)

Erythema dyschromicum perstans (EDP) is a chronic, disfiguring, occasionally pruritic, cutaneous hyperpigmentary disorder. Although

EDP has no age or sex predilection, the majority of patients have been of Central and South American origin. The disorder was once thought to be rare, but a number of investigators now contend that EDP may be more common than previously thought.[19] A number of cases have more recently been reported in light-skinned individuals and it has been further suggested that cases of macular hyperpigmentary disorders described elsewhere in the literature under various other names may, in fact, also have been cases of EDP.

Although large areas of the body may be affected, the trunk, arms, neck, and face are most commonly and symmetrically involved. Individual lesions may be oval, irregular, or even polycyclic and continue to enlarge slowly, varying in size from 3 mm to several centimeters in diameter. Active lesions are typically slate gray or lead-colored (hence the name *ashy dermatosis*) but may have a pale reddish, slightly elevated, border.

Routine laboratory studies are typically either negative or normal. Diagnosis rests upon the history and the exclusion of other macular erythematous or hyperpigmentary disorders. Biopsy findings consisting of follicular hyperkeratosis, decreased basal-layer melanin, and vacuolar alteration of the dermoepidermal junction with melanin incontinence are nondiagnostic but supportive.

Although numerous treatment modalities have been tried, therapy of EDP has been uniformly unsuccessful in either halting the chronic progression of the condition or reversing the hyperpigmentation.

PITYRIASIS ROSEA

Pityriasis rosea (PR) is an acute, inflammatory dermatosis frequently affecting adolescents and young adults. Occurring most often during the spring and autumn, PR is believed, although not proven, to be of viral origin. Although generally asymptomatic, it may vary from mildly to severely pruritic; its onset may occasionally be accompanied by a mild malaise.

The "herald" or "mother" patch, which may appear anywhere on the body and which may go unnoticed in approximately one-third of patients, may range in size from 2 to 6 cm and usually precedes the full eruption of PR by a few days to 2 weeks. The majority of PR lesions, which generally range from 1 to 2 cm in diameter, are confined to the trunk and extremities and typically parallel the rib cage cleavage lines in a so-called fir-tree pattern. Facial lesions may be seen in children. When numerous, lesions may coalesce into large annular patches. They may be salmon-colored, pink, tan, faint brown, or reddish, may possess fine collarettes of scales, and may occasionally be papular, vesicular, or urticarial. Laboratory studies are unhelpful and diagnosis rests upon the history and clinical findings.

Treatment is symptomatic and is generally unnecessary. Erythemogenic doses of ultraviolet B have been found particularly effective for controlling severe pruritus when present. Usually PR resolves spontaneously within 2 to 6 weeks, but it can sometimes persist for several months.

Lymphocytic Infiltrates

PALPABLE MIGRATORY ARCIFORM ERYTHEMA

Palpable migratory arciform erythema, characterized by spontaneous remissions and exacerbations, is an uncommon benign lymphocytic infiltration of the skin, which typically affects the upper back. Lesions may persist and enlarge for months before resolving. Biopsy findings of a normal epidermis and deep perivascular and periappendageal lymphocytic infiltration are supportive. The clinical findings of this dermatosis are summarized in its name.

LYMPHOCYTIC INFILTRATION OF JESSNER-KANOF

Occurring predominantly in men and usually located on the face, ears, and upper back, lymphocytic infiltration of Jessner-Kanof is characterized by spontaneous remissions and exacerbations. Lesions may appear as smooth-surfaced papules, plaques, or annular plaques with central clearing, may vary from pink to reddish brown, and are firm to palpation. Biopsy reveals a moderately dense, superficial and deep, lymphocytic infiltrate, normal epidermis, and mucin deposition between collagen bundles in the reticular dermis.

GRANULOMA FACIALE

Granuloma faciale, which is most often confined to the face—hence its name—usually presents as well-defined oval or polycyclic lesions with an irregular surface. Lesions may be red, bluish red, yellowish, or reddish brown and soft to firm on palpation, depending upon the stage of the lesion. Biopsy of an early lesion reveals a leukocytoclastic vasculitis. Later lesions show a mixed inflammatory cell infiltrate within the dermis with a preponderance of eosinophils. A so-called grenz zone of periappendageal and papillary dermis sparing is characteristic. In later stages fibrosis may supervene.

URTICARIA PIGMENTOSA

Urticaria pigmentosa, the most frequently encountered of the mastocytoses, has been largely reported in white patients, more than 50 percent of whom are children. Lesions usually affect the trunk and extremities, may range in size from a pinhead to several centimeters in diameter, and may be oval or annular. They are reddish brown to orangish and are typically macular but may be papular or even nodular. A positive Darier's sign (lesional urtication upon rubbing) is seen in approximately 90 percent of patients and is virtually pathognomonic. Demonstration of an abundance of mast cells within the mid- to upper dermis using the Giemsa stain is confirmatory.

SARCOIDOSIS

Sarcoidosis is a multisystem, chronic, non-caseating granulomatous disorder, which affects women three times more commonly than men and American blacks nine times more commonly than whites. Cutaneous disease is seen in approximately 30 percent of all sarcoid patients. Plaque lesions, resulting from either the coalescence of nodules or local diffuse skin infiltration, are the most common variety. They are usually symmetrically distributed over the face and extremities but may be solitary and asymmetric. The plaque lesions are irregular in border; they may be annular or serpiginous and vary from purplish to brownish. A variety of other cutaneous sarcoidal lesions may be found, including papules, nodules, erythema nodosum, morbilliform eruptions, lupus pernio, and erythroderma. The diagnosis is supported by the histologic finding in either a biopsy of a cutaneous lesion or a Kveim intradermal test site of noncaseating, so-called hard tubercles, composed of histiocytes and giant cells surrounded by a narrow zone of lymphocytes.

LICHEN PLANUS

Lichen planus (LP) has no racial or sex predilections and generally affects people between the ages of 30 and 60. It may affect any area of the skin, hair, and nails but most commonly symmetrically involves the flexor region of the wrists, ankles, and genitalia. Annular lesions, seen in approximately 10 percent of patients, result from the coalescence of the more typical finely or minimally scaling LP papules. Such lesions are purplish in color, exhibit central clearing, and are more commonly observed on the lower trunk and penis. The annular variant is generally associated with a more chronic variety of LP. Biopsy findings supportive of the diagnosis include a dense, bandlike lymphohistiocytic infiltrate filling the papillary dermis and obscuring the dermoepidermal junction; vacuolar alteration of the dermoepidermal junction; focal hypergranulosis, epidermal hyperplasia, and orthokeratosis; and the presence of Civatte bodies.

NUMMULAR DERMATITIS

Nummular dermatitis is a characteristic, often chronic, reaction pattern generally affecting older individuals. The disorder is associated with xerosis or exposure to irritants, is often related to stress, and typically exhibits remissions and exacerbations. Multifocal, and most often pruritic, lesions of nummular dermatitis most frequently involve the upper and lower extremities and buttocks and are oval to annular in shape. The lesions range from coin size (hence *nummular,* meaning "coin shaped") to occasionally large confluent plaques several centimeters in diameter; they are reddish to reddish brown, scaling, and occasionally vesicular, exudative, or crusted. Diagnosis rests upon the history and clinical picture; biopsy findings of a spongiotic psoriasiform dermatitis are nonspecific.

SEBORRHEIC DERMATITIS

Seborrheic dermatitis is a common subacute dermatosis, which primarily affects those regions having the greatest number of sebaceous glands, namely the scalp, face, and upper trunk. The disorder is unrelated to sebaceous gland secretion, and may be quite localized or may even progress to erythroderma. It is usually characterized by remissions and exacerbations, and pruritus and scaling may be quite pronounced. Annular lesions with central clearing resulting from the confluence of smaller plaques may be particularly pronounced on the chest and back. Lesional borders are often well demarcated, reddish, and covered with fine, greasy yellow scales. Biopsy is seldom necessary; however, the findings of a psoriasiform, spongiotic dermatitis associated with mounds of neutrophil laden scale-crusts at the lips of the follicular ostia are important histologic signs.

APPROACH TO THE PATIENT

Having completed a review of annular erythemas according to etiologies, it would be well to conclude this chapter by outlining a systematic, practical approach for diagnosing the patient who presents with an annular erythematous eruption—an approach useful for diagnosing any cutaneous disorder, for that matter. Table 18-2 summarizes the steps.

First, the overall picture of the patient and his eruption should be assessed through the history, as well as through the overall lesional distribution and configurations. Next, the eruption should be viewed in its specifics (i.e., the morphology, color, and consistency of the individual lesions). Usually at that point enough information has been obtained to enable the formulation of a differential diagnosis, which may be facilitated by systematically examining Table 18-1 for conditions whose history, symptoms, and signs most closely approximate those of the patient's. Finally, appropriate laboratory tests may be ordered to narrow the diagnostic possibilities to a specific disorder. Such an approach, which systematically proceeds from the general to the specific (analogous to the approach of the histopathologist, who first examines a specimen under low-power and then high-power magnifications), will facilitate more rapid and accurate diagnoses of the annular erythemas.

Table 18-2. Approach to the Patient: Annular Erythemas

1. Evaluate background history and symptoms
2. General physical examination
3. Cutaneous physical examination
   a. Distribution of lesions
   b. Overall configuration of lesions
   c. Morphology of individual lesions (annular and variants)
   d. Color and surface characteristics (scaling, crusting, erosion)
   e. Consistency to palpation (induration, atrophy)
4. Formulate differential diagnosis according to possible etiologies (Table 18-1)
5. Order or perform appropriate laboratory and special studies
6. Establish specific diagnosis

REFERENCES

1. Leider M, Rosenblum M: A Dictionary of Dermatological Words, Terms, and Phrases. Dome Laboratories, West Haven, CT, 1976
2. Siemens HW: An Introduction to Dermatology for Students and Physicians. University of Chicago Press, Chicago, 1958
3. Fitzpatrick TB, Eisen AZ, Wolff, K, et al: Dermatology in General Medicine. 2nd Ed. McGraw-Hill, New York, 1979
4. Beare JM: Familial annular erythema. Br J Dermatol 78:59, 1966
5. Braun-Falco O: The initial psoriatic lesion. p. 1. In Farber EM, Cox AJ (eds): Psoriasis: Proceedings of the Second International Symposium. Yorke Medical Books, New York, 1977
6. Emmons CW, Binford CH, Utz JP, et al: Medical Mycology. 3rd Ed. Lea & Febiger, Philadelphia, 1977
7. Sparling PF: Diagnosis and treatment of syphilis. N Engl J Med 284:642, 1971
8. World Health Organization Expert Committee on Leprosy: Fifth Report. World Health Organization, Geneva, 1977
9. Steere AC, Grodzicki RL K, Kornblatt AN, et al: The spirochetal etiology of Lyme disease. N Engl J Med 308:733, 1983
10. Delaney TJ: Tetracycline induced fixed drug eruptions. Br J Dermatol 83:357, 1970
11. Harves AD, Millikan LE: Current concepts of therapy and pathophysiology in arthropod bites and stings. II. Insects, Int J Dermatol 14:621, 1975
12. Shelley WB: Erythema annulare centrifugum due to *Candida albicans*. Br J Dermatol 77:383, 1965
13. Samman PD: The natural history of parapsoriasis en plaques (chronic superficial dermatitis) and prereticulotic poikiloderma. Br J Dermatol 87:405, 1972
14. Edelson RL: Cutaneous T-cell lymphoma. J Am Acad Dermatol 2:89, 1980
15. Leavell UW, Winternitz WW, Black JH: Erythema gyratum repens and undifferentiated carcinoma. Arch Dermatol 95:69, 1967
16. Keil H: The rheumatic erythemas: a critical survey. Ann Intern Med 11:2223, 1938
17. Prystowsky SD, Herndon JH, Gilliam JN: Chronic cutaneous lupus erythematosus (DLE): a clinical and laboratory investigation of 80 patients. Medicine (Baltimore) 55:183, 1975
18. Gilliam JN, Sontheimer RD: Distinctive cutaneous subsets in the spectrum of lupus erythematosus. J Am Acad Dermatol 4:471, 1981
19. Wells, RS, Smith MA: The natural history of granulomas annulare. Br J Dermatol 75:199, 1963
20. Novick NL, Phelps R: Erythema dyschromicum perstans. Int J Dermatol 24:630, 1985

The Perforating Dermatoses

Philip G. Prioleau
Mathew Varghese

The term *perforating disorder of skin* has been applied to a variety of conditions characterized by transepithelial passage of either an altered component of normal body tissue, a product derived from body tissue, or possibly a foreign body. This rather broad, cumbersome definition encompasses many unrelated disorders. These include such varied entities as necrobiotic material in chondrodermatitis nodularis helicis and blood in talon noir ("black heel"). Elimination of deposits of such material as amyloid or calcium has also been included. Neoplastic cells in certain disorders such as malignant melanoma or mycosis fungoides pass through and are eliminated, and these could also conceivably be included.

Some diseases are associated only occasionally with transepidermal elimination, and perforation through the epidermis is considered only a minor characteristic of the disease. Examples of these are granuloma annulare and pseudoxanthoma elasticum.

Four diseases have usually been called the major perforating diseases, since their most prominent microscopic feature is transepidermal elimination of a substance. These include elastosis perforans serpiginosa, perforating folliculitis, reactive perforating collagenosis, and hyperkeratosis follicularis et parafollicularis in cutem penetrans (Kyrle's disease).

To these four we have added a fifth condition, which we term *perforating disorder of renal disease*. All patients with this disorder have renal disease, and most but not all have severe diabetic nephropathy and are on dialysis. This disorder has been variously identified as reactive perforating collagenosis, hyperkeratosis follicularis et parafollicularis in cutem penetrans (Kyrle's disease), and perforating folliculitis. In our opinion none of these terms is apt, since the perforating disorder of renal disease differs significantly from the original descriptions of the other diseases.

Some believe hyperkeratosis follicularis et parafollicularis in cutem penetrans (Kyrle's disease) does not exist. Kyrle's original description is quite detailed and differs considerably from the perforating disorder of renal disease, although it is conceivable that Kyrle's patient, a diabetic, represents one end of the spectrum of the disorder we have observed in renal disease.[1] However, until this can be convincingly demonstrated, we prefer to consider Kyrle's disease a separate but extremely rare entity.

MAJOR PERFORATING DISEASES

Reactive Perforating Collagenosis

History. Mehregan, Schwartz, and Livingood first recorded the classic form of reactive perforating collagenosis in 1967.[2] They described a 6 ½-year-old girl who developed an eruption of her upper and lower extremities at age 9 months and, noting a Koebner phenomenon, postulated that superficial trauma altered the collagenous tissue and precipitated these lesions.

Clinical Features. The classic form of reactive perforating collagenosis is a rare disorder, beginning in early childhood, in which traumatically altered collagen is extruded by the process of transepidermal elimination.

Characteristically, this disorder arises in early childhood as tiny papules on the exposed surfaces, but it may also occur on the trunk. Over a period of several weeks the papules progress to 5- to 10-mm centrally umbilicated papules with erosions, and in 6 to 8 weeks they regress, leaving a small scar with altered pigmentation.[3] The lesions are precipitated by superficial trauma, whereas deep trauma may fail to cause them. At any one time these papules are in varying stages of development. The Koebner phenomenon is characteristic and has been demonstrated experimentally.[4] Lesions have arisen in sites of acne vulgaris.

Males and females are equally affected. Although sporadic cases have been reported, Nair reported a father and three children with reactive perforating collagenosis, which suggests an autosomal dominant mode of inheritance in at least some cases.[5]

Microscopic Findings. In their original description Mehregan, Schwartz, and Livingood studied lesions at different stages of devel-

opment.[2] Early, nonumbilicated papules were characterized by moderately acanthotic epidermis. The central, widened dermal papillae contained connective tissue, which stained a bluish color with hematoxylin and eosin. No inflammatory infiltrate was present, and the epidermis was atrophic and contained a thin layer of parakeratotic cells.

A well-developed lesion shows a dome-shaped papule with a central crater filled with basophilic keratinous and neutrophilic cellular debris as well as neutrophils. Epithelial cells line much of the crater but are often absent at its base. Collagen bundles pass through this epithelium and are easily demonstrable with a Fontana-Masson stain. Collagen bundles also extend from the dermis through the nonepithelialized portion into the base of the crater. Elastic tissue is not seen. Light microscopy fails to detect any abnormalities of collagen. The epidermis adjacent to the crater is moderately hyperplastic, and there is a thickened orthokeratotic layer. These adjacent findings are similar to those of lichen simplex chronicus or prurigo nodularis and indicate that the lesion was probably rubbed. Electron microscopic studies have confirmed the light microscopic findings. However, it is interesting that the collagen fibers being eliminated have a relatively normal configuration and periodicity and do not show substantial alteration.[6]

Treatment. No specific form of therapy has been found to prevent the formation of new lesions. Improvement has been recorded following application of topical 0.1 percent tretinoin cream, corticosteroids under occlusion, and even simple emollients. Methotrexate has also been used with some success.

Prognosis. The disorder lasts for many years and is less active during the summer months. It appears to be primarily a disease of childhood although it has been reported in adults.

Associated Diseases. The classic form has no associated diseases.

Differential Diagnosis. Clinically, this disorder must be differentiated from perforating folliculitis, perforating granuloma annulare, and molluscum contagiosum. Microscopically, perforating folliculitis, Majocchi's granuloma, Kyrle's disease, and elastosis perforans serpiginosa must be considered.

Perforating Disorder of Renal Disease

History. In Kyrle's original description as well as in many subsequent reports, the perforating disorder known as *hyperkeratosis follicularis et parafollicularis in cutem penetrans (Kyrle's disease)* was associated with diabetes mellitus. This disorder has been considered extremely rare; however, a relatively common association of renal failure and/or diabetes mellitus with a perforating disease has been observed.

In 1982 three groups published cases of a perforating disorder associated with diabetes mellitus and/or renal failure. Although the three descriptions were similar clinically and histologically, this disorder was variously identified as reactive perforating collagenosis, Kyrle's disease, and perforating folliculitis.[7–9]

Despite the differing names ascribed to these lesions, we believe that each group of authors was describing the same condition. In retrospect, this disorder might better have been termed *perforating disorder of renal disease,* since it differs either clinically or histologically from the other known types of perforating disease.

Kyrle's report showed a patient with an extremely dense papular eruption with coalescence of papules. The clinical appearance of this sometimes pruritic eruption did not show the typical Koebner phenomenon seen in the chronic dialysis/diabetic population. It is possible, however, that Kyrle's patient, a severe diabetic, did have the same disorder seen in the chronic dialysis/diabetic populus and represented the far end of a spectrum that we have not observed.

The lesions of patients with renal failure appear clinically in a follicular distribution. On rare occasions hair follicles have been reported microscopically. We described this disorder as a form of reactive perforating collagenosis,[7] since it was similar microscopically to the disorder described by Mehregan et al.[2] On close examination we were able to demonstrate strands of collagen perforating the epidermis. Although the perforating disorder of renal disease appears similar clinically to the reactive perforating collagenosis of Mehregan, the latter is an extremely rare disease, which arises in infancy or early childhood and resolves spontaneously in 6 to 8 weeks. In some cases the disorder described by Mehregan appears to be hereditary. Its clinical presentation, therefore, does not resemble the disorder seen in the chronic renal failure/diabetic population.

Clinical Features. All patients with the perforating disease of the chronic renal failure/diabetic population have renal disease and most have had diabetic nephropathy and retinopathy. The disease appears to be relatively common in the dialysis population and has been found in 4.5 to 10 percent of patients undergoing dialysis. Many of the patients are black, and as evidenced by the presence of diabetic retinopathy, have advanced diabetes mellitus. The ages have ranged from the third to the ninth decades, with a median age of 55. The skin lesions consist of numerous umbilicated, hyperpigmented papules, each of which contains a central plug, and their diameters range from 0.2 to 1 cm. They occur mainly on the extensor surfaces of the extremities, particularly around knees and elbows (Fig. 19-1). They may also be present on the trunk and, rarely, the face.

Almost all patients have associated pruritus, which is often intense. The Koebner phenomenon is also common.

Microscopic Findings. Microscopically, there is a dome-shaped papule with a central crater filled with parakeratotic debris and neutrophils. The crater walls are lined by stratified squamous epithelium. The base of the crater

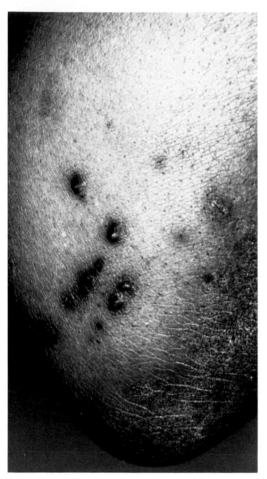

Fig. 19-1. Perforating disorder of renal disease. Hyperpigmented centrally keratotic papules on the elbow of a black patient.

may be lined or there may be a gap in the epithelial lining. There is a sparse to moderately dense, superficial, perivascular, lymphohistiocytic inflammatory infiltrate, and the epidermis adjacent to the crater is moderately hyperplastic and has a thickened, orthokeratotic layer (Fig. 19-2A). In each case we have examined we have seen strands of collagen perforating the epithelium at or near the base of the crater or where there has been a gap, extending into the crater (Fig. 19-2B). This has been confirmed with Masson trichrome stains.

In no cases have we been able to identify either hair shaft or hair follicle differentiation.

Pathogenesis. The pathogenesis of this disorder is unknown. Although these papules are usually pruritic and show clinical and microscopic evidence of rubbing, the microscopic picture differs significantly from that of prurigo nodularis.

It is possible that the perforating disorder of renal disease is an old folliculitis since this group of patients usually have lost much of the hair on their extremities. Hurwitz et al. described hair shafts in the infundibular wall or site of infundibular perforation of nondiabetic patients on dialysis, and they hypothesized that the disorder is a form of perforating folliculitis and that the hair shaft is often removed by rubbing and scratching.[9] This seems unlikely, however, since most other investigators have not been able to demonstrate follicular remnants.

Another possibility may be that the extruded collagen is altered and is therefore being rejected from the dermis. However, microscopically altered collagen cannot be demonstrated.

Treatment. Topical tretinoin cream or gel twice daily results in less pruritus and notable flattening of the lesions in 2 weeks. Ultraviolet light B has also been used successfully.[10]

Prognosis. Without treatment, the lesions tend to persist. Spontaneous resolution does occur, however, and results in atrophic scars.

Associated Diseases. All cases have been associated with renal disease, and almost all of these have had diabetic nephropathy. However, this perforating disorder has been seen in nondiabetic patients with obstructive uropathy and hypertensive nephrosclerosis, anuria, and chronic nephritis.[8] Although usually associated with dialysis, this disorder has also been observed in patients who have never received dialysis.

Differential Diagnosis. In a patient with severe renal disease the lesions are quite characteristic but could possibly be confused clinically with those of perforating folliculitis or Majocchi's granuloma. Microscopically, the same

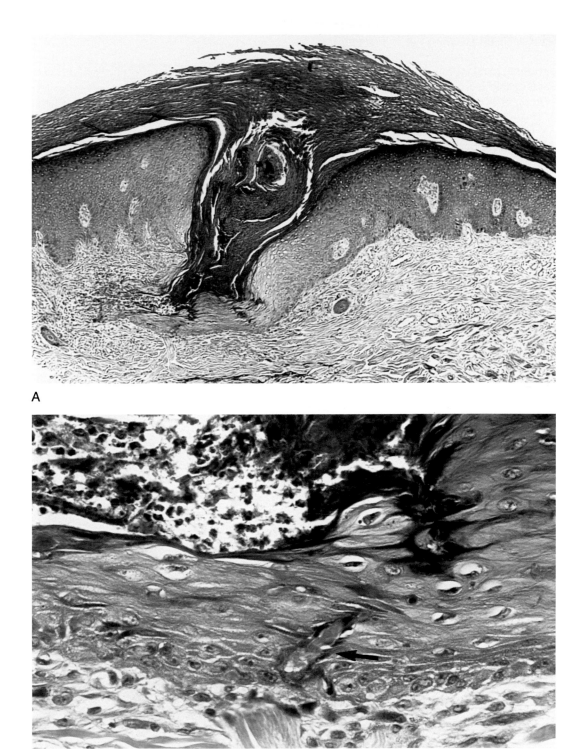

Fig. 19-2. Perforating disorder of renal disease. (**A**) There is a dome-shaped papule with a central crater filled with hyperkeratotic material. The adjacent epidermal hyperplasia and thickened cornified layer indicate that the site has been rubbed. (Low magnification.) (**B**) Note collagen bundle perforating epithelium. See arrow. (High magnification.)

confusion could occur; however, the lack of demonstrable hair shaft or fungi will help exclude these two disorders.

Elastosis Perforans Serpiginosa

History. Elastosis perforans serpiginosa was first clearly described by Lutz as "keratosis follicularis serpiginosa."[11] Baening and Ruiter reported an association with Down's syndrome.[12]

Clinical Features. Elastosis perforans serpiginosa is a not too rare disorder in which abnormal elastic fibers are extruded through the epidermis. It affects males four times more frequently than females, can be familial, and usually presents itself in the third decade, with 90 percent of patients being under age 30.[13]

The lesions of elastosis perforans serpiginosa are usually confined to one anatomic site, with areas of predilection in the following order: (1) nape and sides of the neck (Fig. 19-3); (2) upper extremities; (3) face; (4) lower extremities; and (5) trunk.[13] Disseminated elastosis perforans serpiginosa has been reported.

Characteristically, the lesions start as keratotic papules, which may be skin-colored or erythematous; they measure 2 to 5 mm in diameter and may be in either a circular or serpiginous distribution. Sometimes no arrangement is observed initially. Frequently, there is symmetry of these papules with contralateral involvement, as on both sides of the neck. Satellite lesions may occur. Usually, the lesions are asymptomatic, although mild pruritus may be present. The Koebner phenomenon has been observed. The lesions may last from 6 months to 5 years with appearance of new papules or spontaneous resolution. New lesions may also occur.

Microscopic Findings. Mehregan obtained step sections of the lesions and found areas of perforation in the form of narrow channels.[13] These occur in completely transepidermal, parafollicular, or transfollicular positions and may

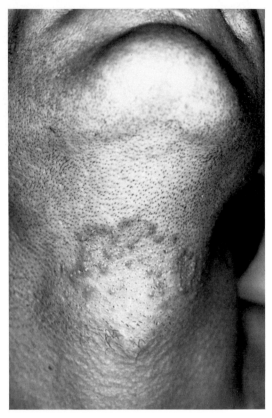

Fig. 19-3. Elastosis perforans serpiginosa. Note annular distribution of papules on the neck. (Photograph courtesy of Steven R. Cohen, M.D., New York, NY.)

have a straight vertical or corkscrew configuration. When transected, they can resemble asbestosis lesions.

Peripherally within the channels there is loose parakeratotic, keratinous material, and centrally there is a basophilic-staining, necrobiotic mass consisting of a mixture of degenerating epithelial cells, nuclei of inflammatory cells, and elastic fibers. Slight adjacent epithelial hyperplasia is present.

Elastic tissue stains show abundant clumped elastic tissue within the upper papillary dermis. These fibers appear thicker than normal and extend across the basement membrane. The fibers of the epidermis stain as elastic tissue but as they enter the perforating channel, they lose their characteristic staining quality. Focal granulomatous inflammation may be present. In some areas there may be strikingly widened dermal papillae containing collections of this abnormal elastic tissue. By electron microscopy the papillary dermis is filled with coarse thick elastic fibers. These large-caliber fibers have an amorphous quality with low electron density[14] and a branching configuration, with numerous fine surface filaments resembling normal embryonic elastic fibers.[15]

Pathogenesis. The exact cause of elastosis perforans serpiginosa is not known; however, there appears to be a primary defect of elastin with alteration of both the chemical composition and the morphologic configuration.

Patterson has reviewed the possible pathogenic mechanisms in detail.[16] He theorizes that elastosis perforans serpiginosa may be the final common pathway for more than one abnormality of elastic fibers, since both genetic and environmental factors have been implicated in some cases but neither have been implicated in all.

It is well documented that copper is essential in the formation of elastin. Penicillamine chelates copper, a necessary cofactor of lysyl oxidase, and the resulting copper deficiency causes a decrease in elastin covalently incorporated into fibers. Patients with Wilson's disease who have been treated with penicillamine occasionally develop a disorder resembling elastosis perforans serpiginosa, but ultrastructural studies show morphologic changes that differ from those of the idiopathic disease.[17] Not all patients with penicillamine-treated Wilson's disease develop this disorder; furthermore, those with Menkes' kinky hair syndrome, a disorder of copper deficiency, do not develop elastosis perforans serpiginosa. Therefore, copper is likely important, but only in combination with other not yet identified factors.

Treatment. No successful form of therapy has been found, although many types have been tried. These include mechanical means such as electrodesiccation with curettage, dermabrasion, and tape stripping. Physical modalities, which include x-radiation, cryotherapy, and ul-

traviolet light, have also been attempted, as well as numerous topical agents such as corticosteroids, vitamins A, B_2, and E, and acids.

Prognosis. Individual lesions last from about 6 months to 5 years and then involute spontaneously, leaving a superficial scar. New lesions often form as older ones resolve, and the condition may be quite persistent.

Associated Diseases. Elastosis perforans serpiginosa has been associated with numerous diseases, Mehregan having noted an association in 26 percent[13] of cases. The most common associations are Down's syndrome. Ehlers-Danlos syndrome, osteogenesis imperfecta, pseudoxanthoma elasticum, and Marfan's syndrome. Less common associated conditions are acrogeria, Rothmund-Thomson syndrome, systemic sclerosis, and morphea.

Differential Diagnosis. The clinical differential diagnosis includes other annular eruptions. Granuloma annulare, sarcoidosis, and tinea corporis are most readily confused with elastosis perforans serpiginosa. Other disorders that can be clinically confusing are porokeratosis of Mibelli, epidermal nevus, and granulomatous secondary syphilis.

Perforating Folliculitis

History. In 1968 Mehregan and Corskey described 25 patients with a discrete, keratotic, follicular eruption involving mainly the extremities. They termed this disorder *perforating folliculitis*.[18]

Clinical Features. Perforating folliculitis is a not uncommon disorder characterized by disruption of the follicular infundibulum with perforation. It appears as slightly elevated erythematous, follicular papules of 2 to 8 mm diameter. A central, keratin-filled crater is present.

The papules are usually on the extremities, especially the hair-bearing areas of the arms, forearms, thighs, and buttocks, and usually are asymptomatic or, less commonly, are associated with mild pruritus. The papules may be widely scattered.

Mehregan's original report included 17 women and 8 men, whose ages ranged from 10 to 64, the average being 29.[18]

Microscopic Findings. By light microscopy the follicular infundibulum is dilated and contains an admixture of keratinous debris and degenerated inflammatory cells. With step sectioning focal perforations of the infundibular lining can be found through which necrotic tissue and elastic fibers can gain access to the follicular cavity. Curled-up hair is often present within the keratinous plug but cannot always be demonstrated. Sometimes the hair is within the dermis, where it incites a foreign body reaction.

The dermis shows a mild, perifollicular, inflammatory infiltrate with degenerative changes of elastic fibers at the perforation site. The adjacent epidermis exhibits slight reactive hyperplasia.

Pathogenesis. The pathogenesis of perforating folliculitis is not known. Mehregan in 1977 noted a great reduction in its prevalence and speculated that the causative factor had been at least partially eliminated.[3] He suspected formaldehyde in clothing and demonstrated its presence in cloth material but could not elicit an allergic reaction in skin tests.

Burkhart believed that the most significant factor is perforation of the follicular epithelium and not the elimination of connective tissue.[19] Since perforating folliculitis is usually located on the extensor surfaces, it is quite possible that friction may be an important causative factor.

Treatment. Various forms of therapy, including topical corticosteroids, topical and systemic antibiotics, oral vitamin A, and keratolytics have been used, but they have generally been unsuccessful. Patterson et al. treated a patient's lesion with retinoic acid, 0.05 percent

cream, twice daily, and noted complete resolution with only atrophic scars 5 months later.[16]

Prognosis. This disorder may last from several months to several years and may show periods of remission and exacerbation.

Associated Diseases. Perforating folliculitis has been associated with psoriasis, juvenile acanthosis nigricans, and arteriosclerotic cardiovascular disease with hypertension. Reports have also linked this disorder with diabetes mellitus and renal failure, but in our opinion this represents a disorder best placed in a separate category.

Differential Diagnosis. Majocchi's granuloma and bacterial folliculitis are most readily confused with perforating folliculitis. Acne vulgaris and oil folliculitis must also be considered in the differential diagnosis. Other perforating diseases, such as reactive perforating collagenosis, in its classic form as well as in the variant that we have termed perforating disorder of renal disease, must be considered, as should lesions of elastosis perforans serpiginosa.

Kyrle's Disease (Hyperkeratosis Follicularis et Parafollicularis in Cutem Penetrans)

History. In 1916 Kyrle described a 22-year-old diabetic woman with numerous papules with central hyperkeratotic plugs, and termed this condition "hyperkeratosis follicularis et parafollicularis in cutem penetrans."[1] Kyrle's illustrations show hundreds of keratotic papules, some discrete and others with coalescence into plaques (Fig. 19-4). The number of papules is far greater than we have observed in the perforating disorder of renal disease. However, Kyrle's microscopic illustrations show changes quite similar to those that we have observed in patients with renal disease.

Whether or not hyperkeratosis follicularis et parafollicularis in cutem penetrans (Kyrle's disease) is a distinct entity has been a source of

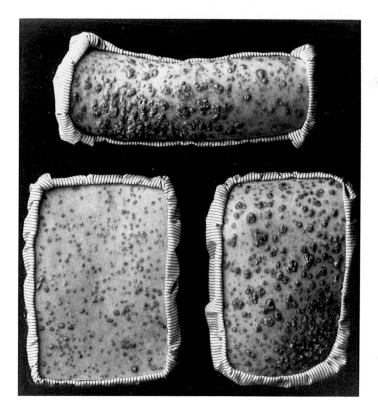

Fig. 19-4. Hyperkeratosis follicularis et parafollicularis in cutem penetrans (Kyrle's disease). Numerous, sometimes coalesced papules, as illustrated in Kyrle's original paper. (Kyrle J: Hyperkeratosis follicularis et parafollicularis in cutem penetrans. Arch Dermatol Syph 123:466, 1916. Copyright 1916, American Medical Association.)

debate. Mehregan in 1977 stated his belief that Kyrle's disease is not a distinctive clinicopathologic entity but represents a histologic pattern of tissue produced by a variety of conditions including perforating folliculitis, hypertrophic Darier's disease, keratosis pilaris and others.[3]

The presence of diabetes mellitus in Kyrle's original patient suggests Kyrle might have been describing the same clinicopathologic condition that has subsequently been observed in patients with renal disease. Abel and Dobson described the first case in the American literature. Their patient, a 36-year-old black male, also had diabetes mellitus, which they described as unregulated, and had numerous related complications.[20]

Clinical Features. The eruption occurs anywhere on the body except for the palms, soles, and mucosae. The primary lesion is a pinhead-shaped papule, which is skin-colored or grayish. Most are follicular, although this is not always the case.

The lesions subsequently develop into dome-shaped papules with central keratotic plugs. Usually they are discrete and scattered, especially over the proximal thighs and around the elbows, but sometimes they are extremely prevalent, with coalescence into plaques. This coalescence has been especially well illustrated by Kyrle[1] and by Aram et al.[21]

The average age of onset is 30 years, and there is no sexual predilection. The eruption may be asymptomatic or pruritic. Most patients have a disturbance of carbohydrate metabolism, and many are diabetic.

A major problem in reviewing reported cases of Kyrle's disease is determining which patients should have been classified as having this disease. In 1968 Carter and Constantine carefully reviewed the previously reported cases and accepted only 12 of the 45 or so designated as such in the literature.[22,23]

Recently, patients have been described as having Kyrle's disease in association with diabetes mellitus and/or renal failure. We believe this group should be placed in the separate category that we have designated as perforating disorder of renal disease.

Microscopic Findings. The lesions of Kyrle's disease, which may be either follicular or parafollicular, have an epithelial invagination filled with a keratotic plug that is partly parakeratotic (Fig. 19-5). In addition, there is basophilic cellular debris, which does not stain with elastic tissue stains. In at least one region of the plug there is abnormal parakeratotic keratinization of all the epithelial cells, including the basal cells. Here there are keratinized cells within the dermis, accompanied by a granulomatous reaction. Parakeratosis is present in the region where the epidermis becomes disrupted.[23]

Constantine and Carter also noted that the epidermis surrounding the keratotic plug was acanthotic. Frequently, there was thinning of the epidermis, with a parakeratotic horny layer. Neutrophils were sometimes observed, and a lymphocytic infiltrate was present.[23]

Pathogenesis. The pathogenesis of Kyrle's disease has been ascribed to an abnormal keratinization process, which forms a keratotic plug. The keratinization proceeds faster than the adjacent normal epithelial proliferation, with resulting abnormal keratinization of the epidermis and all layers of that focus. This causes disruption of the epidermis, release of horny material, and a resulting foreign body reaction.[23]

Because of the improved results with tretinoin, Petrozzi and Warthan hypothesized that the keratinization is excessive in comparison with epidermal proliferation, and that this may

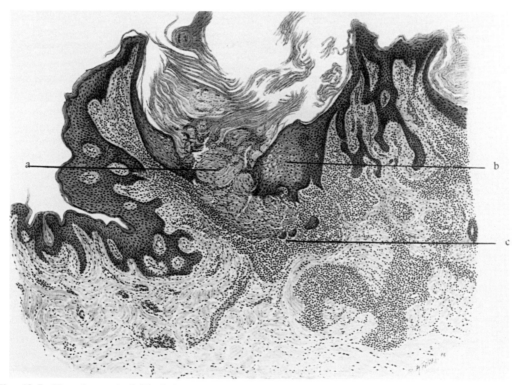

Fig. 19-5. Hyperkeratosis follicularis et parafollicularis in cutem penetrans (Kyrle's disease). Illustration from Kyrle's original paper, showing centrally umbilicated papule filled with keratinous material. (Kyrle J: Hyperkeratosis follicularis et parafollicularis in cutem penetrans. Arch Dermatol Syph 123:466, 1916. Copyright 1916, American Medical Association.)

be important in the pathogenesis of this disorder.[24]

Treatment. Carter and Constantine found aqueous vitamin A (100,000 units per day) effective in five of their six cases. Ultraviolet light, mercurial injections, oral methotrexate, topical fluorouracil, and topical corticosteroids have not been efficacious.[22] Flattening of these lesions has resulted from topical retinoic acid cream in a 0.1 percent concentration.[24]

Prognosis. The disease tends to be persistent. No patients have been recorded as "cured," but correction of the associated systemic disease has resulted in clearing of the cutaneous lesions of Kyrle's disease.[22]

Associated Diseases. The case that Kyrle reported had diabetes mellitus. Carter and Constantine hypothesized that Kyrle's disease might be an unusual manifestation of the diabetic syndrome.[22] Hepatic insufficiency and congestive heart failure have also been associated with Kyrle's disease.

Differential Diagnosis. Clinically and microscopically Kyrle's disease must be differentiated from prurigo nodularis, perforating folliculitis, elastosis perforans serpiginosa, and reactive perforating collagenosis.

DISORDERS ASSOCIATED WITH OCCASIONAL EPIDERMAL PERFORATION

Epithelial perforation with transepidermal elimination has been reported in several other unrelated diseases; however, transepidermal elimination appears as only a minor component of the pathologic process in these. The important disorders with this occasional finding are granuloma annulare and perforating pseudoxanthoma elasticum, although various other disorders also show it occasionally.

Perforating Granuloma Annulare

History. Civette in 1952[25] and Calvan in 1953[26] made the early observation of epidermal perforation in granuloma annulare. Civette described ulcerative forms of granuloma annulare, which he called tuberculoulcerous granuloma annulare. These observations were later confirmed by Owen and Freeman and others.[27–30]

Clinical Features. Most of the reported cases have occurred in children and have been associated with generalized granuloma annulare. The majority of the lesions are on extremities and show a predilection for sun-exposed areas. Seasonal variation, with exacerbation during summer and clearing in winter, has been noticed in some instances. The skin lesions begin as flesh-colored papules, which enlarge and then develop an umbilication and crust at the center. Often there may be a collarette of scale around the crust. Moderate pruritus has been reported in one child[30]; however, the Koebner phenomenon is not present.[29,30] Most of these lesions regress spontaneously over a period of several weeks, leaving scattered punctate, hyperpigmented scars.

Microscopic Findings. Histologic pictures vary with the clinical stage of development of these lesions.[27,30] In well-developed nonumbilicated papules the papillary dermis contains accumulations of necrobiotic tissue surrounded by palisading histiocytes and a lymphocytic inflammatory infiltrate. Multinucleated giant cells may also be seen. The inflammatory cells extend into epidermis in foci, through which transepidermal elimination occurs at a later time.

In well-developed umbilicated papules there are epidermal perforations, which communicate with areas of necrobiosis in the papillary dermis. The perforating channel contains a column of cellular debris, necrotic tissue, and mucinous material. Mild acanthosis and hyperkeratosis are present adjacent to the site of perforation. These necrobiotic areas perforating through the epidermis are located in the superficial dermis and are surrounded by palisading histioctyes.

Similar areas of necrobiosis characteristic of granuloma annulare are present in the deeper dermis. The necrobiotic plug contains no elastic or collagen fibers.[29,30]

Pathogenesis. The pathogenesis of granuloma annulare and its perforating variant is unknown.[29] Ultraviolet light, trauma, diabetes mellitus, thyroiditis, and insect bite have been incriminated as precipitating factors. However, attempts to reproduce these lesions with ultraviolet light and various forms of trauma have been unsuccessful. The relationship of granuloma annulare to diabetes mellitus has not been well established and remains controversial. Papular granuloma annulare secondary to insect bite has been reported; however, the role of insect bite in inducing these lesions is not firmly established.[30]

Treatment. Spontaneous remission occurs in most of these cases. Local application of a corticosteroid under occlusion can result in a good response.[27] Systemic vitamin A, 200,000 units per day, and topical application of liquid nitrogen have been unsuccessful.[29]

Prognosis. Skin lesions usually last for several months to years and then show spontaneous remission.

Associated Diseases. Diabetes has been reported rarely in association with generalized perforating granuloma annulare.[28]

Differential Diagnosis. The lesions of reactive perforating collagenosis are clinically similar. Differential features include the absence of Koebner phenomenon and seasonal variation in generalized perforating granuloma annulare. This form of granuloma annulare is microscopically characterized by palisading granuloma and a necrobiotic plug that contains no collagen fibers.

Perforating Pseudoxanthoma Elasticum

History. In 1976 Lund and Gilbert[31] reported a case of pseudoxanthoma elasticum with focal epidermal perforation by calcified elastic tissue. They also reviewed seven previously reported cases of coexistence of pseudoxanthoma elasticum and elastosis perforans serpiginosa; in only one case was there clear evidence of elastosis perforans serpiginosa, and they concluded that most of the others represented perforating pseudoxanthoma elasticum. This suggests the existence of pseudoxanthoma elasticum alone as a perforating disease.

Clinical Presentation. All reported cases have been in middle-aged multiparous women, who developed solitary hyperpigmented reticulated atrophic patches or plaques.[31-34] Characteristically, they occur in the periumbilical region. Some plaques have a verrucous surface with discrete keratotic papules scattered at their periphery. The plaques may be tender, are usually pruritic, and may discharge purulent material.

Obesity and hypertension are common associations.[32] Angioid streaks of the eye are rarely present. No other clinical manifestation of pseudoxanthoma elasticum has been noted. There is no family history of pseudoxanthoma elasticum in any of the reported cases.

Microscopic Findings. The epidermis shows slight acanthosis with a focal area of perforation and extrusion of altered elastic fibers through the channel.[31-35] The altered elastic fibers are confined to the mid-dermis and are granular, fragmented, curled and frayed, and basophilic and have all the characteristic changes seen in pseudoxanthoma elasticum. The spaces between collagen bundles are widened and contain abundant mucin. The adjacent dermis shows a foreign body reaction, and the papillary dermis is often widened and edematous. Special stains demonstrate calcium content within the fibers.

Pathogenesis. The etiology of this localized disorder is unknown. It appears to be a nonheritable form of pseudoxanthoma elasticum and has only a localized cutaneous manifestation,[34] without associated vascular stigmata as seen in the inherited form. It is possible that multiparity and obesity may damage the elastic fibers in genetically predisposed individuals and produce abnormal fibers, which in turn may induce a foreign-body reaction, with subsequent extrusion through the epidermis. Cutaneous as well as histopathologic changes similar to those of pseudoxanthoma elasticum are seen in individuals exposed to saltpeter (potassium nitrate).[36] This further suggests the acquired nature of the disease.

Treatment. No specific treatment is available. Stripping the surface keratinous material by repeated application of cellophane tape has resulted in clearing of lesions at the margin. Vitamin E at a dose of 400 units twice daily has also been tried.[31]

Prognosis. Skin lesions remain solitary and persist for years without apparent resolution.

Differential Diagnosis. Elastosis perforans serpiginosa is clinically similar.

Miscellaneous Disorders

Goette in 1980 reviewed 17 cases of chondrodermatitis nodularis helicis and in 13 of them found elimination of necrobiotic material from the dermis through transepidermal channels, slits, or erosions overlying the necrobiotic granuloma.[37] Pathogenetically, these granulomas were thought to be actinically induced.

Transepidermal elimination has also been found in necrobiosis lipoidica, and Parra observed elimination of necrotic material and collagen through the follicular opening in three diabetic women.[38] Clinically, these processes presented as comedo-like plugs localized mainly in the periphery of skin lesions of necrobiosis lipoidica.

Similar association of epidermal perforation with necrobiosis has been observed in rheumatoid arthritis as superficial ulcerating necrobiosis, lichen planus,[27] and perforating rheumatoid nodules[39,40] and in lichen nitidus.[41] Elimination of calcium-impregnated connective tissue through epidermal channels has been noted in calcinosis cutis following application of electrode paste containing calcium chloride to the skin. Epidermal necrosis seen in foreign body reactions to silica, beryllium or contents of epidermoid cysts has been thought to represent transepidermal elimination.

Several other disease processes have been theoretically considered among the causes of transepidermal elimination.[42–45] Among these are amyloidosis; subepidermal hemorrhage of black heel; thrombosis of capillary hemangioma; infectious processes such as leprosy, tuberculosis, chromoblastomycosis, histoplasmosis, North American blastomycosis, leishmaniasis, cryptococcosis, and epidermotropism of mycosis fungoides and malignant melanoma.

APPROACH TO THE PATIENT

From a morphologic point of view the perforating disorders can be fairly similar. The primary lesion in many of them is an umbilicated papule, often containing a central keratotic plug. Differentiation between these disorders on morphologic grounds alone can therefore be difficult.

A number of historical elements can occasionally help differentiate between the different syndromes. For example, any of the conditions associated with elastosis perforans serpiginosa should suggest that diagnosis, particularly if the lesions occur in a serpiginous distribution. Onset in childhood is characteristic of reactive perforating collagenosis, and a family history is occasionally helpful in that disorder as well. A history of diabetes or chronic renal failure should alert the clinician to the possibility that

Table 19-1. Approach to the Patient: Clinical Features and Histologic Diagnosis of the Perforating Dermatoses

	History	Physical Examination	Histology
Reactive perforating collagenosis	Onset in childhood, occasionally dominantly inherited	Koebner phenomenon	Cup-shaped invagination of epidermis filled with parakeratotic keratin and perforated by vertical collagen bundles (Fontana-Masson stain)
Perforating disorder of renal disease	Diabetes, renal failure, severe pruritus	Retinopathy, Koebner phenomenon, lesions on extensor surfaces of extremities	Cup-shaped invagination filled with parakeratotic keratin and perforated by vertical collagen bundles (Fontana-Masson stain); histologically identical to reactive perforating collagenosis
Elastosis perforans serpiginosa	Penicillamine; Ehlers-Danlos, Marfan's, and Down's syndromes; osteogenesis imperfecta; pseudoxanthoma elasticum	Serpiginous distribution	Increase in elastic tissue, which perforates the epidermis (Verhoeff-van Gieson stain)
Perforating folliculitis	Minimal pruritus	Extremities, buttocks	Perforation of follicular infundibulum
Kyrle's disease	? Diabetes ? Renal failure	Numerous keratotic papules	Epithelial invagination filled with keratotic plug, parakeratosis over the point of disrupted epidermis

he is dealing with a perforating disorder of renal disease.

Definitive diagnosis relies on pathologic examination of skin biopsy specimens with special stains. Details of the histologic changes are discussed above and enumerated in Table 19-1. Verhoeff-van Gieson stains are useful in examination of elastic tissue, and Fontana-Masson stains are helpful in recognizing collagen. Since a number of diseases have been associated with the perforating dermatoses and different therapeutic modalities have been effective for some of the conditions but not others, definitive diagnosis should help the clinician decide if any further work-up or treatment is needed.

REFERENCES

1. Kyrle J: Hyperkeratosis follicularis et parafollicularis in cutem penetrans. Arch Dermatol Syph 123:466, 1916
2. Mehregan AH, Schwartz OD, Livingood CS: Reactive perforating collagenosis. Arch Dermatol 96:277, 1967
3. Mehregan AH: Perforating dermatoses: a clinicopathologic review. Int J Dermatol 16:19, 1977
4. Bovenmyer DA: Reactive perforating collagenosis. Arch Dermatol 102:313, 1970
5. Nair BKH, Sarojini PA, Basheer AM, Nair CHK: Reactive perforating collagenosis. Br J Dermatol 91:399, 1974
6. Fretzin DF, Beal DW, Jao W: Light and ultrastructural study of reactive perforating collagenosis. Arch Dermatol 116:1054, 1980
7. Poliak SC, Lebwohl MG, Parris A, Prioleau PG: Reactive perforating collagenosis associated with diabetes mellitus. N Engl J Med 306:81, 1982
8. Hood AF, Hardegen GL, Zarate AR, et al: Kyrle's disease in patients with chronic renal failure. Arch Dermatol 118:85, 1982
9. Hurwitz RM, Weiss J, Melton ME, et al: Perforating folliculitis in association with hemodialysis. Am J Dermatopathol 4:101, 1982
10. Cochran RJ, Tucker SB, Wilkin JK: Reactive perforating collagenosis of diabetes mellitus and renal failure. Cutis 31:55, 1983

11. Lutz W: Keratosis follicularis serpiginosa. Dermatologica 106:318, 1953
12. Beening GW, Ruiter M: Keratosis follicularis serpiginosa (Lutz). Dermatologica 110:175, 1955
13. Mehregan AH: Elastosis perforans serpiginosa. Arch Dermatol 97:381, 1968
14. Cohen AS, Hashimoto K: Electron microscopic observations on the lesion of elastosis perforans serpiginosa. J Invest Dermatol 35:15, 1960
15. Meves C, Vogel A: Elektronenmikroskopische Untersuchungen in einem Fall von Elastosis Perforans Serpiginosa. Dermatologica 145:210, 1973
16. Patterson JW: The perforating disorders. J Am Acad Dermatol 10:561, 1984
17. Kirsch N, Hukill PB: Elastosis perforans serpiginosa induced by penicillamine. Arch Dermatol 113:630, 1977
18. Mehregan AH, Coskey RJ: Perforating folliculitis. Arch Dermatol 97:394, 1968
19. Burkhart CG: Perforating folliculitis. Int J Dermatol 20:597, 1981
20. Abele DC, Dobson RL: Hyperkeratosis penetrans (Kyrle's disease). Arch Dermatol 83:277, 1961
21. Aram H, Szymanski FJ, Bailey W: Kyrle's disease. Arch Dermatol 100:453, 1969
22. Carter VH, Constantine VS: Kyrle's disease. Arch Dermatol 97:624, 1968
23. Carter VH, Constantine VS: Kyrle's disease. Arch Dermatol 97:633, 1968
24. Petrozzi JW, Warthan TL: Kyrle's disease. Arch Dermatol 110:762, 1974
25. Civette PA: Les formes tuberculo-ulcereuses et tuberculogommeuses du granuloma annulaire. Ann Dermatol Syph 79:387, 1952
26. Calnan CD: Granuloma annulare. Br J Dermatol 66:254, 1954
27. Owens DW, Freeman EG: Perforating granuloma annulare. Arch Dermatol 103:64, 1971
28. Delaney TJ, Gold SC, Leppard G: Disseminated perforating granuloma annulare. Br J Dermatol 89:523, 1973
29. Izumi AK: Generalized perforating granuloma annulare. Arch Dermatol 108:708, 1973
30. Duncan WC, Smith JD, Knox JM: Generalized perforating granuloma annulare. Arch Dermatol 108:570, 1973
31. Lund HZ, Gilbert CF: Perforating pseudoxanthoma elasticum. Arch Pathol Lab Med 100:544, 1976
32. Hicks J, Carpenter CL, Reed RJ: Periumbilical perforating pseudoxanthoma elasticum. Arch Dermatol 115:300, 1979
33. Schwartz RA, Richfield DF: Pseudoxanthoma elasticum with transepidermal elimination. Arch Dermatol 114:279, 1978
34. Neldner KH, Martinez-Hernandez A: Localized acquired pseudoxanthoma elasticum. J Am Acad Dermatol 1:523, 1979
35. Reed RJ, Clark WH, Mihm MD: The cutaneous elastoses. Hum Pathol 4:187, 1973
36. Neilson AO, Christensen OB, Hentzer B, et al: Saltpeter-induced dermal changes electron-microscopically indistinguishable from pseudoxanthoma elasticum. Acta Derm Venereol (Stockh) 58:323, 1978
37. Goette DK: Chondrodermatitis nodularis chronica helicis: a perforating necrobiotic granuloma. J Am Acad Dermatol 2:148, 1980
38. Parra LA: Transepithelial elimination in necrobiosis lipoidica. Br J Dermatol 96:83, 1977
39. Jorizzo JL, Olansky AJ, Stanley RJ: Superficial ulcerating necrobiosis in rheumatoid arthritis. Arch Dermatol 118:255, 1982
40. Patterson JW, Demos PT: Superficial ulcerating rheumatoid necrobiosis: a perforating rheumatoid nodule. Cutis 36:323, 1985
41. Bardach H: Perforating lichen niditus. J Cutan Pathol 8:111, 1981
42. Mehregan AH: Transepithelial elimination. Curr Probl Dermatol 3:124, 1970
43. Malak JA, Kurban AK: "Catharsis" an excretory function of epidermis. Br J Dermatol 84:516, 1971
44. Batres E, Wolfe JE, Rudolph AH, Knox JM: Transepithelial eliminations of cutaneous chromomycosis. Arch Dermatol 114:1231, 1978
45. Mayoral F, Pennys NS: Disseminated histoplasmosis disorder in an AIDS victim. J Am Acad Dermatol 13:842, 1985

20

Hirsutism

Andrea Dunaif

Hirsutism is the result of androgen action on the hair follicle, which for these hormones is the target tissue in the skin. Both to understand and to treat this most disturbing cosmetic condition it is necessary first to understand the biology of androgen production and action. Androgens are steroid hormones secreted by the gonads and the adrenal glands. They are defined by their ability in bioassay systems to induce the development of the prostate and seminal vesicles and by their capacity to bind tightly to the androgen receptor in the prostatic cytosol. Androgens belong to a larger class of hormones, which includes insulin and growth hormone; all are known as anabolic hormones since all cause nitrogen retention.

The most widely encountered dermatologic manifestation of hyperandrogenism is hirsutism. However, excessive androgen production may also be an important pathogenic factor in a significant proportion of cases of female alopecia and cases of severe acne in both sexes. The specific biochemical abnormalities that lead to the increased production and dermatologic action of androgens are fairly well understood although in the majority of cases the underlying causes of these disturbances are not. Therapies directed at these abnormalities can produce marked improvement in the clinical symptoms of hyperandrogenism. This chapter will review normal and abnormal androgen physiology, the differential diagnosis of hyperandrogenic disorders, and the therapeutic modalities available to the clinician for their control.

THE DERMATOLOGIC SEQUELAE OF ANDROGEN ACTION

Hirsutism

Androgen-sensitive hair follicles are the target tissues whose response produces hirsutism. Not all hair follicles are androgen-dependent. Those in the eyebrows, eyelashes, corona of the scalp, forearm, and lower leg are androgen-independent; it is those on the upper lip, beard, nasal tips, ears, pubis, upper legs, thorax, axillae, and temporal scalp that are androgen-dependent. Further, hair follicle number is genetically and not hormonally determined. Hence certain ethnic and racial groups have greater numbers of hair follicles than others: southern Europeans more than northern Europeans, whites more than Orientals. Indeed, 25 to 30 percent of women of British and non-Scandinavian European origin normally have some terminal hair growth on the upper lip, periareolar area, and linea alba. Hyperandrogenism, however, must be excluded in all women showing terminal hair growth on the sternum, abdomen above the umbilicus, upper back, and shoulders.

The hair follicle produces several types of

hair growth. Lanugo hair is the short, fine, unpigmented hair that is present at birth. In adults the hair follicle may produce either vellus hair, which is short, soft, fine, nonmedullated, and unpigmented, or terminal hair, which is the coarse, pigmented, medullated hair characteristic of the beard area. Androgens act on the androgen-dependent hair follicles to increase the hair diameter, pigmentation, and rate of growth. Hirsutism is defined as vellus-to-terminal hair transformation of androgen-dependent hair follicles. This must be distinguished from hypertrichosis, which is the generalized increase in vellus but not terminal hair growth that may be associated with certain drugs (e.g., dilantin), metabolic disorders (e.g., anorexia nervosa), or malignancies.[1,2]

Alopecia and Acne

Androgens can also act on androgen-dependent hair follicles in the scalp to decrease the rate of hair growth and the hair diameter. This androgen-dependent process leads to hair thinning and eventually to alopecia. Hair thinning can be generalized (Fig. 20-1) and/or localized to the temporal region. The factors that determine this unique response of scalp hair follicles to androgens are incompletely understood. Finally, androgens act on the sebaceous glands of the androgen-dependent hair follicles to increase their secretory rates. The increased production of sebum can lead to acne in susceptible individuals.[3-5]

True Virilization

The signs of true virilization are temporal balding, deepening of the voice, increased muscularity, and clitoromegaly. These changes reflect much more severe androgen excess and suggest that an androgen-secreting neoplasm may be present. However, generalized hair thinning can be seen with mild androgen excess (Fig. 20-1). It is critical to differentiate hirsutism and acne from the changes of true viriliza-

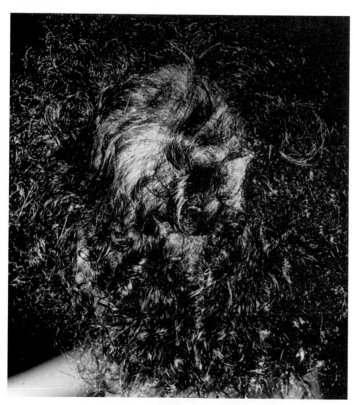

Fig. 20-1. Diffuse alopecia in a hyperandrogenic woman with slight androgen elevations. The patient had no signs of true virilization.

tion because of the different diagnostic implications of these findings.[1]

NORMAL AND ABNORMAL ANDROGEN METABOLISM

There are three determinants of androgen action: (1) androgen production; (2) androgen biologic availability to the target tissue; and (3) androgen clearance and utilization by the target tissue (Fig. 20-2). Although several steroids present in the plasma have androgenic activity in vitro, for practical purposes testosterone (T) is the biologically important extracellular androgen, and its more potent 5-α-reduced metabolite, dihydrotestosterone (DHT), is the biologically important intracellular androgen. Both T and DHT are 17-β-hydroxysteroids, and while the other 17-β-hydroxysteroids, androstenediol and the androstanediols (3-α and 3-β), are also relatively potent androgens, isolated increases in these steroids only rarely result in hirsutism. The other major androgens present in the circulation are the 17-ketosteroids androstenedione (A), dehydroepiandrosterone (DHEA), and dehydroepiandrosterone sulfate (DHEAS); these steroids are androgenic via their eventual conversion to T and DHT. Hence these hormones are considered to be prehormones.

Androgen Production

The ovaries and adrenals each secrete 25 percent of the circulating T. The remaining 50 percent is derived from the extraglandular metabolic conversion of other androgens, mainly A. Androstenedione arises equally from direct ovarian and adrenal glandular secretion. Of the other major T prehormones 80 percent of the DHEA is secreted by the adrenal and 20 percent by the ovary, whereas almost 100 percent of the DHEAS is secreted by the adrenal. In normal women all the circulating DHT is formed from the extraglandular conversion of prehormones, 85 percent from A and 15 percent from T.

Under normal circumstances the major metabolic fate of ovarian androgens is to serve as prehormones for ovarian estrogen synthesis, whereas the metabolic fate of the majority of adrenal androgens is as precursors for adrenal cortisol and aldosterone biosynthesis. Ovarian androgen production is under the control of the pituitary gonadotropin luteinizing hormone (LH). Adrenal androgen production is under the control of adrenocorticotropic hormone (ACTH). Hence the feedback control of both ovarian and adrenal androgen secretion is not direct but occurs via the products of their further metabolism, i.e., estradiol and cortisol, respectively.

In pathologic conditions androgen production can be increased by the increased glandular secretion of the potent androgen T or, rarely, DHT. There can also be increased secretion of the androgen prehormones A, DHEA, and DHEAS. The increased glandular production of androgens can be the result of increased trophic hormone stimulation (i.e., by LH or ACTH), and/or of primary abnormalities within the glands (e.g., enzyme deficiencies or tumors). Moreover, in many hyperandrogenic states both the ovaries and the adrenals contribute to excessive hormone production, even in the presence of androgen-secreting tumors, because of the gonadotropin and steroid biosynthetic enzyme changes that may occur secondary to the abnormal hormonal environment.[1,2]

Androgen Biologic Availability

Most of the T and DHT in the circulation is bound to a specific transport protein, sex hormone–binding globulin (SHBG); most of the remainder of these circulating steroids is loosely associated with albumin; and a very small percentage of each steroid is free. Both T and DHT enter their target tissues by diffusion, and both the steroid that is free and the steroid that is loosely associated with albumin can diffuse into the target tissue and are thus biologically available. Conversely, T and DHT that are bound to SHBG are not available for further metabolism, target tissue action, or eventual excretion via the liver. The SHBG also binds and trans-

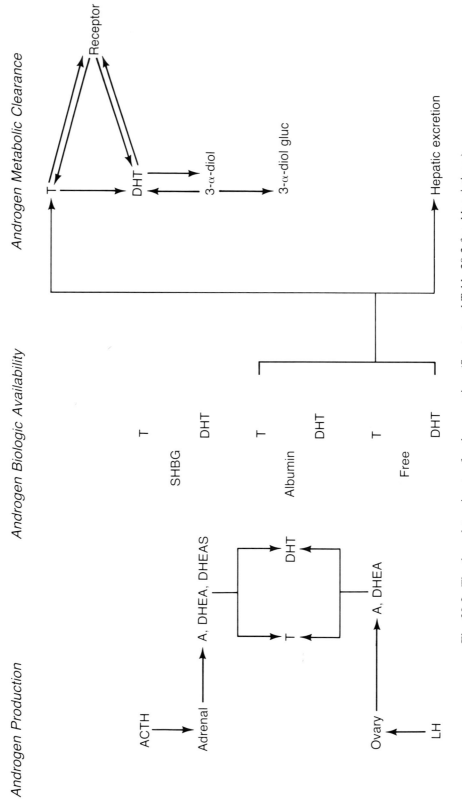

Fig. 20-2. The three determinants of androgen action. (See text and Table 20-2 for abbreviations.)

ports estradiol (E_2) and a number of synthetic androgens and progestins (e.g., levonorgestrel); it binds the steroids that it transports with varying degrees of affinity, DHT having a greater affinity for SHBG than T, which has a greater affinity than E_2. Levonorgestrel, a synthetic progestin, has a yet higher affinity for SHBG and can displace endogenous steroids such as DHT, T, and E_2 from their binding sites, thereby increasing their biologic availability. Synthesis of SHBG occurs in the liver, and androgens decrease SHBG levels whereas estrogens and thyroid hormones increase them.

It follows from the information above that the level of SHBG is a critical modulator of androgen action, decreases in the level increasing the biologic availability of androgens and increases having the opposite effect. Further, the administration of compounds that have a higher affinity for SHBG than endogenous androgens will also increase the biologic availability of those androgens by competitive displacement. The non-SHBG-bound androgens are available not only to enter the target tissue but also to be metabolized by the liver. This results in the increased rate of exit of androgens (metabolic clearance rate) from the plasma compartment that is characteristic of conditions in which SHBG levels are decreased.[6]

Target Tissue Androgen Action

In most androgen target tissues, such as the hair follicle, biologically available T enters by diffusion from the circulation or androgen prehormones are converted intracellularly to T. The intracellular T is metabolized further by the 5-α-reductase enzyme system[7] to the more potent androgen DHT, which then binds to the androgen receptor and initiates the specific molecular events that result in target tissue androgen action. Testosterone may also bind to the androgen receptor and act directly without further conversion to DHT in target tissues such as skeletal muscle. In the hair follicle, however, the conversion of T to DHT by the 5-α-reductase enzyme system appears to be critical for

androgen action.[7,8] Intracellular DHT is further metabolized by *reversible* reduction to 5-α-androstane-3-α, 17-β-diol (3-α-androstanediol). The 3-α-androstanediol is *irreversibly* converted at a variety of sites in the body to 5-α-androstane-3-α,17-β-diol glucuronide (3-α-diol gluc). Both blood and urinary levels of 3-α-diol gluc correlate closely with the actual in vitro measurement of the 5-α-reductase activity androgen target tissue.[7,8]

Target tissue androgen action requires the presence of intracellular androgen receptors, and the absence of such receptors (as in testicular feminization) or the pharmacologic inhibition of androgen binding to them can abolish androgen action. Nevertheless, to date no abnormalities in the androgen receptor have been recognized as etiologies of hyperandrogenism. Indeed normal women, hirsute women, and normal men have similar numbers of target tissue androgen receptors. Enhanced target tissue androgen action must be explained therefore by the increased availability and the increased intracellular utilization of androgens. Hirsute women have been shown to have markedly increased 5-α-reductase activity, greater than that found in normal men, regardless of plasma androgen levels.[7] Further, peripheral levels of 3-α-diol gluc reflect this abnormality and are hence a biochemical marker for target tissue androgen utilization.[8] Alternatively, the finding of increased DHEAS levels in men with severe acne[5] who have otherwise normal androgen levels suggests that DHEAS may have an independent, secretion-stimulating action on the sebaceous gland. This possibility merits further investigation.

Not all hyperandrogenic women have the dermatologic sequelae of hyperandrogenism. This so-called cryptic hyperandrogenism is commonly encountered in adolescents, who may not have been hyperandrogenic long enough to develop the stigmata of the condition. However, this situation is also encountered in adult women who have either very few androgen-sensitive target tissues (as in Orientals with the minimal hair follicle number) or very low levels of the 5-α-reductase enzyme system in their androgen-dependent target tissues. In summary, although the majority of women with the dermatologic sequelae of hyperandrogenism have increased production, biologic availability, and target tissue utilization of androgens, the sine qua non of the dermatologic action of androgens is the presence of the target tissue containing adequate levels of the 5-α-reductase enzyme system.

DIFFERENTIAL DIAGNOSIS OF HYPERANDROGENIC DISORDERS

The majority of cases of hyperandrogenism are caused by one of two relatively benign conditions of unknown etiology that are classified symptomatically[1,2]; these are *idiopathic hirsutism* and the *polycystic ovary syndrome* (PCO). If there is no disturbance of reproductive function associated with the hyperandrogenism, the disorder is classified as idiopathic hirsutism. The term *idiopathic* is, however, a misnomer, since increased target tissue androgen utilization, usually accompanied by increased androgen production and biologic availability, is present in affected individuals. It is the cause of these abnormalities that is not known.

Hyperandrogenism associated with disturbances of ovulatory function is classified as PCO. The ovarian pathology from which the syndrome gains its name consists of varying degrees of ovarian enlargement, thickening of the ovarian cortex, multiple follicular cysts lined by hyperplastic theca cells (the ovarian androgen-secreting cells), and increased follicular atresia. The ovarian morphology, however, is a nonspecific finding, which is the result, and not the cause, of the abnormal hormonal milieu. The so-called ovarian hyperthecosis syndrome represents a subgroup within PCO characterized by clinically more profound hyperandrogenism, often with true virilization, i.e., deepening of the voice, temporal balding, increased muscle bulk, and clitoromegaly. In addition to changes characteristic of PCO, the

ovaries contain islands of luteinized theca cells within the ovarian stroma.

Since the specific causes of these conditions are unknown, their diagnosis remains one of exclusion. A number of potentially life-threatening diseases can present with the dermatologic manifestations of hyperandrogenism. The following conditions must be excluded in *all* women presenting with hyperandrogenism (Table 20-1); androgen-secreting tumors of the ovaries and adrenals; Cushing's syndrome; adult-onset (attenuated or nonclassical) 21-hydroxylase deficiency; and hyperprolactinemia. Very rarely, hypothyroidism can present with the clinical stigmata of hyperandrogenism. Obesity can also increase the production of androgens and decrease SHBG levels for reasons that are not understood, and these changes can produce hirsutism if target tissue utilization of androgens is also increased.

APPROACH TO THE PATIENT: DIAGNOSTIC EVALUATION OF HYPERANDROGENISM

The first question in the approach to the patient is, Who should be evaluated for hyperandrogenism? Any woman who presents with terminal hair growth in androgen-dependent areas on the face or upper trunk should be evaluated. The ethnic background of the individual should be considered since terminal hair growth is found normally in certain areas in various racial and ethnic groups (see above). Terminal hair growth is considered to be pathologic in all women when it occurs on the upper abdomen,

Table 20-1. Differential Diagnosis of Hyperandrogenism

Ovarian and adrenal androgen-secreting tumors
Cushing's syndrome
Adult onset 21-hydroxylase deficiency
Hyperprolactinemia
Hypothyroidism
Idiopathic hirsutism
Polycystic ovary syndrome
Obesity

sternum, back and shoulders. Any perceived increase in terminal hair density in androgen-dependent areas merits further investigation. Women with thinning of scalp hair (Fig. 20-1), even if the pattern does not conform to the classical temporal balding of androgenic alopecia, should have hyperandrogenism excluded.[3] Finally, anyone—female or male—with acne that is resistant to therapy should be evaluated for hyperandrogenism.[5]

Clinical Evaluation

The clinical evaluation must include a detailed history. Particularly important points are the rapidity of onset of the symptoms and the presence of symptoms of true virilization. A rapid onset of hirsutism with virilization is suggestive of an androgen-secreting tumor. Drugs such as anabolic steroids, danazol, and levonorgestrel-containing oral contraceptives may cause androgen-dependent hair growth, whereas agents such as minoxidil, Dilantin, glucocorticoids, and diazoxide may cause hypertrichosis. Metabolic disorders such as anorexia nervosa, juvenile hypothyroidism, and porphyria can also be associated with hypertrichosis. A detailed menstrual and reproductive history is important, since disturbances in menstrual function and fertility suggest the presence of more severe hyperandrogenism.

On physical examination it is important to record carefully the severity of the dermatologic changes of hyperandrogenism in order to monitor the effectiveness of any therapeutic interventions. In addition, stigmata of endocrinopathies such as Cushing's syndrome should be sought. The patient must be examined for signs of true virilization, such as increased muscle bulk and clitoromegaly, since the presence of these is indicative of severe hyperandrogenism, and androgen-secreting neoplasms must be considered in such instances. Galactorrhea as well as abdominal and ovarian masses should be excluded. Acanthosis nigricans may be present, but this dermatologic change is frequently en-countered in obese hyperandrogenic women with PCO and is not a marker for underlying malignancies in such cases.

Laboratory Evaluation

Fortunately, despite the numerous conditions that may cause hyperandrogenism, the laboratory evaluation of this disorder is straightforward. More than 90 percent of women with clinically significant hirsutism will have an elevation of T, biologically available (non-SHBG-bound or free) T, and/or DHEAS in a single random blood sample.[9] Further, over 90 percent of women with acne resistant to therapy will have a T level above the normal mean.[4,10] The percentage of patients with alopecia who will have an abnormality in peripheral androgen levels has not been assessed. In men with severe acne, some workers have found that as many as 80 percent will have an increase in their DHEAS level and decreases in their SHBG levels.[5] It is evident from this information that peripheral levels of T, biologically available T, and DHEAS will be of high diagnostic yield in detecting hyperandrogenism. Androgen levels can fluctuate, and at times pooling of samples or multiple sampling may be necessary to document hyperandrogenism. It is not necessary to obtain A or DHT levels in screening hyperandrogenic women, but such levels can be obtained if repeated assay of other androgen levels has been normal. In addition, since A is a major prehormone of T and DHT, monitoring of its response to therapy may be useful.

Studies in hirsute women indicate that 100 percent of such women will have an elevation in their plasma level of 3-α-diol gluc, the marker of 5-α-reductase activity.[8] Since androgen-dependent alopecia and acne also reflect increased pilosebaceous unit 5-α-reductase activity, 3-α-diol gluc levels would be expected to be consistently elevated in affected patients. Further studies will be required to confirm the specificity of 3-α-diol gluc level as a marker for androgen dependence in these latter disorders. However, 3-α-diol-gluc levels cannot replace T and DHEAS levels in the evaluation of hyperandrogenism since the latter steroid levels are also important markers for androgen-secreting tumors. If T levels are consistently greater than 150 to 200 ng/dl (depending on the sensitivity of the assay employed) and DHEAS levels are greater than 700 μg/dl, androgen-secreting tumors of the ovary or the adrenal *must* be excluded regardless of the clinical presentation. The assay of 3-α-diol gluc levels is difficult, costly, and not widely available at present, so their use is not recommended in the routine screening of hyperandrogenic patients. Such levels can be obtained when repeated measurement of other androgen levels has failed to document hyperandrogenism.

In addition to documenting hyperandrogenism, the laboratory evaluation must exclude other conditions in the differential diagnosis. As discussed above T and DHEAS levels are the required screening tests for androgen-secreting tumors. A prolactin level will exclude hyperprolactinemia, and thyroxine (T_4) and thyroid-binding globulin (TBG) levels will determine thyroid function. Cushing's syndrome must be specifically excluded by an overnight 1 mg dexamethasone suppression test.

Anywhere from a 1 to a 5 percent incidence of adult-onset (also known as attenuated or nonclassical) 21-hydroxylase deficiency has been reported in women presenting with hyperandrogenism.[11] Adult-onset forms of the other adrenal enzyme deficiencies are less well documented. 21-hydroxylase deficiency is inherited as an autosomal recessive trait associated with specific HLA complexes (e.g., HLA-B14, HLA-Bw47), and the gene for the adult-onset form may be allelic to the gene for the more severe childhood-onset form of the disease.[11] The only well-documented way to exclude this diagnosis is by a 1-hour ACTH stimulation test with measurements of basal and stimulated 17-hydroxyprogesterone (17-OHP) levels (the steroid before the enzymatic block).[11] Some workers have advocated the use of a single morning 17-OHP level, but the sensitivity and specificity of such testing remains unvalidated. The homozygous disease state as well as the heterozygous carrier state can be detected by the simulated 17-OHP response. At times basal and stimulated A levels are necessary for more precise genetic classification, but only 17-OHP levels are required to confirm the diagnosis.[11] Patients with PCO may have 17-OHP levels that stimulate into the heterozygous range, but PCO patients can be distinguished from heterozygous carriers on clinical grounds since the latter group have no signs or symptoms of hyperandrogenism. It is important to diagnose 21-hydroxylase deficiency, not

Table 20-2. Approach to the Patient: Initial Evaluation of Hirsutism

Day 1—Androgens
Random blood sample for total T, biologically available T, and DHEAS levels
Other: LH, FSH, prolactin, thyroid function tests
Dexamethasone: 1 mg PO at bedtime (about 11 P.M.)
Day 2—8 A.M.–10 A.M.
Cortisol and 17-OHP (basal value for ACTH test) levels
ACTH test (0.25 mg corsyntropin [alpha 1–24 ACTH]—time 60 minute: 17-OHP level
If menstruating, cycle day 20–25: progesterone level

Interpretation
T > 150–200 ng/dl or DHEAS > 700 μg/dl: exclude ovarian or adrenal androgen-secreting tumor
Morning cortisol > 5 μg/dl: exclude Cushing's syndrome
Elevated prolactin level: exclude prolactinoma
Marked rise 17-OHP with ACTH, i.e., >2,000 ng/dl: compatible with 21-hydroxylase deficiency: treatment: glucocorticoid replacement; screen siblings with 1 hr ACTH test
Normal T, biologically available T and DHEAS levels: repeat, consider pooling several hourly samples and/or obtaining other androgen levels (i.e., A and DHT); if still normal obtain 3-α-diol-gluc level
Normal 3-α-diol-gluc level: hair growth not androgen dependent
Increased T, biologically available T, and/or DHEAS, increased LH:FSH ratio, day 20–25 progesterone in follicular range: consistent with diagnosis of polycystic ovary syndrome
Increased T, biologically available T and/or DHEAS, day 20–25 progesterone in the luteal range: consistent with diagnosis of idiopathic hirsutism

Abbreviations: T, testosterone; DHEAS, dehydroepiandrosterone sulfate; LH, luteinizing hormone; FSH, follicle-stimulating hormone; 17-OHP, 17-hydroxyprogesterone; ACTH, adrenocorticotropic hormone; A, androstenedione; DHT, dihydrotestosterone.

only because this condition can be controlled with glucocorticoid replacement therapy but also because family screening and genetic counseling are indicated for affected women.

All the required studies can be combined into a simple 2-day evaluation (Table 20-2). It is not necessary to perform the testing on 2 consecutive days as long as the dexamethasone is given on the evening before the morning on which the cortisol level is obtained. On day 1 a random blood sample is obtained for T, DHEAS, non-SHBG-bound or free T, prolactin, T_4, TBG, LH, and follicle-stimulating hormone (FSH). The patient then takes 1 mg of dexamethasone at bedtime (approximately 11 P.M.). On the morning following dexamethasone administration, the patient returns for a basal cortisol level and ACTH stimulation test, in which 0.25 mg of Cortrosyn (α 1–24 corticotropin) is administered and 17-OHP level is determined immediately before and again after 60 minutes. A cortisol level of less than 5 μg/dl after dexamethasone excludes the diagnosis of Cushing's syndrome. A stimulated 17-OHP level of 2,000 ng/dl or higher indicates the presence of 21-hydroxylase deficiency.[11] A progesterone level should be obtained in all menstruating women on days 20 to 25 of the menstrual cycle to assess ovulation, since anovulation is usually associated with more severe hyperandrogenism. Furthermore, anovulatory women have an increased chance of having a serious underlying disease.

THERAPY

Therapeutic strategies (Fig. 20-3) are aimed at controlling the biochemical disturbances, since in the majority of hyperandrogenism cases no specific cause can be identified. Hence therapy is directed at decreasing the production, biologic availability, and/or target tissue action of androgens. Once a hair follicle has been transformed under androgenic stimulation to produce terminal hair, it cannot return to producing vellus hair. The rate of hair growth and the caliber of the hair can be decreased, however, by decreasing androgenic stimulation. Only electrolysis can eradicate the hair, but if permanent hair removal is desired, such therapy should be withheld until complete biochemical control of hyperandrogenism has been achieved. Similarly, androgen-stimulated alopecia cannot be reversed but further hair loss can be prevented by control of the hyperandrogenism.

Gonadal Steroids—Oral Contraceptives

MECHANISM OF ACTION

Either estrogen or progesterone in large doses will inhibit pituitary LH secretion and decrease LH-dependent ovarian androgen production.[12] Estrogen will also decrease the biologic availability of androgen by increasing SHBG levels and will decrease adrenal DHEAS production, probably by decreasing ACTH secretion.[13] Progesterone will competitively inhibit 5-α-reductase activity, thus decreasing target tissue androgen utilization. Estrogen and progesterone act synergistically to inhibit LH release, making combined therapy more effective at lower doses than use of either agent alone.

Oral contraceptive preparations are the most convenient modality for administering combined estrogen-progesterone therapy. Oral contraceptives containing 50 μg of ethinyl estradiol (EE_2) or the equivalent (e.g., mestranol) are necessary for complete suppression of LH release, whereas agents containing 35 μg of EE_2 are adequate to increase SHBG levels and suppress DHEAS levels. Biochemical control of hyperandrogenism will occur in 21 days with agents containing 50 μg or more of EE_2 or the equivalent and correlates with suppression of LH secretion.[12] Agents containing 35 μg EE_2 do not consistently suppress total T levels but substantially decrease biologically available T levels. A clinical response can be seen in 3 months with 50 μg EE_2 or its equivalent, but

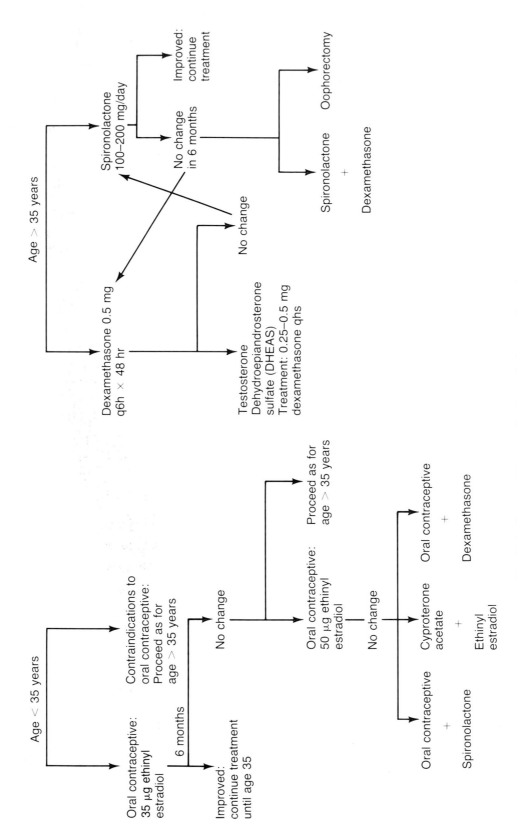

Fig. 20-3. Suggested therapeutic schema for hyperandrogenism.

such a response may require 4 to 5 months with 35 μg EE_2. The type of progestin must be considered when prescribing oral contraceptives since certain progestins, e.g., levonorgestrel, are androgenic and will antagonize the beneficial peripheral effects of the estrogen. Indeed, levonorgestrel has a higher affinity for SHBG than do endogenous steroids and will increase biologically available androgen levels. Oral contraceptives containing androgens such as ethynodiol diacetate or norethindrone are recommended.

RISKS AND SIDE EFFECTS

The major risks of oral contraceptive therapy are thromboembolic phenomena and gallbladder disease. The relationship of these agents to carcinogenesis remains controversial. The risks are directly related to the estrogen dose and the age of the patient. Smoking greatly increases the risk of thromboembolic complications. Oral contraceptives may also cause hypertension, exacerbate migraines, and, very rarely, cause benign liver tumors.

RECOMMENDATIONS

The risks of oral contraceptive agents are low in well-selected patients, and good control of hirsutism and acne can be achieved with agents containing 35 μg EE_2[10]; hence these agents are recommended as a first-line therapy in women under 35 years of age who lack contraindications to their use, such as a strongly positive family history of thromboembolism or breast cancer or a personal history of hypertension or cholelithiasis. The dose can be increased to 50 μg of EE_2 if the clinical and biochemical response is not adequate after 6 months, or another therapy can be instituted. High-dose progesterone in the form of medroxyprogesterone acetate has been recommended by some authors in women who have a contraindication to oral contraceptive use, but other available therapies are more effective.

Glucocorticoids

MECHANISM OF ACTION

Glucocorticoids such as prednisone and dexamethasone decrease adrenal androgen production by suppressing ACTH secretion.[14] There is also evidence suggesting that glucocorticoids may inhibit ovarian androgen production. Glucocorticoid therapy can suppress hyperandrogenism in a significant proportion of patients, even in the absence of DHEAS elevations of identifiable adrenal enzyme abnormalities.[15] Thus, the only way to determine potential therapeutic responsiveness to glucocorticoids is empirically, by suppression testing. Recent studies indicate that a 2-day course of dexamethasone 0.5 mg qid, with measurement of T and DHEAS levels before and the morning after the last dexamethasone dose, accurately predicts patients whose hyperandrogenism will improve with glucocorticoid therapy.[15] If T and DHEAS levels decrease into the normal range during the dexamethasone trial, a prolonged course of glucocorticoid therapy can be initiated. Adrenal androgen production is more sensitive to glucocorticoid suppression than is adrenal cortisol production, and as little as 0.25 mg of dexamethasone at bedtime can suppress adrenal androgens.[14] Clinical improvement in hirsutism can often be seen in 3 months, but occasionally improvement can only be seen after 6 months to 1 year of therapy.

RISKS AND SIDE EFFECTS

The major risk of glucocorticoid therapy is the suppression of the adrenal stress response, resulting in relative hypoadrenalism. Such suppression can be seen with as little as 0.5 mg of dexamethasone at bedtime. Monitoring morning (8 to 9 A.M.) cortisol levels, with titration of the dose to maintain such levels above 2 μg/dl, is necessary to avoid this complication. Iatrogenic Cushing's syndrome is usually not seen from the small doses of glucocorticoids that are employed to control hyperandrogenism, but such symptoms can develop with doses of dexamethasone larger than 0.75 mg per day.

RECOMMENDATIONS

Glucocorticoids can be used in women older than 35 or in women who have failed, or have a contraindication to, oral contraceptive therapy. Glucocorticoids also constitute a well-documented effective therapeutic modality for controlling acne that occurs secondary to elevated DHEAS levels in men.[5] Dexamethasone is the glucocorticoid of choice since it has almost no mineralocorticoid activity and can be given as a single bedtime dose, which effectively decreases the night-time rise in ACTH secretion. As little as 0.25 mg of dexamethasone can be effective in controlling adrenal androgen production.[14] Therapy must be carefully monitored to avoid adrenal oversuppression, and only patients with documented glucocorticoid-suppressible hyperandrogenism should be treated. The clinical response correlates with decreased androgen levels, so therefore therapy should be changed if hyperandrogenism is not controlled with 0.5 to 0.75 mg of dexamethasone per day.

Antiandrogens

Antiandrogens are agents that control hyperandrogenism by inhibiting androgen binding to target tissue androgen receptors; the drugs cimetidine, spironolactone, and cyproterone acetate are all antiandrogens. Cimetidine, also a histamine receptor blocker, is a very weak antiandrogen and is not in widespread clinical use as such.[16] Cyproterone acetate is a very potent antiandrogen, which has been available in Europe and Canada for several years.[17] Spironolactone is also a relatively potent antiandrogen and is widely prescribed as a diuretic.[18,19]

MECHANISM OF ACTION

Spironolactone and cyproterone acetate competitively inhibit endogenous androgen binding to the intracellular androgen receptor. In addition, spironolactone decreases glandular and androgen biosynthesis, thereby decreasing both the production and the action of androgens. Paradoxically, spironolactone also increases biologically available androgen levels by an action on SHBG, but this action does not abolish the beneficial actions of the drug. Cyproterone acetate may also interfere with androgen biosynthesis although the decreased androgen production observed with this agent is secondary mainly to the action of the EE_2 administered with it. Clinical improvement may be seen in 2 to 3 months with both agents.[17,19]

RISKS AND SIDE EFFECTS

The long-term clinical use of both spironolactone and cyproterone acetate has proved safe in humans although spironolactone has been implicated in breast carcinogenesis in rodents. Diuresis and electrolyte disturbances are not major problems with spironolactone therapy. Dysfunctional uterine bleeding can complicate treatment with spironolactone, requiring that the dose be decreased or stopped.[18] Cyproterone acetate is a progestin, and very large doses can cause suppression of the hypothalamic-pituitary-adrenal axis. More commonly, cyproterone acetate causes fatigue, weight gain, and loss of libido; such side effects result in discontinuation of the drug in approximately 10 percent of cases. Both agents are contraindicated for use in pregnancy since their antiandrogenic actions will interfere with the masculinization of a male fetus. Cyproterone acetate is always given in combination with EE_2 in women of reproductive age, both to provide contraception and to prevent dysfunctional uterine bleeding.

RECOMMENDATIONS

Spironolactone in doses of 100 to 200 mg per day (in two divided doses) appears to be the most efficacious therapy available for hirsutism in the United States.[19] However, other agents such as oral contraceptives are adequate in controlling hyperandrogenic symptoms in a large percentage of patients. Cyproterone acetate has been documented to be strikingly effective in controlling both hirsutism and acne. Severely affected patients who have not responded to therapy with spironolactone may consider obtaining cyproterone acetate therapy in countries where it is available.

Bromocriptine (Parlodel)

Bromocriptine is a dopaminergic agonist used in the treatment of hyperprolactinemia. Several groups have reported that bromocriptine can effectively decrease LH and androgen levels, leading to a decrease in hirsutism in a percentage of women with PCO. The mechanism of action is thought to involve central suppression of LH secretion although a peripheral action of bromocriptine on glandular androgen secretion has not been excluded. Prolactin levels are not predictive of a therapeutic response. A dose of 2.5 mg twice daily appears to be required for a therapeutic response, and patients can take up to 6 months to respond. Bromocriptine can cause orthostatic hypotension initially and nausea with gastrointestinal distress. Therapy must be started slowly, usually with a dose of 1.25 mg at bedtime for 2 weeks, which can then be slowly increased to avoid side effects. Further study will define the role of bromocriptine in the management of hyperandrogenism associated with PCO.

Combined Drug Therapy

Additional therapeutic benefit can be obtained by combined therapy with oral contraceptives and glucocorticoids or with either of these and spironolactone.[20] Indications for such therapy are persistent hyperandrogenism or a poor clinical response to a single agent. The risks of such combined therapy are additive but not synergistic.

Other Modalities

Weight reduction in obese hyperandrogenic women will often decrease androgen production and increase SHBG levels, leading to marked reduction in and at times complete resolution of hyperandrogenism. Hence obese hyperandrogenic women should be vigorously encouraged to lose weight, although such exhortations are often fruitless. In women who are not interested in fertility bilateral oophorectomy will abolish ovarian androgen production, but it must be remembered that adrenal androgen hypersecretion frequently occurs in hyperandrogenic women and that this, of course, will not improve with removal of the ovaries. Bilateral ovarian wedge resection causes only transient decreases in androgen levels and is not an effective therapy for hyperandrogenism. Mechanical control of excessive hair growth by shaving, plucking, waxing, depilatories, or electrolysis can prove very satisfactory in controlling the symptoms of hirsutism, particularly in conjunction with oral contraceptive therapy. Such control should always be presented as a serious alternative to more aggressive and potentially harmful medical therapy. Finally, thyroid hormone administration to euthyroid subjects in an effort to increase SHBG levels has no role in the therapy of hyperandrogenism and carries a significant risk of complications.

SUMMARY

Hirsutism, and to a lesser extent acne and alopecia, are the clinical consequences of hyperandrogenism. The development of these disorders requires not only increases in androgen production and availability but also the presence within the target tissue of the enzymatic capacity to respond to androgens. Although a number of serious disorders can present with hyperandrogenism, the majority of cases are the result of the relatively benign conditions of unknown etiology known as idiopathic hirsutism and polycystic ovary syndrome. Understanding the biology of androgen action has permitted the design of therapies that are effective in controlling the dermatologic sequelae of hyperandrogenism. However, a true cure for these troublesome disorders must await further research to identify their specific etiologies.

REFERENCES

1. Maroulis GB: Evaluation of hirsutism and hyperandrogenemia. Fertil Steril 36:273, 1981
2. Hatch R, Rosenfield RL, Kim MH, Tredway D: Hirsutism: implications, etiology, and management. Am J Obstet Gynecol 140:815, 1981
3. Kasick JM, Bergfeld WF, Steck WD, Gupta MK: Adrenal androgenic female-pattern alopecia: sex hormones and the balding woman. Cleve Clin Q 50:111, 1983
4. Steinberger E, Rodriguez-Rigau LJ, Smith KD, Held B: The menstrual cycle and plasma testosterone levels in women with acne. J Am Acad Dermatol 4:54, 1981
5. Marynick SP, Chakmakjian ZH, McCaffree DL, Herndon JH: Androgen excess in cystic acne. N Engl J Med 308:981, 1983
6. Anderson DC: Sex-hormone-binding globulin. Clin Endocrinol (Oxf) 3:69, 1974
7. Mowszowicz E, Melanitou E, Doukani A, et al: Androgen binding capacity and 5-alpha-reductase activity in pubic skin fibroblasts from hirsute patients. J Clin Endocrinol Metab 56:1209, 1983
8. Horton R, Hawks D, Lobo R: 3-Alpha, 17-beta-androstanediol glucuronide in plasma—a marker of androgen action in idiopathic hirsutism. J Clin Invest 69:1203, 1982
9. Wild RA, Umstot ES, Anderson RN, et al: Androgen parameters and their correlation with body weight in one hundred thirty-eight women thought to have hyperandrogenism. Am J Obstet Gynecol 146:602, 1983
10. Palatsi R, Hirvensalo E, Liukko P, et al: Serum total and unbound testosterone and sex hormone binding globulin (SHBG) in female acne patients treated with two different oral contraceptives. Acta Derm Venereol (Stockh) 64:517, 1984
11. New MI, Lorenzin F, Lerner AJ, et al: Genotyping steroid 21-hydroxylase deficiency: hormonal reference data. J Clin Endocrinol Metab 57:320, 1983
12. Givens JR, Anderson RM, Wiser WL, Fish SA: Dynamics of suppression and recovery of plasma FSH, LH, androstenedione and testosterone in polycystic ovarian disease using an oral contraceptive. J Clin Endocrinol Metab 38:727, 1974
13. Wild RA, Umstot ES, Anderson RN, Givens JR: Adrenal function in hirsutism. II. Effect of an oral contraceptive. J Clin Endocrinol Metab 54:676, 1982
14. Rittmaster R, Loriaux DL, Cutler GB Jr: Sensitivity of cortisol and adrenal androgens to dexamethasone suppression in hirsute women. J Clin Endocrinol Metab 61:462, 1985
15. Steinberger E, Smith KD, Rodriguez-Rigau LJ: Testosterone, dehydroepiandrosterone, and dehydroepiandrosterone sulfate in hyperandrogenic women. J Clin Endocrinol Metab 59:471, 1984
16. Vigersky RA, Mehlman I, Calass AR, Smith CE: Treatment of hirsute women with cimetidine. N Engl J Med 303:1042, 1980
17. Hammerstein J, Meckies J, Leo-Rossberg I, et al: Use of cyproterone acetate (CPA) in the steroid treatment of acne, hirsutism and virilism. J Biochem 6:827, 1975
18. Shapiro G, Evron S: A novel use of spironolactone: treatment of hirsutism. J Clin Endocrinol Metab 41:429, 1980
19. Cumming DL, Yang JL, Rebar RW, Yen SSC: Treatment of hirsutism with spironolactone. JAMA 247:1295, 1982
20. Pittaway DE, Maxson WS, Wentz AC: Spironolactone in combination drug therapy for unresponsive hirsutism. Fertil Steril 43:878, 1985

21

Panniculitis

Robert G. Phelps

Panniculitis represents an inflammatory reaction of adipose tissue and can involve cutaneous or extracutaneous sites. Clinically, most panniculitides present primarily in the skin as firm, tender deep-seated nodules more apparent by palpation than by inspection. Many panniculitides have been described with a profusion of terminology but still present problems in classification and understanding.

GROSS AND MICROSCOPIC ANATOMY OF FAT

In order to fully understand panniculitis, knowledge of the gross and microanatomy of the subcutis is essential. The subcutaneous fat is present as a continuous layer beneath the dermis but with considerable regional variation. It is thick and abundant in the abdomen, buttocks, and thigh and thin or absent in penile and eyelid skin. There are age and sex differences as well.[1]

Histologically most subcutaneous adipose tissue is separated by connective tissue septa into discrete lobules. This lobular architecture is most evident in pressure sites such as the palms and soles and may be less apparent at other sites. Within the septa are nutrient vessels, lymphatics, and nerves. The vessels further divide into capillaries, which can occasionally be seen within the lobules.[1]

The inflammatory infiltrate in the panniculitides can preferentially involve the septa or lobules or be equally divided in both. Vessels in the septa may or may not be involved. The precise localization of the inflammatory infiltrate and the presence or absence of vessel disease allows the pathologist to classify the panniculitis.

The classification of panniculitis is listed in Table 21–1. This classification includes both clinical and pathologic criteria.

PANNICULITIS OF INDEFINITE TYPE

Indefinite panniculitides are those in which the diagnosis is often one of exclusion. Most dermatologists agree that in these disorders neither the clinical presentation nor the pathology is sufficiently diagnostic to permit a precise classification. The two that fall into this category are Weber-Christian disease and Rothmann-Makai panniculitis.

Weber-Christian Disease

Weber-Christian panniculitis has evolved in concept but as originally described had a rather classic presentation.[2,3] The patients, usually women, developed crops of tender or nontender nodules on the trunk or extremities. The nodules

Table 21-1. Classification of Panniculitis

Panniculitis of indefinite type
    Weber-Christian disease
    Rothmann-Makai panniculitis
Primary panniculitis
    Erythema induratum
    Erythema nodosum
    Sclerema neonatorum
    Subcutaneous fat necrosis of the newborn
    Cytophagic histiocytic panniculitis
Secondary panniculitis
    Pancreatic panniculitis
    Lupus panniculitis
    Connective tissue panniculitis
Physical panniculitis
    Cold panniculitis
    Factitial panniculitis
    Poststeroid panniculitis
Panniculitis incidental to other diseases
    Scleroderma
    Benign cutaneous periarteritis nodosa
    Superficial thrombophlebitis

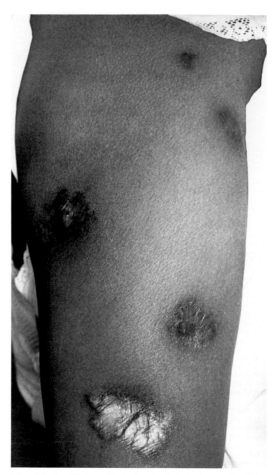

Fig. 21–1. Weber-Christian (indefinite) panniculitis. Flat, atrophic hyperpigmented patches on upper extremity.

would heal spontaneously and leave a depressed atrophic scar and a residue of hyperpigmentation (Fig. 21–1). New lesions arose while others disappeared. The nodules persisted for months and the entire course could last for years, but it was ultimately self-limiting. Systemic signs, particularly fever, were prominent during acute outbreaks. The histopathologic changes consisted of the effects of an intense leukocytic and lymphocytic infiltrate on lobules of fat.

Subsequently, many additional cases of Weber-Christian disease were reported and other features were noted. Even though Weber-Christian panniculitis was originally called nodular nonsuppurative panniculitis, several authors described variants with similar clinical presentation and pathology, in which nodules spontaneously suppurated and discharged an oily fluid.[4] Cases of Weber-Christian panniculitis were also reported with involvement of both cutaneous adipose tissue and visceral adipose tissue.[5,6] Hence, Weber-Christian was expanded to include both suppurative and nonsuppurative variants and localized and systemic forms.

Furthermore, Weber Christian panniculitis or Weber-Christian-like syndromes were found to occur in association with or as a consequence of a multitude of inciting agents. Among those described are pancreatic disease,[7] factitial panniculitis,[8] α_1-antitrypsin deficiency[9,10] and immunologic abnormalities.[11] This broad etiologic association has led some authors to question whether this panniculitis is a separate entity at all.[12]

Most of the nosologic confusion in Weber-Christian disease centers around what is essential for establishing the diagnosis, the so-called diagnostic histopathology. Pathologically Weber-Christian disease is said to evolve through three phases[12]: (1) an acute inflammatory stage, in which lobules of fat are replaced by neutrophils, lymphocytes, and histiocytes

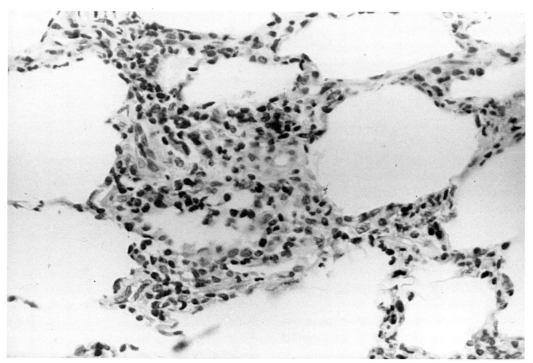

Fig. 21–2. Lobular panniculitis. Lobules of adipocytes with minimal injury invaded by an infiltrate of small lymphocytes and larger histiocytes.

(Fig. 21–2); (2) an intermediate lipophagic phase, in which the degenerated fat is ingested by uninucleate and multinucleate foam cells; and (3) a fibrotic late phase, in which fibrosis replaces the foam cells. Other changes, such as endothelial proliferation and vascular swelling, have been described.[13] The second stage is claimed to be the most diagnostic.

Despite this rather characteristic evolution, many investigators have shown that the pathology of Weber-Christian disease can be mimicked by other panniculitides. Forstrom and Winklemann[14] studied 34 cases that had been diagnosed as acute panniculitis. Patients had sudden onset of nodose lesions, which were biopsied shortly after their inception. All biopsies showed a dense, primarily polymorphonuclear leukocytic infiltrate replacing fat lobules; in some, foam cells were present as well. The clinical course, laboratory data, and additional clinical findings in these patients suggested panniculitis of diverse types (erythema nodosum,

erythema induratum, traumatic infections) other than Weber-Christian disease. The study suggested that acute panniculitis, rather than being diagnostic for the first stage of Weber-Christian disease, may be the initial phase in multiple types of panniculitides. The second stage with preponderance of foam cells may occur, but to a lesser degree, in trauma[8,15] or as a nonspecific response to injury.[16]

Rothmann-Makai Panniculitis

Rothmann-Makai panniculitis is of uncertain nosology as well and is considered by some to be a variant of Weber-Christian panniculitis. In the cases appraised by Laymon and Peterson, the patients, usually children, presented with multiple small, nontender nodules on the lower extremity or trunk. Old nodules resolved with atrophy and hyperpigmentation, and new lesions arose singly rather than in crops. Systemic signs and symptoms, notably fever, were conspicuously absent. The disorder was self-limited and improved within 6 to 12 months.[17]

The pathology was said to evolve through the same three phases as Weber-Christian disease: an acute necrotic phase, a lipophagic phase, and a fibroblastic phase.[17] Granuloma formation and microcyst formation have been said to be prominent features.[18,19]

Other authors, however, have described other clinical presentations and pathology. It has been suggested that Rothmann-Makai be designated as a nonspecific or indefinite panniculitis that does not fit into the other predetermined categories.

PRIMARY PANNICULITIS

Primary panniculitides are those in which the primary insult or injury is in the panniculus. An accompanying systemic disease may be present but is not essential for the diagnosis.

Erythema Induratum

Erythema induratum is a panniculitis about which there is general agreement with respect to pathology and clinical presentation, but not with respect to etiology and pathogenesis.

Clinically, erythema induratum presents as multiple, grouped, deep nodules on the calves of young women. The nodules are usually, but not necessarily, painless, and they commonly ulcerate. Individual lesions persist for weeks to months and heal with irregularly shaped atrophic scars. A history of cold sensitivity and exacerbation during winter months is often elicited. The disease can last for months to years.

In cases of otherwise typical clinical erythema induratum, the pathology can vary depending on whether an early or late lesion is biopsied. Early lesions may display only an acute leukocytic lobular panniculitis with focal granuloma formation.[14] Later lesions show varying degrees of one of the three following changes: (1) large-vessel vasculitis; (2) epithe-

lioid cell granulomas; and (3) caseation necrosis.[20-22] Medium-sized subcutaneous arteries and veins show a dense inflammatory infiltrate in their walls, with subsequent luminal thrombosis and occlusion. The surrounding adipose tissue shows a lobular panniculitis with numerous mononuclear cells interspersed between adipocytes. Clusters of typical epithelioid cells and giant cells may be seen surrounding normal or involved vessels or scattered throughout the fat. Often that fat undergoes a granular, eosinophilic necrosis, referred to as *caseation necrosis*. Other features described include an extensive fibrosing reaction in a granulomatous infiltrate[23] or palisading granulomas.[22]

The pathogenesis of erythema induratum is controversial. Ever since the original description by Bazin it has long been assumed to be a tuberculid (i.e., a reaction to tubercle bacilli in patients with a high degree of immunity to mycobacteria). This was supported by its "tuberculoid" histopathology. Many cases, however, were described subsequently in which there was a similar clinical presentation and pathology and no tuberculosis. Hamilton[23] separated erythema induratum into two categories: nontuberculous erythema induratum, or nodular vasculitis, and tuberculous erythema induratum. Clinical and pathological differences were said to exist between the two: nodular vasculitis occurred on the calves of older women, did not ulcerate, and did not exhibit caseation, whereas erythema induratum (Bazin) occurred on the calves of younger women, often ulcerated, and did involve caseation necrosis. Both types exhibited a medium-vessel vasculitis. Despite these apparent differences, Hamilton and others[20] confirmed that these distinctions were not absolute and that considerable overlapping occurred.

What is the evidence that some types of erythema induratum are etiologically related to tuberculosis? Many but not all patients with erythema induratum exhibit high sensitivity to old tuberculin or purified protein derivative.[20,21] Some investigators have demonstrated positive guinea pig inoculations or acid-fast bacilli.[23] Mycobacterial antigens have been found in blood vessels of patients with nodular vasculitis,[24] and excellent response to antituberculous therapy has often been noted.[20,25,26] The incidence of erythema induratum has been said to be declining in parallel with that of tuberculosis.[20]

Despite this compelling evidence, other facts do not support a tuberculous etiology. First, tuberculin reactivity is endemic in many populations, and its presence does not prove cause and effect. Second, most cultures, guinea pig inoculations, and acid-fast stains from tissue of erythema induratum do not yield organisms. Third, the mechanism of action of antituberculous therapy may not be related to antibacillary action but rather to effects on metabolism. Fourth, many patients respond to other medications (e.g., systemic steroids).

Erythema Nodosum

Erythema nodosum is the most common type of panniculitis seen in clinical practice. Two types have been described, the acute "classical" type and a variant chronic form.

In the acute classical type, a young adult patient, most commonly a female, presents with multiple, bilateral, slightly ecchymotic, tender nodules on the shins (Fig. 21–3) or occasionally on the thighs or forearms. The nodules are discrete, 1 to 5 cm in diameter, and sharply demarcated. Lesions may occur in crops. Individual lesions last for weeks and the eruption can last for months, but generally the condition resolves without sequelae. Accompanying the outbreak, fever, arthralgia and malaise may be present.

The chronic form of erythema nodosum, known as *erythema nodosum migrans* or *nodular migratory panniculitis*,[27–29] also appears primarily on the extensor tibial surfaces. It differs from the acute form in several aspects. Instead of multiple bilateral small nodules, one or more large unilateral nodules appear, which then undergo gradual clearing while peripheral "migratory" satellite nodules appear. Scarring, ulceration, and tenderness are absent. The eruption can last for years rather than months. Accompa-

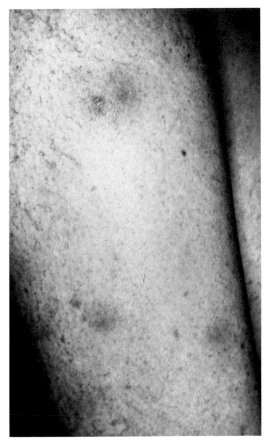

Fig. 21–3. Erythema nodosum. Tender, erythematous nodules on the calf.

nying systemic signs or symptoms are less frequent than with acute forms, but despite this apparent difference considerable overlap with acute forms can occur.

Acute erythema nodosum, and less commonly chronic erythema nodosum, are known for their association with infectious and systemic diseases. This association most likely represents an immunologically mediated hypersensitivity reaction. Erythema nodosum may follow β-hemolytic streptoccoccal infections, tuberculosis, yersinia infection, histoplasmosis, blastomycosis, coccidioidomycosis, and other infections. Perhaps the best known association is with sarcoid and hilar adenopathy (Lofgren's syndrome). Systemic immunologic disorders, inflammatory bowel disease, and Behçet's syn-

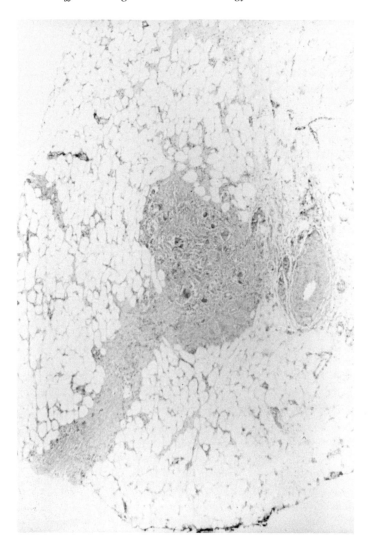

Fig. 21–4. Erythema nodosum. Subcutaneous fat showing widened, fibrotic interlobular septum infiltrated by multinucleated giant cells.

drome can precipitate erythema nodosum. Drug-induced erythema nodosum is most commonly secondary to use of oral contraceptives.

The pathology of classic erythema nodosum is that of a septal panniculitis. Initially, an acute inflammatory infiltrate occupies edematous, thickened subcutaneous septae and small veins and venules may show wall infiltration. Later, fibrosis supervenes, as well as a granulomatous infiltrate (Fig. 21–4). The granulomas consist primarily of multinucleate giant cells, with few epithelioid cells and no caseation. The granulomas and inflammatory infiltrate encroach on the periphery of the fat lobules but spare the lob-

ules. In chronic erythema nodosum the histopathology is similar to that of the acute form, although it may be more granulomatous or involve greater vessel changes.[27]

Panniculitis in Children: Sclerema Neonatorum and Subcutaneous Fat Necrosis of the Newborn

Sclerema neonatorum and subcutaneous fat necrosis of the newborn are two panniculitides that occur in the perinatal period and have markedly different prognoses. A clear-cut distinction between the two can usually but not always be made.

Hughes and Hammond[30] in 1948 first clearly delineated sclerema neonatorum, and their classic description remains valid today. Sclerema neonatorum, although ostensibly a panniculitis, presented quite differently from other panniculitides. Instead of firm discrete nodules the patients who were neonates or young infants would develop a "tallowlike" induration, which could remain localized to the extremities or buttocks or spread rapidly to involve most of the body surface. The skin was described as immobile, "bound down" to underlying structures, and cold to touch. Almost any body site could be involved, although palms, soles, and genitalia were often spared.

Sclerema neonatorum carried an ominous prognosis because of its association with other underlying disease. The infants, at or shortly after birth, exhibited signs or symptoms of a serious underlying illness; that is, they had severe diarrhea, intestinal obstruction, respiratory distress, convulsions, pneumonitis, or shock. The infants were often of low birth weight but not necessarily premature. Simultaneously with or following these signs and symptoms, the patients would develop sclerema. Almost invariably the patients would succumb to the concurrent illness, but in those who survived, the sclerema could resolve without sequelae.

Despite the rather dramatic clinical presentation, biopsies and autopsies of patients with sclerema often demonstrated minimal changes. The most common was the presence of fibrous bands in a thickened subcutis.[30] Cellular infiltration and fat necrosis were absent to minimal. Occasional adipocytes were "engorged" with fat or replaced by fine, needle-shaped crystals.[31]

Subcutaneous fat necrosis of the newborn is a self-limited disease afflicting healthy neonates and young infants (Fig.21–5). They present with multiple violaceous or firm nodules on the buttocks, shoulders, or trunk, which tend to be discrete rather than confluent. Liquefaction and secondary calcification are common occurrences.[32] A useful diagnostic adjunct is the aspiration of a viscous gray material from

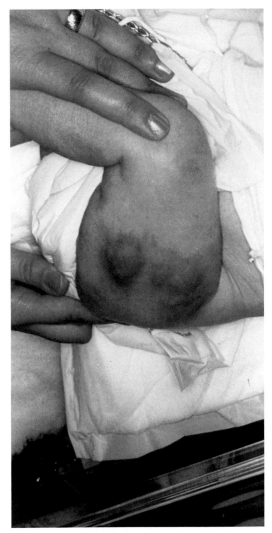

Fig. 21–5. Subcutaneous fat necrosis of the newborn. Multiple fluctuant erythematous nodules on upper thigh of a neonate.

individual lesions. The nodules resolve spontaneously within a period of several months.

The pathology is similar to that of sclerema neonatorum, but there are important differences. Both show enlarged lipocytes replaced by radially arrayed needle-shaped crystals, but in subcutaneous fat necrosis there is a much more florid inflammatory reaction.[33] Degenerated adipocytes are surrounded by macrophages and foreign-body giant cells (Fig. 21–6). Dys-

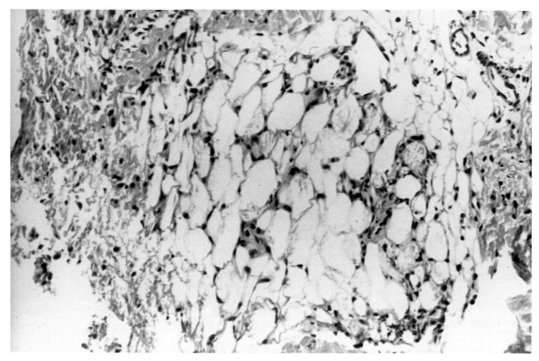

Fig. 21–6. Subcutaneous fat necrosis of the newborn. Degenerated lipocytes replaced by needle-shaped crystals and surrounded by multinucleated giant cells.

trophic calcification may ensue. Broad fibrous bands are not commonly seen.

Cytophagic Histiocytic Panniculitis

Cytophagic histiocytic panniculitis was delineated in 1981 by Crotty and Winkelmann.[34] This unique, complex clinicopathologic syndrome showed features of a systemic panniculitis, a histiocytosis, and a systemic disease with hematopoietic and hepatic failure. The five patients described died as a consequence of their disease.

The patients presented with a several-month to several-year history of multiple, recurrent large (2 to 10 cm) subcutaneous nodules. The nodules occurred most commonly on the lower extremities, but trunk, forearm, and forehead involvment were also present. The nodules were confluent, tender, and ecchymotic in later stages of the disease. When resolution occurred, usually there were no or minimal sequelae.

Simultaneously with or preceding their pannicultis the patients developed signs and symptoms of a systemic disease, fever and leukopenia being the two most common associations. Evidence of infiltration of the reticuloendothelial system (i.e., hepatosplenomegaly) was present in three patients. Later in the course of the disease all patients exhibited a rapid downhill course characterized by progressive liver dysfunction or a coagulopathy. All patients died with, or as a consequence of, intravisceral hemorrhage.

Pathologic examination revealed an extensive and destructive lobular panniculitis with numerous lymphocytes and histiocytes located between adipocytes. Foci of fat necrosis, nuclear debris and hemorrhage were present. The diagnostic feature, however, was the presence of numerous cytologically benign histiocytes, which showed extensive phagocytic activity. Their cytosols were replaced by erythrocytes, lymphocytes, or nuclear debris; they were therefore referred to as "bean bag" cells.

In other organ systems, such as the liver, spleen, lymph node, and bone marrow, similar histiocytes showing prominent lymphohistiocytosis and erythrophagocytosis were seen. These cells were often abundant and in some tissues, such as the lung, obliterated the architecture. Since erythrophagocytosis and lymphophagocytosis have been seen in malignant histiocytosis,[35] T-cell lymphomas,[36] and certain genetic disorders,[37] the question arises as to whether this is a panniculitis or rather a systemic histiocytosis in which the panniculus is primarily involved.[38]

SECONDARY PANNICULITIS

Secondary panniculitides occur as a consequence of, or are related to, underlying disease.

Panniculitis and Pancreatic Disease

The association of panniculitis or subcutaneous fat necrosis with pancreatic disease (pancreatitis, pancreatic carcinoma) is well established in the literature. Characteristic clinical and dermatopathologic findings may be present and may allow the dermatologist to suggest the possibility of pancreatic disease.[39–41]

The classic patient is a middle-aged or elderly man who presents with multiple nodose lesions of the lower extremities. The nodules may vary from 2 to 5 cm in diameter, are erythematous, tender or nontender, and may occur on the buttocks or trunk as well. Spontaneous liquefaction and drainage may occur. An associated large-joint arthritis is present in up to 65 percent of cases and may affect almost any large joint (e.g., knee, wrist, elbow), but the most common site is the ankle. Because of the association of tender nodules and arthralgias, this type of panniculitis is often mistaken for erythema nodosum.

Other systemic signs and symptoms and laboratory abnormalities may also be present. Patients with pancreatitis, and less often those with pancreatic carcinoma, often have concomitant or antecedent abdominal pain. Ascites and pleural or pericardial effusions may be present and augur a poor prognosis.[39] Peripheral eosinophilia is seen, especially in patients with pancreatic carcinoma. Serum amylase, lipase, and other proteolytic enzymes are invariably elevated. Some patients may exhibit only panniculitis, and the underlying pancreatic disease may be clinically silent.[41]

The histopathology of panniculitis with pancreatic subcutaneous fat necrosis is pathognomonic. The adipocytes become shrunken and anuclear, and their cell membranes thicken—the result is so-called ghost cells. Surrounding the cell membranes and in the adjacent connective tissue is a basophilic granular material, which stains for calcium. Identical changes may be seen in peripancreatic tissue, serosa, and periarticular fat.

The pathogenesis of pancreatic subcutaneous fat necrosis is primarily enzymatic. A damaged pancreas or an acinar type of carcinoma of the pancreas releases large amounts of lipolytic and proteolytic enzymes. These enzymes presumably are relayed to distant sites by lymphatic or hematogenous spread and act in concert on peripheral fat deposits. The result is lipolysis and saponification of fat, with the formation of calcium-triglyceride complexes.

Lupus Panniculitis

Lupus panniculitis is the subject of several recent reviews and will be covered here briefly.[42–44] Essentially, lupus panniculitis or lupus profundus is a rather broadly defined category, which includes most nodular fat proliferations or panniculitides that occur with systemic lupus erythematosus (SLE) or discoid lupus erythematosus (DLE).

Lupus panniculitis presents as large, deep-seated, sometimes tender nodules on the deltoids, face, neck, back, or buttocks. It occurs primarily in middle-aged females (ages 40 to 60) and usually follows many years of DLE or SLE but, rarely, may be the initial manifestation. The overlying skin may be normal or erythematous or may exhibit atrophy or poikilodermatous changes of lupus. Individual lesions may persist for months, and recurrences of nodules in adjacent sites or scars is common. Ulceration or atrophy can occur secondarily and can produce a large, irregularly shaped lesion.

Lupus panniculitis is a rare manifestation of lupus. In several large series of SLE and DLE patients, no more than 2 to 3 percent had histories of nodular lesions. Contrary to earlier reports, two-thirds of patients with lupus panniculitis have DLE, not SLE. Since most cases occur with DLE, there are few associated signs and symptoms. Nephritis appears to be less common in patients with SLE and lupus panniculitis. Serositis and arthritis may accompany the nodules.

The pathology of lupus panniculitis can be suggestive or nonspecific. If there are epidermal changes, the usual findings of lupus may be seen, namely, vacuolar alteration, epidermal atrophy, or dermal mucinosis. The panniculitis is lobular and lymphocytic. Germinal centers and lymphoid nodules may appear at the periphery of the fat lobules, and this infiltration can produce a peculiar hyalinization and necrobiosis of the fat and connective tissue. Secondary calcification, elastosis, or mucin deposition can occur. Vessel damage may be present but is infrequent. In some instances only a mildly patchy lymphocytic or nonspecific panniculitis is present, and other signs and symptoms are necessary for the diagnosis.

In lupus panniculitis a useful diagnostic adjunct is immunofluorescence. Approximately two-thirds of lesions will exhibit linear basement membrane zone fluorescence overlying the lesions, most commonly for IgM or C3. This occurs irrespective of whether or not epidermal changes are present and of whether the patient has SLE or DLE. Other serologic studies including the VDRL test and tests for antinuclear, anti-double-stranded DNA, anti-Sm, and anti-RNP (ribonucleoprotein) antibodies, should be performed as necessary.

Connective Tissue Panniculitis

Recently, Winkelmann and Padilla-Gonçalves[45] described an atypical panniculitis occurring in two young women, who presented with a several-month history of large, tender subcutaneous nodules on the upper trunk and arms. The nodules resolved with atrophy. Biopsy specimens showed an extensive, lobular panniculitis with numerous mononuclear cells between fat lobules, and were initially interpreted as lymphoma, erythema induratum, erythema nodosum, or other panniculitides. Extensive laboratory work-up showed findings suggestive of but not diagnostic for a connective tissue disease: anemia, leukopenia, hypergammaglobulinemia, and antibodies to native DNA and to SS-B. Both patients responded to antimalarial therapy. Because of the similarity of this entity to connective tissue disease and morphea and its response to antimalarial therapy, it was labeled *connective tissue panniculitis*.

PHYSICAL PANNICULITIS

Physical panniculitis refers to panniculitis induced by external agents. Almost any blunt trauma, injection, or temperature change can induce a panniculitis. The types most encountered by clinical dermatologists are cold panniculitis, factitial panniculitis, and poststeroid panniculitis.

Cold Panniculitis

Cold panniculitis occurs primarily, but not exclusively, in children less than 3 years of age. The precise reason for this is unknown but may involve biochemical differences in fat composition. The panniculitis follows a rather characteristic evolution. Within 12 to 24 hours following exposure to intense (usually subfreezing) cold the patients develop erythema in exposed areas, which becomes indurated and plaquelike within days. The most common locations are uncovered areas (cheeks, chin), although covered areas can be affected. The lesions persist for weeks and disappear without sequelae. A burning sensation or discomfort may precede the eruption. Lesions often can be induced by topical ice application. Cases have been described in adults, particularly horseback riders.

Histopathologic studies have been performed on induced lesions at various stages of development. The earliest change is a lymphohistiocytic infiltrate appearing at the dermal subcutaneous junction. Later, adipocytes rupture, and the inflammatory infiltrate extends into the subcutaneous fat. The infiltrate consists primarily of mononuclear cells, although neutrophils and eosinophils may also be present. The infiltrate is primarily lobular, but small and medium-sized vessels may show a perivascular infiltrate.

Factitial Panniculitis

Factitial (self-induced) panniculitis is often the most difficult to diagnose. The patients present with multiple painful subcutaneous nodules in scattered random locations. The nodules may drain spontaneously and persist, or they may remit and recur. Systemic signs, such as fever and tachycardia, may be seen during acute episodes. History is of little value, as the patient may deny self-induced injury.

Often the only clue to the diagnosis is an index of suspicion by the clinician. The lesions may show a bizarre distribution or configuration that does not conform to any known panniculitis. The patient may exhibit signs of psychiatric disease such as egocentrism, immaturity, dependency, or depression. A history of multiple prior unexplained hospitalizations or surgical procedures is often obtained.

Biopsy specimens, similarly, do not conform to usual histologic patterns. A Weber-Christian-like histopathology, an acute inflammatory infiltrate, a fibrosing reaction, and a foreign body reaction all may be present. A useful clue is foreign material that can be detected by polarizing microscopy or routine x-ray.

Factitial panniculitis can be induced by any means. The most common pattern is self-injec-tion of foreign substances, usually pharmaceuticals. Organic materials including oil, silicone, and feces have been injected. Trauma should be suspected, especially if the lesions are ecchymotic, and in women and children abuse should always be suspected.

Poststeroid Panniculitis

Poststeroid panniculitis occurs in young children who have received a prolonged course of systemic steroids for renal or rheumatologic disease.[46] Once the steroids are discontinued, within 1 to 2 weeks the patients develop tender 0.5 to 4.0 cm subcutaneous nodules. The overlying skin is erythematous and warm, but ulceration or atrophy never occurs. The nodules resolve without sequelae within weeks to months.

The histopathologic changes are similar to those of sclerema neonatorum and subcutaneous fat necrosis of the newborn. Many adipocytes are replaced by needle-shaped clefts in radial array. Foam cells, giant cells, and lymphocytes may be scattered through the fat. No septal infiltrate is present.

PANNICULITIS AS AN INCIDENTAL FINDING

In many connective tissue disorders or large-vessel vasculitides, the panniculus may be secondarily involved, although this is not part of the primary pathology or clinical presentation.

Scleroderma

In scleroderma of all types the earliest changes occur in the panniculus.[47] A lymphohistiocytic infiltrate or germinal centers[48] are present within thickened subcutaneous trabeculae. The infiltrate may contain plasma cells or extend around eccrine coils. The subcutaneous fat is gradually replaced by a hyalinized collagen. In later stages the fibrosis becomes more acellular, with fewer inflammatory cells.[47]

Benign Cutaneous Periarteritis Nodosa

Benign cutaneous periarteritis nodosa presents as multiple tender erythematous nodules on the legs. Associated arthralgias, myalgias, and fever may occur, but there is no evidence of systemic disease. The nodules occur in crops and may either resolve spontaneously or ulcerate. Clinically, it resembles other types of panniculitis.[49]

Histologically, the primary pathology is a panarteritis of muscular arteries. Deep dermal or subcutaneous arteries show transmural inflammation, fibrinoid necrosis, or fragmentation of elastica. In the vicinity of the vessels, a focal mild panniculitis may be present. This lack of adipose inflammation distinguishes benign cutaneous periarteritis nodosa from other nodular panniculitides.[49]

Superficial Thrombophlebitis

Superficial thrombophlebitis also presents as multiple tender nodules, primarily on the lower extremities. An important clinical difference is that the lesions can be palpated as linear cords rather than discrete nodules. Systemic signs and symptoms are absent. Histology demonstrates thrombosis of medium and large veins, with subsequent destruction and degeneration of vessel walls. Periphlebitis and panniculitis may be associated but are usually minimal.

APPROACH TO THE PATIENT

Any patient with subcutaneous nodules should receive a thorough diagnostic workup. Panniculitis may be the first clue to an underlying systemic disease.

A complete history is of paramount importance. The patient should be queried as to the duration of the eruption, the life span of individual nodules, their locations, changes with climate, exacerbations or remissions, and the presence or absence of suppuration. Accompanying systemic signs and symptoms must be looked for. In particular, the patient should be asked about fever, sore throat, respiratory distress, joint pains, gastrointestinal disturbances, visual difficulties, or spontaneous bleeding. A personal or family history of tuberculosis or a past exposure to tuberculosis should be investigated. Drug history, use of oral contraceptives, and other habits should be evaluated.

Once the history has been obtained, a biopsy examination, except in clear-cut cases, is essential. A fully evolved lesion several weeks old, not a new or resolving lesion, should be selected. A fusiform incisional biopsy with adjacent normal skin and a depth to fascia should be taken. The specimen obtained must be serially sectioned, as histopathologic changes may be focal.

After the biopsy specimen has been examined, the panniculitis can be further subclassified. The pathologist should state whether it is primarily septal or lobular, whether a vasculitis is present or absent, whether foam cells are abundant, if caseation is present, and if other changes (e.g., ghost cells or needlelike clefts) are observed. A scheme for the pathologic evaluation of panniculitis is given in Figure 21–7.

If any pathognomonic features are present, such as acicular clefts, ghost cells, or hyaline necrobiosis, the diagnostic work-up is rather limited. The evaluation becomes complicated in two circumstances, a panniculitis of the indefinite type and erythema nodosum.

If the biopsy shows a preponderance of foam cells, an acute panniculitis, or features that do not allow a precise categorization, an extensive diagnostic work-up is indicated. Indefinite panniculitis probably represents a response to a variety of insults or injuries. Recommended baseline screens are shown in Table 21–2. If there is evidence of systemic disease, it is recommended that the patient have multiple biopsies, even of lymph nodes, to rule out systemic lymphoproliferative diseases (e.g., cytophagic panniculitis or malignant histiocytosis). If the features are those of a septal panniculitis (i.e., erythema nodosum), a rather extensive work-up is again indicated. This is listed in Table 21–3.

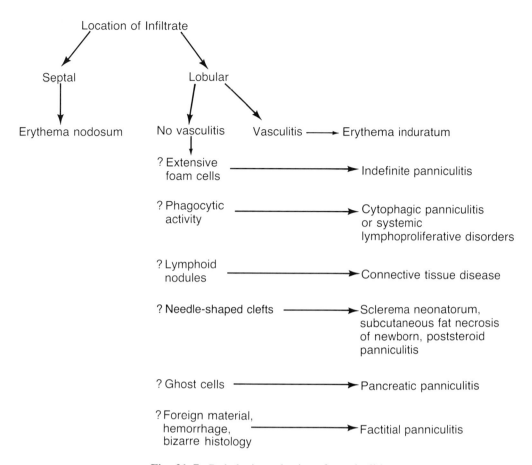

Fig. 21–7. Pathologic evaluation of panniculitis.

Tables 21–2 and 21–3 are intended to provide the clinician with a rough guide to the work-up of the patient with panniculitis. Clinical features should direct the work-up further. For example, in a patient with chronic diarrhea the gastrointestinal series with small bowel follow-through and barium enema are particularly important, since inflammatory bowel disease is a strong consideration. Similarly, a patient who comes from an endemic area for coccidioidomycosis should be investigated for that condition. The tests listed in these tables provide only a basic diagnostic approach to the patient with panniculitis. More detailed evaluation should be directed by initial test results.

Table 21-2. Approach to the Patient: Suggested Investigation for Indefinite Panniculitis

Complete blood count
Liver function tests
Amylase, lipase
α_1 antitrypsin
Polarization of biopsy specimen/history of abuse or trauma
Antinuclear antibodies
Lymph node biopsy or biopsy of other lesions if systemic panniculitis is present

Table 21-3. Approach to the Patient: Suggested Investigation in Patients with Septal Panniculitis

Chest x-ray
Gastrointestinal series with small bowel follow through
Barium enema
Complete blood count
Erythrocyte sedimentation rate
Antistreptococcal titers
Intradermal coccidiodin or histoplasmin
Careful drug history
Microbiologic studies as indicated (*Mycoplasma, Yersinia, Trichophyton, Streptococcus*, etc.)

REFERENCES

1. Ham AW, Cormack DH: Histology. 8th ed. JB Lippincott, Philadelphia, 1979
2. Weber FP: Relapsing nonsuppurative nodular panniculitis showing phagocytosis of subcutaneous fat by macrophages. Br J Dermatol 37:301, 1925.
3. Christian HA: Relapsing febrile nodular nonsuppurative panniculitis. Arch Intern Med 42:338, 1928
4. Hoyos N, Shaffer B, Beerman H: Liquefying nodular panniculitis. Arch Dermatol 94:436, 1965
5. Ciclitra PJ, Wigit DGD, Dick AP: Systemic Weber-Christian disease. Br J Dermatol 103:685, 1980
6. Steinberg B: Systemic nodular panniculitis. Am J Pathol 29:1059, 1953
7. DeGraciansky P: Weber-Christian syndrome of pancreatic origin. Br J Dermatol 79:278, 1967
8. Ackerman AB, Mosher DJ, Schwumin HA: Factitial Weber-Christian syndrome. JAMA 198:731, 1966
9. Bleunick E, Klokke HA: Protease-inhibitor deficiencies in a patient with Weber-Christian panniculitis. Arch Dermatol 120:936, 1984
10. Breit SW, Clark PC, Robinson JP, et al: Familial occurrence of α_1 antitrypsin deficiency and Weber-Christian disease. Arch Dermatol 119:198, 1983
11. Iwatsuk K, Tagami H, Yamacker M: Weber-Christian panniculitis with immunological abnormalities. Dermatologica 164:181, 1982
12. MacDonald A, Feiwel I: A review of the concept of Weber-Christian panniculitis with a report of five cases. Br J Dermatol 80:355, 1968
13. Cummins LJ, Lever WF: Relapsing febrile nodular nonsuppurative panniculitis. Arch Dermatol Syph 38:415, 1935
14. Forstrom L, Winkelmann RK: Acute panniculitis: a clinical and histopathologic study of 34 cases. Arch Dermatol 113:909, 1977
15. Winklemann RK, Burker JM: Factitial traumatic panniculitis. J Am Acad Dermatol 13:988, 1985
16. Tedeschi G: Pathological anatomy of adipose tissue. p. 141. In Renold AE, Cahill GF: Handbook of Physiology, vol. 5. Williams & Wilkins, Baltimore, 1965
17. Laymon CW, Peterson WL: Lipogranulomatosis subcutanea (Rothmann-Makai). An appraisal. Arch Dermatol 90:288, 1964
18. Chan HL: Panniculitis (Rothmann-Makai), with good response to tetracycline. Br J Dermatol 92:351, 1975
19. Ackerman BA: Histologic diagnosis of inflammatory skin disease: a method by pattern analysis. Lea & Febiger, Philadelphia, 1978
20. Fleiwel M, Munro DD: Diagnosis and treatment of erythema induratum (Bazin). Br Med J 2:1109, 1965
21. Forstrom L, Winkelmann RK: Granulomatous panniculitis in erythema nodosum. Arch Dermatol 111:335, 1975
22. Niemi KW, Forstrom L, Hannuksela M, et al: Nodules on the legs. A clinical, histological, and immunohistological study of 82 patients representing different types of nodular panniculitis. Acta Derm Venereol (Stockh) 57:145, 1977
23. Montgomery H, O'Leary PA, Barker NW: Nodular vascular diseases of the legs. Erythema induratum and allied conditions. JAMA 128:335, 1945
24. Parish WE, Rhodes EL: Bacterial antigens and aggregated gamma globulin in the lesions of nodular vasculitis. Br J Dermatol 79:131, 1967
25. Anderson SLC: Erythema induratum (Bazin) treated with isoniazid. Acta Derm Venereol (Stockh) 50:55, 1970
26. Forstrom L, Hannuksela M: Antituberculosis treatment of erythema induratum bazin. Acta Derm Venereol (Stockh) 50:143, 1970
27. Fine, RM, Meltzer HD: Chronic erythema nodosum. Arch Dermatol 100:33, 1969
28. Hannuksela M: Erythema nodosum migrans. Acta Derm Venereol (Stockh) 53:313, 1973
29. Rostas A, Lowe D, Smout MS: Erythema nodosum migrans in a young woman. Arch Dermatol 116:325, 1980
30. Hughes WE, Hammond ML: Sclerema neonatorium. J Pediatr 32:676, 1948
31. Kellum RE, Ray TL, Brown GK: Sclerema neonatorum. Report of case and analysis of subcutaneous and epidermal-dermal lipids by chromatographic methods. Arch Dermatol 97:372, 1968
32. Martin MM, Steven EM: Subcutaneous fat necrosis of the newborn with calcification of the tissues. Arch Dis Child 32:146, 1957.
33. Tsuji T: Subcutaneous fat necrosis of the newborn. Light and electron microscopic studies. Br J Dermatol 95:407, 1976
34. Crotty CP, Winkelmann RK: Cytophagic histiocytic panniculitis with fever, cytopenia, liver failure, and terminal hemorrhagic diathesis. J Am Acad Dermatol 4:181, 1981

35. Wick MR, Sanchez WP, Crotty CP, Winkelmann RK: Cutaneous malignant histiocytosis: a clinical and histopathologic study of eight cases, with immunohistochemical analysis. J Am Acad Dermatol 8:50, 1983

36. Spritz RA: The familial histiocytoses. Pediatr Pathol 8:43, 1985

37. Kadis ME, Kamain M, Lambery J: Erythrophagocytic T-gamma lymphoma—a clinicopathologic entity resembling malignant histiocytosis. N Engl J Med 304:648, 1981

38. Barron DR, Davis BR, Pomeranz JR, et al: Cytophagic histiocytic panniculitis: a variant of malignant histiocytosis. Cancer 55:2538, 1985

39. Potts DE, Mass MF, Iseman MD: Syndrome of pancreatic disease, subcutaneous fat necrosis and polyserositis. Case report and review of literature. Am J Med 58:417, 1975

40. Hughes PSH, Apisarnthanarox P, Mullins JF: Subcutaneous fat necrosis associated with pancreatic disease. Arch Dermatol 111:506, 1975

41. Bennet RB, Petrozzi JW: Nodular subcutaneous fat necrosis. A manifestation of silent pancreatitis. Arch Dermatol 111:896, 1975

42. Winkelmann RK, Peters MJ: Dermatol Update 135, 1982

43. Winkelmann RK: Panniculitis in connective tissue disease. Arch Dermatol 119:336, 1983

44. Izumi A, Takiyuchi P: Lupus erythematosus panniculitis. Arch Dermatol 119:61, 1983

45. Winkelmann RK, Padilla-Gonçalves A: Connective tissue panniculitis. Arch Dermatol 116:291, 1980

46. Roenigk HH, Haserick JR, Arundell FD: Poststeroid panniculitis. Arch Dermatol 90:387, 1964

47. Fleischmajer R, Newdich A: Generalized morphea. Histology of the dermis and subcutaneous tissue. Arch Dermatol 106:509, 1972

48. Harris RB, Duncan SC, Eicker RJ, Winkelmann RK: Lymphoid folliculitis subcutaneous inflammatory disease. Arch Dermatol 115:442, 1979

49. Diaz-Perez SL, Winkelmann RK: Cutaneous periarteritis nodosa. Arch Dermatol 110:407, 1974

22

Photosensitivity

Jeffrey D. Bernhard

Even when a patient knows that sunlight has contributed to the appearance of a rash, the precise diagnosis of a light-provoked or light-exacerbated disorder is usually not easy. When the patient is completely unaware that light exposure may be involved, it is even more difficult to establish a diagnosis. Only rarely are the physical findings by themselves pathognomonic, as they may be, for example, in solar urticaria. In few other areas of dermatology is the acquisition of a detailed history so important, and in few other areas of medicine is it likely to be so rewarding. In classical polymorphous light eruption (PMLE), for example, the history may be so characteristic that a presumptive diagnosis can occasionally be made on that basis alone. On the other hand, the history in certain types of chronic actinic dermatitis, such as actinic reticuloid, may occasionally be so vague, multifaceted, or misleading that only biopsy examination, phototesting, exclusion of other possibilities, and time will confirm the diagnosis.

Drugs are an important cause of photosensitivity and may produce a wide variety of cutaneous manifestations. Since the relationship between drug ingestion and rash is not always obvious, since the chronology is often not clearcut, and since there are no uniformly reproducible and safe ways to confirm drug involvement short of rechallenge, definitive diagnosis of drug-related photosensitivity is also difficult.

Since the photosensitive state in some instances may persist for some time even after a drug has been discontinued, the problem is confounded. Here again, time (as well as patience) becomes a critical diagnostic tool. Drug ingestion must be considered, reconsidered, and considered again in the differential diagnosis of any photosensitive eruption. Atypical presentations due to well-known photosensitizing drugs, as well as photosensitization by drugs that only rarely cause such problems, must be constantly borne in mind.

Tables 22-1 and 22-2 present a provisional listing and classification of abnormal reactions to light in humans.[1] The idiopathic photodermatoses present the greatest diagnostic challenge, and it is upon these that this chapter will concentrate. Disorders in the other categories will be considered only insofar as they pertain to the differential diagnosis of the idiopathic photodermatoses; further information on diagnoses not covered in detail here may be found in more exhaustive sources, such as Bernhard et al,[1] Harber and Bickers,[2] and Frain-Bell.[3]

It is customary to consider a group of medical disorders by considering the particular attributes of each disease in sequence. The utility of such an approach to the clinician faced with a diagnostic problem is predicated upon a presumed level of familiarity with the possibilities, the generation of a ranked differential diagnosis, and the subsequent matching of pertinent posi-

Table 22-1. Abnormal Reactions to Light in Humans

I. Genetic and metabolic disorders
  A. Light alone
    1. Ephelides (freckles)
    2. Xeroderma pigmentosum
    3. Bloom's syndrome
    4. Cockayne's syndrome
    5. Rothmund-Thomson syndrome
    6. Melanin deficiency syndromes
      a. Albinism
      b. Phenylketonuria
      c. Vitiligo
      d. Hypomelanotic individuals (skin type I)
  B. Light plus endogenous metabolite
    1. Certain porphyrias
    2. Disorders of tryptophan metabolism
      a. Hartnup syndrome
      b. Hydroxykynurenuria
      c. Carcinoid syndrome
      d. Pellagra
  C. Light plus exogenous chemical
    1. Hexachlorobenzene-induced porphyria turcica
    2. Alcohol- or estrogen-induced porphyria cutanea tarda

II. Idiopathic photodermatoses
  A. Acute intermittent photodermatoses (occurring or recurring within minutes to hours of single exposure)
    1. Polymorphous light eruption, and variants
    2. Solar urticaria
  B. Chronic persistent photodermatoses (chronic actinic dermatitis: acute exacerbations may occur)
    1. Photosensitive eczema
    2. Actinic reticuloid

III. Chemical photosensitivity
  A. Phototoxicity (acute and chronic; see Table 22-8)
  B. Photoallergy (acute and chronic; see Table 22-8)
  C. Persistent light reaction
  D. Phytophotodermatitis
  E. Certain genetic and metabolic disorders

IV. Degenerative and neoplastic disorders
  A. Dermatoheliosis
  B. Actinic keratoses
  C. Stucco keratoses
  D. Actinic granuloma
  E. Bowen's disease
  F. Squamous cell carcinoma
  G. Basal cell carcinoma
  H. Melanoma
  I. Idiopathic guttate hypomelanosis

V. Other disorders that can be precipitated or exacerbated by light—see Table 22-2.

(Modified from Bernhard JD, Pathak MA, Kochevar I, Parrish JA: Abnormal reactions to ultraviolet radiation. p. 1481. In Fitzpatrick TB, Eisen AZ, Wolff K, et al. (eds): Dermatology in General Medicine. 3rd ed. McGraw-Hill, New York, 1987. Reproduced with permission.)

Table 22-2. Other Disorders that Can Be Precipitated, Provoked, or Exacerbated by Light

Acne vulgaris
Atopic eczema
Bullous pemphigoid
Darier-White disease
Erythema multiforme
Hailey-Hailey disease
Herpes simplex labialis (recurrences)
Lichen planus
Lupus erythematosus
Pemphigus erythematosus
Pemphigus foliaceus
Pemphigus vulgaris
Physical occlusion of skin (increased susceptibility to sunburn)
Pityriasis alba
Pityriasis rubra pilaris
Pseudoporphyria
Psoriasis
Reticular erythematous mucinosis syndrome
Rosacea
Seborrheic dermatitis
Transient acantholytic dermatosis (Grover's disease)
Viral infections of the skin
Vitiligo

(Modified from Bernhard JD, Pathak MA, Kochevar I, Parrish JA: Abnormal reactions to ultraviolet radiation. p. 1481. In Fitzpatrick TB, Eisen AZ, Wolff K, et al. (eds): Dermatology in General Medicine. 3rd ed. McGraw-Hill, New York, 1987. Reproduced with permission.)

tive and negative findings to the standard descriptions. The major textbooks of dermatology and a number of monographic sources (e.g., Bernhard et al.[1] and Harber et al.[2]) are readily available and already provide the information required to follow such an approach to the photodermatoses. I therefore propose to consider the differential diagnosis of the patient who presents with photosensitivity or a photodistributed eruption, not by going through the usual systematic litany of disorders but by elaborating what I hope will be a clinically practical approach.

The main objective of the following approach is not only to arrive at the correct diagnosis but also to consider and exclude the most serious possibilities, such as lupus erythematosus (LE), expeditiously. Rather than giving a customary decision tree format, I propose to consider the problem of the patient who presents with presumed photosensitivity through a series of leading questions.

Is photosensitivity truly present, or is there an alternative explanation?

The dermatologist may consider photosensitivity in the differential diagnosis for one of several reasons. These include

1. Distribution of abnormal changes of the skin on exposed areas (i.e., photodistribution) (Fig. 22-1)
2. Complaint of sun sensitivity in the absence of such changes
3. Patient's statement that his or her problem is related to sunlight exposure

Any one or more of these possibilities permits entry into the photodermatosis algorithm. None is entirely specific, however. For example, an airborne or other contact dermatitis could lead to an apparent photodistribution. A complaint of sun sensitivity may be a misinterpretation of discomfort due to other causes, such as heat, or the patient could be mistaken in a conviction that sunlight exposure is the cause of his or her problem.[4] Therefore, the first order of business is to establish that the problem is in fact light-related. Criteria to support the proposition that photosensitivity is indeed present are listed in Table 22-3.

If no apparent pathologic changes of the skin can be observed and are said not to occur but the patient's chief complaint is one of burning or other strange sensations due to sun exposure, the diagnosis of erythropoietic protoporphyria (EPP) should be considered and excluded. The differential diagnosis of conditions that cause cutaneous symptoms without physical findings is given in Table 22-4, as it frequently arises in this context. If no changes are detectable on first glance, however, the skin should be examined even more closely. In EPP, for example, wrinkling and "weathering" of the skin in exposed areas may be detected on close inspection. In other instances the presence of telangiectasia may point to one of the congenital telangiectatic syndromes that may be associated with photosensitivity, such as Bloom's syn-

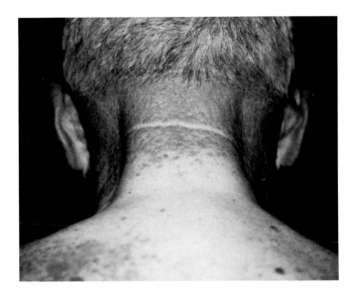

Fig. 22-1. Photoallergic eruption provoked by hydrochlorothiazide. Note spared areas behind the earlobes (Wilkinson's triangles) and in the deeply recessed skin folds ("bare bands") of the neck. (Bernhard JD, Pathak MA, Kochevar I, Parrish JA: Abnormal reactions to ultraviolet radiation. p. 1501. In Fitzpatrick TB, Eisen AZ, Wolff K, et al. (eds): Dermatology in General Medicine. 3rd ed. McGraw-Hill, New York, 1987. Reproduced with permission.)

Table 22-3. Criteria to Establish that a Problem is Presumptively Light Related

Historical grounds

Patient who is a reliable observer is able to provide a history in which features of the symptoms and signs, as well as exposure parameters, point clearly to specific light exposures.

The history (and physical findings) fail to provide any more likely explanation.

Objective grounds

The patient has abnormal findings on light-exposed skin, such as the nonshielded areas of the face, neck, hands, forearms, dorsa of feet, and V-area of chest. Additional findings on nonexposed areas may be present, and do not exclude possibility of light relatedness.

If such changes are absent on presentation they can be provoked by a controlled outdoor exposure and can then be observed by the physician.

Provocative light testing with artificial light sources produces observable abnormal responses.

Table 22-4. Differential Diagnosis of Conditions That May Cause Cutaneous Symptoms on Sun-Exposed Skin without Objective Physical Changes

Erythropoietic protoporphyria
Prodrome of herpes zoster
Prodrome of herpes simplex
Metabolic disorders (e.g., diabetes)
Flushing syndrome
Neurologic disorders
Dysesthesias/paresthesias due to contactants (e.g., synthetic pyrethroids, solvents)
?Subclinical drug sensitivity
?Subclinical chemical phototoxicity
Pruritus (due to systemic or other causes (e.g., aquagenic pruritus)
Delusional parasitosis (e.g., monosymptomatic hypochondriacal psychosis)

drome and Rothmund-Thomson syndrome. These disorders and their most prominent clinical features are listed in Table 22-5. An early age at onset and other related features should raise the index of suspicion and prompt referral to other sources of information.

If a rash is present on typical sun-exposed areas but is also present on usually shaded areas such as the submental region, the triangular areas shielded by the pinna of the ears, and the skin folds of the posterior neck, one must consider alternative possibilities, such as airborne or other contact dermatitis before too much time, energy, and money have been expended in exploring the photodermatoses route. This problem is severely confounded, however, by the likelihood that some airborne contact sensitizers may contribute to photosensitivity as well and by the fact that changes "spill over" on to covered skin in several photodermatoses, such as actinic reticuloid. In such circumstances observation after a controlled outdoor or artificial ultraviolet exposure may be required to confirm that photosensitivity is at play. A partial differential diagnosis of cutaneous eruptions that occur commonly on exposed areas but in which light exposure is not usually an important etiologic factor is given in Table 22-6. The differential diagnosis of facial edema, which may occur in photosensitive states but may also be due to many other causes, is given in Table 22-7.

Table 22-5. Hereditary Telangiectatic Syndromes with Photosensitivity[a]

Syndrome	Sites	Cutaneous Features	Other Features
Rothmund-Thomson syndrome	Face, arms, legs, buttocks	Erythema Mottled pigmentation Poikiloderma	Moderate dwarfism Sparse hair Cataracts
Bloom's syndrome	Butterfly area of face, forehead, ears, forearms	Erythema Papulosquamous lesions	Moderate dwarfism Neoplasia
Cockayne's syndrome	Butterfly area of face	Erythema Bullae Mottled pigmentation Atrophic scars	Physical and mental retardation Loss of subcutaneous fat on face Mickey Mouse ears

[a] The differential diagnosis includes the collagen-vascular disorders and the following hereditary telangiectatic syndromes not associated with photosensitivity: focal dermal hypoplasia, hereditary hemorrhagic telangiectasia, ataxia telangiectasia, and generalized essential telangiectasia.

(Modified from Rook A: Genetics in dermatology. p. 121. In Rook A, Wilkinson DS, Ebling FSG (eds): Textbook of Dermatology. 3rd ed. Blackwell Scientific Publications, Oxford, 1979.)

Table 22-6. Differential Diagnosis of Cutaneous Eruptions in Exposed Areas in which Light Exposure Is Not Usually an Important Factor

Acne vulgaris[a]
Rosacea
Seborrheic dermatitis
Contact dermatitis (allergic and irritant)
Impetigo
Erysipelas
Cellulitis
Eczematous dermatoses (e.g., atopic)
Erythema infectiosum
Physical urticarias other than solar
Angioedema
Other causes of facial edema (See Table 22-7)

[a] On occasion, acne can be exacerbated by sunlight exposure—so-called acne aestivalis.

Table 22-7. Differential Diagnosis of Facial Edema

Congenital
    Facial hemihypertrophy
    Infantile cortical hyperostosis
    Apert's syndrome
    McCune-Albright syndrome
    Hurler's syndrome; other storage diseases
    Sturge-Weber syndrome
Infectious
    Erysipelas
    Herpes zoster
    Leprosy
    Tuberculosis (lupus vulgaris)
    Trichinosis
Malignant
    Angiosarcoma
    Lymphoma
    Lymphosarcoma
    Mycosis fungoides
    Leukemia (particularly chronic lymphocytic leukemia)
Inflammatory
    Acne rosacea
    Lupus erythematosus
    Sarcoidosis (Heerfordt's syndrome)
    Angioedema
    Melkersson-Rosenthal syndrome
    Acne vulgaris
    Connective tissue panniculitis
    Allergic contact dermatitis
    Phototoxicity
    Photoallergy
Miscellaneous
    Myxedema
    Superior vena cava syndrome

(Modified from Connelly MG, Winkelmann RK: Solid facial edema as a complication of acne vulgaris. Arch Dermatol 121:87, 1985. Copyright 1985, American Medical Association.)

Is the patient taking any medications or are any potentially photosensitizing substances being used topically?

A list of some of the most commonly used photosensitizing chemicals is given in Table 22-8.[5] Since this table is not all-inclusive, the reader is advised to check on other specific medications as each case may require. Some medications act through phototoxic mechanisms, some through photoallergic mechanisms, and some probably through both. Given a sufficient dosage of chemical and an adequate exposure to ultraviolet radiation of the appropriate wavelength, drugs that act through a phototoxic mechanism will lead to an exaggerated sunburn-like reaction in any individual. In contrast, an element of individual susceptibility (specific immunologic responsiveness) is involved in abnormal reactions that appear to be due to a photoallergic mechanism. The practical importance of such a differentiation lies in its implications for treatment and prognosis. Broadly speaking, the treatment for a phototoxic reaction is to eliminate the offending chemical, provide appropriate symptomatic and supportive measures as required, and avoid the offending agent in the future, at least at dosages that caused the initial problem. The prognosis is good; there is little likelihood of persistent photosensitivity or rash provided the offending agent can be avoided. Although the treatment for a photoallergic reaction is similar, the potential for persistent photosensitivity and a slower response to treatment is greater.

While phototoxic reactions can be best likened to an exaggerated sunburn in which the cutaneous changes are continuous within exposed areas, photoallergic reactions most often present with discontinuous (nonconfluent) changes. These may consist of papules, papulovesicles, eczematous patches, and other changes that, at least at the outset, tend to be nonconfluent. Rubbing, scratching, and further evolution of the eruption may lead to areas of confluence, so it is important to learn from the history if the patient's rash started with discrete lesions that eventually became confluent or as a continuous confluent eruption.

Table 22-8. Some Commonly Used Drug Photosensitizers

Drug	Clinical Manifestations
Amiodarone	Delayed erythema, slate grey pigmentation
Benoxaprofen	Pruritus, delayed erythema, photo-onycholysis
Coal tar derivatives Anthralene Methylanthra- cene Acridine Phenathrene Benzo(a)pyrene	"Tar smarts," pricking sensation, erythema, melanosis
Furocoumarins Psoralen 5-methoxypsora- len 8-methoxypsora- len (methox- salen) 4,5,8-trime- thylpsoralen (trioxsalen)	Delayed erythema, phytophotodermatitis
Halogenated salicylanilides	Photoallergic contact dermatitis
Musk ambrette	Eczematous reaction
Nalidixic acid	Bullae, fragility, milia
Phenothiazines Chlorpromazine Thioridazine Promethazine Trimeprazine	Delayed erythema, eczematous reaction, slate gray pigmentation
Piroxicam	Bullae, delayed erythema
Quinidine	Delayed erythema
Sulfonamides	Delayed erythema, eczematous reaction
Sulfonylureas	Delayed erythema, eczematous reaction
Tetracyclines	Delayed erythema; photo-onycholysis, bullae, fragility, milia
Thiazides	Delayed erythema, eczematous reaction, lichenoid eruption, bullae
Quindoxin (quinoxa-line 1,4-dioxide)	Eczematous reaction
6-Methylcoumarin	Eczematous reaction

(Modified from Epstein JH, Wintroub BV: Photosensitivity due to drugs. Drugs 30:42, 1985.)

Unless the history, review of systems, and physical examination point to an alternative diagnosis, the patient who presents with photosensitivity and who is using one of the drugs or chemicals listed probably ought to be considered to have chemically induced photosensitivity until proven otherwise. The putatively culpable agent(s) should be discontinued insofar as possible. Unfortunately, improvement cannot be expected immediately. Not only does the initial acute insult require time to heal but some agents appear to induce sensitivity that may take weeks or even months to resolve. This seems to be the case particularly with photosensitivity induced by thiazides[6] (Fig. 22-1) and in the context of changes comprising the pseudoporphyria syndrome[7] (Fig. 22-2). The latter consists of abnormal skin fragility and bulla formation in sun-exposed areas in a pattern that closely resembles porphyria cutanea tarda but without any detectable abnormality in heme metabolism or porphyrin excretion. Pseudoporphyria has been associated with oral medications such as nalidixic acid, furosemide, and tetracycline, with systemic disease (diabetes mellitus or renal failure), and with hemodialysis. In addition, photosensitive eruptions with clinical, histologic, and serologic features of subacute lupus erythematosus were recently attributed to hydrochlorothiazide therapy in five patients whose eruptions cleared when the drug was discontinued.[8]

Photosensitivity due to a photocontact dermatitis can occasionally be confirmed by photopatch testing if the guilty antigen is part of the standard collection for photopatch testing or can be obtained. Photopatch testing is a fairly complex undertaking; details can be found in the references, particularly Bernhard et al.[1] and Harber and Bickers.[2] In this technique selected chemicals or products in question are applied as in standard patch testing but in duplicate and under opaque dressings to prevent light exposure. After 24 hours one set is examined for reactions and then exposed to either a standard dose of 10 joules/cm^2 ultraviolet A light (UVA) or less if the patient is abnormally sensitive to UVA alone. Both sets are examined subse-

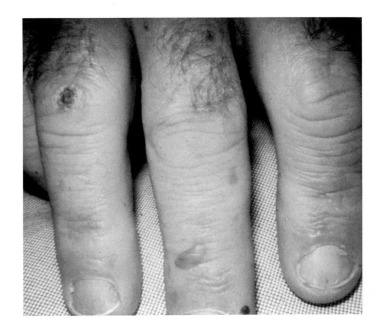

Fig. 22-2. Pseudoporphyria. Erosions and blisters on dorsum of the hand in a diabetic patient with renal failure.

quently for abnormal reactions that may occur as much as 7 days later. There are several variations of this technique, and individual modifications may be required for testing with certain chemicals, such as 6-methylcoumarin, which may show reactions more quickly over a period of hours. In addition to photopatch tests, routine phototesting for the minimal erythema dose and for abnormal immediate and delayed reactions to ultraviolet B light (UVB), UVA, and visible radiation may be performed.

In *phytophotodermatitis* a phototoxic reaction occurs after skin exposed topically to photosensitizing chemicals from certain plants has been additionally exposed to sunlight. One variant of phytophotodermatitis provoked by exposure to limes was recently dubbed "Club Med dermatitis,"[9] and an epidemic among produce handlers caused by furocoumarin exposure from celery was recently reported as well.[10] Although an acute reaction with vesicles and bullae may occasionally occur, an acute phase is often absent or undetected, and the patient may present merely with hyperpigmentation.

Unfortunately, no safe, standardized in vivo or in vitro tests are routinely available for the confirmation of chemical photosensitivity due to ingested drugs. Intradermal tests followed by irradiation and in vitro tests that utilize the patient's own lymphocytes have been reported from research centers and may be helpful in some cases, but these have not yet been perfected for routine clinical use.

Does the history point directly to a diagnosis of polymorphous light eruption, solar urticaria, or erythropoietic protoporphyria?

Although PMLE, solar urticaria, and EPP are certainly three very different disorders, they will be considered together at this point because the history in each can occasionally, if not frequently, be so distinctive that a presumptive diagnosis can be made almost immediately. Since polymorphous light eruption is the most common photodermatosis and since the history is often very typical, it is reasonable to approach the patient by considering it first in the differential diagnosis. Although solar urticaria is far less common (in fact, it is rare), the history, description of previous episodes, and physical findings are so distinctive that it deserves early consideration as well. As with other forms of hives, the cardinal feature of solar urticaria is evanescence. Solar urticaria usually occurs within minutes of sun exposure, whereas PMLE is more often delayed by hours.

As discussed earlier, a distinctive history, particularly smarting, stinging, or burning sensations of the face and hands during or immediately after sun exposure, is often elicited in EPP. Physical findings may remain rather subtle, but eventually waxy scars over the nose and dorsa of the hands, skin thickening in exposed areas, and weathering of the knuckles may become apparent. Since EPP is an autosomal dominant disorder, the family history may be helpful. A personal or family history of cholelithiasis can often be obtained in EPP as well. Acute skin reactions in EPP may consist of edematous plaques, erythema, purpura, and occasionally urticarial lesions; EPP must be considered in the differential diagnosis of all cases of solar urticaria and can be evaluated by appropriate porphyrin analyses of urine (normal porphyrins), feces (elevated protoporphyrin), and red blood cells and plasma (elevated protoporphyrin and fluorescence of red cells in a fresh preparation).

Typically, PMLE presents as an eruption of papules or papulovesicles on exposed areas following sun exposure. Perhaps because of chronic ambient UV exposure and "hardening," the face is often spared. Patients can frequently remember the specific time and place at which their first episode took place, often on a trip to sunny regions in the lower latitudes. Some people experience recurrences only on returning to such places; others begin to have episodes during subsequent springs and summers even at home. In many patients solar sensitivity and the intensity of the eruption seem to worsen over the years. In most the problem is worse in spring and early summer and diminishes as hardening occurs during the remainder of the summer. The rash usually occurs after a latent interval (lag time) of between 2 hours and 5 days after exposure and subsides over the next 7 to 10 days. In contrast, the lag time

for appearance of solar urticaria is usually much shorter, with lesions most often appearing while the patient is outdoors and persisting for only minutes to hours. In both, itching is almost always present and occasionally precedes the eruption. Differentiation between the more persistent papules of PMLE and the more evanescent wheals of solar urticaria should not be difficult on either physical examination or historical grounds.

Although it may be possible to arrive at a presumptive diagnosis from the history, every effort must be made to see the eruption. Depending on the patient's observational abilities, what sounds like PMLE or solar urticaria to the clinician could turn out to be recurrent sun-provoked herpes labialis or miliaria. Other possibilities, such as a contact reaction to a sun screen or cosmetic product have to be considered as well. If the patient comes in after an episode but with no eruption, it is often possible to reproduce solar urticaria by sending the patient outdoors to return within a few hours. If the history indicates PMLE, the patient can be instructed to try to provoke the rash before a follow-up visit in a few days. If this approach is not feasible, it may be desirable to try to elicit the rash by provocative light testing. In this technique, the minimal erythema doses of UVB and UVA are determined by administering gradually increasing doses of each to small (about 1 cm^2) squares on the back, buttocks, or previously involved areas (which probably have the highest yield) and then administering multiples of this dose. As much as 50 to 100 joules of UVA may be required.[11] Especially in PMLE, however, provocative light testing with artificial UV sources can be time-consuming and difficult. In any event it is usually worthwhile to obtain a biopsy of the provoked eruption for final confirmation of the diagnosis and for exclusion of other possibilities. Despite the designation polymorphous, PMLE is usually monomorphous in a single patient. The existence and nature of so-called plaque-type and eczematous PMLE is problematic; it is not difficult to imagine such changes resulting as secondary consequences of rubbing and scratching.

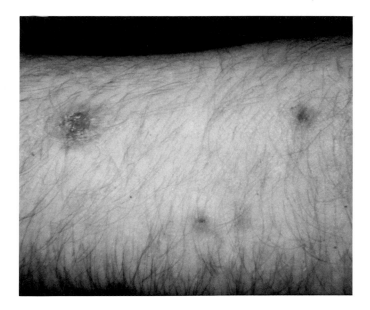

Fig. 22-3. Hydroa vacciniforme. Papules, papulovesicles, and excoriated papules which heal with scarring in an adolescent boy.

If the history or physical findings do not support the proposition that the initial lesions were papular or papulovesicular, one must seriously consider alternative diagnoses, such as subacute cutaneous LE [antinuclear antibody-negative, Ro-positive lupus]. A number of other idiopathic photodermatoses are sometimes regarded as variants of PMLE. These include Hutchinson's summer prurigo (prurigo aestivale), actinic prurigo, hydroa vacciniforme (Fig. 22-3), and hereditary PMLE of American Indians. Except for certain areas in which the latter may be seen with some frequency, the others are so rare that they are not often seen even at referral clinics for light-related disorders, and further information about them should be sought in the references.

Does the patient have lupus?

To put it quite simply, it is my practice to exclude the possibility of systemic LE by appropriate serological testing in any patient who presents with the complaint or findings of photosensitivity (Figs. 22-4 to 22-6). I obtain an ANA test in every case and when appropriate, perform tests for ANA-negative LE as well (anti-Ro and anti-La antibodies). Photosensitive

dermatitis is an important presenting complaint of so-called ANA-negative, Ro-positive, subacute cutaneous LE, which may occur on the malar area of the face and in which distinctive annular lesions also occur (Fig. 22-6). All patients with photosensitivity should be questioned about other signs and symptoms associated with lupus. Solar urticaria is said to be a rare presentation of lupus; some cases of so-called plaque-type PMLE should also be followed carefully for that possibility. Lesions of discoid LE are often most prominent on sun-exposed areas; these lesions, which include erythema, telangiectasia, pigmentary changes, follicular plugging, scaling, atrophy, and scarring, are easily recognized by the trained observer (Fig. 22-5).

Are scarring, milia, hypertrichosis, or bullae present?

If scarring, milia, hypertrichosis or bullae are present, porphyrin studies of urine, blood, and stool should be considered to exclude porphyria cutanea tarda (PCT) (Fig. 22-7), variegate porphyria (VP), EPP, and other members of the porphyria group. It is critical to remember that PCT and VP can be clinically indistinguish-

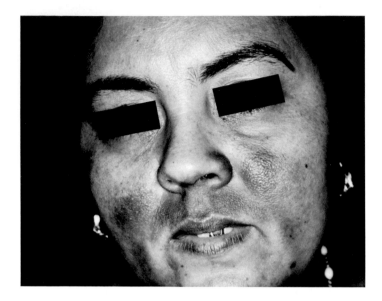

Fig. 22-4. Systemic lupus erythematosus. Photosensitive malar eruption.

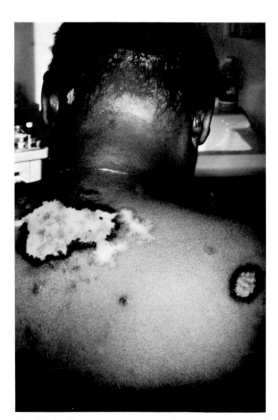

Fig. 22-5. Cutaneous lupus erythematosus. Typical discoid lesions.

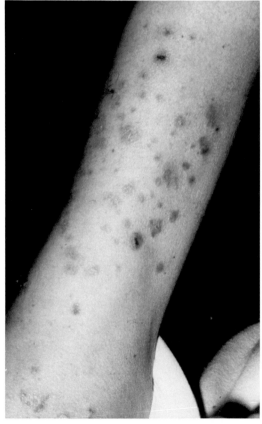

Fig. 22-6. Subacute cutaneous lupus erythematosus in a patient who had anti-Ro antibodies but whose ANA determination was negative.

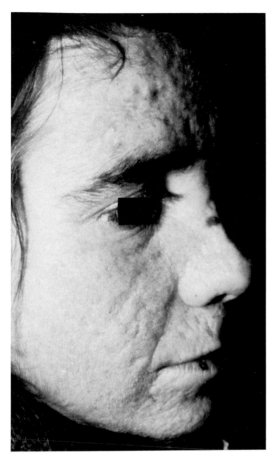

Fig. 22-7. Porphyria cutanea tarda provoked by excessive ethanol ingestion and oral contraceptive agents in a young woman.

able, so that stool porphyrin analysis must be performed in addition to quantitative analysis of 24-hour urinary porphyrin excretion. At the bedside laboratory Wood's lamp examination of a random urine sample acidified by adding a few drops of 10 percent hydrochloric or acetic acid will often confirm the diagnosis of PCT by revealing orange-red fluorescence. It is also important to recognize that patients are often unaware that sunlight plays a role in producing the lesions of PCT and VP.

Aside from the cutaneous findings, other features may point toward one or another of the various porphyrias. These include, for example, the family history (e.g., autosomal dominance in VP), a detailed history of drug and/or chemical exposure (e.g., alcohol or oral contracep-

tives in PCT), and the presence of abdominal pain or neurologic changes (e.g., acute attacks of gastrointestinal symptoms in VP). The specific diagnosis can then be made by appropriate assessment of biochemical parameters, including abnormal excretory patterns and enzymatic defects. For a thorough approach to the diagnosis of porphyria, the reader is referred to Bickers and Pathak.[12]

Scarring, atrophy, pigmentary changes, follicular plugging, and telangiectasia, especially when all present together, point to a diagnosis of discoid lesions of LE (Fig. 22-5).

Bullae in sun-exposed areas are also noted in phototoxic reactions, phytophotodermatitis, and the pseudoporphyria syndrome (which may also be drug-induced). One must, of course, also consider the entire range of non-sun-induced bullous disorders in the differential diagnosis, with the following proviso: Several classic bullous diseases that are not usually conceptualized as photosensitive (for example, pemphigus, especially pemphigus erythematosus, pemphigoid, and Hailey-Hailey disease) can be exacerbated by UV radiation exposure.

Is telangiectatic erythema present?

The presence of telangiectatic erythema again raises the question of a collagen-vascular disorder, particularly lupus or dermatomyositis. Telangiectases, often "matted" or collected prominently in polyangular macules, are notable in scleroderma and may be more pronounced in sun-exposed areas.

On the other hand, telangiectasia and erythema may point merely to rosacea, dermatoheliosis (the term used to describe the constellation of findings in chronic actinic damage to the skin), or the hereditary telangiectatic syndromes listed in Table 22-5.

Are eczematous or infiltrated plaques present?

The differential diagnosis of eczematous lesions in sun-exposed areas ranges from simple atopic eczema to photoexacerbated atopic eczema, from simple contact dermatitis to photocontact dermatitis, and from photosensitive eczema to actinic reticuloid. The physical examination may provide very helpful clues. The presence of lesions in non-sun-exposed areas may point away from light involvement, but not reliably so. Lesions of a photoexacerbated eruption do not require sunlight exposure and so may be present in any location in which they are prone to occur for other reasons. Furthermore, the eruptions of photosensitive eczema and actinic reticuloid frequently spill over to non-sun-exposed areas. These two chronic persistent photodermatoses tend to occur in older men. Along with persistent light reactivity caused by antecedent drug or chemical exposure, they form a group, sometimes labeled *chronic actinic dermatitis,* with a number of features in common, including eczematous morphology and a tendency to acute exacerbations.

In actinic reticuloid clinical and histologic changes resemble those seen in cutaneous T-cell lymphoma (mycosis fungoides). Photosensitive eczema seems to develop in some older men after many years of eczema of various types. Its action spectrum lies in the UVB range, and patients tend to have a lowered minimal erythema dose on exposure to UVB. In actinic reticuloid the action spectrum is usually broader and often includes not only UVB but also UVA and visible radiation. Patients whose photosensitivity was originally provoked by chemicals but who remain photosensitive for months to years despite careful avoidance are called *persistent light reactors.* These patients are often markedly sensitive to UVA and UVB. Cases in which transitions from photosensitive eczema or persistent light reactivity to actinic reticuloid occur have been reported. Especially when there are infiltrated plaques, the diagnosis of actinic reticuloid must be considered, and a biopsy should be performed. In the setting of eczematous changes in a photodistribution, not only the histopathology but also the history is indispensable. Only the most detailed and painstaking history, going back to antecedent skin disorders and to every conceivable exposure, will permit progress through the complicated maze of interacting possibilities (e.g., atopic eczema eventuating in photosensitive eczema, photocontact dermatitis or persistent light reactivity eventuating in actinic reticuloid, and/or drugs or even sun screens complicating the entire clinical picture.)

Is photosensitivity acute and intermittent, with clearing between episodes, or is it chronic, with acute exacerbations and a tendency for skin changes to persist between exacerbations?

Within minutes of meeting the patient the distinction of acute intermittent photosensitivity, with clearing between episodes, from chronic photosensitivity, with acute exacerbations and a tendency for skin changes to persist between exacerbations, may be apparent. This distinction is most helpful in classifying the idiopathic photodermatoses, as indicated in Table 22-1. For example, solar urticaria and PMLE fall clearly into the acute intermittent group, in which the skin returns to normal between episodes, which may occur every summer. On the other hand, the skin tends to remain abnormal between acute exacerbations of actinic reticuloid, although clearing may occur.

APPROACH TO THE PATIENT WITH PHOTOSENSITIVITY

The most important components of the history, physical examination, and laboratory evaluation are summarized in Table 22-9. If the approach outlined here is not sufficient to lead to a reasonably likely diagnosis, one is probably dealing with a case that is either sufficiently complex or sufficiently rare that further investigation at a referral center specializing in photosensitivity disorders may be assumed to be warranted. Such a center would be equipped to undertake more sophisticated phototesting. Furthermore, the rarity of some of the photodermatoses has prohibited the collection of series large enough to provide a sufficiently practical approach to their diagnosis.

Table 22-9. Approach to the Patient with Photosensitivity

History

Age at onset of photosensitivity (e.g., early age-at-onset may imply genetic component)

Occupation, leisure activities, and possible chemical exposures

Topical applications (including cosmetic products, sunscreens, contact with plants, chemicals)

Past history of response to sun exposure (susceptibility to sunburn; skin type)

Medications: topical or oral

Family history (photosensitivity, atopy; gallstones and cholecystitis can occur in erythropoietic protoporphyria)

Exposure parameters

Minimum duration of sun exposure to elicit reaction

Lag period between exposure and eruption

Seasonal and geographic variation in incidence and severity (results of provocation tests with artificial light sources if indicated/required)

Eruption (physical features and additional historical aspects)

Morphology (e.g., hives, blisters, papules, papulovesicles, eczematous lesions)

Distribution (exposed versus nonexposed; absence in shaded areas)

Accompanying or premonitory symptoms (itching, burning sensation, swelling, dizziness)

Is the morphology that of an exaggerated sunburn, or of a discontinuous eruption?

Does the rash appear without sunlight exposure?

Are findings typical for any of the diseases listed in the tables (such as lupus erythematosus or disseminated superficial actinic porokeratosis) present?

Laboratory investigation (as indicated)

Antinuclear antibody determination

Anti-Ro (SSA) and anti-La (SSB) antibodies

Skin biopsy

Direct immunofluorescence on biopsy specimen

Porphyrin analyses

Phototesting and photopatch testing

REFERENCES

1. Bernhard JD, Pathak MA, Kochevar I, Parrish JA: Abnormal reactions to ultraviolet radiation. p. 1481. In Fitzpatrick TB, Eisen AZ, Wolff K, et al. (eds): Dermatology in General Medicine. 3rd ed. McGraw-Hill, New York, 1987

2. Harber LC, Bickers DR: Photosensitivity Diseases. Principles of Diagnosis and Management. WB Saunders, Philadelphia, 1981

3. Frain-Bell W (ed): Photodermatoses. Semin Dermatol 1:153, 1982

4. Bernhard JD, Parrish JA: Nonrashes. 2. Solatics. Cutis 29:253, 1982

5. Epstein JH, Wintroub B: Photosensitivity due to drugs. Drugs 30:42, 1985

6. Robinson HN, Morison WL, Hood AF: Thiazide diuretic therapy and chronic photosensitivity. Arch Dermatol 121:522, 1985

7. Harber LC, Bickers DR: Porphyria and pseudoporphyria. J Invest Dermatol 82:207, 1984

8. Reed BR, Huff JC, Jones SK, et al: Subacute cutaneous lupus erythematosus associated with hydrochlorothiazide therapy. Ann Intern Med 103:49, 1985

9. White W: Club Med Dermatitis. N Engl J Med 314:319, 1986

10. Berkley SF, Hightower AW, Beier RC, et al: Dermatitis in grocery workers associated with high natural concentrations of furanocoumarins in celery. Ann Intern Med 105:351, 1986

11. Hozle E, Plewig G, Hofmann C, Roser-Maass E: Polymorphous light eruption. Experimental reproduction of skin lesions. J Am Acad Dermatol 7:111, 1982

12. Bickers DR, Pathak MA: The porphyrias. p. 1666. In Fitzpatrick TB, Eisen AZ, Wolff K, et al. (eds): Dermatology in General Medicine. 3rd ed. McGraw-Hill, New York, 1987

23

The Dermatoses of Pregnancy

George B. Winton[*]

The specific dermatoses of pregnancy are a confusing group of diseases, which are presumably unique to pregnancy and the puerperium and which share many overlapping features. Over the years a total of 10 entities have been described; however, it has become clear that not all of them are distinct and some of them may not be specific to the gestational state. A provisional classification of these diseases and review of their diagnostic features will aid the clinician in making a difficult diagnosis.

The complete list of these 10 dermatoses of pregnancy is as follows:

1. Herpes gestationis (HG)
2. Impetigo herpetiformis (IH)
3. Pruritus gravidarum (PG)
4. Autoimmune progesterone dermatitis of pregnancy (Bierman[1])
5. Pruritic urticarial papules and plaques of pregnancy (PUPPP)
6. Pruritic folliculitis of pregnancy
7. Prurigo of pregnancy (Besnier/Nurse[2])
8. Toxemic rash of pregnancy (Bourne[3])
9. Papular dermatitis of pregnancy (PDP) (Spangler[4])
10. Prurigo annularis (Davies[5])

The last four of these diseases have been particularly troublesome for clinicians, as there was no histologic data in their original descriptions, and their clinical features are similar both to each other and to those of the more recently described PUPPP. Two other diseases, IH and pruritic folliculitis of pregnancy, are considered by some clinicians to occur coincidentally in pregnancy rather than to have a specific relation to the gestational period. And finally, autoimmune progesterone dermatitis of pregnancy has been seen in only the single patient reported by Bierman.[1]

It was considerations such as these that in 1979 led Fitzpatrick et al.[6] to remark that the practical differential diagnosis of the eruptions of pregnancy only includes four diseases, namely, HG, IH, PG, and PUPPP, and that the other previously described entities must await more solid clinical and histologic description to be useful diagnostic concepts. Suggestions for grouping certain of the five overlapping dermatoses under a single title were made almost 20 years ago by Nurse,[2] who felt that prurigo of pregnancy and toxemic rash were

[*]The opinions expressed are those of the author and are not to be construed as official or as reflecting the views of the Department of the Army or the Department of Defense.

419

Table 23-1. Classification of the Dermatoses of Pregnancy

Clearly defined entities
    Herpes gestationis
    Pruritic urticarial papules and plaques of pregnancy
    Pruritus gravidarum
    Impetigo herpetiformis
    Autoimmune progesterone dermatitis of pregnancy
Provisionally classified entities
    Prurigo of pregnancy
    Pruritic folliculitis of pregnancy
Classification uncertain
    Papular dermatitis of pregnancy

(Modified from Holmes RC, Black MM: The specific dermatoses of pregnancy. J Am Acad Dermatol 8:405, 1983.)

the same disease and that papular dermatitis of pregnancy might well be the same except for its associated high fetal mortality. Sasseville et al.[5] more recently suggested that all five diseases could effectively be unified under the name prurigo gestationis.

Certain questions arise. Are these simplified classifications suggested by Fitzpatrick, Nurse, and Sasseville still valid in the light of current knowledge? Is there a straightforward approach to the diagnosis of these diseases? What new information is available regarding controversies about certain of these entities?

Table 23-1 provides a current classification of the specific dermatoses of pregnancy. For completeness, all diseases not known to be duplicates of others have been included.

OLDER ENTITIES EXCLUDED FROM CLASSIFICATION

Prurigo Annularis

Prurigo annularis was described in 1941 by Davies,[5] who noted an eruption consisting of scaly, hyperpigmented rings varying in diameter from 7 to 38 cm and distributed over the trunk and proximal limbs. The lesions occurred either early or late in pregnancy and could persist for years thereafter. No histology or laboratory data were reported, and Davies' two cases constitute the only report of this disease in the

literature; therefore, if this disorder is being seen today it is probably being called by some other name. Lack of a biopsy means that certain coincidental causes of annular skin lesions in pregnancy, such as erythema annulare centrifugum, sarcoidosis, and subacute cutaneous lupus erythematosus, were not ruled out.

Toxemic Rash of Pregnancy

In 1962 Bourne[3] described an intensely pruritic rash occurring late in pregnancy in 22 women. His description of pruritic red wheals and papules so closely resembles the more recently reported PUPPP that it is very likely that these two diseases are the same.[5,7]

Late-Onset Prurigo of Pregnancy

Prurigo gestationis was first described by Besnier in 1904 and reviewed by Nurse in 1962 under the name *prurigo of pregnancy*.[2] Nurse divided the eruption into two types, one affecting extensor surfaces of the extremities and occurring in the second trimester and the other occurring on the abdomen and proximal extremities late in the third trimester. The late form is clinically indistinguishable from PUPPP in the original description, while the early form may be a separate disease entirely, as will be seen.

CLEARLY DEFINED DERMATOSES

Herpes Gestationis

Herpes gestationis is a pruritic, vesiculobullous skin disease of pregnancy and the puerperium, which so closely resembles bullous pemphigoid that the name *pemphigoid gestationis* is favored by some dermatologists.[7] Although herpetiform vesicular skin lesions can be seen in some patients, there is no evidence of a viral etiology.

Clinical Presentation. Onset may occur any time between the ninth week of gestation and the first week postpartum but is most frequent in the second trimester. Many patients experience a prodrome of fever, malaise, nausea, headache, and burning or itching of the skin. Lesions usually begin as patchy erythema and urticarial edema, with severe pruritus localized initially to the abdomen and spreading subsequently to the buttocks, the remainder of the trunk, and the extremities. Within a few days, papules, vesicles, and bullae develop (Figs. 23-1 and 23-2). The oral mucosa is generally spared.[8] Even in mild cases a predilection for the umbilicus can be seen (Fig. 23-3). Recently, a pustular presentation of HG was described in which clear vesicles were not seen.[9]

Histology. Urticarial lesions demonstrate a superficial and deep perivascular infiltrate of lymphocytes, histiocytes, and eosinophils. There is spongiosis, upper dermal edema, and necrosis of basal cells at the dermal papillae. Eosinophils are sometimes seen in spongiotic foci. Vesicles and bullae also show subepidermal separation of the blister due to necrosis of basal cells. Ultrastructurally, the plane of blister formation is in the lamina lucida.

Immunofluorescence. Direct immunofluorescence usually demonstrates a bandlike deposit of complement component C3 with or without IgG at the basement membrane zone (BMZ). Deposits seen less commonly include IgA, IgM, Clq, C4, C5, and properdin.[5,10] Conventional indirect immunofluorescence is positive in only 20 to 25 percent of cases; however, circulating HG factor, an avid complement-fixing IgG autoantibody, is usually present in the serum at low titer.[5,7,10] Its presence can be detected by indirect immunofluorescence microscopy with use of a complement fixation technique.[11]

Laboratory Tests. An elevated white blood count with eosinophilia as high as 50 percent may be present.[12] Of great current interest are reports of HLA typing both in patients with HG and in their mates. Patients have an increased frequency of the HLA-DR3 and DR4 combination.[13,14] This association extends to black women with the disease, in whom both HG and HLA DR4 are quite uncommon.[15] Mates of patients with HG have a higher frequency of HLA-DR2, and antibodies to this antigen can be detected is some patient sera.[15,16]

Course. The disease waxes and wanes throughout pregnancy, with clearing usually occurring within 3 months after delivery. The patient of Fine and Omura,[17] who experienced persistent disease activity for 11 years postpartum, is a notable exception. A return of pruritus or skin lesions with menstruation or with the use of oral contraceptives can occur.[18] A recurrence of disease in subsequent pregnancies with earlier onset and a more severe course is typical, although occasional patients have no subsequent disease at all.[18] The occurrence of "skip" pregnancies does not completely correlate with the HLA type of the father.[14]

The prognosis for the fetus in HG-affected gestations has been debated for many years. Kolodny reviewed the literature in 1969 and could find no solid evidence of poor fetal outcome.[19] However, Lawley et al.,[20] adding immunologic criteria to the diagnosis of 40 cases, found increased rates of stillbirth and prematurity. Holmes et al.[21] found similar rates of prematurity but no fetal deaths among 24 patients. Shornick et al.[18] could find no increased morbidity or mortality in their 28 patients but noted a transient skin eruption morphologically similar to HG in 5 percent of neonates.

Differential Diagnosis. Herpes gestationis is the only specific dermatosis of pregnancy that produces blisters; however, its early papular or urticarial stage can easily be confused with PUPPP. If a patient presents with the rare pustular form of HG, it is necessary to rule out IH.

A secondary differential diagnosis may be

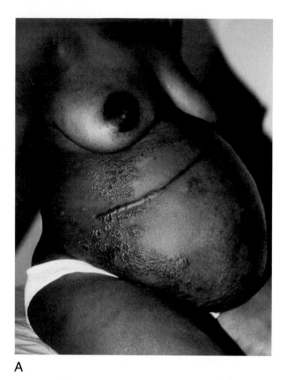

A

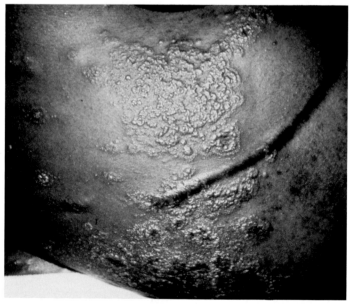

B

Fig. 23-1. **(A)** Several types of skin lesions are scattered over the abdomen in this rare case of herpes gestationis in a black patient. **(B)** A closer view shows vesicles and bullae arranged in a polycyclic configuration. Several lesions are targetoid in appearance, and a few urticarial papules can be seen. (Photographs courtesy of Robert T. Horn, M.D., Ithaca, NY.)

of greater importance and would include blistering diseases coincidentally occurring in pregnancy, such as pemphigus vulgaris, pemphigus foliaceus, dermatitis herpetiformis, and bullous drug eruption.[22] Appropriate biopsies and direct and indirect immunofluorescence studies should allow differentiation of these diseases. In rare instances, vesicular viral eruptions such as

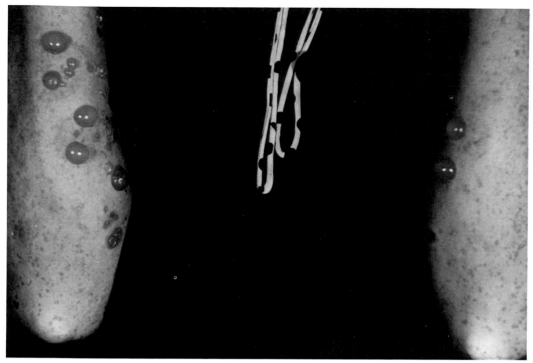

Fig. 23-2. Tense blisters on the forearms can be seen in this patient with severe herpes gestationis. (Photograph courtesy of Charles W. Lewis, M.D., San Antonio, TX.)

herpes zoster, herpes simplex, or varicella might cause confusion; however, smears or cultures should distinguish them.

Pruritic Urticarial Papules and Plaques of Pregnancy

Pruritic urticarial papules and plaques of pregnancy is a benign, pruritic eruption of late pregnancy described by Lawley and coworkers[23] in 1979. It was believed by them to be a distinctive entity; however, there is a growing consensus that the disease is the same as Bourne's toxemic rash and the late form of Nurse's prurigo of pregnancy.[5,7,24,25] Descriptions have appeared in the literature under various titles, including polymorphic eruption of pregnancy, toxic erythema of pregnancy, and erythema multiforme of pregnancy.[7] It is the most common of the dermatoses of pregnancy, with an incidence of 1/200 to 1/300.[7,21,24]

Clinical Presentation. The disease occurs most commonly in primagravidas: 76 percent in two major series.[21,26] The skin eruption usually begins after the thirty-fourth week of gestation with the sudden appearance of pruritic, erythematous papules and urticarial plaques over the abdomen. Lesions often begin within periumbilical striae distensae and soon spread to involve the thighs, buttocks, upper inner arms, lower back, and occasionally the breasts, hands, or feet (Fig. 23-4). Blanched halos are seen at the periphery of some lesions,[26] and vesiculation has been reported.[21,26,27]

Histology. In the superficial dermis there is a mild to moderate perivascular infiltrate of lymphocytes, histiocytes, and occasional eosinophils. Upper dermal edema is usually present. The epidermis may be normal or may show focal parakeratosis, spongiosis, and acanthosis.[7,21,23,27]

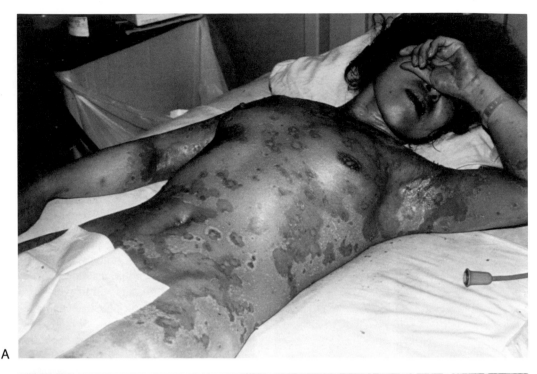

A

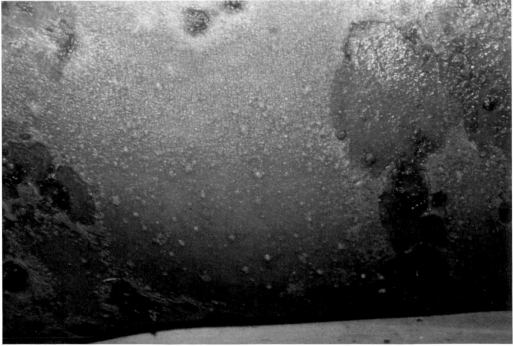

B

Fig. 23-5. (A) The characteristic skin lesions of impetigo herpetiformis are seen in this Oriental woman. Widespread patches of erythema, some with crusting and impetiginization, can be seen. The axilla is most severely affected. Elsewhere, individual, scattered pustules are also visible. **(B)** A closer view better demonstrates the typical small pustules characteristic of the disease. (Photographs courtesy of Eric W. Kraus, M.D., San Antonio, TX.)

sometimes tetany secondary to hypocalcemia. Dehydration, prostration, and convulsions can occur.

Initial skin lesions consist of patches of erythema with tiny pustules at the margins. Intertriginous areas are preferentially involved, sometimes with subsequent peripheral extension until the entire body is affected. (Fig. 23-5). As pustules break down, crusting and impetiginization occur centrally. Vegetating plaques may develop in flexural areas, and onycholysis secondary to subungual pustule formation can occur.

Histology and Immunofluorescence. The histologic changes are identical to those of pustular psoriasis. The spongiform pustule of Kogoj, a collection of neutrophils arising within a focus of spongiotic epidermis, is characteristic[12] (Fig. 23-6). Other changes include parakeratosis, regular elongation of the rete ridges, and exocytosis of mononuclear cells. Immunofluorescent studies are negative.

Laboratory Tests. An elevated white blood cell count and sedimentation rate are common in severe cases. Hypocalcemia secondary to hypoparathyroidism can also be seen. Bacterial cultures of skin lesions and blood are negative.

Course. Without modern supportive care many patients in the past succumbed to renal or cardiac failure, hyperthermia, or prostration. Correction of hypocalcemia or of fluid and electrolyte imbalance and the use of systemic corticosteroids now make maternal death rare, although the fetal mortality rate is still significant.[35] The skin eruption clears postpartum, usually without residual psoriatic plaques but may recur in subsequent pregnancies. The case of Oumeish et al,[34] in which IH recurred

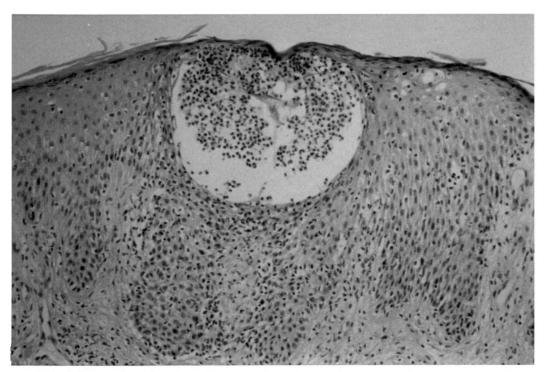

Fig. 23-6. The spongiform pustule of Kogoj is the characteristic histologic finding in impetigo herpetiformis. A collection of neutrophils arises within an area of spongiotic epidermis. (Photograph courtesy of Donald E. Clemons, M.D., Johnson City, TN.)

in nine successive pregnancies, none of which produced a viable offspring, illustrates the devastating consequences of severe disease.

Differential Diagnosis. The combination of a pustular eruption and severe constitutional symptoms are unique to IH. Mild forms might be confused with pustular or impetiginized HG, but biopsy and immunofluorescent studies should distinguish the two disorders. Bierman's autoimmune progesterone dermatitis also produces pustules; however, both the morphology and histology of the lesions are different from those of IH lesions.

Candidiasis[36] and subcorneal pustular dermatosis of Sneddon and Wilkinson[35] can also resemble IH. The former can be ruled out by smears and cultures. The latter is usually seen in middle-aged to elderly patients, is not hormonally modulated, and usually responds to sulfonamides.

Autoimmune Progesterone Dermatitis of Pregnancy

In 1973 Bierman[1] described an acneiform eruption with associated arthritis in successive pregnancies of an East Indian woman. Although a detailed investigation was performed and an association with the hormonal changes of pregnancy was established, there have been no subsequent reports of similar disease in other patients. Until confirmatory data are available, some authors prefer to exclude this disease from the group of pregnancy-related skin disorders.

Clinical Presentation. A 25-year-old East Indian woman developed an explosive, acneiform eruption within 2 weeks of conception in successive pregnancies. The eruption began on the fingers, arms, and legs and rapidly spread to involve the buttocks. Individual lesions consisted of follicular and perifollicular comedones, papules, and pustules. As the disease progressed, the pustules became large, firm, and turbid, and an arthritis of the wrists, knees, ankles, and metacarpophalangeal joints developed.

Histology and Immunofluorescence. Acanthosis, spongiosis, and exocytosis of lymphocytes and histiocytes were seen in the epidermis of a clinical lesion. An eosinophil-predominant, perivascular and interstitial infiltrate was present throughout the dermis. In the subcutis there was a lobular panniculitis, with abscess formation and numerous eosinophils. In some specimens intraepidermal abscesses composed almost entirely of eosinophils were seen. Immunofluorescent studies were negative.

Laboratory Tests. Serum IgG and IgM were elevated. Skin tests to three concentrations of aqueous progesterone produced painful abscesses with histologic features of primary skin lesions. Skin tests to estrogen were negative. Cultures of a pustule grew *Escherichia coli* and *Staphylococcus aureus*.

Course. Spontaneous abortion in the first trimester terminated both pregnancies, and the skin eruption cleared over a period of several weeks. An attempt to use progesterone-containing oral contraceptives led to recurrence of the rash.

Differential Diagnosis. The clinical features of this disease combined with the association with pregnancy are unique. Acne fulminans and halogenoderma can produce similar lesions,[5] but the clinical setting should establish the correct diagnosis.

PROVISIONALLY CLASSIFIED DERMATOSES

Prurigo of Pregnancy

In 1904 Besnier described a prurigo-like eruption on the extensor sides of the hands and feet, which began in the third and fourth months of pregnancy.[25] Nurse's review[2] of this entity in 1968 described two types of eruptions, an early form compatible with Besnier's description and a late form more similar to PUPPP. Today it seems best to consider these two variants separate diseases,[7] grouping the late form with PUPPP and retaining the term prurigo of pregnancy for the other. It is also possible that prurigo of pregnancy is a variant of PG.

Clinical Presentation. Skin lesions appear between the twenty-fifth and thirtieth weeks of pregnancy and consist of small, closely grouped papules, which become excoriated and crusted. Extensor surfaces of the limbs are predominantly affected, sometimes with spread to the upper trunk or abdomen (Fig. 23-7). Among the eight cases reported by Holmes et al.,[7] a personal or family history of atopy was common.

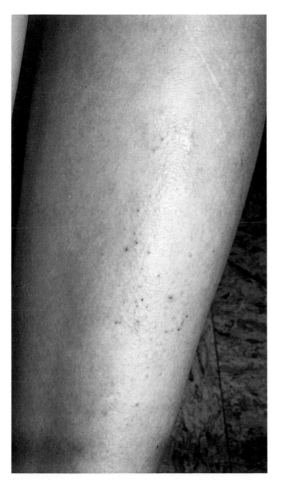

Fig. 23-7. Dry, excoriated papules on the extensor surface of the lower legs are seen in this patient early in the second trimester of pregnancy. Similar lesions were present on the arms, and together these findings suggest a diagnosis of prurigo of pregnancy.

Histology. Biopsy of a lesion demonstrates parakeratosis and acanthosis, sometimes associated with a full-thickness excoriation and serous crusting. A perivascular dermal infiltrate of lymphocytes and occasional areas of fibroplasia are also found.[7]

Laboratory Tests. Patients with a clinically evident atopic diathesis may have elevated levels of IgE.[7]

Course. The skin eruption is benign both to mother and fetus but may persist up to 3 months postpartum.[7]

Differential Diagnosis. Prurigo of pregnancy differs from PUPPP in several aspects:

1. The eruption is most prominent on the extremities rather than on the abdomen.
2. Onset is earlier in pregnancy.
3. Urticarial plaques are absent.
4. There is frequently a history of atopy, and the disease may represent PG or subclinical liver dysfunction in a patient with an atopic diathesis.[7]

Other coincidental causes of itching in pregnancy should also be considered (see pruritus gravidarum).

Pruritic Folliculitis of Pregnancy

In 1981 Zoberman and Farmer[37] reported six cases of a pruritic, papular eruption of pregnancy, which proved histologically to be a folliculitis. Without careful examination the disease could be confused with PUPPP or papular dermatitis of pregnancy. Whether the disease should be considered a specific dermatosis of pregnancy or merely a form of hormonally induced acne is debatable.[7]

Clinical Presentation. Some time between the fourth and ninth months of gestation, 3- to 5-mm pruritic, erythematous papules appear on the arms and abdomen. Occasionally, spread to a generalized distribution can be seen.

Table 23-2. Approach to the Patient: Clinical Features and Diagnostic Findings of the Dermatoses of Pregnancy

Diagnosis	Incidence	Etiology	Trimester of Onset	Characteristic Eruption
Herpes gestationis	1/50,000–1/60,000 (ref. 16)	Unknown	Usually 2nd but can occur anytime from 9 weeks gestation to 6 days postpartum	Erythema and urticarial edema, followed by papules, vesicles, and bullae on abdomen, buttocks, back, forearms, and occasionally palms and soles
Pruritic urticarial papules and plaques of pregnancy (PUPPP)	1/200–1/300	Unknown	Usually 3rd	Erythematous papules and urticarial plaques on abdomen, thighs, arms, and buttocks
Pruritus gravidarum	0.02–2.4%	Cholestasis	Usually 3rd; severe cases can start in 1st	Excoriations in well-developed cases
Impetigo herpetiformis	Rare	Unknown; has features resembling pustular psoriasis	Usually 3rd	Sterile pustules appear first in flexures and folds, spreading centrifugally; verrucous plaques can occur in intertriginous areas; mucosa, tongue, and esophagus can be involved
Autoimmune progesterone dermatitis of pregnancy	Only one patient is reported	Probable hypersensitivity to endogenous progesterone	1st	Acneiform eruption of extremities and buttocks consisting of nonpruritic follicular papules, turbid pustules, comedones, and crusts
Prurigo of pregnancy	2%	May represent pruritus gravidarum (mild cholestasis) in an atopic individual	Usually 2nd	Small, closely grouped papules that become excoriated and crusted usually appearing on extensor surfaces of the extremities
Pruritic folliculitis of pregnancy	Unknown	May represent hormonally induced acne	Usually 2nd	3–5 mm erythematous papules occur on the arms and abdomen; can also become generalized
Papular dermatitis of pregnancy	1/2400	May represent hypersensitivity to placental antigens	Any trimester	Pruritic, soft, erythematous papules with central crust appear a few at a time starting on the trunk and spreading to the extremities

(Modified from Winton GB, Lewis CW: Dermatoses of pregnancy. J Am Acad Dermatol 6:977, 1982; and Winton GB: Dermatoses of pregnancy. J Assoc Milit Dermatol 7:20, 1981.)

Systemic Symptoms	Histology	Laboratory Findings	Complications
Prodromata include malaise, fever, nausea, headache, hot and cold sensations, burning, and pruritus	Perivascular infiltrate of lymphocytes, histiocytes, and eosinophils; subepidermal bulla with separation above basement membrane zone (BMZ); direct immunofluorescence; bandlike deposit of C3 and IgG at BMZ; indirect immunofluorescence: "HG factor," occasionally anti-BMZ IgG	Leukocytosis with 50% eosinophilia; increased HLA-DR3, -DR4	Maternal: secondary infection; fetal: prematurity, transient blisters in the newborn
None	Superficial, perivascular, lymphohistiocytic infiltrate with either normal epidermis or with parakeratosis and focal spongiosis; immunofluorescence is negative	Normal urinary chorionic gonadotropin	None
Pruritus	Not reported	In severe cases elevated serum alkaline phosphatase, SGOT, and bilirubin	Icteric form is associated with low birth weight and postpartum hemorrhage
Malaise, delirium, diarrhea, vomiting, tetany	Spongiform pustule of Kogoj	Leukocytosis, elevated erythrocyte sedimentation rate, hypocalcemia	Maternal: hyperthermia, prostration, renal failure, cardiac failure; fetal: abortion, stillbirth, neonatal death
Arthritis	Acanthosis, focal spongiosis, exocytosis of lymphocytes and histiocytes; perivascular and interstitial infiltrate with predominance of eosinophils; lobular panniculitis with abscess formation	Eosinophilia, hyperglobulinemia, intradermal skin testing with progesterone is positive	Spontaneous abortion
None	Parakeratosis, acanthosis, sometimes full-thickness excoriation; perivascular lymphocytic infiltrate; occasional areas of fibroplasia	IgE may be elevated	None
None	Mild focal spongiosis, patchy parakeratosis, exocytosis of mononuclear and occasional polymorphonuclear leukocytes; pustule formation within hair follicles; occasional dermal abscesses	Cultures are negative	None
None	Acanthosis, parakeratosis, spongiosis, crust formation, perivascular lymphohistiocytic infiltrate in upper dermis, dermal edema	Elevated urinary chorionic gonadotropin, low urinary estriol, low plasma hydrocortisone half-life; positive skin test to patients' own placental extract	Probably benign

Histology. The epidermis shows mild focal spongiosis with exocytosis of mononuclear cells and occasional polymorphonuclear leukocytes. There may be patchy parakeratosis. Involved hair follicles contain an intraluminal pustule filled with neutrophils, lymphocytes, mononuclear cells, and eosinophils. Destruction of follicular walls with abscess formation in the dermis sometimes occurs. Immunofluorescence is negative.

Laboratory Tests. Cultures of lesions are negative. Urinary human chorionic gonadotropin and estriol levels have not been reported.

Course. Skin lesions may respond to topical acne medications such as 10 percent benzoyl peroxide.[7] They usually resolve within several weeks of delivery but may recur in subsequent pregnancies. There are no fetal complications.

Differential Diagnosis. This disorder most closely resembles PUPPP and Spangler's papular dermatitis of pregnancy. A biopsy demonstrating folliculitis should establish the diagnosis. Elevated urinary chorionic gonadotropin levels are seen in papular dermatitis during the last trimester and also help to differentiate that disease.

Pruritic folliculitis also resembles the monomorphic acne seen in patients taking systemic corticosteroids and in occasional patients taking progestational agents. For this reason, the disease may not be specific to pregnancy and is given only a provisional classification here.[7]

DERMATOSIS OF UNCERTAIN CLASSIFICATION: PAPULAR DERMATITIS OF PREGNANCY

Spangler's papular dermatitis of pregnancy (PDP), described in 1962,[4,38] is perhaps the most controversial of the dermatoses of pregnancy. Spangler described another pruritic, papular skin eruption, presumably distinguished by a set of peculiar laboratory abnormalities and a high fetal mortality rate. His study has

been criticized for ill-defined diagnostic criteria, a lack of histologic data, misinterpretation of his own fetal mortality figures, and his recommendation that the disease be treated with diethylstilbestrol,[7,39] a recommendation that he later repudiated.[40] Despite these criticisms the recent case report by Michaud et al.[41] tends to confirm the existence of this disease, which otherwise might be considered a variant of PUPPP.

Clinical Presentation. Skin lesions may erupt at any time during gestation and consist of 3- to 5-mm, intensely pruritic, soft erythematous papules surmounted by a smaller central papule or crust. Papules appear a few at a time, beginning on the trunk and spreading to the extremities. Severe cases may be widespread, with rare involvement of the face and scalp.

Histology and Immunofluorescence. Biopsies were not performed by Spangler and his co-workers; however, a subsequent histologic report of 16 cases by Rahbari[42] and the report of Michaud et al.[41] show the histology to be similar to that of PUPPP. Acanthosis, parakeratosis, spongiosis, and crust formation can be seen in the epidermis. There is a perivascular lymphohistiocytic infiltrate in the upper dermis, with occasional neutrophils and eosinophils. Edema of the dermis may also be present. Immunofluorescence microscopy is negative.

Laboratory Tests. Urinary chorionic gonadotropin is elevated in the last trimester. Low urinary estriol, plasma hydrocortisone, and plasma hydrocortisone half-life are also reported. If patients are skin-tested to their own placental extracts or with extracts of other PDP patients, a marked inflammatory response is seen. No reaction is produced with skin tests from normal placenta.

Course. No maternal complications are reported. The skin clears promptly postpartum, although retained placental fragments may prolong the disease.[4] Half of Spangler's cases suffered a recurrence in subsequent pregnancies, and both Spangler and Michaud reported difficulty in controlling the disease without systemic corticosteroids.

Spangler[4] reported 27 percent fetal mortality in his original series of patients, a figure that requires reassessment.[7,39] He studied 12 patients, who had a total of 37 current or previous pregnancies. There were 10 fetal deaths, including both stillbirths and spontaneous abortions, among the 37 pregnancies, giving Spangler's figure of 10/37, or 27 percent, fetal mortality. However, closer examination of Spangler's data reveals that only 24 of the 37 pregnancies were accompanied by skin disease, and in this group there were only three fetal deaths, giving an incidence of 3/24, or 12.5 percent, a figure very close to the average spontaneous abortion rate in a healthy population.[43] A later series of 16 patients treated with diethylstilbestrol suffered a similar fetal loss of 12 percent.[38]

Differential Diagnosis. Possibly, PDP is similar to PUPPP, except that the skin eruption lacks urticarial plaques, tends to be more widespread, is difficult to control without systemic corticosteroids, and is accompanied by several laboratory abnormalities. The fetal risk in PDP is probably overstated.

If PDP exists as a separate entity, it will undoubtedly be difficult to distinguish from severe cases of PUPPP. The most useful and available of laboratory tests for making the diagnosis is determination of urinary chorionic gonadotropin. Only by performing this test on large numbers of patients with PUPPP-like disease will the existence of papular dermatitis be verified. Until such data are available, it is probably best to classify the disease separately.

CONCLUSION

Despite continuing research into the nature and pathogenesis of the dermatoses of pregnancy, information is still incomplete. Although some simplification of the classification of these diseases has been achieved, the diagnosis in certain cases may not be straightforward. Table 23-2 summarizes the salient features of each entity.

ACKNOWLEDGMENTS

The author wishes to thank Kim B. Yancey, M.D., who reviewed the manuscript and provided invaluable guidance, and Mrs. Sheila Braer for her excellent assistance in preparing the manuscript.

REFERENCES

1. Bierman SM: Autoimmune progesterone dermatitis. Arch Dermatol 107:896, 1973
2. Nurse DS: Prurigo of pregnancy. Australas J Dermatol 9:258, 1968
3. Bourne G: Toxemic rash of pregnancy. Proc R Soc Med 55:462, 1962
4. Spangler AS, Reddy WA, Bardawil WA, et al: Papular dermatitis of pregnancy. JAMA 181:577, 1962
5. Sasseville D, Wilkinson RD, Schnader JY: Dermatoses of pregnancy. Int J Dermatol 20:223, 1981
6. Fitzpatrick TB, Parrish JA, Rhodes AR (eds): Sorting out the pruritic dermatoses of pregnancy. Dermatologic Capsule Comment 1(6):1 (Aug. 1979)
7. Holmes RC, Black MM: The specific dermatoses of pregnancy. J Am Acad Dermatol 8:405, 1983
8. Hertz KC, Katz SI, Maize J, Ackerman AB: Herpes gestationis, a clinicopathologic study. Arch Dermatol 112:1543, 1976
9. Bercovitch L, Bogaars HA, Murray DO: Pustular herpes gestationis. Arch Dermatol 119:91, 1983
10. Katz SI, Hertz KC, Yaoita H: Herpes gestationis: immunopathology and characterization of the HG factor. J Clin Invest 57:1434, 1976
11. Dahl MV: Clinical Immunodermatology. Year Book Medical Publishers, Chicago, 1981, p. 248
12. Fitzpatrick TB, Eisen AZ, Wolf, et al: p. 1363. Dermatology in General Medicine. McGraw-Hill, New York, 1979
13. Shornick JK, Stasny P, Gilliam JN: High frequency of histocompatibility antigens HLA-DR3 and DR4 in herpes gestationis. J Clin Invest 68:553, 1981

14. Holmes RC, Black MM, Jurecka W, et al: Clues to the aetiology and pathogenesis of herpes gestationis. Br J Dermatol 109:131, 1983

15. Shornick JK, Meek TJ, Nesbitt LT, et al: Herpes gestationis in blacks. Arch Dermatol 120:511, 1984

16. Shornick JK, Stastny P, Gilliam JN: Paternal histocompatibility (HLA) antigens and maternal anti-HLA antibodies in herpes gestationis. J Invest Dermatol 81:407, 1983

17. Fine J, Omura EF: Herpes gestationis: persistent disease activity 11 years postpartum. Arch Dermatol 121:924, 1985

18. Shornick JK, Bangert JL, Freeman RG, et al: Herpes gestationis: clinical and histological features of twenty-eight cases. J Am Acad Dermatol 8:214, 1983

19. Kolodny KC: Herpes gestationis, a new assessment of incidence, diagnosis, and fetal prognosis. Am J Obstet Gynecol 104:39, 1969

20. Lawley TJ, Stingl G, Katz SI: Fetal and maternal risk factors in herpes gestationis. Arch Dermatol 114:552, 1978

21. Holmes, RC, Black MM, Dann J, et al: A comparative study of toxic erythema of pregnancy and herpes gestationis. Br J Dermatol 106:499, 1972

22. Honeyman JF, Eguiguren G, Pinto A, et al: Bullous dermatoses of pregnancy. Arch Dermatol 117:264, 1981

23. Lawley TJ, Hertz KC, Wade TR, et al: Pruritic urticarial papules and plaques of pregnancy. JAMA 241:1696, 1979

24. Noguera J, Moreno A, Moragas JM: Pruritic urticarial papules and plaques of pregnancy (PUPPP). Acta Derm Venereal (Stockh) 63:35, 1983

25. Faber WR, Van Joost T, Houseman R, et al: Late prurigo of pregnancy. Br J Dermatol 106:511, 1982

26. Yancey KB, Hall RP, Lawley TJ, et al: Pruritic urticarial papules and plaques of pregnancy: clinical experience in 25 patients. J Am Acad Dermatol 10:473, 1984

27. Schwartz RA, Hansen RC, Lynch PJ: Pruritic urticarial papules and plaques of pregnancy. Cutis 27:425, 1981

28. Holzbach RT: Jaundice in pregnancy—1976. Am J Med 61:367, 1976

29. Editorial: Itching in pregnancy. Br J Med 3:608, 1975

30. Furhoff A: Itching in pregnancy. Acta Med Scand 196:403, 1974

31. Bynum TE: Hepatic and gastrointestinal disorders in pregnancy. Med Clin North Am 61:129, 1977

32. Stewart AF, Battaglini-Sabetta J, Millstone L: Hypocalcemia-induced pustular psoriasis of von Zumbusch. Ann Intern Med 100:677, 1984

33. Sauer GC, Gecha BJ: Impetigo herpetiformis. Arch Dermatol 83:119, 1961

34. Oumeish OY, Farrej SE, Bataineh AS: Some aspects of impetigo herpetiformis. Arch Dermatol 118:103, 1982

35. Beveridge GW, Harkness RA, Livingstone JRB: Impetigo herpetiformis in two successive pregnancies. Br J Dermatol 78:106, 1966

36. Baker H, Wilkinson DS: Psoriasis, p. 1362. In Rook A, Wilkinson DS, Ebling FJG (eds): Textbook of Dermatology. Blackwell Scientific Publications, Oxford, 1979

37. Zoberman E, Farmer ER: Pruritic folliculitis of pregnancy. Arch Dermatol 117:20, 1981

38. Spangler AS, Emerson K: Estrogen levels and estrogen therapy in papular dermatitis of pregnancy. Am J Obstet Gynecol 110:534, 1971

39. Winton GB, Lewis CW: Dermatoses of pregnancy. J Am Acad Dermatol 6:977, 1982

40. Spangler AS: Letter to the Editor. Am J Obstet Gynecol 113:570, 1972

41. Michaud RM, Jacobsen D, Dahl MV: Papular dermatitis of pregnancy. Arch Dermatol 118:1003, 1982

42. Rahbari H: Pruritic papules of pregnancy. J Cutan Pathol 5:347, 1978

43. Williams JW: Abortion. p. 484. In Pritchard JA, MacDonald PC (eds): Obstetrics. Appleton & Lange, East Norwalk, CT, 1976

44. Winton, GB: Dermatoses of pregnancy. J Assoc Milit Dermatol 7:20, 1981

Index

Page numbers followed by *f* represent figures; those followed by *t* represent tables.